T0183151

Lecture Notes in Computer Science 9699

Commenced Publication in 1973
Founding and Former Series Editors:
Gerhard Goos, Juris Hartmanis, and Jan van Leeuwen

More information about this series at http://www.springer.com/series/7412

Anders Tingberg · Kristina Lång
Pontus Timberg (Eds.)

Breast Imaging

13th International Workshop, IWDM 2016
Malmö, Sweden, June 19–22, 2016
Proceedings

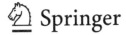 Springer

Editors
Anders Tingberg
Lund University and Skåne University
 Hospital
Malmö
Sweden

Pontus Timberg
Lund University and Skåne University
 Hospital
Malmö
Sweden

Kristina Lång
Lund University and Unilabs
Malmö
Sweden

ISSN 0302-9743   ISSN 1611-3349 (electronic)
Lecture Notes in Computer Science
ISBN 978-3-319-41545-1   ISBN 978-3-319-41546-8   (eBook)
DOI 10.1007/978-3-319-41546-8

Library of Congress Control Number: 2016943320

LNCS Sublibrary: SL6 – Image Processing, Computer Vision, Pattern Recognition, and Graphics

Printed on acid-free paper

This Springer imprint is published by Springer Nature
The registered company is Springer International Publishing AG Switzerland

Preface

This volume of Springer's *Lecture Notes in Computer Science* series comprises the scientific proceedings of the 13th International Workshop on Breast Imaging (IWDM 2016), which was held June 19–22 in Malmö, Sweden. This workshop was formerly called the International Workshop on Digital Mammography, IWDM for short. Although the term "Digital Mammography" was changed to "Breast Imaging" starting at the meeting in 2012, we still kept the familiar abbreviation "IWDM." This new name was chosen to recognize clearly the movement in breast imaging from mammography toward recent emerging technologies and multimodality imaging solutions.

The IWDM meetings traditionally bring together a diversity of researchers (physicists, mathematicians, computer scientists, and engineers), clinicians (radiologists, surgeons, radiographers), and representatives of industry, who are jointly committed to developing technology for the early detection of breast cancer and subsequent patient management. The conference series was initiated at a 1993 meeting of the SPIE in San Jose, with subsequent meetings hosted every two years. Previous meetings have been held in York (1994), Chicago (1996), Nijmegen (1998), Toronto (2000), Bremen (2002), Durham (2004), Manchester (2006), Tucson (2008), Girona (2010), Philadelphia (2012), and Gifu (2014).

A total of 89 papers from around 20 countries were submitted to IWDM 2016. Each of the abstracts along with the four-page supporting documents was reviewed in a double-blinded process by two members of the Scientific Committee, which led to a final selection of 35 oral presentations and 50 posters during the two- and- a- half days of sequential scientific sessions. Six invited speakers gave excellent lectures on the current state of the art in their respective field of expertise. The 85 peer-reviewed papers in this proceedings volume (LNCS 9699) constitute a comprehensive state of the art in breast imaging today.

Invited speakers who are working as radiologists, medical physicists at hospitals, and researcher in universities or companies were chosen. Dr. Sophia Zackrisson of Lund University at Skåne University Hospital, Sweden, discussed the results from the Malmö Breast Tomosynthesis Screening Trial, which included 15,000 women investigated separately with breast tomosynthesis and with digital mammography. Prof. Nico Karssemeijer at Radboud University Medical Centre, The Netherlands, gave a lecture on texture analysis and CAD of breast images. Dr. Savannah Partridge, at the University of Washington in Seattle, USA, summarized the current state of the art in breast MRI and quantitative breast imaging. Prof. Per Hall at Karolinska Institutet in Stockholm, Sweden, described the possibilities to perform individualized breast cancer screening based on the experiences from the KARMA study. Dr. Eva Maria Fallenberg from Charité Universitätsmedizin Berlin, Germany, discussed the new diagnostic possibilities of spectral mammography. Finally, Prof. Marco Stampanoni, ETH Zürich, Switzerland, gave a lecture on X-ray phase contrast mammography.

Finally, a meeting as large and successful as IWDM 2016 is only possible through the efforts and commitment of many people. First, I would like to acknowledge the excellent work of the Scientific Committee in guaranteeing scientific significance by means of providing feedback to the authors for the final papers. Second, special thanks to Kristina Lång and Pontus Timberg for making this meeting a reality, and to Johanna Søger and Anna Zetterholm at Malmö Kongressbyrå for taking care of all the practicalities around the workshop. Third, thanks go to the local committee: Magnus Dustler, Daniel Förnvik, Hannie Petersson, Aldana Rosso, and Sophia Zackrisson. Finally, grateful acknowledgment goes to the research funds, academic partners, cooperating organizations, and industrial partners for their enthusiastic support of the scientific progress in breast imaging.

June 2016   Anders Tingberg

Organization

Program Chairs

Anders Tingberg   Lund University and Skåne University Hospital, Sweden

Kristina Lång   Lund University and Unilabs, Sweden

Program Committee

Andrew Maidment   University of Pennsylvania, USA

Ulrich Bick   Charité - Universitätsmedizin Berlin, Germany

Etta Pisano   Medical University of South Carolina, USA

Hannie Petersson   Lund University, Sweden

Sophia Zackrisson   Lund University and Skåne University Hospital, Sweden

Martin Yaffe   Sunnybrook Research Institute, Canada

Nico Karssemeijer   Radboud University Medical Center, The Netherlands

Elizabeth Krupinski   Emory University, USA

Anders Tingberg   Lund University and Skåne University Hospital, Sweden

Reyer Zwiggelaar   Aberystwyth University, UK

Aldana Rosso   Lund University and Skåne University Hospital, Sweden

Susan Astley   University of Manchester, UK

Maryellen Giger   The University of Chicago, USA

Hilde Bosmans   University Hospital Leuven, Belgium

Pontus Timberg   Lund University and Skåne University Hospital, Sweden

Hiroshi Fujita   Gifu University, Japan

Daniel Förnvik   Lund University and Skåne University Hospital, Sweden

Martin Tornai   Duke University, USA

Joan Marti   University of Girona, Spain

Ioannis Sechopoulos   Radboud University Medical Center, The Netherlands

Kristina Lång   Lund University and Unilabs, Sweden

Magnus Dustler   Lund University, Sweden

Contents

Mammography, Tomosynthesis and Breast CT

Novel Technology

Density Assessment and Tissue Analysis

Dose and Classification

Image Processing, CAD, Breast Density and New Technology

Contrast-Enhanced Imaging

Phase Contrast Breast Imaging

Simulations and Virtual Clinical Trials

Screening

Agreement Between Radiologists' Interpretations of Screening Mammograms

Robert M. Nishikawa[1]([⊠]), Christopher E. Comstock[2],
Michael N. Linver[3], Gillian M. Newstead[5], Vinay Sandhir[4],
and Robert A. Schmidt[5]

[1] Department of Radiology, University of Pittsburgh, Pittsburgh, USA
nishikawarm@upmc.edu
[2] Memorial Sloan-Kettering Cancer Center, New York, USA
[3] X-Ray Associates of New Mexico, P.C., Albuquerque, USA
[4] American College of Radiology, Washington, D.C., USA
[5] Department of Radiology, The University of Chicago, Chicago, USA

Abstract. We performed a preliminary investigation to determine how similar radiologists' interpretations of screening mammograms are. Our dataset consisted of 50 cancer cases and 50 normal cases that were read by 50 radiologists. We computed sensitivity, specificity, and interpretation on a case-by-case basis to study similarity between pairs of radiologists. We failed to find any pairs of radiologists who read all the cases, only the normal cases, or only the cancer cases the same. There were very few radiologists who read both cancer cases and normal cases in a similar manner. Even radiologists who had similar sensitivities or similar specificities differed substantially on the interpretation of individual cases. Our data indicate that there may be an underlying variability between radiologists in terms of image features used to detect cancers and when a false detection is made. This underlying variability may make the development and implementation of model observers more difficult.

Keywords: Screening · Mammography · Radiologist performance · Model observer · Virtual clinical trials

1 Introduction

There are several research areas where predicting radiologists' behavior when reading screening mammograms is essential or would be useful. Virtual clinical trials, for example, require a model observer to mimic a radiologist. The model observer must be developed using individual radiologists. In developing computer-aided detection systems, the goal is to help radiologists. Therefore, it would be useful to know or predict which cancers and what false lesions a radiologist would detect, and flag, or not flag, lesions appropriately.

For example, if one is trying to optimize an imaging system to detect microcalcifications, it is important to know if radiologists would have higher performances with images that were sharp, but noisy, or is it better to suppress the noise (and lose some sharpness) and by how much. If different radiologists were affected differently by image noise, a single model observer would not be appropriate.

© Springer International Publishing Switzerland 2016
A. Tingberg et al. (Eds.): IWDM 2016, LNCS 9699, pp. 3–10, 2016.
DOI: 10.1007/978-3-319-41546-8_1

It is well known that there is substantial variability between radiologists reading screening mammograms. This makes developing a single model observer to represent all radiologists difficult. It may be possible, however, to categorize radiologists into a small number of groups that cover the reading skills of most radiologists.

In this study, we examined how similar radiologists' interpretations of screening mammograms on individual cases are. We examined both the detection of positive lesions on cases with a path-proven cancer and false lesions on normal mammograms. The goal was to determine if there were sub-groups of radiologists with similar reading patterns.

2   Method

2.1   Observer Study

This was a preliminary study with 50 radiologists, and 50 cancer cases and 50 normal cases. All cases were collected retrospectively from four different medical centers and were considered "good" teaching cases. All images were de-identified. The images were randomly selected from the first five American College of Radiology (ACR) Mammography Boot Camp (currently called Breast Imaging Boot Camp). The Boot Camp was an intensive 3-day course on how to read screening mammograms. Each radiologist read screening mammograms under the direct supervision of five course instructors. All radiologists consented to have their de-identified readings used in research studies.

From the 236 radiologists who read up to 356 cases, we found 80 radiologists who read the same 299 cases. From those, we randomly selected 50 radiologists, 50 cancer cases, and 50 normal cases for use in this preliminary study. For each case, the radiologist marked the location of suspicious lesions: those that they would recall for diagnostic workup. We used that information to score each breast as the radiologist having a true positive, false positive, true negative, or false negative, based on whether a lesion was located in the breast with a malignant lesion. The exact lesion location was not used in this study.

We computed each radiologist's sensitivity and specificity. To compare radiologists, we computed correlation in their binary scores (recall or no recall) between all pairs of radiologists. We also determined the absolute difference in sensitivity and in specificity between all pairs of radiologists, and the number of differences in the 50 interpretations for all pairs of radiologists, once for the cancer cases and once for the normal cases. We then looked for radiologists with similar reading patterns based on these data. Note that sensitivity and specificity were measured on a 0.0 to 1.0 scale.

3   Results

3.1   Characteristics of Cases and Readers

Figure 1 shows the sensitivity (cancer cases) or specificity (normal cases) for each case. There is a distribution of sensitivities and specificities indicating the general difficulty of the cases. There were 29 cases where more than 90 % of the radiologists detected the cancer, but there were three cases where more than 50 % of radiologists missed the cancer. The average sensitivity of the 50 cancer cases was 0.84 (standard deviation of +/−0.19).

There were 20 cases where more than 90 % of the radiologists correctly called the case normal and three normal cases where more than 50 % of the radiologists detected a false lesion. The average specificity was 0.83 (standard deviation of +/−0.16). Not discernible from the plots is that there were 9 cancer cases where all radiologists correctly called the case abnormal and only 2 normal cases that all radiologists recalled.

Figure 2 shows the distribution of sensitivity and specificity for the 50 radiologists. While there is some variation in performance, there are radiologists who have similar performance values. The spread in performances is not unexpected and is similar to what has been reported in other studies [1].

Figure 3 shows two color maps that indicate correct and incorrect interpretations of the 50 radiologists (along the rows) for the cancer and normal cases running along the columns. Each of the maps is sorted by the cases with the most correct interpretations on the left and least on the right. Both maps are sorted by the radiologist with the highest sensitivity on top to lowest on bottom. It is apparent that the radiologists with the highest sensitivity (cancer cases) do not have the highest specificity (normal cases).

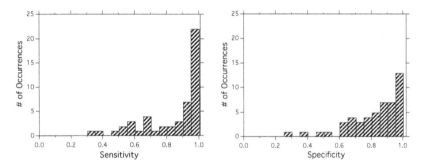

Fig. 1. The distribution of the case sensitivity for the 50 cancer cases and the distribution of the case specificity for 50 normal cases. These distributions are based on the readings from 50 radiologists.

3.2   Agreement Between Radiologists

Figure 4 compares the number of discrepancies between two radiologists for the cancer cases versus for the normal cases. Radiologists who tended to agree on cancer cases (small differences) did not necessarily agree on the interpretation of normal cases. There was only one pair of radiologists (out of 1225 pairs) who agreed on more than 90 % of the cancer cases and more than 90 % of the normal cases – more than 90 % is five or fewer cases. Whereas 90 % agreement on the cancer cases could lead to as much as 40 % disagreement on normal cases, and vice versa.

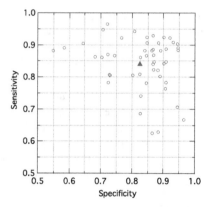

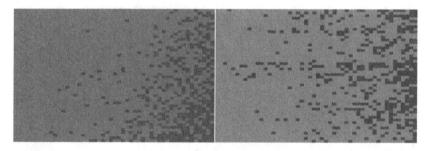

Fig. 2. (Left) shows a plot of sensitivity versus specificity for the 50 radiologists (circles). Note a small amount of random jitter was added to all the points to avoid completely overlapping points. The triangle is the average for the 50 radiologists.

Fig. 3. Color maps of the correct (red) and incorrect (blue) interpretations of the 50 radiologists (running from the radiologist with the highest sensitivity to lowest from top to bottom) on the cancer cases (left) and the normal cases (right). The cases are sorted from the case with the most correct interpretations on the left and least on the right, separately for the cancer and normal cases. (Color figure online)

We next examined whether radiologists with similar sensitivities or similar specificities had good agreement. In Fig. 5, we plotted the number of differences in their binary scores (recall or do not recall) for the cancer cases (top) and for the normal cases (bottom) versus the absolute value of their differences in sensitivities (top) or specificities (bottom) between all possible pairs of two radiologists. While there was a trend for increasing difference in interpretation with increasing difference in sensitivity or specificity (correlations of $r = 0.62$ for sensitivity and $r = 0.65$ for specificity) in the plots, there were wide variations in values at given differences in sensitivity/specificity values. That is, radiologists who have the same performance values are not necessarily detecting the same cancers and false detections.

Finally, we computed Cohen's kappa for each pair of radiologists separately for the cancer cases and for the normal cases. Figure 6 clearly shows that agreement between radiologists is not high, in general. Further, radiologists who had good agreement on

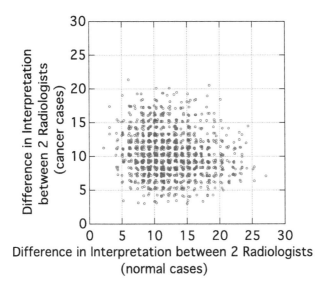

Fig. 4. (Left) compares the number of discrepancies between two radiologists for the cancer cases versus for the normal cases.

the cancer cases rarely had good agreement on the normal case and vice versa. In fact, it is more likely that two radiologist who had kappa > 0.5 on cancer cases had low or even negative kappa than kappa > 0.5 on normal cases.

In addition, there was better agreement among pairs of radiologists on cancer cases than normal cases. The average kappa was 0.24 for cancer cases and 0.17 for normal cases. The standard deviation for both was 0.16. This can be seen qualitatively in Fig. 3 where the false positive detections are more sporadic in the normal cases than the false negatives in the cancer cases.

4 Discussion

We could not identify any subgroups of readers. In all of the 1225-paired comparisons, no two radiologists read exactly the same. The best similarity was eight differences in 100 cases or a kappa of 0.8. There was little similarity between radiologists who had the same sensitivities or who had the same specificities. Further, radiologists who read somewhat similarly on cancer cases did not necessarily read normal cases similarly.

Our premise was that since false detections appear to be similar to a cancer as judged by the radiologist, then whatever characteristics of the lesion that is used by the radiologist to make the decision to recall or not recall would be the same whether the lesion was a cancer or a false detection. This would imply that radiologists who tend to agree on cancers would tend to agree on normal cases. We found no such relationship. That is, the features of the cancers that were used by two radiologists to detect a cancer were not necessarily the same features that caused a false detection.

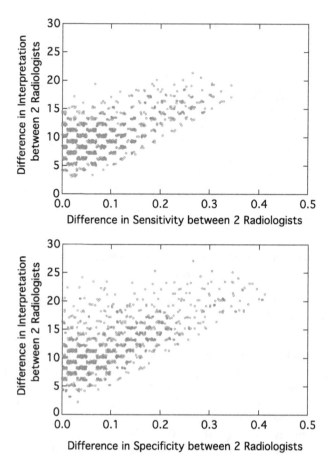

Fig. 5. Shows the relationship between the number of differences in their binary scores (recall or do not recall) on the cancer cases (top) and the normal cases (bottom) versus their differences in sensitivities (top) or specificities (bottom) between all possible pairs of two radiologists. Absolute values for differences in sensitivity and specificity are plotted. We added a small amount of random positive jitter to avoid the overlap of a large number of data points.

However, while there is poor agreement on a case-to-case basis, there were radiologists who had similar sensitivity/specificity values. Approximately 10 % (127/1225) of all pairs of radiologists had both sensitivity and specificity values agree to within +/−0.05. Also, if the goal is to find radiologists who are equally adept at detecting cancer, then 30 % (373/1225) of pairs of radiologists agree to within +/−0.05.

The two main limitations of this study are that we did not use location information when scoring whether radiologists detected the lesion in the breast. It is likely that agreement will be lower when we require radiologists to detect the same lesion (by location). Second, we did not perform any statistical analyses for this preliminary study, as we were only looking for trends that would be studied in more detail in our future work. Specifically, we treated cases as a fixed effect. We plan to estimate 95 %

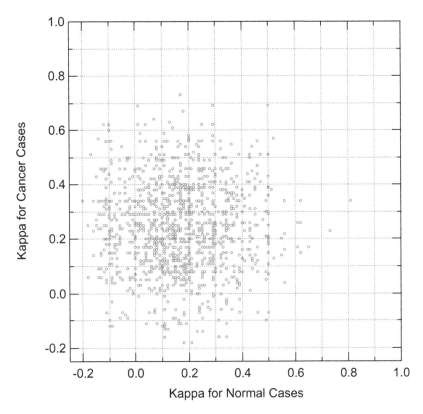

Fig. 6. Plots, for each pair of radiologists, the kappa coefficient for cancer cases versus the kappa coefficient for the normal cases. The 95 % confidence intervals on each point typically spans a range of +/−0.07.

confidence intervals using bootstrapping when we expand the data set to include more cases and radiologists. This will allow us to treat cases as a random effect and thus generalize our result to a population of cases.

Also as future work, we will determine whether a group of radiologists can statistically match a single radiologist's interpretation. Similarly, we will determine if there are image features that are used by pairs or groups of radiologists to detect cancer and when they identify a false detection.

5   Conclusions

In conclusion, our data show that no two radiologists read the same for either cases with a cancer or for normal cases. It is well known that there is large inter-reader variability in performance (sensitivity and specificity). Our data suggests that there is an underlying variability in features that radiologists use to detect a cancer or a false positive, and the variability is not simply a choice of decision threshold. Further, the image features used to detect a cancer by two radiologists are not necessarily the same features used when a false positive is detected. This underlying variability may make the development and implementation of model observers more difficult.

Acknowledgments. The work was supported in part by a grant from the National Institutes of Health, National Institute of Biomedical Imaging and Bioengineering, grant R01EB013680.

Reference

1. Beam, C.A., Layde, P.M., Sullivan, D.C.: Variability in the interpretation of screening mammograms by US radiologists. Findings from a national sample. Arch. Intern. Med. **156** (2), 209–213 (1996)

Quality Control of Breast Tomosynthesis for a Screening Trial: Preliminary Experience

Aili Maki[1(✉)], James Mainprize[1], Gordon Mawdsley[1], and Martin Yaffe[1,2]

[1] Sunnybrook Research Institute, Toronto, Canada
aili.maki@sri.utoronto.ca
[2] University of Toronto, Toronto, Canada

Abstract. The Tomosynthesis Mammography Imaging Screening Trial (TMIST) Lead-In Study is a randomized screening trial that aims to compare the performance of standard two-dimensional full-field digital mammography (FFDM) and tomosynthesis at five sites in Canada, with multiple vendors' platforms and a target enrollment of 6300 women. To characterize and monitor the image quality of the tomosynthesis systems in the trial, a quality control (QC) program has been developed, including semi-annual physics tests, and daily tests performed on a phantom imaged by the radiographer.

Here we describe the test regimen and phantoms and present initial results. The physics tests include measurement of image quality parameters in the reconstructed tomographic slices and evaluation of the AEC performance by measuring signal difference to noise ratio (SDNR) of a low contrast simulated lesion. The physics tests have been performed on a GE Senoclaire, two Hologic Selenia Dimensions and two Siemens Mammomat Inspiration units. In addition to the physics tests, we have remotely collected 15 months of daily QC data on the GE unit and 2 and 3 months on the Hologic units.

Keywords: Breast tomosynthesis · Image quality · Quality control · Modulation transfer function · Artefact spread function · Radiation dose

1 Introduction

The efficacy of tomosynthesis mammography as a screening modality has yet to be determined with a large, multi-vendor, multi-center randomized screening trial in North America. The TMIST Lead-In Study is a randomized screening trial to compare the performance of FFDM and tomosynthesis at five sites in Canada, with a protocol designed to roll into the full TMIST trial (148,054 women at approximately 70 sites in the United States and Canada). To characterize and monitor the image quality of the tomosynthesis systems in a harmonized manner, a QC program has been developed that includes semi-annual tests and performance measures and daily tests to monitor system stability.

© Springer International Publishing Switzerland 2016
A. Tingberg et al. (Eds.): IWDM 2016, LNCS 9699, pp. 11–19, 2016.
DOI: 10.1007/978-3-319-41546-8_2

2 Method

2.1 Philosophy

A comprehensive quality control program, including specially designed phantoms and automated analysis software was developed to monitor different aspects of image quality on the different manufacturer's tomosynthesis systems. Wherever possible, image quality is assessed in views most relevant to the radiologists (*i.e.* the reconstructed tomographic slices). The radiographer's tests were set up to be automated as much as possible using a client-server methodology, automatic image analysis and report generation. The tests were designed to be as universal as possible, such that they could be implemented on any system, and ideally, could be compared across systems. Because this was a developmental program, extra tests were performed to determine which tests are most effective.

2.2 Phantoms

Four phantoms were developed for QC tests: the *Wire Phantom*, the *Daily QC Phantom*, the *Uniform Phantom*, and the *Modular Phantom*. The latter three are semi-circular in shape.

The 40 mm thick daily QC Phantom incorporates a 12.7 mm (0.5 in.) polyethylene sphere for measurement of signal difference to noise ratio (SDNR), calcification clusters ($\sim$0.57 mm diameter calcifications arranged in a 6.3 mm diameter circle) at heights of 10, 20 and 30 mm for assessment of geometric localization (reconstruction accuracy) and a 0.79 mm (1/32 in.) aluminum BB for the assessment of the artefact spread function (ASF) and slice sensitivity profile (SSP) (Fig. 1). A "chest wall" backing plate facilitates placement on the table.

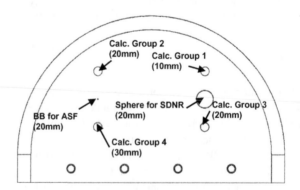

Fig. 1. Schematic of the daily QC phantom with test objects indicated. Heights are given in parentheses.

The modulation transfer function (MTF) is evaluated with the Wire Phantom, a slanted 35 μm diameter taut tungsten wire embedded in a 4 cm thick uniform resin block. The wire is slanted 1:10 with respect to the x and z directions to allow pre-sampling estimation of the point-spread function (PSF) [2].

The Modular Phantom (MP) is used for assessment of geometric reconstruction accuracy and the performance of the automatic exposure control. The phantom consists of semicircular slabs, 1 cm thick. The top and bottom slabs have rounded edges to minimize image processing artefacts by avoiding non-breast-like transitions in x-ray beam transmission. The phantom thickness can be adjusted between 2 and 8 cm in 1 cm increments. A thin plastic sheet supporting a grid of 0.79 mm aluminum BBs, spaced 4 cm apart in the x direction and 2 cm apart in the y direction can be positioned at different heights in the phantom. A 2 cm thick insert containing a polyethylene sphere can be added to measure how the SDNR varies with phantom thickness. Blank slabs are used to create uniform regions for evaluation of the noise power spectrum (NPS).

2.3 Tests

The QC program includes tests to be performed daily (QC phantom) and monthly (monitor lag) by the radiographer, and semi-annually by the medical physicist (Table 1). Initial tolerances on the test results are given for the daily QC tests (Table 2). Because of limited experience with the wide variety of different technologies available, the tolerances are given with respect to the reference operating levels (ROL) established after acceptance testing of the unit. Note here the "x" direction refers to the direction parallel to the chest-wall edge of the breast-support. The "z" direction is perpendicular to the plane of the breast support plate.

Table 1. Performance metrics evaluated during semi-annual physics testing. MP = Modular Phantom, FS = Foam Spacers

Test	Phantom	Parameters evaluated
Resolution (MTF)	Wire Phantom	MTF in x and z directions
Noise power spectrum (NPS)	Uniform Phantom	NPS in x and y directions
Artefact spread function (ASF), Slice sensitivity profile (SSP)	MP + BB-grid insert	FWHM of ASFs (x and y) and SSPs (z)
Reconstruction fidelity	MP + BB-grid insert	Spacing between BBs (x-y) average height of BBs (z)
Mean glandular dose	MP + SDNR insert + FS	Dose at equivalent 21, 45, 75 and 103 mm thick breasts
Collimation	NA	Collimator blades not visible in projection images.
Automatic exposure control (AEC) evaluation	MP + SDNR insert + FS	SDNR
Ghosting evaluation	MP + SDNR insert	Visual assessment in projections and volumes

Table 2. Parameters measured on the Daily QC phantom, and preliminary tolerances

Test	Preliminary tolerance
SDNR	Within 10 % of ROL
Geometric localization	Within 1 slice of ROL
ASF and SSP	FWHM in x, y and z' directions within 10 % of ROL
Normalized NPS (NNPS)	Radial NNPS within 10 % of ROL at 1, 2 and 4 mm^{-1}

The semi-annual physics tests include an assessment of the MTF and the NPS, which can be combined to assess the noise equivalent quanta (NEQ).

2.4 Analysis

SDNR. The SDNR is measured in a polyethylene sphere embedded in PMMA. It is calculated as $SDNR = (I_{bkd} - I_{sphere})/\sigma_{bkd}$, where I_{bkd} is the mean voxel value in a region of interest (ROI) adjacent to the sphere, I_{sphere} is the mean voxel value in an ROI within the sphere and σ_{bkd} is the standard deviation among the voxels in the background ROI. For the Daily QC Phantom, the slice where the BB (which is in the same plane as the centre of the sphere) has its peak intensity voxel was selected for SDNR measurement. This method ensures a robust yet fully automatic method of segmenting the appropriate ROIs.

MTF. The MTF is assessed in the x-z plane. First the pre-sampled PSF is obtained from x-z plane cross-sections of the reconstructed volume. Because the wire is so fine (35 microns), the slight oval-shape of the cross sections through the wire and the size of the wire can be neglected. The Fourier transform of the PSF yields the 2D MTF. The non-linear nature of most manufacturers' reconstruction algorithms gives peaks at frequencies other than zero. On the system for which we have the most data (GE) we found the MTF at low frequencies to be unstable over time. We suspect this is due to non-linearity in the artefact suppression algorithm. To mitigate this, the MTFs are set to 1.0 at $f_x = 1$ cycle/mm.

NNPS. The NNPS is measured in projections and different x-y planes in the reconstructed volume using the multi-taper method described by Wu et al. [3]. The NNPS is calculated at 3 different heights within the modular phantom – 1, 2 and 3 cm above the breast support plate and radially averaged for comparison over time.

ASF and SSP. The artefact spread function (ASF in x and y) and slice-sensitivity profile (SSP, in z) are assessed for 0.79 mm (1/32 in.) aluminum BBs. As per Bouwman et al. [4] the SSP is calculated as shown in Eq. (1). A Gaussian is fit to the ASF or SSP used to estimate full-width half maximum (FWHM) value.

$$SSP = \frac{P_{obj}(z) - P_{bkd}(z)}{P_{obj}(z_0) - P_{bkd}(z_0)} \tag{1}$$

P_{obj} and P_{bkd} are the voxel values at slice z in the object and the background and z_0 is the slice with the peak voxel value.

Most systems report DICOM volumes in a Cartesian coordinate system (CCS) and the out-of-plane artefacts are naturally angled towards the focal spot of the central projection, causing the slice sensitivity profile (SSP) to be dependent on the position of the object with respect to the central ray on the detector. To reduce the effect of object position on SSP, the volumes in CCS can be transformed to a "cone-beam coordinate system" (CBCS) in which the (x, y, z) positions correspond to points on a cone, effectively creating an alternative coordinate system in which the focal spot is moved to infinity thus making the SSPs parallel [1].

Reconstruction Fidelity. The relative locations of the BBs are assessed for constancy of spacing in x and y. Because the grid of BBs is imaged at different heights within the modular phantom, the z locations of the BBs are compared between the different configurations to determine the dimensional accuracy of the z direction.

Mean Glandular Dose. The mean glandular dose is estimated for typical breasts of 2, 4.5, 7.5 and 10.3 cm. Measurements of Half-Value Layer and entrance exposure made in 2D (FFDM) mode for the different technique factors selected by the unit when imaging the SDNR phantom for AEC performance are used. The dose is calculated as per Dance et al. [5], using a "t-factor" to adjust for the difference between tomosynthesis geometry and the conventional FFDM measurement conditions. These calculated doses are then compared with the estimate of dose in the DICOM header.

AEC Performance. The performance of the AEC was assessed by imaging the modular phantom with the SDNR insert in the configurations given in Table 4, with foam spacers added to achieve compression paddle heights such that the attenuation of the PMMA matches the attenuation of breasts of different compressed thickness, as per the work by Dance et al. [6]. The SDNR between a region inside the sphere and adjacent background regions was calculated for the slices passing through the middle of the sphere.

3   Results

Routine QC data was gathered on a GE Essential Senoclaire for 15 months, and on two Hologic Selenia Dimensions systems for 2 and 3 months. The semi-annual physics data was also collected on all three units, as well as on two Siemens Inspiration units.

Plots of SDNR over time for the GE system and the Hologic system are shown in Fig. 2. The control limits of ± 10 % are shown. New baselines were calculated when the units had gain calibrations and hardware upgrades.

As shown in Fig. 3, GE and Siemens use CCS geometry whereas Hologic employs CBCS. All volumes were transformed to CBCS to evaluate MTF, ASF and SSP. Typical MTFs in the x-direction for the three system types are plotted in Fig. 4. The z-direction response is not shown, as the nature of the tomosynthesis reconstruction results essentially in a delta-function dictated by slice thickness. Typical 2D MTFs in the x-z plane obtained from the Wire Phantom are shown in Fig. 5 (top).

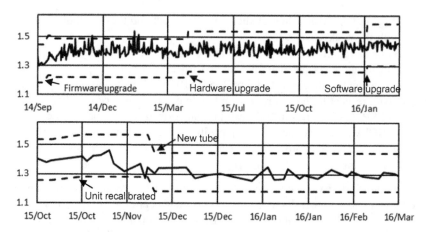

Fig. 2. Daily SDNR measurements over time on the GE Essential (top) and Hologic Dimensions (bottom)

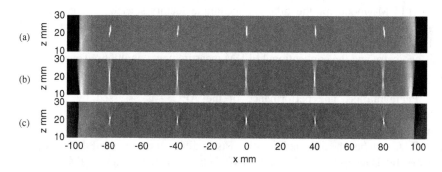

Fig. 3. Cross plane (x-z) slices through the reconstructed volumes of the modular phantom with a grid of BBs inserted at 2 cm above the breast support for (a) GE, (b) Hologic, (c) Siemens.

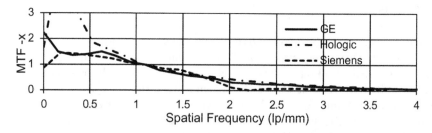

Fig. 4. Typical MTF measured from the wire phantom in the x-direction. These curves have been adjusted to 1.0 at 1 cycle/mm.

Figure 5 (bottom) illustrates typical 2D normalized NPS for the x-y plane in the middle of the reconstructed volume for the different systems.

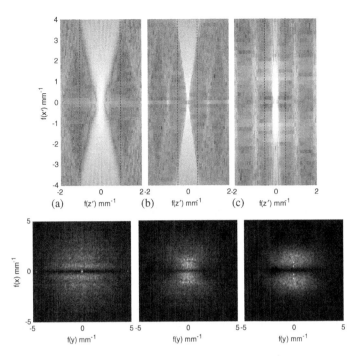

Fig. 5. Typical x-z plane pre-sampled MTFs (top, log-scaled) and NNPS (bottom) for (a) GE, (b) Hologic and (c) Siemens. Dashed lines indicate the Nyquist frequency in the z-direction. Each NNPS is scaled to show best detail for display.

Table 3 gives the typical FWHM values measured for the artefact spread functions in x and y and the slice-sensitivity profiles for all 3 systems.

Table 3. Typical average FWHMs in mm for the ASF and SSP of the BBs when the BB insert is 2 cm above the breast support plate. The standard deviation is given in brackets.

Unit	ASF x	ASF y	SSP z
GE	0.77 (0.04)	0.75 (0.03)	5.65 (0.2)
Hologic	0.65 (0.03)	0.77 (0.05)	8.72 (0.4)
Siemens	0.59 (0.02)	0.63 (0.02)	2.93 (0.03)

Mean glandular doses for the different phantom thicknesses imaged to characterize AEC and dose are given in Table 4.

Table 4. Typical mean glandular dose values as calculated from physicist's measurements (C) and reported in the DICOM header (D).

PMMA/Equiv. breast (cm)	2/2		4/4.5		6/7.5		8/10.3	
Composition (% Fibroglandular)	97		41		9		3	
Dose (mGy)	C	D	C	D	C	D	C	D
GE	1.2	0.8	1.3	1.2	1.9	2.0	4.4	5.3
Hologic	1.3	1.1	1.8	1.5	3.7	3.3	4.5	4.6
Siemens	1.0	1.0	1.7	1.4	2.7	2.3	5.0	4.2

4   Discussion

The measured SDNR values are reasonably stable over time. Upgrades to the equipment resulted in marked shifts in the operating levels. The MTF measurements are very sensitive to background correction and normalization making serial monitoring difficult. The MTFs are very different between systems.

The differences in the angular range used for acquisition of the tomosynthesis images are clearly seen in the differences in the SSP FWHM values. The Siemens system, which has the greatest angular range, has the smallest z FWHM values (best z direction resolution), while the Hologic system, which has the smallest angular range of the three, has the largest z FWHM values.

Examining the reconstructions of the modular phantom with the grid of BBs in the x-z plane is informative. The directionality of the artefacts, angled towards the focal spot, and varying with the position in the phantom relative to the perpendicular beam, are clearly visible in the GE and Siemens images. No evidence of this is seen in the Hologic images. This suggests their reconstruction algorithm assumes a parallel beam geometry (such as the basic shift and add technique).

Some discrepancies between the manufacturer's calculated doses (reported in the DICOM header) and the physicist's calculated doses were noted. These may be due to different assumptions regarding the composition of the breast being imaged. It is possible that the homogeneous nature of the PMMA phantom used to simulate a patient breast confused the AEC software. Future work to explore this further by calculating the doses to actual patients is planned.

Acknowledgements. The authors wish to thank Moira Pearson and Joseph Yang for their assistance with this project and the Canadian Breast Cancer Foundation for funding through the 2012 Earlier Detection of Breast Cancer grant.

References

1. Maki, A.K., Mainprize, J.G., Yaffe, M.J.: Robust measurement of the slice-sensitivity profile in breast tomosynthesis. Med. Phys. (2016, accepted)
2. Fujita, H., Tsai, D.Y., Itoh, T., Doi, K., Morishita, J., Ueda, K., Ohtsuka, A.: A simple method for determining the modulation transfer function in digital radiography. IEEE Trans. Med. Imaging **11**, 34–39 (1992)

3. Wu, G., Mainprize, J., Yaffe, M.: TU-A-301-05: spectral analysis of breast images using multitaper method. Med. Phys. **38**, 3745 (2011)
4. Bouwman, R.W., Visser, R., Young, K.C., Dance, D.R., Lazzari, B., van der Burght, R., Heid, P., van Engen, R.E.: Daily quality control for breast tomosynthesis. In: Proceedings of the SPIE, vol. 7622, 762241-1–9 (2010)
5. Dance, D.R., Young, K.C., van Engen, R.E.: Estimation of mean glandular dose for breast tomosynthesis: factors for use with the UK, European and IAEA breast dosimetry protocols. Phys. Med. Biol. **56**, 453–471 (2011)
6. Dance, D.R., Skinner, C.L., Young, K.C., Beckett, J.R., Kotre, C.J.: Additional factors for the estimation of mean glandular breast dose using the UK mammography dosimetry protocol. Phys. Med. Biol. **45**, 3225–3240 (2000)

Summary of Outcomes from Consecutive Years of Tomosynthesis Screening at an American Academic Institution

Emily F. Conant[1($\boxtimes$)], Andrew Oustimov[1], Samantha P. Zuckerman[1],
Elizabeth S. McDonald[1], Susan P. Weinstein[1], Andrew D.A. Maidment[1],
Bruno Barufaldi[1], Marie Synnestvedt[2], and Mitchell Schnall[1]

[1] Department of Radiology, Perelman School of Medicine, University of Pennsylvania,
Philadelphia, PA, USA
emily.conant@uphs.upenn.edu
[2] Division of General Internal Medicine, Perelman School of Medicine,
University of Pennsylvania, Philadelphia, PA, USA

Abstract. Digital breast tomosynthesis (DBT) screening outcomes are sustainable over consecutive years with significant reductions in recall and increasing cancers per recalled patients compared to screening with digital mammography alone (DM). There is a prevalence effect with a reduction in cancer detection at the second round of screening that is no longer present at the third round. There is a non-statistically significant trend of decreased interval cancers with DBT compared to DM alone screening. Early data on the implementation of synthetic 2D (s2D) imaging coupled with DBT shows maintenance of screening outcomes with reduction in radiation dose compared to DM/DBT screening .

Keywords: Breast cancer · Screening · Mammography · Digital breast tomosynthesis

1 Introduction

Screening with a combination of digital mammography and digital breast tomosynthesis (DBT) has been shown to reduce false positives and improve cancer detection compared to screening with digital mammography (DM) alone. The bulk of the evidence on the improved outcomes achievable with DBT has come from first round screening in either limited prospective trials [1–3] or retrospective studies, mostly from single sites [4–7]. Questions remain whether the improved outcomes are sustainable over multiple rounds of screening and whether the implementation of synthetic 2D imaging as a method to reduce the dose of DBT screening will have similarly improved outcomes. There are also few reports on the rate of false negative DBT screens.

At the University of Pennsylvania, we are entering our 5th year of screening all patients with DBT and therefore have the data to analyze the "prevalence effect" of screening with this new modality. We also have tumor registry follow-up from the first few years of screening to begin to evaluate false negative rates. Finally, over the last year of screening, we have implemented synthetic 2D images and removed the DM

© Springer International Publishing Switzerland 2016
A. Tingberg et al. (Eds.): IWDM 2016, LNCS 9699, pp. 20–24, 2016.
DOI: 10.1007/978-3-319-41546-8_3

acquisition of the combination DM/DBT mode of screening. A summary of our DBT screening outcomes will be reviewed [8].

2   Method

An IRB approved, retrospective analysis of DBT screening metrics is ongoing at our institution. Screening outcomes were evaluated for a total of 44468 examinations attributable to 23,958 women over a 4 year period (year 0 cohort (DM0) n = 10728, year 1 cohort (DBT1) n = 11007, year 2 cohort (DBT2) n = 11157, year 3 cohort (DBT3) n = 11576. For women screened with DBT, 21,395 women were screened at least once, 9316 women were screened at least twice and 3023 women underwent 3 rounds of screening. Outcome metrics (recall and cancer detection rates and PPV1) were calculated for all patients presenting for screening over 4 consecutive years (DM, year 0; DBT, years 1–3). Interval cancer rates for DM0 and DBT1, defined as cancer presenting as symptomatic within one year of a negative screen, were calculated after linkage with the state cancer registry thru June 2014 [8].

In addition, preliminary data on recall and cancer detection rates and average glandular dose from the first 6 months (January 1 – June 30th, 2015) of screening with synthetic 2D combined with DBT (s2D/DBT) were compared with similar published metrics from DBT year 1 [9].

3   Results

There was no practical difference in the patient characteristics including age, breast density, race and screening volumes race across the years 0–3. Additionally, we have previously demonstrated no statistically significant difference in calculated breast cancer risk between DM year 0 and the first 18 months of screening with DBT [5].

Table 1 demonstrates that at the site level, recall rates rose slightly for DBT1–3 years (88, 90, 92/1000 screened, respectively) but remained significant reduced compared to DM0 rate of 104/1000 screened. There was also no statistically significant difference in the recall rate across the three DBT years (p = 0.549). Cancer detection rate continued to increase at 4.6, 5.5, 5.8, and 6.1/1000 screened for years 0, 1, 2, and 3 respectively, but was not significantly different from that of DM (DM vs DBT1 p = 0.370, DM vs DBT2 p = 0.196, DM vs DBT3 p = 0.110), and was not significantly different across three DBT years (p = 0.796). Although, the rate of invasive cancers detected per 1000 screened increased slightly over time (DM = 3.2, DBT1 = 3.8, DBT2 = 4.1, DBT3 = 4.1), the increase, in any DBT year compared with DM, or across the DBT years, was not significant. The positive predictive value for recalls (PPV1) continued to rise from DM0 rate of 4.4 % to 6.2 % (p = 0.06), 6.5 % (p = 0.03), 6.7 % (p = 0.02) for DBT1–3 (Table 1). The biopsy rate in each DBT year did not significantly differ from that of DM (DM vs DBT1 p = 0.167, DM vs DBT2 p = 0.606, DM vs DBT3 p = 0.597) and did not differ significantly over three DBT years (p = 0.600). Complete cancer registry data were only available to assess DM0 and DBT 1 years. The change in interval cancer rates/1000 screened across these years showed a downward trend (DM = 0.7, DBT1 = 0.5) but was not statistically significant (p = 0.603).

Table 1. Site level analysis of screening outcomes comparing each digital breast tomosynthesis year (DBT1–3) with the digital mammography year (DM0), as well as across the three DBT years (modified from Reference [8])

Characteristic	DM 0	DBT 1	P	DBT 2	P	DBT 3	P	P (DBT)
Recall, n/1000	104	88	<0.0001	90	0.0005	92	0.0025	0.549
Biopsy, n/1000	18	20	0.167	19	0.606	19	0.597	0.600
Cancer, n/1000	4.6	5.5	0.370	5.8	0.196	6.1	0.110	0.796
PPV 1, %	4.4	6.2	0.063	6.5	0.034	6.7	0.020	0.915
Invasive cancer, n/1000	3.2	3.8	0.420	4.1	0.243	4.1	0.269	0.929
In-situ cancer, n/1000	1.4	1.5	0.779	1.3	0.914	1.8	0.440	0.668
Interval cancer, n/1000	0.7	0.5	0.603	NA	NA	NA	NA	0.069

Note— Ps represent Pearson chi-square and Fisher's exact test p-values, comparing proportions across each of the DBT years (1–3) with the baseline DM0 year. The P (DBT) column contains the p-values for testing null hypothesis that values are not significantly different across DBT 1–3 years. The NAs in the interval cancer line (bottom row) indicate that adequate cancer registry follow up was not available for DBT years 2 and 3. PPV1 is defined as cancers/recalled cases.

Table 2 demonstrates at the individual level, the outcomes for women screened with DBT at a first, second and third round. Recall rate decreased at each consecutive round of screening from 103 to 69 to 59/1000 screened, from the first round to third, respectively. Cancer detection rates were 6.3, 4.2 and 7.3/1000 screened at the first, second and third rounds of screening, respectively. The decrease in the cancer detection rate in the second round suggests a prevalence or, first round screening effect that was no longer evident at the third round. PPV1 showed a similar reduction at the second round and an increase at the third round.

Table 2. Recall, cancer detection, and PPV 1 for first, second, and third round of digital breast tomosynthesis (DBT) screening **(modified from Reference [8])**

	One screen	Two screens	Three screens
	21395 (100 %)	9316 (44 %)	3023 (14 %)
Recall, n/1000	103	69.2	59
Cancer, n/1000	6.3	4.2	7.3
PPV 1, %	6.1	6.1	12.4
Recall, n	2201	645	177
Cancer, n	135	39	22

When comparing the screening metrics from the first six months of implementing s2D with DBT compared to DBT year 1, there was a reduction in recall from 88 to 71/1000 screened (p < 0.001). The cancer detection rate for s2D/DBT was not significantly different from DBT1: 5.03 vs 5.5/1000 women screened, respectively (p = 0.72). The reduction in recalls and maintenance of the overall cancer detection rate was accompanied by a 39 % reduction in average glandular radiation dose (4.88 mGy vs 7.99 mGy, p < 0.001).

4   Discussion

The continued controversy surrounding mammographic screening revolves mainly around the so-called "harms" of a false positive screen. Incorporating DBT in screening has clearly shown that the new modality can reduce false positives while increasing cancer detection, specifically invasive cancers [1, 4]. Our study demonstrates that while there may be a small prevalence effect with the first round of screening, the improved outcomes achieve with DBT screening are sustainable and associated with a trend of decreasing interval cancers. However, the improved outcomes achieved with DM/DBT screening are obtained with an increase in radiation dose. Reconstructed or, "synthetic 2D DM" images offer the opportunity to significantly reduce patient dose over a lifetime of screening. In addition, our preliminary results with synthetic 2D imaging suggest that s2D is a non-inferior replacement of the DM portion of combination DM/DBT imaging. Screening with s2D/DBT allows for the benefits of DBT with a significant decrease in increased radiation dose compared to DM/DBT.

References

1. Skaane, P., Bandos, A.I., Eben, E.B., Jebsen, I.N., Krager, M., Haakenaasen, U., Ekseth, U., Izadi, M., Hofvind, S., Gullien, R.: Two-view digital breast tomosynthesis screening with synthetically reconstructed projection images: comparison with digital breast tomosynthesis with full-field digital mammographic images. Radiology **271**(3), 655–663 (2014)
2. Ciatto, S., Houssami, N., Bernardi, D., Caumo, F., Pellegrini, M., Brunelli, S., Tuttobene, P., Bricolo, P., Fanto, C., Valentini, M., Montemezzi, S., Macaskill, P.: Integration of 3D digital mammography with tomosynthesis for population breast-cancer screening (STORM): a prospective comparison study. Lancet Oncol. **14**(7), 583–589 (2013)
3. Gilbert, F.J., Tucker, L., Gillan, M.G., et al.: The TOMMY trial: a comparison of TOMosynthesis with digital MammographY in the UK NHS breast screening programme–a multicentre retrospective reading study comparing the diagnostic performance of digital breast tomosynthesis and digital mammography with digital mammography alone. Health Technol. Assess. **19**(i–xxv), 1–136 (2015)
4. Friedewald, S.M., Rafferty, E.A., Conant, E.F.: Breast cancer screening with tomosynthesis and digital mammography-reply. JAMA **312**, 1695–1696 (2014)
5. McCarthy, A.M., Kontos, D., Synnestvedt, M. et al.: Screening outcomes following implementation of digital breast tomosynthesis in a general-population screening program. J. Natl. Cancer Inst. **106**, 1–7 (2014)
6. Rose, S.L., Tidwell, A.L., Bujnoch, L.J., et al.: Implementation of breast tomosynthesis in a routine screening practice: an observational study. AJR Am. J. Roentgenol. **200**, 1401–1408 (2013)
7. Haas, B.M., Kalra, V., Geisel, J., et al.: Comparison of tomosynthesis plus digital mammography and digital mammography alone for breast cancer screening. Radiology **269**, 694–700 (2013)

8. McDonald, E.S., Oustimov, A., Weinstein, S.P., Synnestvedt, M., Schnall, M., Conant, E.C.: Effectiveness of tomosynthesis in combination with digital mammography: outcomes analysis from three years of breast cancer screening. JAMA Oncol. (2016, in press)
9. Zuckerman, S.P., Conant, E.F., Weinstein, S.P., Synnestvedt, M., Korhonen, K.E., McDonald, E.S.: Early implementation of synthesized 2D in screening with digital breast tomosynthesis: a pictorial essay of early outcomes. Presented at the 101st RSNA Annual Meeting, Chicago, IL, 29 November – 4 December 2015

CAD

LUT-QNE: Look-Up-Table Quantum Noise Equalization in Digital Mammograms

Alessandro Bria[1(✉)], Claudio Marrocco[1], Jan-Jurre Mordang[2],
Nico Karssemeijer[2], Mario Molinara[1], and Francesco Tortorella[1]

[1] DIEI, University of Cassino and Southern Latium, Cassino, FR, Italy
{a.bria,c.marrocco,m.molinara,tortorella}@unicas.it
[2] DIAG, Radboud University Nijmegen Medical Centre, Nijmegen, The Netherlands
{jan-jurre.mordang,nico.karssemeijer}@radboudumc.nl

Abstract. Quantum noise is a signal-dependent, Poisson-distributed noise and the dominant noise source in digital mammography. Quantum noise removal or equalization has been shown to be an important step in the automatic detection of microcalcifications. However, it is often limited by the difficulty of robustly estimating the noise parameters on the images. In this study, a nonparametric image intensity transformation method that equalizes quantum noise in digital mammograms is described. A simple Look-Up-Table for Quantum Noise Equalization (LUT-QNE) is determined based on the assumption that noise properties do not vary significantly across the images. This method was evaluated on a dataset of 252 raw digital mammograms by comparing noise statistics before and after applying LUT-QNE. Performance was also tested as a preprocessing step in two microcalcification detection schemes. Results show that the proposed method statistically significantly improves microcalcification detection performance.

Keywords: Digital mammography · Quantum noise · Nonparametric · Noise equalization · Microcalcification detection

1 Introduction

Digital mammography is the standard tool for breast cancer screening today [1]. To help radiologists in the difficult task of interpreting screening mammograms, computer-aided detection (CADe) systems have been proposed and demonstrated to improve the detection of cancer [2]. However, the presence of intensity-dependent quantum noise in the image may hamper the detectability of subtle lesions such as microcalcifications. It has been shown that suppressing [3] or equalizing [4] quantum noise in digital mammograms has a significant influence on the success of automated microcalcification detection and, thus, a number of image preprocessing techniques have been proposed with this aim [3–7]. These methods, however, require either to robustly estimate the noise properties from one or more mammogram images [3–6], or to characterize the imaging transfer function from a set of phantom images [7]. A nonparametric, easy-to-implement

© Springer International Publishing Switzerland 2016
A. Tingberg et al. (Eds.): IWDM 2016, LNCS 9699, pp. 27–34, 2016.
DOI: 10.1007/978-3-319-41546-8_4

solution that reduces the quantum noise negative effect on microcalcification detection performance has been missing.

In this work, we adopt a *quasi-uniform* noise model in which we hypothesize that if the noise properties do not vary significantly across the images, then a suboptimal yet effective nonparametric noise equalization that enables improved microcalcification detection can be obtained. Based on this assumption, we propose a Look-Up-Table for Quantum Noise Equalization (LUT-QNE) that rescales pixel intensities to a scale with non-intensity-dependent quasi-uniform noise level. Then, we provide and validate an analytical formulation for the noise inhomogeneity on the transformed images.

Our method can be easily and directly embedded in any existing automatic microcalcification detection scheme to boost detection performance without additional computational load. We show this for two microcalcification detection methods, namely the Haar-like feature based cascade of boosting classifiers (Cascade) [8] and the weighted Difference-of-Gaussian (DoG) filter [9].

2   Method

2.1   Quasi-Uniform Square-Root Noise Model

Quantum noise is caused by fluctuations in photon fluence at the detector. These fluctuations can be described by a Poisson distribution and the standard deviation σ_q in which the number of detected photons fluctuate around the mean detected number of photons λ is equal to $\sqrt{\lambda}$ [6]. Since in digital mammography a linear relationship exists between pixel intensity y and exposure, quantum noise standard deviation σ_q can be estimated by [4,6]:

$$\sigma_q(y) = c\sqrt{y} \tag{1}$$

where c is a noise level parameter which we hypothesize uniform in one mammogram and distributed with mean $\bar{c}$ and standard deviation σ_c in a set of N mammograms, with $\sigma_c \ll \bar{c}$ (hence the term '*quasi-uniform*').

2.2   LUT-QNE

Let us first consider the case of a single mammogram image that has to be transformed to a scale with uniform noise level β. Then, the desired scale transform $\tilde{y} = T(y)$ should satisfy the following differential equation:

$$dT(y) = \frac{\beta}{\sigma_q(y)}dy \tag{2}$$

where the denominator $\sigma_q(y)$ eliminates the dependency of the differential dy on the noise variation and, thus, realizes the noise equalization, whereas the numerator β determines the constant noise level on the transformed scale.

After applying the square-root model of Eq. 1 and adding border conditions, we obtain the following boundary value problem (BVP):

$$
\begin{cases}
\frac{dT(y)}{dy} = \frac{\beta}{c\sqrt{y}} \\
T(0) = 0 \\
T(2^b - 1) = 2^b - 1
\end{cases}
\tag{3}
$$

where we supposed, without loss of generality, that the transformation does not alter the original image bitdepth b. The BVP so obtained is clearly overdetermined since there are two boundary conditions and a differential equation of first order. Specifically, after solving the differential equation, we obtain the following overdetermined system:

$$
\begin{cases}
T(y) = \frac{2\beta}{c}\sqrt{y} + k \\
T(0) = 0 \\
T(2^b - 1) = 2^b - 1
\end{cases}
\tag{4}
$$

which has no solution since there is only one unknown (k). In order to obtain a well-determined system, we consider β as the second unknown. Intuitively, this means that we allow the noise level β on the transformed image to depend on the noise parameter c of the original image, i.e. $\beta = \beta(c)$. After applying the two border conditions, we get:

$$
\beta = \frac{c}{2}\sqrt{2^b - 1}
\tag{5}
$$

which yields the following noise-equalizing transform:

$$
\tilde{y} = T(y) = \sqrt{y(2^b - 1)}
\tag{6}
$$

Since this transform only depends on the pixel intensity y, it can be implemented with a LUT for Quantum Noise Equalization (LUT-QNE) whose elements $\{LUT_i\}_{i=0,1,\dots,2^b-1}$ are:

$$
LUT_i = \left\lfloor \sqrt{i(2^b - 1)} + 0.5 \right\rfloor
\tag{7}
$$

We now want to apply the LUT-QNE to a set of N mammograms under the hypothesis of quasi-uniform model described in Sect. 2.1. According to Eq. 5, this means that each image $j = 1, \dots, N$ will be equalized to a different noise level β_j that is well approximated by:

$$
\beta_j \approx c_j \sqrt{2^{b-2}}
\tag{8}
$$

which is the quantum noise level $\sigma_q(y)$ of the jth image at the intensity level $y = 2^{b-2}$ (see Eq. 1). For the Central Limit Theorem, if N is large (usually $N > 30$), the 95 % confidence interval in which β varies is given by:

$$
\beta^{95\%} = \bar{\beta} \pm 2\sigma_\beta = \bar{c}\sqrt{2^{b-2}} \pm 2\sigma_c\sqrt{2^{b-2}}
\tag{9}
$$

where the term $\sigma_\beta \triangleq \sigma_c \sqrt{2^{b-2}}$ describes the variation of equalized noise level β among the mammograms and, thus, provides an analytical formulation for the noise level inhomogeneity in the transformed scale. In an ideal noise equalization scheme, σ_β should be close to zero and should not depend on σ_c, meaning that all images are equalized to the same noise level independently from their original noise level. In our framework, however, we allow the transformed noise level to vary in a rather small range ($\sigma_\beta \ll 10$ since $\sigma_c \ll \bar{c}$ and $\bar{c} < 1$ as it will be shown next) and hypothesize that this suboptimal noise equalization is effective enough to improve microcalcification detection.

In the following subsection, we theoretically validate our proposed scheme to confirm its effectiveness under the framework adopted.

2.3   Theoretical Validation

In the nonequalized raw mammogram, the Poisson-distributed quantum noise causes the intensity y to fluctuate in the range $y \pm c\sqrt{y}$. Then, if we apply the scale transform of Eq. 6, the transformed intensity $\tilde{y}$ will fluctuate in the range:

$$\sqrt{(y \pm c\sqrt{y})(2^b - 1)} \tag{10}$$

which can be rearranged in:

$$\sqrt{y(2^b - 1)}\sqrt{1 \pm \frac{c}{\sqrt{y}}} \tag{11}$$

Since c is close to zero in practice [4–6], we can approximate the second multiplicative term with the first-order McLaurin series centered in $c = 0$:

$$f(c) \triangleq \sqrt{1 \pm \frac{c}{\sqrt{y}}} \approx f(0) + f'(0)c = 1 \pm \frac{c}{2\sqrt{y}} \tag{12}$$

which substituted in Eq. 11 yields:

$$\sqrt{y(2^b - 1)} \pm \frac{c}{2}\sqrt{2^b - 1} \tag{13}$$

where the first term is the transformed intensity $\tilde{y}$ as in Eq. 6, and the second term is the intensity fluctuation (i.e. the noise level) β as in Eq. 5. This confirms that the proposed scale transform effectively equalizes the noise in a single mammogram and also theoretically validates the analytical formulation for noise level inhomogeneity σ_β derived in Eq. 9.

3   Results

3.1   Dataset

The assessment of the proposed noise equalization method was performed on 252 raw DICOM 'FOR PROCESSING' digital mammograms extracted from a private database containing more than $40,000$ cases obtained in routine screening. Specifically, the 252 mammograms were taken from 129 abnormal cases (70 benign and 59 malignant) extracted by selecting all the available images with individual microcalcifications manually labeled by an experienced reader ($7,758$ in total). The 252 images were acquired during a period spanning years 2003-2008 with three full field direct digital mammography systems (163 the first, 52 the second, 37 the third), all from Hologic and with a resolution of $70\,\mu m$ per pixel and 14-bit grayscale pixel depth. The combination of anode target and filter materials was molybdenum/molybdenum in 103 acquisitions, molybdenum/rhodium in 112 acquisitions, and unknown in the remaining 37 acquisitions made with the third mammography system.

3.2   Experimental Validation

Experimental validation of the proposed noise equalization scheme was performed by comparing noise statistics before and after applying LUT-QNE to the images. Noise statistics in each image were calculated with a slightly modified version of the truncated distribution method proposed by McLoughlin et al. [4], and later improved by Schie and Karssemeijer [6]. In short, it consisted of the following steps: (i) the breast-air boundary was eroded by half of the breast thickness to discard the inner peripheral zone where noise estimates are overwhelmed by thickness changes; (ii) the image was convolved with a high-pass Gaussian filter of s.d. $100\,\mu m$ and the local contrast $l_i = y_i - y'_i$ was computed at each location i, with y'_i being the pixel value of the smoothed image; (iii) the grayscale of the smoothed image was divided into 10 equally populated bins, each associated to its weighted mean intensity $\overline{y}_k$, $k = 1, ..., 10$; (iv) for every bin, local contrast distributions were obtained by mapping l_i to the bin of y'_i; (v) Gaussian fitting with truncation of the values below the 20 % of the maximum was applied to each local contrast distribution to estimate the noise level σ_k.

The noise parameter c was estimated for each nonequalized image by least squares fitting of the noise sample points $(\sigma_k, \overline{y}_k)$ to the model $\sigma_q(y) = c\sqrt{y}$ and it varied in the range $\overline{c} \pm \sigma_c = 0.397 \pm 0.044$ (average goodness-of-fit $\overline{R^2} = 0.974$). Scatter plots of noise sample points taken from the 252 images before and after applying the LUT-QNE are shown in Fig. 1 along with the predicted 95 % confidence intervals. In both cases, at least 95 % of the data points were in the predicted range, thus validating the proposed noise equalization model and the analytical formulation for noise level inhomogeneity σ_β (see Eq. 9). This was equal to 2.82, corresponding to 11 % of the average noise level $\overline{\beta} = 25.2$.

3.3   Microcalcification Detection

Effectiveness of the proposed LUT-QNE method was tested on two microcalcification detectors, namely the Haar-like feature based cascade of boosting classifiers (Cascade) [8] and the weighted difference-of-Gaussian (DoG) filter [9]. Detectors with and without LUT-QNE were evaluated on the 252 mammograms

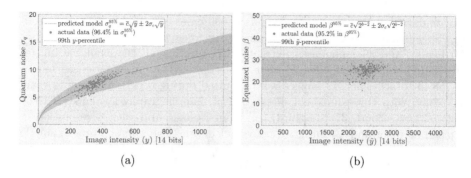

Fig. 1. Scatter plots of noise level in 252 raw digital mammograms before (a) and after (b) applying the proposed noise equalization scheme.

at $7,758$ pixel locations centered on labeled microcalcifications (positive samples) and at $25,190,476$ pixel locations on background tissue (negative samples), using a subwindow of size 13×13 pixels ($0.9\,\mathrm{mm} \times 0.9\,\mathrm{mm}$).

The Cascade detector was trained and tested with 10-fold cross validation considering 9 folds for training set, validation set and pool and the remaining fold as test set. In each cross validation step we used 6,982 positive samples equally parted between training and validation sets and 22,751,429 negative samples subdivided in 20,000, 60,000 and 22,671,429 respectively for training set, validation set and pool. The configuration of the cascade was the same as in [8], with node detection rate equal to 0.99 and node false positive rate equal to 0.3. After the 10-fold cross validation, the confidence degrees obtained for each sample in the test sets were pooled together.

For the DoG detector, we used commonly adopted parameter values [10] after validation with grid search. The values of the kernel width used for the positive and negative Gaussian kernels were 0.75 and 4, respectively, and the weight associated with the positive kernel was 0.8. At every pixel location, a confidence degree was calculated by taking the maximum DoG filter response in the subwindow centered on that pixel.

Detection performance of both the detectors was evaluated in terms of Receiver Operating Characteristics (ROC) curve by plotting True Positive Rate (TPR) against False Positive Rate (FPR) for a series of thresholds on the confidence degree associated to each sample. We considered as performance measure the *Partial Area Under the ROC Curve* (PAUC) defined as $\mathrm{PAUC}(x) = \int_0^x TPR \ dFPR$ where $[0, x]$ is the range of interest for FPR [11].

To determine if LUT-QNE provided statistically significantly better microcalcification performance, we applied the bootstrap procedure. The test set was sampled with replacement 2,000 times so that each new set of sampled data contained the same number of examples as the original set. For each FPR range and detector considered, the difference ΔPAUC in PAUC between the detector with and without LUT-QNE was computed. Resampling 2,000 times resulted in 2,000 values for ΔPAUC. p-values were defined as the fraction of ΔPAUC values that were negative or zero, corresponding to cases in which LUT-QNE

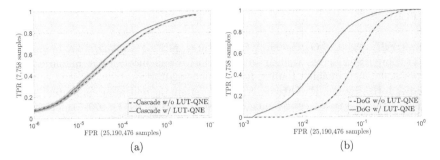

Fig. 2. Average ROC curves for Cascade (a) and DoG (b) microcalcification detectors with and without LUT-QNE obtained from 2,000 bootstrap samples. Confidence bands indicate 95 % confidence intervals along the TPR axis.

did not provide any improvement. The statistical significance level was chosen as $\alpha = 0.05$ and, thus, performance differences were statistically significant if $p < 0.05$.

Average ROC curves for the two detectors are reported in Fig. 2. For the Cascade detector, LUT-QNE yielded an increase in PAUC of 4 % ($p < 0.05$), 10 % ($p < 0.05$), and 6 % ($p = 0.11$) at $FPR = 10^{-3}, 10^{-4}$ and 10^{-5}, respectively. For the DoG detector, LUT-QNE yielded an increase in PAUC of 8 % ($p < 0.05$), 120 % ($p < 0.05$), and 1085 % ($p < 0.05$) at $FPR = 1, 10^{-1}$ and 10^{-2}, respectively.

4 Discussion

In this work we have investigated the use of a nonparametric scale transform to equalize signal-dependent quantum noise in raw digital mammography images to improve microcalcification detection performance. We hypothesized that a suboptimal yet effective nonparametric noise equalization can be obtained if noise properties do not vary significantly across the images. However, this does not hold if the gain factor determining the linear relationship between intensity and exposure changes, which may happen when the images are acquired with systems from different manufacturers or running substantially different software.

Both theoretical and experimental validation of the proposed equalization model were provided and showed that the noise level on the transformed scale was no more signal-dependent and varied in a rather small range among the mammograms. When embedded in two microcalcification detection schemes, the proposed method always yielded statistically significantly better performance. It is important to note, however, that these schemes did not include clustering of the microcalcifications, nor benign vs. malignant characterization, nor false-positive reduction. We expect that since results show an improvement in these relatively simple detection schemes, our method will also be effective in more complex detection algorithms. This is also confirmed by the results obtained in [12], where our method was employed in a complete CADe system that revealed to be competitive with the state-of-the-art commercial CADe systems.

34 A. Bria et al.

References

1. Ekpo, E.U., Egbe, N.O., Egom, A.E., McEntee, M.F.: Mammographic breast density: comparison across women with conclusive and inconclusive mammography reports. J. Med. Imaging Radiat. Sci. **1**, 55–59 (2015)
2. Eadie, L.H., Taylor, P., Gibson, A.P.: A systematic review of computer-assisted diagnosis in diagnostic cancer imaging. Eur. J. Radiol. **81**(1), e70–e76 (2012)
3. Romualdo, L., Vieira, M., Schiabel, H., Mascarenhas, N., Borges, L.: Mammographic image denoising and enhancement using the anscombe transformation, adaptive wiener filtering, and the modulation transfer function. J. Digit. Imaging **26**(2), 183–197 (2013)
4. McLoughlin, K.J., Bones, P.J., Karssemeijer, N.: Noise equalization for detection of microcalcification clusters in direct digital mammogram images. IEEE Trans. Med. Imaging **23**(3), 313–320 (2004)
5. Veldkamp, W.J.H., Karssemeijer, N.: Normalization of local contrast in mammograms. IEEE Trans. Med. Imaging **19**(7), 731–738 (2000)
6. van Schie, G., Karssemeijer, N.: Detection of microcalcifications using a nonuniform noise model. In: Krupinski, E.A. (ed.) IWDM 2008. LNCS, vol. 5116, pp. 378–384. Springer, Heidelberg (2008)
7. Tromans, C.E., Cocker, M.R., Brady, S.M.: Quantification and normalization of x-ray mammograms. Phys. Med. Biol. **57**(20), 6519 (2012)
8. Bria, A., Marrocco, C., Molinara, M., Tortorella, F.: Detecting clusters of microcalcifications with a cascade-based approach. In: Maidment, A.D.A., Bakic, P.R., Gavenonis, S. (eds.) IWDM 2012. LNCS, vol. 7361, pp. 111–118. Springer, Heidelberg (2012)
9. Dengler, J., Behrens, S., Desaga, J.: Segmentation of microcalcifications in mammograms. IEEE Trans. Med. Imaging **12**, 634–642 (1993)
10. El Naqa, I., Yang, W.M.N., Galatsanos, Y.N.P., Nishikawa, R.M.: A support vector machine approach for detection of microcalcifications. IEEE Trans. Med. Imaging **21**(12), 1552–1563 (2002)
11. Yousef, W.A.: Assessing classifiers in terms of the partial area under the ROC curve. Comput. Stat. Data Anal. **64**, 51–70 (2013)
12. Bria, A., Karssemeijer, N., Tortorella, F.: Learning from unbalanced data: a cascade-based approach for detecting clustered microcalcifications. Med. Image Anal. **18**(2), 241–252 (2014)

Automatic Microcalcification Detection in Multi-vendor Mammography Using Convolutional Neural Networks

Jan-Jurre Mordang[1]([envelope]), Tim Janssen[1], Alessandro Bria[2], Thijs Kooi[1],
Albert Gubern-Mérida[1], and Nico Karssemeijer[1]

[1] Department of Radiology and Nuclear Medicine,
Radboud University Nijmegen Medical Center, Nijmegen, The Netherlands
jan-jurre.mordang@radboudumc.nl
[2] Department of Electrical and Information Engineering,
University of Cassino and Southern Lazio, Cassino, Italy

Abstract. Convolutional neural networks (CNNs) have shown to be powerful for classification of image data and are increasingly used in medical image analysis. Therefore, CNNs might be very suitable to detect microcalcifications in mammograms. In this study, we have configured a deep learning approach to fulfill this task. To overcome the large class imbalance between pixels belonging to microcalcifications and other breast tissue, we applied a hard negative mining strategy where two CNNs are used. The deep learning approach was compared to a current state-of-the-art method for the detection of microcalcifications: the cascade classifier. Both methods were trained on a large training set including 11,711 positive and 27 million negative samples. For testing, an independent test set was configured containing 5,298 positive and 18 million negative samples. The mammograms included in this study were acquired on mammography systems from three manufactures: Hologic, GE, and Siemens. Receiver operating characteristics analysis was carried out. Over the whole specificity range, the CNN approach yielded a higher sensitivity compared to the cascade classifier. Significantly higher mean sensitivities were obtained with the CNN on the mammograms of each individual manufacturer compared to the cascade classifier in the specificity range of 0 to 0.1. To our knowledge, this was the first study to use a deep learning strategy for the detection of microcalcifications in mammograms.

Keywords: Mammography · Calcifications · Deep learning · Convolutional neural networks · Computer aided detection

1 Introduction

Convolutional Neural Networks (CNNs) [9,12] have been shown to be very powerful in the classification of large image databases [7,8]. Moreover, CNNs are

© Springer International Publishing Switzerland 2016
A. Tingberg et al. (Eds.): IWDM 2016, LNCS 9699, pp. 35–42, 2016.
DOI: 10.1007/978-3-319-41546-8_5

also increasingly applied in medical image analysis, e.g. included in CADe systems, and have shown to achieve cutting edge performances [3,4,6]. Another great advantage of applying CNNs is that the networks themselves determine the most descriptive features to separate the positive from the negative class while current CADe systems use pre-determined features which can lead to a loss of information or an increase of processing time. Therefore, CNNs might be very suitable for detecting microcalcifications in mammograms.

One of the main difficulties in the detection of microcalcifications in mammograms is that the positive class, i.e. pixels belonging to microcalcifications, is very small compared to the negative class, i.e. other breast tissue. This large class imbalance is a big impediment for most classification strategies and make them unsuitable for this task. A previous study about applying CNNs to a class imbalanced dataset yielded very good results [3]. Additionally, a single mammogram consists of millions of pixels to be analyzed. Therefore, a CADe system should operate very fast. A CADe system with high-complexity classifiers and/or features can lead to a very slow system and consequently become useless to process millions of images. An additional benefit of CNNs is that they can be applied with a very high computation speed.

The purpose of this study is to implement and study the performance of a deep learning approach with CNNs to detect microcalcifications in mammograms. The proposed system is compared to a current state-of-the-art microcalcification detection approach. Another important aspect for a CADe system to be applicable in breast cancer screening is their compatibility with mammograms acquired with mammographic units developed by different vendors. Each vendor has its own detector type for making mammograms which can result in a substantial variation in noise characteristics and appearance. Therefore, we used a heterogeneous dataset consisting of mammograms acquired with mammographic units developed by three different manufacturers.

2   Methods

2.1   Materials

For this study, we collected a multi-vendor and multi-center dataset consisting of 490 mammograms acquired with Hologic digital mammography systems (Hologic, Bedford, Massachusetts, United States), 1044 mammograms acquired with GE Senographe systems (GE, Fairfield, Connecticut, United States), and 72 mammograms acquired with Siemens Mammomat Inspiration systems (Siemens, Erlangen, Germany). In the dataset all available medio-lateral oblique and cranial caudal views of the left and right breast were included. All mammograms were acquired with standard clinical settings and unprocessed raw FFDM images were used in this study. The data acquired with the Hologic digital mammography systems were obtained from women whom participated in a national screening program (Bevolkings Onderzoek Midden-West, The Netherlands) and were referred for diagnostic follow up. The other mammograms were acquired in our own institution after referral in screening. An overview of the dataset is shown

Table 1. Overview of the dataset.

Dataset configuration			
Manufacturer	# cases	# exams	# mammograms
Hologic	104	132	490
GE	255	268	1044
Siemens	23	23	72

in Table 1. In all mammograms, individual microcalcifications were annotated based on the diagnostic reports. Annotations were made by marking the center of each microcalcification.

2.2 Convolutional Neural Networks

The general aim for a microcalcification detector is to classify each pixel in the mammogram in one of two classes: microcalcification or non-microcalcification. We propose a hard negative mining strategy to overcome the large class imbalance between the microcalcification and non-microcalcification classes. First, a CNN is trained on a small dataset. Second, the trained CNN is applied to the whole dataset to remove the easy samples. Finally, a second CNN is trained on a larger dataset which contains the hard negative samples, i.e. samples that are more difficult to differentiate from microcalcification pixels than easy classifiable samples. For new samples such as those in the test set, only the second CNN is applied.

To train a CNN, patches, sub-images centered around the pixel of interest, are obtained from both the positive and negative class. These patches are then fed into the first convolutional layer. In each layer, filters are trained to divide the data in separate classes. This approach uses all information within the patch that is supplied to the CNN and determines its most descriptive features between the two groups by itself. Training of the CNN is an iterative process, where in each iteration (or epoch) network parameters and discriminative parameters are optimized. In each epoch, the CNN minimizes a cost function by updating its parameters via back-propagation.

A CNN consist of several layers, the most commonly used layers are the convolutional layers, the pooling layers and the fully connected layers. The convolutional layers consist of a set of learnable 2D rectangular filters. These filters are convolved with the input patch and the activations are passed through an activation function. The pooling layers reduce the spatial size of the input by sub-sampling the output of the previous layer. Commonly, the maximum activation is taken over a sub window with a specified stride and are called max-pooling layers. The third type of mainly used layers are the fully connected layers. These layers have full connections to all activations in the previous layer. This type of layers are commonly used in regular neural networks. The final layer is a fully connected layer with two output neurons, one for each class.

The CNN structure in our study is inspired by the OxfordNet [13]. This structure consists of repetitions of two convolutional layers, with 32 filters each, followed by a max-pooling layer of size 2×2 and a stride of 2. Additionally, fully connected layers are used as final layers and a soft-max function calculates the final output. The two CNNs used in this study consist of 2 repetitions followed by three fully connected layers. An overview of the CNN architecture used for both CNNs used in this study is shown in Table 2. To reduce over fitting, dropout is applied for each fully connected layer during training of the CNNs [14].

Table 2. Overview of the convolutional neural network architecture. The input for the convolutional layers are zero padded to preserve the input size.

CNN Architecture				
Layer	Layer type	Filter size	Input size	Output size
1	Convolutional	3×3	$1 \times 13 \times 13$	$32 \times 13 \times 13$
2	Convolutional	3×3	$32 \times 13 \times 13$	$32 \times 13 \times 13$
3	Max-pooling	2×2 (stride $= 2$)	$32 \times 13 \times 13$	$32 \times 6 \times 6$
4	Convolutional	3×3	$32 \times 6 \times 6$	$32 \times 6 \times 6$
5	Convolutional	3×3	$32 \times 6 \times 6$	$32 \times 6 \times 6$
6	Max-pooling	2×2 (stride $= 2$)	$32 \times 6 \times 6$	$32 \times 3 \times 3$
7	Fully connected	256	$32 \times 3 \times 3$	256
8	Fully connected	256	256	256
9	Fully connected	2	256	2

2.3 Cascade Classifier

A current state-of-the-art method for the detection of microcalcifications is the cascade classifier [2]. This cascade classifier consist of a sequence of nodes where in each node an independent, single classifier classifies the patches. In each node, patches with a classification score below a specific threshold, which is determined during training, are filtered out and receive a final score of zero. Patches which remain in the last node receive the score of the last classifier. Gentle-Boost classifiers are used as single classifiers and regression stumps are used as weak classifiers [15]. These GentleBoost classifiers are trained on straight [16] and 45° rotated [10] Haar-like features.

During training, each GentleBoost classifier is optimized on a validation set. This optimization is based on two criteria: the detection and false positive rate on the validation set. The validation set is classifier by the GentleBoost classier after adding a weak classifier. If the criteria are not met, another weak classifier is added to the GentleBoost classifier. Training of the node finishes when the criteria are met or the maximum number of weak classifiers is reached. After each node, all samples in the training set are classified by the newly formed node and samples are removed when they received a classification score below the trained threshold. Training of the whole cascade is stopped when there are too few negative samples left in the training set.

2.4   Experiments and Evaluation

From the dataset two sets were created, a training set and a test set. For each annotation, a patch was extracted from the mammogram and were considered as positives. Each patch had a size of 13×13 pixels with the individual microcalcification centered in the patch. From the Hologic and GE data 80 % of these positives were included in the training set. The remaining 20 % of the Hologic and GE positives together with all positives obtained from the Siemens data were included in the test set. Additionally, negative patches were randomly taken from all mammograms (excluding the positive locations). For the training set, up top 35,000 negative patches were extracted from each mammogram in the Hologic data and up to 17,500 from each mammogram of the GE data. For the test set, up to 70,000 negative patches were extracted per mammogram in the Hologic and Siemens data and 35,000 per mammogram in the GE data. An overview of all samples in each training and test set is shown in Table 3.

Table 3. Overview of the training and test sets.

Samples per dataset				
Manufacturer	Training set		Testing set	
	# Positives	# Negatives	# Positives	# Negatives
Hologic	5,744	13,321,334	1,868	7,244,003
GE	5,967	14,625,465	1,652	6,842,428
Siemens	-	-	1,778	4,234,545
Total	11,711	27,946,799	5,298	18,320,976

The CNNs were trained on the training set. During training, the learning rate was initially set to 0.01 and linearly decreased to 0.0001 over the maximum number of epochs. For the first CNN, the maximum number of epochs was set to 1500 and to 750 for the second CNN. However, an early stopping criterion was set to prevent the CNN from over fitting: when the validation loss did not change over 100 epochs, training of the first CNN was stopped. For the second CNN early stopping was set to 50 epochs.

Training of the first CNN was performed on a balanced dataset containing 10 times the number of positives (each positive was taken 10 times) and an equal amount of negatives randomly sampled from the training set. In total, 117,110 negatives and 117,110 positives were used to train the first CNN. The second CNN was trained on a dataset containing 1 million samples. All 11,711 positive samples were included in this set together with 988,289 negative samples. The negative samples were obtained by weighted sampling of the whole training set according to the classification scores obtained with the first CNN. Furthermore, to create more positive samples for training the second CNN, positive samples were augmented. Augmentation was performed by flipping the positive samples horizontally and vertically and by rotating the patches 90°, 180°, and 270°. In each mini-batch the number of positives and negatives were balanced.

For evaluation, the performance of the (second) CNN was compared to a current state-of-the-art method for microcalcification detection: the cascade classifier [2]. The cascade classifier consists of several nodes with one single GentleBoost classifier. For training of the cascade classifier, all positives and all negatives in the training set were used. Subsequently, both systems were applied to the test set and Receiver Operating Characteristics (ROC) analysis was performed to compare the two systems. Furthermore, the mean sensitivity of the ROC curve in the specificity range on a logarithmic scale was calculated and compared. The mean sensitivity is defined as:

$$\overline{S}(i,j) = \frac{1}{ln(j) - ln(i)} \int_i^j \frac{s(f)}{f} \mathrm{d}f \tag{1}$$

where i and j are the lower and upper bound of the false positive fraction and were set to 0.000001 to 0.1, respectively, and $s(f)$ is the sensitivity at the false positive fraction f.

Statistical comparison was performed by means of bootstrapping [5]. On the test set, average ROC curves were calculated over 1000 bootstraps. Additionally, the mean sensitivity was calculated for each bootstrap and p-values were computed for testing significance [1,11]. Differences were considered to be significant for p-values < 0.05.

3   Results

The mean sensitivity obtained from the ROC analysis are shown in Table 4. In this table, the mean sensitivity is shown for each individual vendor as well as on the whole test set. For each dataset, the CNN obtained a higher mean sensitivity for all datasets. On the complete test set, containing Hologic, GE, and Siemens data, the CNN achieved a significantly higher mean sensitivity compared to the cascade, 0.6914 ± 0.0041 (mean±stdev) versus 0.6381 ± 0.0038 ($p < 0.001$). ROC curves were calculated on the whole test set for both methods and are shown in Fig. 1. The ROC curves are plotted on a logarithmic scale to show the difference between the two methods at high specificity. In Fig. 1, it can be seen that the CNN yields a higher sensitivity over the whole specificity range. All positive samples were detected at a specificity of 0.71 by the CNN while the cascade detects all positive samples at a specificity of 0.02. At a false positive fraction of 0.1, 0.01, 0.001, and 0.0001, the CNN detected 99.92 %, 99.58 %, 95.17 %, and 74.63 % of the positive samples, respectively. At the same false positive fractions, the cascade classifier detected 98,90 % 95.79 %, 90.85 %, and 63.89 % of the positives, respectively.

4   Discussion

Automated computer aided detection systems of microcalcifications in mammography have the potential to aid radiologists in reading mammograms. These

Table 4. Mean sensitivities in the false positive fraction range of 0.000001 and 0.1 for the individual datasets.

Mean sensitivities			
Dataset	CNN	Cascade	p-value
Hologic	0.7035 ± 0.0068	0.6534 ± 0.0062	$<0.001^\dagger$
GE	0.7015 ± 0.0069	0.6499 ± 0.0069	$<0.001^\dagger$
Siemens	0.6726 ± 0.0069	0.6180 ± 0.0064	$<0.001^\dagger$
Hologic + GE + Siemens	0.6914 ± 0.0041	0.6381 ± 0.0038	$<0.001^\dagger$

†Results are significantly different between the CNN and the cascade classifier ($p < 0.05$).

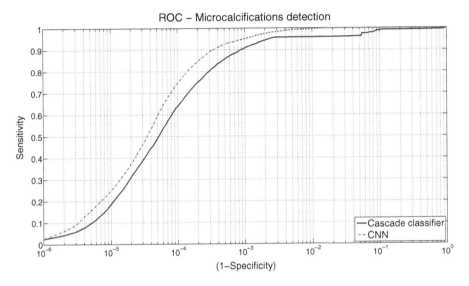

Fig. 1. Average ROC curves of the microcalcification detection with the cascade classifier and the convolutional neural network of 1,000 bootstraps. The ROC curves are plotted on a logarithmic scale.

systems are often designed into two stages: (1) detection of microcalcification candidates in the whole mammogram and (2) classifying microcalcification groups into benign and malignant. In this study, we focused on the detection of microcalcification candidates and we implemented a convolutional neural network for this task. To our knowledge, this is the first study where a deep learning strategy is developed for this task. The convolutional neural network was compared to a current state-of-the-art method, the cascade classifier. The comparison showed that the CNN outperforms the cascade classifier in terms of sensitivity in the whole specificity range. Additionally, the mean sensitivity in a false positive fraction range of 0.000001 to 0.1 was significantly higher with the CNN in the classification of all datasets acquired with three different mammography unit manufacturers.

References

1. Bornefalk, H., Hermansson, A.B.: On the comparison of FROC curves in mammography CAD systems. Med. Phys. **32**, 412–417 (2005)
2. Bria, A., Karssemeijer, N., Tortorella, F.: Learning from unbalanced data: a cascade-based approach for detecting clustered microcalcifications. Med. Image Anal. **18**, 241–252 (2013)
3. Cireşan, D.C., Giusti, A., Gambardella, L.M., Schmidhuber, J.: Mitosis detection in breast cancer histology images with deep neural networks. In: Mori, K., Sakuma, I., Sato, Y., Barillot, C., Navab, N. (eds.) MICCAI 2013, Part II. LNCS, vol. 8150, pp. 411–418. Springer, Heidelberg (2013)
4. Cruz-Roa, A.A., Arevalo Ovalle, J.E., Madabhushi, A., González Osorio, F.A.: A deep learning architecture for image representation, visual interpretability and automated basal-cell carcinoma cancer detection. In: Mori, K., Sakuma, I., Sato, Y., Barillot, C., Navab, N. (eds.) MICCAI 2013, Part II. LNCS, vol. 8150, pp. 403–410. Springer, Heidelberg (2013)
5. Efron, B., Tibshirani, R.J.: An Introduction to the Bootstrap, vol. 57. CRC Press, Boca Raton (1994)
6. Guo, Y., Wu, G., Commander, L.A., Szary, S., Jewells, V., Lin, W., Shen, D.: Segmenting hippocampus from infant brains by sparse patch matching with deep-learned features. In: Golland, P., Hata, N., Barillot, C., Hornegger, J., Howe, R. (eds.) MICCAI 2014, Part II. LNCS, vol. 8674, pp. 308–315. Springer, Heidelberg (2014)
7. He, K., Zhang, X., Ren, S., Sun, J.: Delving deep into rectifiers: Surpassing human-level performance on imagenet classification (2015). arXiv:150201852v1
8. Krizhevsky, A., Sutskever, I., Hinton, G.E.: Imagenet classification with deep convolutional neural networks. Adv. Neural Inf. Process. Syst. **25**, 1097–1105 (2012)
9. LeCun, Y., Bengio, Y., Hinton, G.: Deep learning. Nature **521**(7553), 436–444 (2015)
10. Lienhart, R., Maydt, J.: An extended set of Haar-like features for rapid object detection. In: Proceedings of 2002 International Conference on Image Processing, vol. 1, pp. I-900–I-903 (2002)
11. Samuelson, F., Petrick, N.: Comparing image detection algorithms using resampling. In: IEEE International Symposium on Biomedical Imaging, pp. 1312–1315 (2006)
12. Schmidhuber, J.: Deep learning in neural networks: an overview. Neural Netw. **61**, 85–117 (2015)
13. Simonyan, K., Zisserman, A.: Very deep convolutional networks for large-scale image recognition (2014). arXiv:14091556
14. Srivastava, N., Hinton, G., Krizhevsky, A., Sutskever, I., Salakhutdinov, R.: Dropout: a simple way to prevent neural networks from overfitting. J. Mach. Learn. Res. **15**(1), 1929–1958 (2014)
15. Torralba, A., Murphy, K., Freeman, W.: Sharing visual features for multiclass and multiview object detection. IEEE Trans. Pattern Anal. Mach. Intell. **29**, 854–869 (2007)
16. Viola, P., Jones, M.: Rapid object detection using a boosted cascade of simple features. In: Proceedings of IEEE Conference on Computer Vision and Pattern Recognition, vol. 1, pp. I-511–I-518 (2001)

Similar Image Retrieval of Breast Masses on Ultrasonography Using Subjective Data and Multidimensional Scaling

Chisako Muramatsu[1](✉), Tetsuya Takahashi[1], Takako Morita[2],
Tokiko Endo[3,4], and Hiroshi Fujita[1]

[1] Department of Intelligent Image Information, Gifu University, Gifu, Japan
{chisa,tetsuya,fujita}@fjt.info.gifu-u.ac.jp
[2] Department of Breast Surgery, Nagoya Medical Center, Nagoya, Japan
takako@rose.sunnet.ne.jp
[3] Department of Advanced Diagnosis, Nagoya Medical Center, Nagoya, Japan
[4] Department of Breast Surgery, Higashi Nagoya National Hospital, Nagoya, Japan
endot@e-nagoya.hosp.go.jp

Abstract. Presentation of images similar to a new unknown lesion can be helpful in medical image diagnosis and treatment planning. We have been investigating a method to retrieve relevant images as a diagnostic reference for breast masses on mammograms and ultrasound images. For retrieval of visually similar images, subjective similarities for pairs of masses were determined by experienced radiologists, and objective similarity measures were computed by modeling the subjective similarity space using multidimensional scaling (MDS). In this study, we investigated the similarity measure for masses on breast ultrasound images based on MDS and an artificial neural network and examined its usefulness in image retrieval. For 666 pairs of masses, correlation coefficient between the average subjective similarities and the MDS-based similarity measure was 0.724. When one to five images were retrieved, average precision in selecting relevant images, i.e., pathology-matched images for benign/malignant index image, was 0.778, indicating the potential utility of the proposed MDS-based similarity measure.

Keywords: Image similarity · Image retrieval · Breast ultrasound · Breast masses · Mass classification · Multidimensional scaling

1 Introduction

Breast cancer is the most frequently diagnosed and one of the leading causes of cancer deaths for women in the United States, some European countries, and Japan [1–3]. Early detection and proper treatment can reduce the number of cancer deaths and improve patients' quality of lives. Mammography is considered the most effective method for screening breast cancers in general population with normal risk [4–6]. When an abnormality is found, additional image examinations, such as ultrasonography, are generally performed for diagnosis. Breast ultrasound is not only useful for differential diagnosis but also for screening in young women and/or women with dense breasts [7–10]. With

© Springer International Publishing Switzerland 2016
A. Tingberg et al. (Eds.): IWDM 2016, LNCS 9699, pp. 43–50, 2016.
DOI: 10.1007/978-3-319-41546-8_6

the approval of use of automated breast ultrasound system for screening by the Food and Drug Administration, ultrasound screening in adjunct to mammography is expected to increase. Therefore, computer-aided diagnosis system that can support an efficient multimodality reading may be useful.

We have been investigating a computer-aided diagnosis system that provides the similar images with known pathologies as a reference in the diagnosis of breast lesions on mammograms [11–14]. For retrieval of images that are diagnostically relevant and also visually similar, subjective similarity data by experienced radiologists for pairs of lesions on mammograms were obtained and used as the gold standard for training the system in our previous studies. The results of these studies indicated the potential usefulness of the method for determination of similarity measures using the subjective data. In general, masses with the same pathologies were considered more similar than those with different pathologies in terms of malignancy and benignity. However, it was more difficult to distinguish subcategories, such as cysts and fibroadenomas, on mammograms. It is expected that some lesions are more easily distinguished on ultrasound. Thus, an image retrieval system for ultrasound images can be useful. However, it is not known that our previous method can be effectively applied to ultrasound images. In this study, we investigated the method for determination of similarity measure for masses on breast ultrasound images and examined its usefulness in image retrieval.

2   Database

Breast ultrasound images used in this study was obtained at Nagoya Medical Center, Nagoya, Japan. This study was approved by the institutional review board. Ultrasonography examinations were performed as screening, follow-ups, or diagnostic work-ups using EUB-8500 (Hitachi Medical Corporation, Tokyo, Japan) or Aplio XG (Toshiba Medical Systems Corporation, Otawara, Japan) by diagnostic physicians or technologists together with physicians. When an abnormal lesion was found, two orthogonal views were generally captured. In some cases, two views were saved in a single image (Fig. 1(a)), whereas in others each view was saved in a single image (Fig. 1(b)). In this study, 14 images of benign masses, including 5 cysts, 6 fibroadenomas (FAs), and 3 benign phyllodes tumors, and 23 images of malignant masses, including 15 invasive

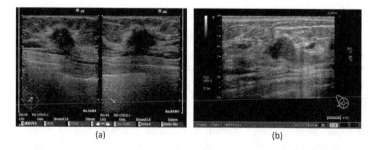

(a)   (b)

Fig. 1. Breast ultrasound images. (a) An image of orthogonal views of a scirrhous carcinoma (invasive ductal carcinoma) and (b) an image of a single view of a ductal carcinoma in situ

ductal carcinomas (IDCs) with 3 subtypes, 3 ductal carcinomas in situ (DCISs), 3 invasive lobular carcinomas, and 2 mucinous carcinomas, were selected as typical examples. They were employed in the observer study to establish the gold standard of subjective similarities of ultrasound masses.

3   Methods

3.1   Acquisition of Subjective Similarity Data

An observer reading study was performed for obtaining subjective similarity ratings for mass images. Using the 37 images, all possible pairs constitute 666 paired comparisons. Nine radiologists or breast surgeons who are certified for breast ultrasound reading by Japan Central Organization on Quality Assurance of Breast Cancer Screening participated in the study. Pairs of images were presented one by one as shown in Fig. 2, and each reader individually provided the similarity ratings on the continuous scale based on the overall assessment of shape, density and margin with respect to the anticipated diagnosis. The average ratings by the nine readers were considered as the gold standard (GS-A).

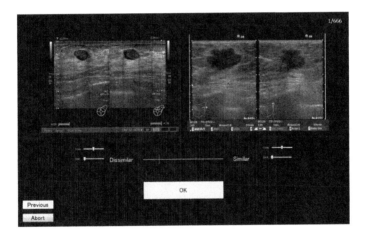

Fig. 2. User interface for obtaining subjective similarity ratings

Clinicians are not accustomed to evaluating similarities of lesions. Although some training cases were provided in the beginning, determination of similarity is not an easy task. In addition, reading of 666 pairs is a laborious task. There could be some pairs with large variations in their ratings. Thus, we also investigated the removal of outliers. For each pair, the ratings larger or smaller than 1.5 times the standard deviation from the average were excluded, and the average of the remaining ratings was considered as the alternative gold standard (GS-B).

3.2 Similarity Measure Based on Multidimensional Scaling

Multidimensional scaling (MDS) is a multivariate statistical technique which can display the dissimilarity relationship of data as a distance in lower dimensional space [15, 16]. It is a useful tool for visualization of the relationship with respect to the similarity between the subjects. In this study, the MDS was applied to the average dissimilarity (1- similarity) ratings for modeling the subjective similarity space reflecting the similarity relationship between the masses as illustrated in the top of Fig. 3. The number of dimensions was experimentally set to three in this study. Using the determined coordinates, a three-layered artificial neural network (ANN) with the back propagation algorithm was trained to estimate each dimension with image features as input data as illustrated in the bottom of Fig. 3.

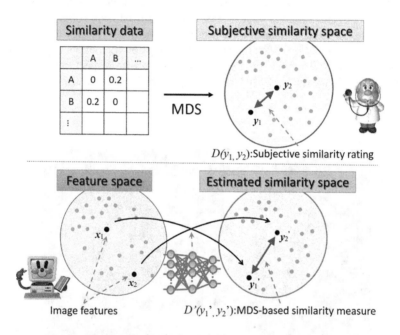

Fig. 3. Illustration of similarity space modeling

Eight image features characterizing the mass shape and four features related to the echo level were determined. The shape features included the ratio of height and width, circularity, irregularity, the degree of outline complexity, the number of dents in mass outline, the fraction of dented part in outline, the degree of dents, and the number of corners in outline. The height and width is determined as those of the rectangle enclosing the mass. The circularity is defined as the fraction of overlapped area of a mass and a circle placed at the center of the mass, whose area is equivalent to the mass. The irregularity is the ratio of the perimeter of the circle to the outline of the mass. The degree of outline complexity is the standard deviation of distances between points on the outline and the mass center. The number of dents is determined using the convex hull enclosing the mass. The degree of dents is defined as the ratio of areas of dents and the mass. The corners in outline are determined by sliding a circle on the outline and finding the area of overlap between the circle and the mass. Echo level features include the mean and standard deviation of pixel values, contrast, and posterior echo. The contrast is the difference of average pixel values in adjacent areas inside and outline the outline. The posterior echo is the ratio of average pixel values in the area posterior to the mass and the surrounding area. For the images with the combined two views such as in Fig. 1(a), the features were determined from both views and averaged. In the reconstructed space (MDS-based similarity space), MDS-based dissimilarity measure was determined by the Euclidean distance, which was then transformed to the similarity measure ranging from 0 to 1.

The MDS-based similarity measure was compared with the gold standard, and the usefulness of the measure for image retrieval was evaluated by the precision and recall. The precision is defined as the fraction of relevant images in the retrieved images whereas the recall is the fraction of relevant images that are retrieved to the total number of relevant images in the database. The images with the matched benignity or malignancy to an index image were considered relevant in this study. The similarity space modeling using MDS and ANN and the image retrieval test were performed by a leave-one-out cross validation test method. The performance was evaluated using GS-A and GS-B. For comparison, a conventional similarity measure based on the Euclidean distance (ED) in the feature space was also determined.

4   Result

Using all features, the subjective similarity space modelled by MDS was estimated by the ANN. The correlation coefficient between the GS-A and the MDS-based similarity measure was 0.724. When the GS-B was used in the space modelling, the correlation coefficient between the GS-B and the MDS-based similarity measure was 0.663. The correlation coefficient between the GS-A and ED-based measure was 0.514.

Using the MDS-based similarity measure, the most similar images for an index ("unknown") image were retrieved from the dataset (in this case from the 36 images). Figure 4 shows the precision and recall curves by using the GS-A, GS-B, ED-based measure, and the MDS-based measures using the GS-A and GS-B. The average precision at retrieving one to five most similar images was slightly higher when the GS-B was used than that using the GS-A (0.89 for the GS-B vs 0.88 for the GS-A).

When one to five most similar images were selected on the basis of the MDS-based similarity measure, the average precision was 0.78 and 0.81 using the GS-A and GS-B, respectively, for the training. They were not as high as those by the subjective ratings but higher than that using the ED-based similarity measure (0.70).

5   Discussion

It was expected that the subjective similarity ratings provided by experts were useful in selecting visually similar and diagnostically relevant images. Our previous study indicated the potential usefulness of the presentation of similar images in distinction between

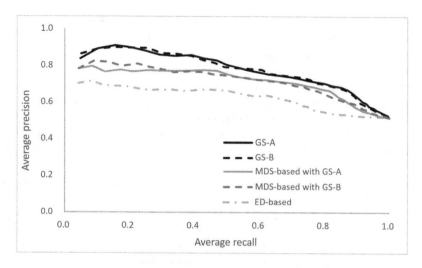

Fig. 4. Precision and recall curves for image retrieval using the gold standard and ED-based and MDS-based similarity measures

benign and malignant masses on mammograms [17, 18]. The high precision using the gold standard (GS-A and GS-B) for image retrieval in this study indicates the potential utility of the reference images selected on the basis of the image similarity by the experts for diagnosis of new lesions.

It was expected that the removal of outliers of subjective similarities may provide more reliable gold standard and improve the training process. The estimation of subjective rating using the ANN was more successful when the GS-A was used, which was suggested by the higher correlation. On the other hand, the average precision was slightly higher by using the GS-B when less than 5 images were retrieved, although it can be observed in Fig. 4 that the two curves are almost equivalent. These results may be due to the non-optimized parameters. Better parameter optimization process and the evaluation with an independent dataset are needed in the future. Also the usefulness of the presentation of images for the diagnosis of breast ultrasound images in clinical practice must be evaluated.

Overall, the result indicated that the MDS was effectively applied to model the subjective similarity space, and the similarity space was successfully estimated using ANN. Relatively high correlation coefficient between the gold standard and the MDS-based similarity measure and the high precision for image retrieval indicate the potential usefulness of the proposed similarity measure for selection of reference images that can be helpful in the diagnosis of breast masses on ultrasound images.

Acknowledgements. Authors are grateful to Mikinao Oiwa, MD, PhD and Misaki Shiraiwa, MD, PhD for their contribution in this study. This study was supported in part by the Grant-in-Aid for Scientific Research for Young Scientists (no. 26860399) by Japan Society for the Promotion of Science and Grant-in-Aid for Scientific Research on Innovative Areas (no. 26108005) by Ministry of Education, Culture, Sports, Sciences and Technology in Japan.

References

1. American Cancer Society: Cancer Facts & Figures 2016. American Cancer Society, Atlanta (2016)
2. Ferlay, J., Soerjomataram, I., Ervik, M., Dikshit, R., Eser, S., Mathers, C., Rebelo, M., Parkin, D.M., Forman, D., Bray, F.: GLOBOCAN 2012 v1.0, Cancer incidence and mortality worldwide: In: IARC CancerBase No. 11 [Internet], International Agency for Research on Cancer, Lyon (2013). http://globocan.iarc.fr
3. National Cancer Center, Center for Cancer Control and Information Services: Monitoring of Cancer Incidence in Japan MCIJ 2011. National Cancer Center (2015)
4. Tabar, L., Fagerberg, G., Duffy, S.W., Day, N.E., Gad, A., Grontoft, O.: Update of the Swedish two-county program of mammographic screening for breast cancer. Radiol. Clin. North Am. **30**, 187–210 (1992)
5. Shapiro, S., Venet, W., Strax, P., Venet, L., Roeser, R.: Selection, follow-up, and analysis in the health insurance plan study: a randomized trial with breast cancer screening. J. Natl. Cancer Inst. Monogr. **67**, 65–74 (1985)
6. Humphrey, L.L., Helfand, M., Chan, B.K.S., Woolf, S.H.: Breast cancer screening: a summary of the evidence for the U.S. preventive services task force. Ann. Intern. Med. **137**, E-347–E-367 (2002)
7. Berg, W.A., Zhang, Z., Lehrer, D., Jong, R.A., Pisano, E.D., Barr, R.G., Bohm-Velez, M., Mahoney, M.C., Evans III, W.P., Larsen, L.H., Morton, M.J., Mendelson, E.B., Farria, D.M., Cormack, J.B., Marques, H.S., Adams, A., Yeh, N.M., Gabrielli, G.G.: ACRIN 6666 investigators: detection of breast cancer with addition of annual screening ultrasound or a single screening MRI to mammography in women with elevated breast cancer risk. JAMA **307**, 1394–1404 (2012)
8. Chae, E.Y., Kim, H.H., Cha, J.H., Shin, H.J., Kim, H.: Evaluation of screening whole-breast sonography as a supplemental tool in conjunction with mammography in women with dense breasts. J. Ultrasound Med. **32**, 1573–1578 (2013)
9. Brem, R.F., Lenihan, M.J., Lieberman, J., Torrente, J.: Screening breast ultrasound: past, present, and future. AJR **204**, 234–240 (2015)
10. Ohuchi, N., Suzuki, A., Sobue, T., Kawai, M., Yamamoto, S., Zhang, Y.F., Shiono, Y.N., Saito, H., Kuriyama, S., Tohno, E., Endo, T., Fukao, A., Tsuji, I., Yamaguchi, T., Ohashi, Y., Fukuda, M., Ishida, T.: J-START investigator groups: Sensitivity and specificity of mammography and adjunctive ultrasonography to screen for breast cancer in the Japan Strategic Anti-cancer Randomized Trial (J-START): a randomized controlled trial. Lancet **387**, 341–348 (2016)
11. Muramatsu, C., Li, Q., Suzuki, K., Schmidt, R.A., Shiraishi, J., Ewstead, G.M., Doi, K.: Investigation of psychophysical measure for evaluation of similar images for mammographic masses: preliminary result. Med. Phys. **32**, 2295–2304 (2005)
12. Muramatsu, C., Li, Q., Shiraishi, J., Doi, K.: Investigation of similarity measures for selection of similar images in the diagnosis of clustered microcalcifications on mammograms. Med. Phys. **35**, 5695–5702 (2008)
13. Muramatsu, C., Schmidts, R.A., Shiraishi, J., Li, Q., Doi, K.: Presentation of similar images as a reference for distinction between benign and malignant masses on mammograms: analysis of initial observer study. J. Digit. Imaging **23**, 592–602 (2010)
14. Muramatsu, C., Nishimura, K., Endo, T., Oiwa, M., Shiraiwa, M., Doi, K., Fujita, H.: Represenattion of lesion similarity by use of multidimensional scaling for breast masses on mammograms. J. Digit. Imaging **26**, 740–747 (2013)
15. Kruskal, J.B., Wish, M.: Multidimensional Scaling. Sage Publication, Beverly Hills (1978)

16. Shepard, R.N., Romney, A.K., Nerlove, S.B.: Multidimensional Scaling: Theory and Applications in the Behavioral Sciences. Seminar Press, New York (1972)
17. Muramatsu, C., Schmidt, R.A., Shiraishi, J., Endo, T., Fujita, H., Doi, K.: Usefulness of presentation of similar images in the diagnosis of breast masses on mammograms comparison of observer performances in Japan and the USA. Radiol. Phys. Technol. **6**, 70–77 (2013)
18. Muramatsu, C., Endo, T., Oiwa, M., Shiraiwa, M., Doi, K., Fujita, H.: Effect of reference image retrieval on breast mass classification performance: ROC analysis. In: Breast Image Analysis MICCAI, pp. 50–57 (2013)

A Comparison Between a Deep Convolutional Neural Network and Radiologists for Classifying Regions of Interest in Mammography

Thijs Kooi[1(✉)], Albert Gubern-Merida[1], Jan-Jurre Mordang[1], Ritse Mann[1], Ruud Pijnappel[2], Klaas Schuur[2], Ard den Heeten[3], and Nico Karssemeijer[1]

[1] Department of Radiology, Radboud University Medical Center, Nijmegen, The Netherlands
Thijs.Kooi@radboudumc.nl
[2] Dutch Reference Centre for Screening, Nijmegen, The Netherlands
[3] Department of Radiology, University of Amsterdam, Amsterdam, The Netherlands

Abstract. In this paper, we employ a deep Convolutional Neural Network (CNN) for the classification of regions of interest of malignant soft tissue lesions in mammography and show that it performs on par to experienced radiologists. The CNN was applied to 398 regions of 5×5 cm, half of which contained a malignant lesion and the other half depicted suspicious regions in normal mammograms detected by a traditional CAD system. Four radiologists participated in the study. ROC analysis was used for evaluating results. The AUC of CNN was 0.87, which was higher than the mean AUC of the radiologists (0.84), though the difference was not significant.

1 Introduction

Computer Aided Detection and Diagnosis (CAD) systems are being developed for a variety of modalities and pathologies. Mammography has traditionally been on the fore front of this endeavor and commercial CAD systems are widely used in clinical practice. Unfortunately, progress has mostly stagnated in the past decade and the merit of contemporary systems is strongly questioned, with studies showing no significant improvements in the sensitivity for invasive breast cancer [1]. Therefore, there is a strong need to continue the development of mammography CAD.

The culmination of several decades of research into statistical learning methods, in particular *deep learning* [2,3], is recently making headlines [4,5], with many Artificial Intelligence (AI) systems claiming human or even superhuman performance in a variety of tasks, previously thought to be insurmountably complicated. Deep Convolutional Neural Networks (CNN) have emerged as the de-facto standard for vision based AI tasks and form the basis for face and object detection and autonomous vehicles. Traditional CAD systems employ features

© Springer International Publishing Switzerland 2016
A. Tingberg et al. (Eds.): IWDM 2016, LNCS 9699, pp. 51–56, 2016.
DOI: 10.1007/978-3-319-41546-8_7

such as spiculation, texture and contrast which are subsequently fed to a statistical learning machine. Rather than relying on engineers that mold medical knowledge into a set of features, deep architectures learn relevant features from data and the system is trained end-to-end. In essence, these ideas are not new and have been around since the late seventies. Their success in recent years can largely be attributed to more efficient training, advances in hardware and employment of many core computing and most importantly, sheer amounts of annotated training data.

In this paper, we employ a CNN for the classification of soft tissue lesions (e.g. masses and architectural distortions). We operate on square regions of 5×5 cm extracted from mammograms at suspicious locations identified by a traditional CAD system. This system outperforms a traditional CAD system we developed previously. In this study we compare the performance of this system to radiologists.

2   Deep Convolutional Neural Networks

To get a label for every sample, the image is convolved with a set of filter kernels, not unlike Gaussian derivative filters used in many traditional CAD systems, generating feature maps, which again are subjected to several transformations. Unlike traditional systems, however, most transformations are learned from data rather than handcrafted, allowing the algorithm to focus on information relevant for the classification problem and not predefined by the engineer. After the convolutional layers, several fully connected layers, where each activation is associated with a weight, are typically added, the exact benefit of which is still an open research question. Most people report an increase in performance when added, however. After the fully connected layers, the activations are fed to a softmax function, which generates a posterior probability over the labels. The parameters in the network are learned using maximum likelihood and backpropagation in combination with Stochastic Gradient Descent (SGD).

Pooling layers are typically added in between convolutional layers to reduce the size of the feature maps and induce some degree of translation invariance. Apart from this, these models do not exhibit any inherent invariances, although work is being done to incorporate this. Data augmentation, making new samples by means of deformations that one would expect to model possible variations in the data, is typically performed to make the networks robust and prevent overfitting.

For training the CNN, we used raw images and only applied a log transform. Images were scaled from 70 micron to 200 for faster processing. We employed a previously developed candidate detector designed for mammographic lesions [6] to generate candidate locations. It operates by extracting five features based on first and second order Gaussian kernels, two designed to spot the center of a focal mass and two looking for spiculation patterns, characteristic of malignant lesions. A final feature indicates the size of optimal response in scale-space.

To generate the pixel based training set, we extracted positive samples from a disk of constant size inside each annotated malignant lesion in the training set, to sample the same amount from every lesion size and prevent bias for larger areas. To obtain normal pixels for training, we randomly sampled 1 in 300 pixels from normal tissue in normal images, resulting in approximately 130 negative samples per normal image. The resulting samples were used to train a random forest [7] (RF) classifier. RFs can be parallelized easily and are therefore fast to train, are less susceptible to overfitting and easily adjustable for class-imbalance and therefore suitable for this task.

Centered at each location, we extracted patches of size 250×250 (5×5 cm). The pixel values in the patches were scaled using simple min-max scaling, with values calculated over the whole training set. Since some candidates occur at the border of the imaged breast, we padded the images with zeros. Negative samples were only taken from normal images. Annotated benign samples such as cysts and fibroadenomae were removed from the training set. However, not all benign lesions in our data are annotated and therefore some may have ended in the train or validation set as negatives. An overview of the data is provided in Table 1. The train, validation and test set were split on a patient level. We augmented all positive samples by translating and scaling each patch 16 times. All patches were subsequently flipped randomly during training. After augmentation, the train set consisted of 334752 positive patches and 853800 negatives. When combining the train and validation set, this amounts to 379632 positive and 931640 negative patches.

We used a VGG-like architecture [8] with 5 convolutional layers of $\{16, 32, 64, 128, 128\}$ with 3×3 kernels and 2×2 max-pooling on all but the fourth convolutional layer. A stride of 1 was used in all convolutions. Two fully connected layers of 300 each were added. The network architecture was chosen in a similar fashion as described by Simonyan et al. [8]. An illustration is provided in Fig. 1. To learn the model, we used RMSProp [9], an adaption of R-Prop for SGD with Nesterov momentum. We used Drop-out [10] on the fully connected layers with $p = 0.5$ as a regularizer and employed the MSRA [11] weight filler, with a uniform distribution. A learning rate of 5×10^{-5} with a weight decay of 5×10^{-5} was used. To battle the strong class imbalance, positive samples were presented multiple times during an epoch, keeping a 50/50 positive/negative ratio in each minibatch. All hyperparameters were optimized on a validation set and the CNN was subsequently retrained on the full training + validation set using the found parameters.

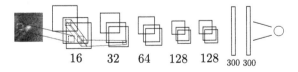

Fig. 1. Illustration of the employed architecture.

3   Reader Study

The mammograms used were collected from a screening program in The Nether-lands (Bevolkingsonderzoek Mid-West) and were recorded with a Hologic Selenia mammography device. All tumors are biopsy proven malignancies and annotated by an experienced reader. The test set consisted of 199 biopsy proven malignant lesions and an equal amount of normals taken from normal cases, that were considered the most difficult by the candidate detector, resulting in 398 patches. This gives a representative set of difficult samples and allows for larger differences between readers and the CNN.

The group of readers comprised four experienced and certified breast radiol-ogists. Since the CNN was trained with patches at 200 micron, we provided the two first readers with this resolution (reader one and three). This resolution was considered acceptable by the readers for analysis of mass lesions, but does not allow detection of microcalcifications. Since we excluded cases with microcalci-fications this was not an issue. However, to assess whether the downsampling affected the reading, the other two radiologists read the patches at the original resolution.

The patches used in the reader study were the same as those fed to the CNN except that the standard processing algorithm provided by the manufacturer was applied for the images read by the radiologists. The radiologists were provided with a slider and instructed to score the patch between zero and one hundred based on their assessment of the suspiciousness of the patch.

Statistical analysis was performed with the DBM MRMC method [12] in which radiologists and the CNN are considered as two modalities (e.g. each radiologist was paired with the CNN in the analysis of variance).

4   Results

The ROC curve of the CNN and mean curve of the readers are shown in Fig. 2. The CNN obtained an AUC of 0.87, the radiologists a mean AUC of 0.845. We found no significant difference between the network and the radiologist ($p = 0.2530$). The invididual AUC values of the readers were: reader $1 = 0.845$, reader $2 = 0.8774$, reader $3 = 0.8411$ and reader $4 = 0.8274$. The first two readers were given patches at 200 micron and the last two at 70. There is clearly no significant difference between the readers performance at different resolutions.

Table 1. Overview of the data the network is trained with. Pos refers to the amount of malignant lesions and neg to the amount of normals.

	Cases		Exams		Images		Candidates	
	Pos	Neg	Pos	Neg	Pos	Neg	Pos	Neg
Train	296	6433	358	11780	634	39872	634	213450
Validation	35	710	42	1247	85	4218	85	19460

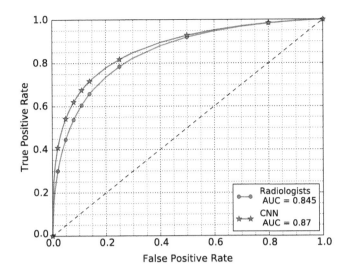

Fig. 2. Comparison between the CNN and the mean of the radiologists.

5   Discussion

In this paper, we have shown that a deep Convolutional Neural Network (CNN) trained on a large dataset of patches, centered around locations of interest is performing comparable to experienced radiologists. The patch based system is a sub problem and is clearly not the way radiologist read a mammogram in the clinic. We are currently exploring the incorporation of context information inside one view, addition of CC/MLO correlation, symmetry and temporal information.

We believe deep CNNs or similar statistical learning methods show great promise, have potential to advance the interest of Computer Aided Diagnosis (CAD) and that these algorithms can ultimately not only *aid* the physician but will eventually be able to read mammograms independently.

Acknowledgements. This research was funded by grant KUN 2012-5577 of the Dutch Cancer Society and supported by the Foundation of Population Screening Mid West.

References

1. Fenton, J.J., Abraham, L., Taplin, S.H., Geller, B.M., Carney, P.A., D'Orsi, C., Elmore, J.G., Barlow, W.E.: Effectiveness of computer-aided detection in community mammography practice. J. Natl. Cancer Inst. **103**, 1152–1161 (2011)
2. LeCun, Y., Bengio, Y., Hinton, G.: Deep learning. Nature **521**(7553), 436–444 (2015)
3. Krizhevsky, A., Sutskever, I., Hinton, G.E.: Imagenet classification with deep convolutional neural networks. Adv. Neural Inf. Process. Syst. **25**, 1097–1105 (2012)

4. Mnih, V., Kavukcuoglu, K., Silver, D., Rusu, A.A., Veness, J., Bellemare, M.G., Graves, A., Riedmiller, M., Fidjeland, A.K., Ostrovski, G., et al.: Human-level control through deep reinforcement learning. Nature **518**, 529–533 (2015)

5. Silver, D., Huang, A., Maddison, C.J., Guez, A., Sifre, L., van den Driessche, G., Schrittwieser, J., Antonoglou, I., Panneershelvam, V., Lanctot, M., et al.: Mastering the game of go with deep neural networks and tree search. Nature **529**(7587), 484–489 (2016)

6. Karssemeijer, N., te Brake, G.M.: Detection of stellate distortions in mammograms. IEEE Trans. Med. Imaging **15**, 611–619 (1996)

7. Breiman, L.: Random forests. Mach. Learn. **45**(1), 5–32 (2001)

8. Simonyan, K., Zisserman, A.: Very deep convolutional networks for large-scale image recognition (2014). arXiv:14091556

9. Dauphin, Y.N., de Vries, H., Chung, J., Bengio, Y.: RMSProp and equilibrated adaptive learning rates for non-convex optimization (2015). arXiv:150204390

10. Srivastava, N., Hinton, G., Krizhevsky, A., Sutskever, I., Salakhutdinov, R.: Dropout: a simple way to prevent neural networks from overfitting. J. Mach. Learn. Res. **15**(1), 1929–1958 (2014)

11. He, K., Zhang, X., Ren, S., Sun, J.: Delving deep into rectifiers: Surpassing human-level performance on imagenet classification (2015). arXiv:150201852v1

12. Hillis, S.L., Berbaum, K.S., Metz, C.E.: Recent developments in the Dorfman-Berbaum-Metz procedure for multireader ROC study analysis. Acad. Radiol. **15**, 647–661 (2008)

Mammography, Tomosynthesis and Breast CT

Diagnostic Usefulness of Synthetic MMG (SMMG) with DBT (Digital Breast Tomosynthesis) for Clinical Setting in Breast Cancer Screening

Nachiko Uchiyama[1(✉)], Mari Kikuchi[1], Minoru Machida[1], Yasuaki Arai[1],
Ryusuke Murakami[2], Kyoichi Otsuka[3], Anna Jerebko[4], Michael Kelm[4],
and Thomas Mertelmeier[4]

[1] Department of Radiology, National Cancer Center, Tokyo, Japan
{nuchiyam,markikuc,mmachida,yaarai}@ncc.go.jp
[2] Department of Radiology, Nippon Medical School, Tokyo, Japan
rywakana@nms.ac.jp
[3] Siemens Healthcare K.K., Tokyo, Japan
Kyoichi.otsuka@siemens.com
[4] Siemens Healthcare GmbH, Erlangen, Germany
{anna.jerebko,michael.kelm,thomas.mertelmeier}@siemens.com

Abstract. We evaluated the diagnostic performance of a novel image processing technique of synthetic MMG (SMMG) as 2D-like visualization approach with and without DBT slice images (DBT) compared with that of 2D MMG (MMG) alone. With one-view MMG and DBT, the radiation doses, utilizing the ACR phantom 156, were 1.20 mGy and 1.80 mGy. The number of the cases was 108. MMG, SMMG, and DBT slice images were evaluated independently by 4 readers utilizing ROC analysis and diagnostic performance. SMMG plus DBT demonstrated higher area under the curve (AUC) and superior diagnostic accuracy with sensitivity, specificity, and NPV compared with SMMG and MMG alone ($p < 0.05$). In addition, a 40 % decrease of radiation dose with SMMG plus DBT compared with MMG plus DBT as the current setting will enable us to apply a two-view SMMG plus DBT in breast cancer screening instead of MMG.

Keywords: Digital mammography · Tomosynthesis · Synthetic mammogram

1 Introduction

Digital breast tomosynthesis (DBT) provides an advantage in detection of breast masses compared to 2D MMG since it allows the separation of the tissue layers and the noticeable reduction of occlusions caused by overlapping anatomical structures. While DBT slice images provide advantages for detecting mass lesions, it is more difficult to get an overview and evaluate the distribution of microcalcifications in comparison with the 2D MMG image. Thus, concurrent usage of 2D MMG and DBT slice images currently is inevitable in clinical diagnostic usage. However, in the screening setting, using both 2D MMG and DBT is not an acceptable option due to the increased patient dose which would not comply with regulations on radiation dose in breast cancer screening, such

© Springer International Publishing Switzerland 2016
A. Tingberg et al. (Eds.): IWDM 2016, LNCS 9699, pp. 59–67, 2016.
DOI: 10.1007/978-3-319-41546-8_8

as the EUREF guidelines. The reprocessing of the tomosynthesis data to generate a 2D MMG-like image from DBT image data is an opportunity to obtain the information provided with 2D MMG and DBT but at the dose level of a single DBT scan. In this study, we evaluated a novel image processing technique for generating synthetic MMG (SMMG) for 2D-like visualization. We evaluated the diagnostic accuracy of SMMG with or without DBT slice images (DBT) and compared those with 2D MMG (MMG).

2 Materials and Methods

The clinical data sets were acquired with a DBT system (MAMMOMAT Inspiration, Siemens, Germany). A two-view DBT (rotation angle interval $\pm 25°$) was performed with the same compression pressure as with the MMG. The combination of the target and the filter was W/Rh. The DBT slice images were reconstructed into 2 mm thick slices with 1 mm slice distance and high in-plane resolution of 0.085 mm $\times$ 0.085 mm using a novel iterative reconstruction method based on super-resolution theory [1]. The reconstruction technique of SMMG is based on a 3D volume ray casting method. In order to obtain the exact same distribution of micro-calcifications and the same tissue structures as in the MMG, the exact X-ray geometry of the employed DBT system is simulated in the ray casting. The SMMG reconstruction process is optimized to ensure detectability of microcalcifications and masses and to resolve overlapping tissue structures that would, for example, mask lesions in dense breasts. The SMMG images were reconstructed together with the DBT slices from the 25 raw projection images acquired with the DBT system (Fig. 1). With one-view MMG and DBT, the radiation doses, utilizing the ACR phantom 156, were 1.20 mGy and 1.80 mGy. One hundred eight females were selected and enrolled in this study in May, in 2015. The clinical study was approved by the ethics committee. Informed consent was obtained from all patients. The mean age of the women was 57.0 years old (Raging from 19.0 to 81.0 years old). MMG and SMMG, and MMG and SMMG plus DBT images, from 108 cases with 216 breasts (38 cases of breast cancer and 70 cases of normal or benign) were analyzed for this study. Thirty-eight cancers were diagnosed using a core or vacuum-assisted biopsy procedure under ultrasound or stereotactic imaging guidance, and final histopathologic diagnoses were obtained at surgery. Pathological diagnosis regarding lesions were IDC (n = 27), DCIS (n = 6), ILC (n = 3), Muc Ca (n = 1), and IDC Pred DCIS (n = 1). Radiological findings were microcalcifications-dominant (n = 4), mass-dominant (n = 27), and mass with microcalcifications (n = 7). A Partial mastectomy or a total mastectomy was conducted in 35 cases. Radiofrequency ablation was conducted in 3 cases with IDC (n = 2) and DCIS (n = 1). Neoadjuvant chemotherapy was conducted in seven out of 35cases before surgery. In twenty three cases, the average lesion size regarding invasive component by pathological findings was 20.6 mm (ranged from 0.5 mm to 52 mm). In this study, all patients received a full two-view (CC and MLO) MMG and DBT and in addition, two view SMMG and DBT were interpreted in combination for diagnostic purposes. Prior mammograms were not available for comparison in this study. The two-view MMG and SMMG, and the two-view MMG and SMMG plus DBT images were evaluated independently by four readers utilizing ROC analysis with the BI-RADS scale and POM (Probability of Malignancy) scale. At first, MMG from group A (54 cases) and SMMG with and without DBT from group B (54 cases) were evaluated. Second, SMMG with or without DBT from group A and MMG from group B were evaluated. Each participant completed two reading sessions spaced 4 weeks apart to minimize recall bias. Each of the readers had more than ten years of experience of interpreting MMG. The experience of the readers interpreting the images of DBT ranged from one to five years utilizing the same DBT system. Readers 1, 2, and 4 had more than 1000 cases interpreting DBT images for diagnostic purpose. Reader 3 had less experience and the number of cases was less than 200 cases. The reader-specific area under the curve (AUC) for BI-RADS and POM (Probability of Malignancy) was analyzed and the average AUC were calculated. In addition, diagnostic performance (sensitivity, specificity, PPV, and NPV) was also calculated. In addition, variability regarding inter-diagnostic procedures and inter-reader performance was analyzed by multiple comparison with Tukey method.

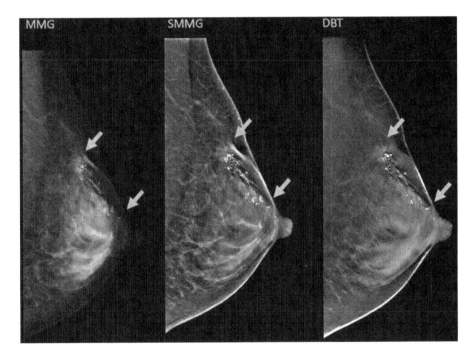

Fig. 1. The images of MMG, SMMG, and DBT slice image

A spiculated mass with pleomorphic calcifications with linear structure is visualized in each image (Arrow). Pathological findings were IDC (Sci Ca) with non-invasive ductal component (Comedo).

3   Results

The average breast thicknesses were 46.4 mm (22.0–85.0 mm) in CC view and 44.3 mm (19.0–89.0 mm) in MLO view. The AGDs (Average Glandular Dose) with MMG were 1.08 mGy (0.70–2.62 mGy) in CC view and 1.07 mGy (0.68–2.00 mGy) in MLO view. With DBT, the AGDs were 1.65 mGy (0.98–3.93 mGy) in CC view and 1.59 mGy (1.02–3.00 mGy) in MLO view (Figs. 2a and 2b). With the BI-RADS scale, AUC for MMG, SMMG, and SMMG plus DBT were 0.863, 0.850, and 0.972 by Reader 1, 0.808, 0.811, and 0.911 by Reader 2, 0.784, 0.803, and 0.815 by Reader 3, and 0.819, 0.796, and 0.895 by Reader 4. With the POM scale, AUC for MMG, SMMG, and SMMG plus DBT were 0.865, 0.853 and 0.977 by Reader 1, 0.807, 0.815, and 0.918 by Reader 2, 0.786, 0.785, and 0.795 by Reader 3, and 0.833, 0.802 and 0.876 by Reader 4. Regarding inter-reader performance variability, between Reader 1 and 3, there was significant difference ($p < 0.05$) and there was no significant difference between the other comparisons among readers. The average AUC for MMG, SMMG, and SMMG plus DBT were 0.817, 0.813, and 0.892. With POM scale, the average values of AUC for MMG, SMMG, and SMMG plus DBT were 0.822, 0.813, and 0.889. Regarding inter-diagnostic procedure's variability, DBT plus SMMG demonstrated superior diagnostic accuracy compared with MMG and SMMG alone ($p < 0.05$) (Fig. 3 and Table 1). On the other hand, between SMMG and MMG alone, there were no statistical differences in each ($p > 0.05$).

Table 1.   The average AUC with BIRADS and POM

	Average AUC with BIRADS	Average AUC with POM
MMG	0.817	* 0.822
SMMG	0.813	* 0.813
SMMG+DBT	0.892	0.889

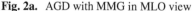

*: p<0.05

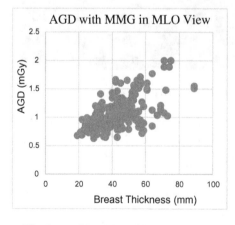

Fig. 2a.   AGD with MMG in MLO view

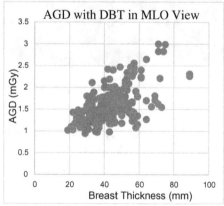

Fig. 2b.   AGD with DBT in MLO view

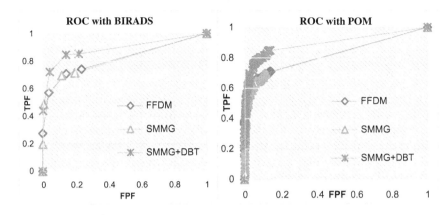

Fig. 3. ROC curve with BIRADS and POM

Diagnostic performance of SMMG plus DBT demonstrated superior diagnostic performance with sensitivity, specificity, and NPV compared with SMMG and MMG alone ($p < 0.05$). Between SMMG and MMG, there was no statistical difference with sensitivity, PPV, and NPV. Regarding specificity, SMMG demonstrated superior performance ($p < 0.01$) (Table 2).

Table 2. Overall diagnostic performance in reading study of MMG, SMMG alone and SMMG plus DBT with BI-RADS

MMG	Disease(+)	Disease(−)	Total	Sensitivity	0.717
Positive	109	103	212	Specificity	0.831
Negative	43	609	652	PPV	0.514
Total	152	712	864	NPV	0.934
SMMG	Disease(+)	Disease(−)	Total	Sensitivity	0.697
Positive	106	83	189	Specificity	0.851
Negative	46	629	675	PPV	0.561
Total	152	712	864	NPV	0.932
SMMG+DBT	Disease(+)	Disease(−)	Total	Sensitivity	0.847
Positive	129	100	229	Specificity	0.858
Negative	23	612	635	PPV	0.563
Total	152	712	864	NPV	0.964

	Sensitivity	Specificity	PPV	NPV
SMMG+DBT vs. MMG	$p < 0.01$	$p < 0.01$	$p > 0.05$	$p < 0.01$
SMMG+DBT vs. SMMG	$p < 0.01$	$p < 0.05$	$p > 0.05$	$p < 0.01$
SMMG vs. MMG	$p > 0.05$	$p < 0.01$	$p > 0.05$	$p > 0.05$

4 Discussion

Our study was conducted as a feasibility study to determine if two-view SMMG plus DBT can be applied and replace two-view MMG for screening purpose. The primary endpoint was a comparison of diagnostic accuracy between two-view SMMG plus DBT and two-view MMG. We evaluated whether two-view SMMG plus DBT could provide higher diagnostic accuracy compared with two-view MMG. The secondary endpoint was to compare the diagnostic accuracy of MMG and the new imaging of SMMG. Because of the limitation of radiation dose, we needed to skip taking MMG and we needed to utilize SMMG that was reconstructed from DBT image data instead. We needed to verify the image quality of SMMG and the reconstruction algorithms of SMMG. According the background of this study, our population was organized from many malignant cases that were recalled for diagnosis compared to actual screening population [2–4]. In accordance with previous studies, Gur et al. reported that SMMG +DBT resulted in lower sensitivity with comparable specificity in comparison with MMG+DBT [5]. Zuley et al. reported that the diagnostic performance regarding SMMG with or without DBT is comparable in diagnostic performance in comparison with MMG with or without DBT [6]. Van Schie et al. reported that AUC regarding the diagnostic accuracy with SMMG was comparable, but higher in comparison with MMG [7]. In this study, we assessed the evaluation of diagnostic performance between the following: (1) SMMG with DBT and MMG, (2) SMMG with DBT and SMMG, and (3) SMMG and

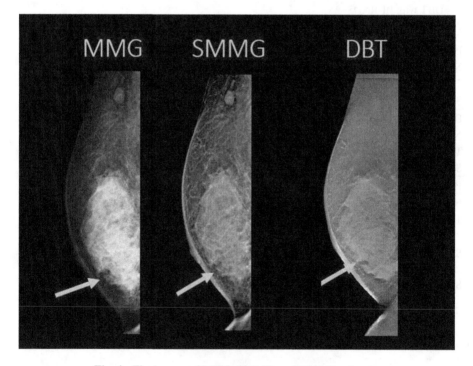

Fig. 4. The images of MMG, SMMG, and DBT slice image

MMG. Regarding inter-diagnostic procedure variability, DBT plus SMMG demonstrated superior diagnostic accuracy compared with MMG and SMMG alone ($p < 0.05$). On the other hand, between SMMG and MMG alone, there were no statistical differences in each ($p > 0.05$) with ROC analysis. Regarding inter-reader variability, between Reader 1 and 3, there was significant difference ($p < 0.05$) and there was no significant difference between the other comparisons among readers. The difference of experience utilizing DBT images with diagnostic feedback could affect the results. The average diagnostic performance of SMMG with DBT was higher regarding sensitivity, specificity, and NPV with comparable PPV in comparison with single usage of MMG and SMMG in each. Regarding the comparison between SMMG and MMG, SMMG resulted in comparable, but lower sensitivity in comparison with MMG with higher specificity (Table 1). In addition, the AGDs with SMMG with DBT were 1.65 mGy in CC view and 1.59 mGy in MLO view with acceptable radiation dose level. The average breast thicknesses were 46.4 mm in CC view and 44.3 mm in MLO view. Regarding the comparison between SMMG and MMG, in accordance with Zuley et al., the difference between SMMG and MMG in AUC was smaller than that reported previously for an experimental version of SMMG. In addition, the diagnostic performance was not specifically related to the detection of microcalcification clusters. Furthermore, they reported that five out of eight readers' performances with the SMMG images alone were comparable, but slightly better than with the original MMG images alone and suggested that diagnostic performance was dispersed depending on the readers' interpretation. As well as their study, our study also resulted in the fact. Two out of four readers' AUC with SMMG were comparable, but slightly better than MMG. The other two out of four readers' AUC with MMG were comparable, but slightly better than SMMG (Table 2). The results came from the different image impressions with SMMG images compared to MMG images with not only microcalcifications, but with masses also. Depending on the image reconstruction algorithms regarding SMMG, in some cases, the images were depicted having different density patterns of the masses, background breast densities, and different densities and morphologies of the microcalcifications in comparison with MMG (Figs. 4 and 5). According to our preliminary clinical results, the results can be different depending on the algorithms and image acquisition systems we used regarding SMMG. If we will apply SMMG plus DBT for screening, there will be some necessity to redesign the reconstruction algorism with SMMG to adjust MMG, or we require clinical case trainings to adjust diagnostic criteria for SMMG. Because the image acquisition and reconstruction are quite different between SMMG and MMG and there are limitations to assimilate the SMMG image to the MMG image completely.

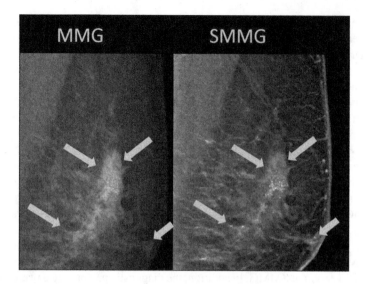

Fig. 5. The images of MMG and SMMG

5   Conclusion

SMMG plus DBT will offer the benefit of increased diagnostic accuracy compared with MMG. In addition, the AGDs with SMMG and DBT were 1.65 mGy in CC view and 1.59 mGy in MLO view with the average breast thicknesses being 46.4 mm in CC view and 44.3 mm in MLO view with acceptable level. A 40 % decrease of radiation dose with SMMG plus DBT compared with MMG plus DBT as the current setting will enable us to apply SMMG plus DBT in screening instead of MMG clinically.

An indistinct mass with cutaneous thickening is visualized in DBT slice image (Arrow). In comparison with MMG, the densities of the lesion and background breast tissue give quite different impressions in comparison with SMMG (Arrow). Pathological findings were IDC (Sci Ca).

An indistinct mass with clustered pleomorphic calcifications is visualized in each image (Arrow), but the densities and morphology of the microcalcifications give different impressions between MMG and SMMG. Pathological findings were IDC pred DCIS.

Disclaimer. The concepts and information presented in this paper are based on research and are not commercially available.

References

1. Abdurahman, S., Dennerlein, F., Jerebko, A., Fieselmann, A., Mertelmeier, T.: Optimizing high resolution reconstruction in digital breast tomosynthesis using filtered back projection. In: Fujita, H., Hara, T., Muramatsu, C. (eds.) IWDM 2014. LNCS, vol. 8539, pp. 520–527. Springer, Heidelberg (2014)

2. Skaane, P., Bandos, A.I., Gullien, R., et al.: Comparison of digital mammography alone and digital mammography plus tomosynthesis in a populationbased screening program. Radiology **267**(1), 47–56 (2013)
3. Bernardi, D., Caumo, F., Macaskill, P., et al.: Effect of integrating 3D-mammography (digital breast tomosynthesis) with 2D-mammography on radiologists' true-positive and false-positive detection in a population breast screening trial. Eur. J. Cancer **50**(7), 1232–1238 (2014)
4. Lång, K., Andersson, I., Rosso, A., et al.: Performance of one-view breast tomosynthesis as a stand-alone breast cancer screening modality: results from the Malmö Breast Tomosynthesis Screening Trial, a population-based study. Eur. Radiol. **26**, 184–190 (2016)
5. Gur, D., Zuley, M.L., Anello, M.I., et al.: Dose reduction in digital breast tomosynthesis (DBT) screening using synthetically reconstructed projection images: an observer performance study. Acad. Radiol. **19**(2), 166–171 (2012)
6. Zuley, M.L., Guo, B., Catullo, V.J., et al.: Comparison of two-dimensional synthesized mammograms versus original digital mammograms alone and in combination with tomosynthesis images. Radiology **271**(3), 664–671 (2014)
7. Van, S.G., Mann, R., Imhof-tas, M., et al.: Generating synthetic mammograms from reconstructed tomosynthesis volumes. IEEE Trans. Med. Imaging **32**(12), 2322–2331 (2013)

Development of Digital Phantom for Digital Mammography with Soft-Copy Reading

Norimitsu Shinohara[1,2], Katsuhei Horita[2(✉)], and Tokiko Endo[2,3(✉)]

[1] Department of Radiological Technology, Faculty of Health Sciences,
Gifu University of Medical Science, Seki, Japan
shinohara@u-gifu-ms.ac.jp

[2] The Japan Central Organization on Quality Assurance of Breast Cancer Screening,
Hamada, Japan
horita@onyx.ocn.ne.jp

[3] Department of Radiology, National Hospital Organization Higashi Nagoya National Hospital,
Nagoya, Japan
endot@hosp.go.jp

Abstract. In Japan, soft-copy diagnoses shift rapidly, and the method for facilities applying it is necessary for soft-copy diagnosis. Digital mammography has high resolution and a large matrix size. On a monitor, the image is either displayed partially at 1:1 pixel mapping or narrowed to fit the screen, resulting in loss of image quality. Therefore, we developed a digital phantom for soft-copy diagnosis in digital mammography. This phantom is like the Contrast Detail Phantom and comprises 12 different shapes and eight different brightness levels. It becomes one group of nine, and each signal is located at the prime number coordinate from a central signal coordinate. Visual evaluation refers to the visibility of the nine signal coordinates when the image is adjusted to fit the monitor's display. Although digital phantoms have been implemented at 120 facilities, at two other facilities, viewer problems were detected.

Keywords: Digital phantom · Soft-copy diagnosis · Mammography · Visual evaluation

1 Background

In Japan, the number of breast cancer patients is on the rise, and the incidence and mortality rates are extremely high [1]. Breast cancer in particular is the most common type of cancer in women, who are at greater risk of dying from their 30s through to their 60s than from any other form of cancer. In recent years, a rising number of women have been developing breast cancer in their 40s, and improved methods of breast cancer screening are under consideration [2]. The technology of mammography in Japan is lagging in terms of digitizing diagnostic radiography. However, systems Equipmented with flat-panel detectors are spreading rapidly, and although only 4.0 % were Equipmented with flat-panel detectors in 2005 [3], more than 14.8 % (675 machines) had them as of December 31, 2011 [4]. Moreover, due to revision of the medical payment system in April 2010, a large number of facilities are transitioning to soft-copy diagnosis.

© Springer International Publishing Switzerland 2016
A. Tingberg et al. (Eds.): IWDM 2016, LNCS 9699, pp. 68–74, 2016.
DOI: 10.1007/978-3-319-41546-8_9

Spatial resolution in mammography requires a high spatial frequency depending on the characteristics of the lesion visualized. The digital mammography detectors currently used in Japan feature pixel sizes of 25–100 μm [5] with a matrix size that increases accordingly. Some detectors have a matrix size as large as 7080 × 9480. In contrast, a 5 MP monitor, which has the highest resolution of any monitor, has a resolution of only 2560 × 2028.

Soft-copy diagnosis in mammography requires the following: (1) recognition of the lesion characteristics by displaying it in as much detail as possible; and (2) recognition of bilateral symmetry and structural continuity by displaying the entire breast. In criterion (1), displaying the mammography information in its entirety requires observation with 1:1 pixel mapping [6] in which a single pixel corresponds to a single pixel on the display. However, in 1:1 pixel mapping, observing the entire breast requires shifting of the effective field of view and other cumbersome tasks. In criterion (2), even if the facility is able to conduct a soft-copy diagnosis with a 5 MP monitor, if the detector uses a matrix size of 2560 × 2048 or greater, the image must be decreased in size to observe the entire breast. This means that the entire breast image fits the screen using the maximum monitor display size [5]. Reducing functions for the image interpreting workstation (hereafter "viewer") includes the nearest neighbor algorithm, linear interpolation, bicubic interpolation, and data thinning. It is widely known in engineering that reducing images via these functions results in signal loss. However, medical professionals have little interest in reduction functions and little understanding of the differences in image visibility [7]. Furthermore, there is currently no established method or tool for assessing this. Therefore, we developed a digital phantom for soft-copy diagnosis in digital mammography and describe it here.

2   Methods

The objective of visual evaluation is to evaluate the viewer rather than the monitor quality alone. Therefore, display systems are defined as "monitors" and "viewers"; the objective is to evaluate various conditions related to display systems, such as image interpolation, display libraries, OpenGL, and video cards. What is assessed here is whether the imaging device can display the recorded signals without deficiencies. This is determined by the correlation between monitor resolution (pixel count) and mammogram pixel count. In particular, the disappearance of high-frequency signals (determination of microcalcifications) in a full-image display necessitates the development of a tool for determining image scope and the establishment of a visual evaluation method. However, since images shot on film are subjected to shooting conditions and various other factors, the present method evaluates the response (output) from when the digital images are inputted (physical quantity).

2.1   Digital Phantom

For our digital phantom, we used C to create signals, which we converted to DICOM (tagging information such as secondary capture and spacing) using Osirix. In doing so, we used a window center (0028, 1050) and window width (0028, 1051) of 2048 and 4096, respectively. However, to avoid display problems in the viewer, the tags for the detector used in the mammography were analyzed, and the DICOM tags for imager pixel spacing (0018, 11164), detector element physical size (0018, 7020), detector element spacing (0018, 7022), rows (0028, 0010), columns (0028, 0011), pixel spacing (0028, 0030), bits allocated (0028, 0100), bits stored (0028, 0101), and high bit (0028, 0102) were set to be identical to these detector tags. The vertical and horizontal components of the digital phantom include 12 different signal shapes (A, B, C, D, E, F, G, H, J, K, L, and M) (Fig. 1) and eight different signal brightness values (1, 2, 3, 4, 5, 6, 7, 8); a single group comprises nine signals in a dot shape. The dots for A, B, C, D, E, F, G, H, J, K, L, and M connote different signal sizes (different pixel sizes) according to the individual detector. Therefore, a different digital phantom is prepared for each individual detector used for mammography. The digital phantoms that have been created to date are shown in Table 1. The digital phantom is tailored to the matrix size of the detector used in mammography; thus, it is possible to perform evaluations per detector used at a given facility.

Table 1. Relation between Equipments and the pixel size of each signal

Equipment	1	2	3	4	5	6
Pixel size	25um	50um	70um	85um	85um	100um
Matrix X	9480	4740	3328	2816	2812	2294
Matrix Y	7080	3540	2560	2016	2012	1914

A	25x25	50x50	70x70	85x85		100x100
B	25x50	50x100	70x140	85x170		100x200
C	50x25	100x50	140x70	170x85		200x100
D-G	50x50	100x100	140x140	170x170		200x200
H,J	75x75	150x150	210x210	255x255		300x300
K	100x100	200x200	280x280	340x340		400x400
L	125x125	250x250	350x350	425x425		500x500
M	150x150	300x300	420x420	505x505		600x600

An overview of the digital phantom is shown in Fig. 2. The basic form of a digital phantom resembles a contrast detail phantom in which the steps are annotated on the left margin and C1, C3, C5, and C7 are annotated in the four corners. We created 20 steps, with a step increased every 51 pixel value. To prevent signal loss at a specified reduction rate, the nine signal coordinates in a group were placed on prime number coordinates (Fig. 3). Therefore, although the signal configuration is distorted, this configuration avoids problems with reduction functions and rates.

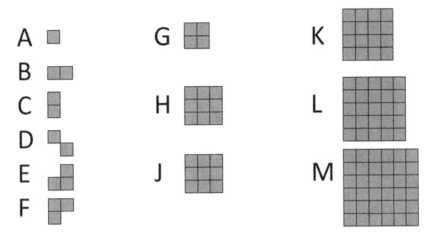

Fig. 1. The shape of the signal on digital phantom for evaluation. A, B, C, D, E, F, G, J, and K are signals. H, L, M are reference signals.

Fig. 2. An over view of the digital phantom

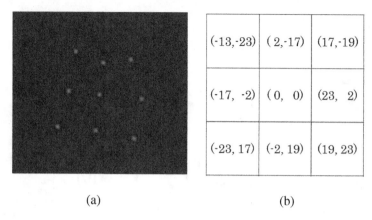

(-13,-23)	(2,-17)	(17,-19)
(-17, -2)	(0, 0)	(23, 2)
(-23, 17)	(-2, 19)	(19, 23)

(a)   (b)

Fig. 3. Nine signal coordinates in a group. (a) Image of a group (b) coordinates of a group

2.2 Preparations for the Evaluation

Evaluation preparation consists of the following four steps:

1. Load the digital phantom into the viewer.
2. Resize the full-screen display to fit the monitor's maximum display.
3. Confirm that C1, C3, C5, and C7 are displayed on the screen.
4. When adjusting window width (WW) and window level (WL), they must be displayed in a way that enables visual confirmation of the differences in brightness in the 20-step grayscale. Essentially, WW and WL do not require adjustment.

Digital phantoms can be loaded easily in most viewers. However, there may be demands for non-type 1 DICOM tags depending on the viewer, so some DICOM tags may require modification.

2.3 Visual Evaluation

Visual evaluation refers to the visibility of the nine signal coordinates when the image is adjusted to fit the monitor's display. At this time, visibility is both a sensory and a subjective index; therefore, using the relatively large digital phantom signals H, L, and M as reference signals, if the above-mentioned nine signal coordinates are equivalent to H, L, and M, they are considered visible. Thus, visual evaluation is the selection of dots deemed equivalent to H, L, and M (i.e. visible dots). Depending on the reduction rate and function, some dots are easily visible, while others have weak signal values and some even disappear due to the reduction. A sample visual evaluation is shown in Fig. 4. Visible signals are circled, while signals that have disappeared are not marked. We chose not to use expansion tools or perform gradation processing for the visual confirmations.

A total of 96 signal groups and the display systems that feature reduction functions can be compared by confirming the visibility of signals of the same size. The correlation between the sampling pitch of a detector and the signal size of the digital phantom using

Fig. 4. Example of the visual evaluation

a 5 MP monitor is shown in Table 2. For example, when the actual size of the micro-calcification to be detected is 100 µm based on a radiology consultation, a comparison can be made by evaluating the visibility at an equivalent of 100 µm in a digital phantom.

Table 2. The correlation between Equipments and the signal size of the digital phantom using a 5 MP monitor

	Pixel size	Maximum length of the signal [mm]					
		0.025	0.05	0.1	0.2	0.3	0.5
Equipment 1	25 um	A–C	D–G	K	L, M	–	–
Equipment 2	50 um	–	A–C	G	H–K	L, M	–
Equipment 3	70 um	–	A	B, C	H–K	L, M	–
Equipment 4	85 um	–	A	B, C	H–K	L, M	–
Equipment 5	85 um	–	A	B, C	H–K	L, M	–
Equipment 6	100 um	–	–	A	B–G	H–J	L

3   Results and Discussion

A digital phantom is useful not only for evaluating display systems that feature reducing functions and monitor resolution but also for educational purposes such as confirming the effects of the monitor's resolution and reducing functions as well as for precision management with regard to deterioration and malfunction.

Although digital phantoms have been implemented at 150 facilities, 47 facilities are unsuited for its implementation. At 44 facilities, the evaluator did not receive a sufficient explanation of the evaluation methods and tools described above. However, at three other facilities, viewer problems were detected. Therefore, while the visual image eval-uation was mostly subjective, it has become possible to replace some of these subjective elements with certain objective evaluations.

The digital phantom proposed in the present study is currently being adopted for soft-copy image evaluations and put into practical use by the nonprofit organization Facility Image Evaluation Committee of the Japan Central Organization on Quality Assurance of Breast Cancer Screening. However, because the visual evaluation technique proposed in the present study is self-assessed, a proper evaluation may not be possible if the group composed of nine signals shown in Fig. 3 is presented as-is. Therefore, this assessment must be made accurately, not by creating a model that uses fixed signal values for the nine signal values that comprise a digital phantom group but rather by creating (1) a model that combines weak and strong signal values and changes the balance, or (2) a partial disappearance model in which some of the nine signal values are changed to 0.

In future, we intend to evaluate the differences between specific monitor resolutions and reduction functions using a digital phantom.

4   Conclusion

Here we reported the development of a digital phantom for soft-copy diagnosis in digital mammography as well as the involved evaluation method. Many facilities have transitioned to soft-copy diagnosis to date. In addition, there have been many instances of image interpretation by remote diagnosis as well as the interpretation of images from multiple devices with a viewer. Therefore, we anticipate that the present study's findings will contribute to the precision management of these new breast cancer diagnostic methods.

References

1. Office for Cancer Control, Health Services Bureau, Ministry of Health, Labour and Welfare, JAPAN: Basic Plan to Promote Cancer Control Programs. http://www.mhlw.go.jp/english/wp/wp-hw4/dl/health_and_medical_services/P74.pdf. Accessed 20 June 2015. (In Japanese)
2. Minami, Y., Tsubono, Y., Nishino, Y., Ohuchi, N., Shibuya, D., Hisamichi, S.: The increase of female breast cancer incidence in Japan: emergence of birth cohort effect. Int. J. Cancer 108(6), 901–906 (2004). (In Japanese)
3. List of facilities with mammography in Japan. Mon. New Med. 36(10), 177–183 (2009). (In Japanese)
4. The modality installation number deciphered from data. Rad Fun. 10(6), 67–69 (2012). (In Japanese)
5. Bick, U., Diekmann, F.: Digital Mammography. Medical Radiology-Diagnostic Imaging. Springer, Heidelberg (2010)
6. Quality assurance programme for digital mammography. IAEA Human Health Series, vol. 17, pp. 79–115. IAEA, Austria (2011)
7. Ihori, A., Fujita, N., Yasuda, N., Sugiura, A., Kodera, Y.: Phantom-based comparison of conventional versus phase-contrast mammography for LCD soft-copy diagnosis. Int. J. Comput. Assist. Radiol. Surg. 8(4), 621–633 (2013)

Improving the Quality of Optimisation Studies Undertaken in Mammography and General Radiology Using High Level Blended Teaching

Alistair Mackenzie[1(✉)], Kenneth C. Young[1,2], Saartje Creten[3],
Nelis Van Peteghem[4], and Hilde Bosmans[4]

[1] National Coordinating Centre for the Physics of Mammography,
Royal Surrey County Hospital, Guildford GU2 7XX, UK
alistairmackenzie@nhs.net
[2] Department of Physics, University of Surrey, Guildford GU2 7XH, UK
[3] Educational Development Unit,
KU Leuven, Kapeldreef 62 box 5206, 3001 Leuven, Belgium
[4] Medical Physics and Quality Control,
KU Leuven, Herestraat 49, bus 7003, 3000 Leuven, Belgium

Abstract. The EU funded project EUtempe-RX to develop 12 modules for training of medical physics experts (MPEs) in diagnostic and interventional radiology. Each course module provided 80 h of blended learning (a mixture of online and face-to-face training). The effectiveness of high-level blended learning for training MPEs up to EQF level 8 was tested on optimisation in mammography and general radiology. The training methods were evaluated using a questionnaire (89 % response rate) and reviewing participants' proposed optimisation studies. The online training was the most highly rated part of the module. The participants produced a wide range of feasible and interesting optimisation proposals. All questionnaire responders intend to undertake their study. Overall, the proposals showed a good understanding of the process of optimisation, but some showed weaknesses in applying the results clinically. The blended learning approach showed potential for training MPEs to undertake successful optimisation projects.

Keywords: Medical physics expert · Optimisation · Education · Mammography · General radiography

1 Introduction

The role of the Medical Physics Expert (MPE) was defined in the EU Basic Safety Standards (BSS) [1] to ensure the optimal use of ionising radiation in healthcare. The MPE requires sufficient training and experience to be able to introduce new developments and best practice into healthcare. Thus, it was determined that an MPE needs the highest level of knowledge, skills and competencies (KSCs) associated with an EQF level 8 (equivalent to PhD) by the EU funded 'Guidelines for the MPE' project [2]. The guidelines cover the use of radiation in radiotherapy, nuclear medicine and diagnostic and interventional radiology (D&IR).

© Springer International Publishing Switzerland 2016
A. Tingberg et al. (Eds.): IWDM 2016, LNCS 9699, pp. 75–82, 2016.
DOI: 10.1007/978-3-319-41546-8_10

It can be difficult to ensure that MPEs have sufficient high-level training particularly in many countries with financial restrictions and/or have enough expert physicists to train the next generation of medical physicists to achieve the highest level of expertise. The EUtempe-RX project (www.eutempe-rx.eu) was formed to provide high level training in D&IR to reach EQF level 8 [3]. A European network of partners was brought together in an FP7 EC project to ensure sufficient expertise in all fields of study and to create a harmonized programme of courses. The project has 12 modules covering the diverse areas within D&IR including professional skills (e.g. leadership, communication), dosimetry, imaging technologies and image quality. The target groups for this project are medical physicists in hospitals, medical devices industry and in regulatory authorities. It is hoped that the method will be expanded to other areas of medical physics.

A blended learning process was used, where learning is undertaken using a mixture of e-learning techniques and face-to-face training. This method has a number of benefits:

- It supports medical physicists who cannot spend significant time away at a course either due to personal or work commitments. This was considered a major part of a gender action plan for the profession.
- Much of the learning can be undertaken at the pace of the student.
- Traditional high level training faces the challenge of a heterogeneous audience. An e-learning course prior to a face-to-face meeting provides a more homogenous audience and so allows training at a higher level.
- The face-to-face training can focus on practical aspects and more in-depth discussion.
- The variety of teaching techniques aids learning.

During the e-learning phase, the participant must actively interact with the material and the course tutors. It is a challenge and a big task for course organisers to provide high level material that allows high-level interactions. E-learning has been used successfully in medical physics for many years [4], while blended learning has been shown to have benefits for medical education generally and in particular for countries that are economically disadvantaged [5, 6]. However, much of the training evaluated is aimed at EQF level 6 (BSc equivalent) or 7 (MSc equivalent). The effectiveness of blended learning methods undertaken by EUtempe-RX to reach EQF level 8 has not been tested in medical physics expert courses, as far as we know. This study evaluates the effectiveness of the training for the optimisation of imaging in diagnostic radiology for both mammography and general radiography. This topic covered approximately half of the topics in EUtempe-RX Module 7, entitled 'Optimisation of X-ray imaging using standard and innovative techniques', while the other half covered quantitative analysis methods (e.g. detective quantum efficiency (DQE)).

The ability to undertake a successful optimisation study is a key competency of being an MPE. As properly optimised imaging systems will provide maximum benefit to the patients. The aim of this study is to show whether high level blended training has the potential to help future MPEs successfully plan and undertake an optimisation study. Very importantly, they must know how to implement the conclusions of their study into an imaging department and thus maximize the clinical benefit of imaging to the patients.

2 Method

2.1 Choice of Participants

The process for accepting the participants to the module was based on their curriculum vitae (CV) and a motivation statement; in addition the selection process gave some bias to women, candidates from Eastern Europe and had to ensure a spread of nationalities. There were 47 applications for module 7 and 23 candidates were chosen, 3 of whom withdrew before the face-to-face course. Of the remaining 20 participants, 13 were women, and there were 16 different nationalities.

2.2 Module 7 Design

Each module in EUtempe-RX was designed to cover 80 h of training. Module 7 was designed to have 60 h of online training and 20 h of face-to-face training, while the other modules split the time equally between the face-to-face and the online parts. In module 7, the participants were given over 2 months for the online phase.

A list of the knowledge, skills and competencies (KSCs) required by an MPE are in Annex 1 of the EC guidelines for medical physics experts [7]. This module was designed to fully or partially cover 11 skills (out of 43) and 18 knowledge requirements (out of 118) listed in the report for the specific KSCs for D&IR. The EUtempe-RX modules were accredited by the European Federation of Medical Physics (EFOMP).

We used a blended learning technique for the high level training, where the method included flipped learning where the participants undertook learning using a variety of teaching modules online primarily in their own country at their own pace and then attended a course in a central location. This variety of teaching methods potentially provides better learning outcomes [8]. An innovative part of the training was that participants were informed at the beginning of the module that they had to produce a plan for an optimisation study in mammography or general radiography. The proposed study would be examined. Participants were encouraged to talk with colleagues both from physics and radiology departments to find the topic of their study. The proposed study had to be original and not simply be a repetition of previous work.

The training methods used as part of this module were:

- E-learning: content was provided by means of text documents, videos, webcast lectures, scientific papers and quizzes (both multi-choice and open questions).
- Online discussion: The organisers and participants placed questions and topics on a discussion board.
- Tutorial: there was an online tutorial of up to 5 participants for up to 1 h per session using online teleconferencing
- Assignment: Each participant provided an outline of their proposed optimisation study ($\sim$500 words) and received feedback on their assignment.
- Contact with tutors: the participants had the opportunity to email questions to the tutors.
- Face-to-face training: lectures and seminars including a radiologist's talk and training in optimisation techniques.

- Practicals: There were three practicals at the face-to-face training; Case studies of situations requiring optimisation, undertaking an observer study, analysis of observer study data.
- Examination: The examination was an open book exam (i.e. notes and internet could be used) based on their planned optimisation study.

This part of the module was designed to develop 5 out of 32 competencies listed in the EC guidelines for medical physics experts [7]. The knowledge and skills were demonstrated by examination on the last day of the face-to-face meeting. The development of competencies will be demonstrated if they can successfully implement their study or use their training to develop a new project. Ultimately, the results of the study should be implemented clinically and, ideally, the results published in a peer-reviewed journal. It is this final stage that would truly demonstrate the competency of an MPE.

2.3 Evaluation of Training Methods

The effectiveness of the training was judged by reviewing the assignments and the examination papers. Following the face-to-face course, a questionnaire was sent to the 19 participants who had sat the exam. The questionnaire asks how the various parts of the module influenced their proposal and also if they plan to undertake the study that they proposed.

3 Results

3.1 Proposed Optimisation Studies

It was clear that most of the proposed optimisation studies covered areas that were of genuine concern or of interest for a clinical department. There were a number of reasons for the justification of the proposed studies: poor image quality for specific examinations or for specific subgroups such as large breasts, dose audit, legislative changes or the introduction of new technology. There were a range of factors that were proposed for investigation during the optimisation studies: tube voltage, use of filters, image processing, automatic exposure control (AEC) set up, use of grid, use of virtual grid, use of synthetic view in digital breast tomosynthesis and use of imaging technology. The optimisation plans intended to use a number of different techniques: contrast-to-noise ratio, contrast detail tests, DQE, effective DQE (eDQE), visual grading analysis (absolute and relative), observer studies, model observers, anthropomorphic phantoms, simulated images, adaption of real clinical images and clinical audit.

3.2 Questionnaire About Preparation of Optimisation Study

Each of the participants was sent a questionnaire after the module had finished. The questionnaire included:

- Rate how this module affected the preparation for your optimisation study plan (from 0 to 4), where 0: 'No difference', 1: 'Slightly', 2: 'Helpful', 3: 'Very helpful', 4: 'Essential'.

One participant decided not to sit the exams and so there were only 19 studies. All the other participants passed the optimisation exam. The training methods are listed in Table 1 with the average score given by the participants. Seventeen out of 19 questionnaires were returned. All responders stated that they hope to undertake the study that they designed. The counts of scores for each training method used in the module are shown in Fig. 1.

Table 1. Questionnaire about module training methods and the average score given by the participants

Training methods	Average score
Online training material	3.5
Teleconference tutorial	2.1
Assignment	3.3
Discussion & email correspondence with module tutors	2.9
Face-to-face training: Seminars & lectures	3.4
Face-to-face training: Practicals	2.9
Examination of optimisation plans	3.3
Overall	3.5

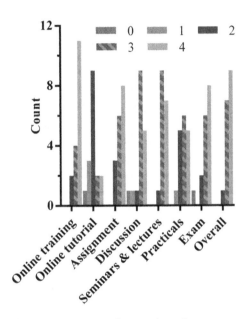

Fig. 1. Summary of questionnaire response (Color figure online)

3.3   Summary of Issues Found in the Assignments and Examination

The common weaknesses in some of the optimisation proposals in the assignment and to a lesser extent in the examination papers were:

- Use of entrance dose to the patient or the detector rather than a risk based dose measure e.g. organ dose or effective dose
- Lack of justification of the optimisation study, i.e. it was not clear why they were undertaking the study and this affected the quality of the proposal.
- Lack of a link between measurements and the clinical task.
- Weak ideas on how to implement the results in a clinical department.
- A lack of understanding of the limitations of their study.

Some of the strengths of the proposals were:

- Structured proposals involving technical measurements and task based studies.
- Good involvement with clinical staff; it was clear that the justification for many projects must have originated from discussion with clinical staff
- Clear plan to implement the results of the study in the clinical department.
- Inclusion of clinical audit within the proposal.
- The participants were pragmatic in their choice of study methodologies that were achievable within their available resources.

3.4   Wider Issues Highlighted About the Implementation of Optimisation Studies

A number of common challenges arose in the assignments and during discussions during the face-to-face training. The following are five main issues and the thoughts of the group:

1. A key stage of undertaking optimisation is to understand the clinical task and what the radiologists need to be able to see. However, many physicists working in D&IR have very little clinical contact with radiologists and radiographers. The MPEs must make an effort to create formal or even informal relationships with both radiologists and radiographers. Physicists need to demonstrate that they can contribute to improving the imaging within a department.
2. The link between the effect of image quality and clinical outcomes is difficult to quantify. The participants are aware that any dose reduction and associated change in image quality must not adversely affect the clinical outcome which may have a net increase in risk to the patient due to an increase in misdiagnosis.
3. Anthropomorphic phantoms are very useful for many optimisation techniques. However, they are expensive and few departments own one and only a few large centres would own a wide range of phantoms. It is necessary to create relationships with departments that own phantoms or for national bodies to create a phantom library. During the module, an arrangement was made between participants about the loan of an anatomical phantom.
4. Some large scale projects [9, 10] use complex software that were developed to create images for optimisation studies. Access to such complex software could allow smaller scale projects to be undertaken. However, the programs are not currently in a distributable form and collaboration will be needed between the groups and ideally should be shareable in the future.
5. Participants are busy and are generally time pressured. Optimising imaging systems is an integral part of the MPE role and they need adapt current practice to make time or find extra resources.

Clearly, MPEs require not only with good scientific skills, but that the MPE also needs leadership and soft skills to build relationships with clinical staff and other physicists world-wide. They also need time management skills and the ability to prioritize and critically appraise the work that they undertake.

4 Discussion

The training in this module was rated highly with an average score of 3.5 out of 4. The online course was rated the highest in terms of helping with the proposal, as this included the principles of optimisation and taught the participants about the wide range of options for optimisation studies. The online teleconferencing tutorial helped the least in the preparation of the optimization plan, though it must be noted that this part covered a range of topics (including quantitative measurements) and not just the optimisation studies.

The participants were highly motivated and worked hard during the online and face-to-face stages. They demonstrated that they could produce scientifically sound and original optimisation study plans. It is interesting to note the wide range of methods, clinical examinations and parameters included in the optimisation plans. Although, the course has given the participants the skills and knowledge, it is still too early to judge if the course will actually help the participants to successfully undertake an optimisation study. The participants were also very aware of constraints due to their available time and tailored their studies to be achievable. They ensured that the proposals were clinically relevant and realized that they need to develop their leadership and personal skills to be able to implement these studies clinically.

Training at a high educational level such as EQF8 requires high level experts for teaching and low student to teacher ratios. Therefore, it would not have been financially viable to create the modules without EU funding, as there are a limited number of potential participants. However, funding has allowed the modules to be developed and in the future each module will have to be self-financing. The EUtempe-RX consortium has developed an excellent mix of traditional and e-learning training. We can further utilize the available technology to provide the best training opportunities for future MPEs and in particular participants from further afield. In the future, an e-learning only option could be offered alongside the current module. This could enlarge the pool of students for this module. A challenge will be to convert the current face-to-face content to an e-learning environment. The conversion of lectures may be relatively simple, but ensuring the quality of training using practicals, in-depth discussion and case studies in an online environment is challenging. Examining participants also presents potential pitfalls. One of successes of this module was the interaction between the teachers and participants and this needs to continue for an e-learning only course.

5 Conclusions

The high level blended learning approach enhanced the participants' skills and knowledge to be able to write clinically relevant and scientifically sound optimisation plans. They all have the potential to undertake a successful optimisation study.

Acknowledgements. This project was funded by the European Commission from a 2012 FP7 EC call for European fission training schemes (EFTS) in 'Nuclear fission, safety and radiation protection' grant (grant agreement number: 605298). We thank our colleagues who prepared material, lectured and helped to run the module. We also thank the participants of this module for their hard work and enthusiasm during the module and their co-operation with this paper.

References

1. European Commission: Council Directive 2013/59/Euratom of 5 December 2013 Laying Down Basic Safety Standards for Protection against the Dangers Arising from Exposure to Ionising Radiation. L13 57, 1977-0677 (2014)
2. European Commission: Guidelines on Medical Physics Expert. Radiation Protection report 174 (2014)
3. Bosmans, H., Bliznakova, K., Padovani, R., et al.: EUtempe-RX, an EC supported FP7 project for the training and education of medical physics experts in radiology. Rad. Prot. Dosim. **165**, 518–522 (2015)
4. Jönsson, B.-A., Tabakov, S.D., Aitken, V., et al.: EMERALD and EMIT-worldwide computer aided education and training packages in medical physics. Int. J. InnovSci. Math. **13**, 10–15 (2012)
5. Pinto, A., Brunese, L., Pinto, F., et al.: E-learning and education in radiology. Eur. J. Radiol. **78**, 368–371 (2011)
6. Frehywot, S., Vovides, Y., Talib, Z., et al.: E-learning in medical education in resource constrained low-and middle-income countries. Hum. Resour. Health **11**, 1–15 (2013)
7. European Commission: European Guidelines on Medical Physics Expert: Inventory of learning outcomes for the MPE in Europe. Radiation Protection report 174 Annex 1 (2014)
8. Lage, M.J., Platt, G.J., Treglia, M.: Inverting the classroom: a gateway to creating an inclusive learning environment. J. Econ. Educ. **31**, 30–43 (2000)
9. Elangovan, P., Warren, L.M., Mackenzie, A., et al.: Development and validation of a modelling framework for simulating 2D-mammography and breast tomosynthesis images. Phys. Med. Biol. **59**, 4275–4293 (2014)
10. Moore, C.S., Beavis, A.W., Saunderson, J.R.: Investigation of optimum X-ray beam tube voltage and filtration for chest radiography with a computed radiography system. Brit. J. Radiol. **81**, 771–777 (2014)

Simplified Method for FROC Observer Study to Evaluate the Diagnostic Accuracy of a Digital Breast Imaging System by Using a CDMAM Phantom

Rie Tanaka[1](✉), Fujiyo Akita[2], Daisuke Fukuoka[3], Yusuke Bamba[4], and Junji Shiraishi[5]

[1] School of Health Sciences, College of Medical,
Pharmaceutical and Health Sciences, Kanazawa University, Kanazawa, Japan
rie44@mhs.mp.kanazawa-u.ac.jp
[2] Department of Diagnostic Imaging, Shizuoka Cancer Center, Sunto-gun, Japan
f.akita@sccsr.jp
[3] Department of Technology Education,
Faculty of Education, Gifu University, Gifu, Japan
dfukuoka@gifu-u.ac.jp
[4] R&D, Visual Technologies (ASIC), EIZO Corporation, Hakusan, Japan
yusuke.bamba@eizo.com
[5] Faculty of Life Sciences, Kumamoto University, Kumamoto, Japan
j2s@kumamoto-u.ac.jp

Abstract. We propose a simplified method for performing an FROC observer study by using regions of interest (ROIs) of CDMAM phantom images as case sample images. This new method would help researchers to plan and perform FROC observer studies in shorter time, with smaller errors and reduced complexity. As examples of experimental procedure, the digital images obtained by a direct-conversion flat-panel detector (FPD) system in three imaging conditions with different levels of patient dose were used to compare the diagnostic accuracies for low-contrast signal detection. There was a high correlation between the average figure of merit (FOM) obtained by our proposed method and inverse image quality figure (inv. IQF) calculated by CDMAM Analyser 1.55 in each dose level ($r = 0.98$).

Keywords: FROC observer study · CDMAM · Digital mammography · Jackknife free-response receiver operating characteristic (JAFROC)

1 Introduction

CDMAM phantom images have been used widely for evaluating the image quality of digital breast imaging systems [1]. To avoid inter- and/or intra-reader variations and reduce the time taken by human observers to read the phantom images, a number of computer software applications for automatic reading of the CDMAM phantom images have been developed and utilized for mammography image quality assurance [2–8]. Although automatic computer reading can evaluate reproducibly the image quality

© Springer International Publishing Switzerland 2016
A. Tingberg et al. (Eds.): IWDM 2016, LNCS 9699, pp. 83–88, 2016.
DOI: 10.1007/978-3-319-41546-8_11

without human errors, the diagnostic accuracy of the radiologic images should be evaluated by taking into account various factors due to human observers as well as the characteristics of the display used in the interpretation.

A free-response receiver operating characteristic (FROC) observer study has been employed to evaluate the diagnostic accuracy of radiologic images. The FROC observer study is superior to the ROC observer study because it allows for multiple lesions in any single case and multiple responses of a human observer for all possible lesions. This leads to an increased complexity when performing an FROC observer study, such as determining the degrees of subtlety of the lesions on an image, collecting confidence ratings for all case samples together with their locations, judging true positive and false positive findings, and so on.

The aim of this study is to propose a simplified method for performing an FROC observer study by using regions of interest (ROIs) of the CDMAM phantom images as case sample images. The method is outlined in the next section, followed by a discussion of the results in Sect. 3, and finally the study is summarized in Sect. 4.

2 Methods and Materials

Figure 1 shows the experimental procedure for an FROC observer study that is commonly used for evaluating the diagnostic accuracy of radiologic images. By using our new method, a number of improvements were accomplished. These include a simplified and standardized preparation procedure of case samples (with signals of appropriate degrees of visual perception difficulty), avoidance of human error by using computer software to collect confidence rating scores with location data, and time savings in classifying the computer-outputs of rating scores obtained from a number of observers. The latter are transformed into true/false positives for the jackknife alternative FROC (JAFROC) analysis [9].

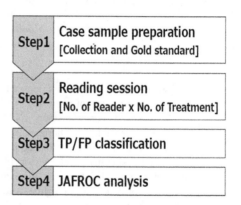

Fig. 1. Experimental procedure for the FROC observer study.

2.1 Case Sample Preparation

We employed a direct-conversion flat-panel detector (FPD) system (Amulet, Fuji Film Co. Ltd., Japan) to produce case sample images (matrix size = 3540 × 4740, pixel size = 50 μm) of a CDMAM phantom (version 3.4, Nijmegen) [1]. Three imaging conditions with different levels of patient doses (60, 80, and 100 % of the average glandular dose obtained during a routine examination, 30 kV, W/Rh) were used to compare the diagnostic accuracies for low-contrast signal detection. We produced three phantom images for each imaging condition and calibrated an average 50 % threshold contrast based on the analysis results of CDMAM analyzer [6, 10]. Then, as shown in Fig. 2, fourteen ROIs (matrix size 270 × 270) were selected manually based on the predicted threshold contrast. Each ROI image is cropped from the cross section of four cells, which contain gold disk(s) of varied sizes and at varied depths. This was used as a case sample image for the FROC observer study. The predicted degree of difficulties of the ROI images for the FROC observer study was determined in advance based on the results obtained by using a CDMAM Analyser [3]. From the 126 (42 × 3 conditions) ROI images obtained without and with various number of signals (the maximum number of signals per case is 3), 120 case sample images with 153 signals (0–3 signals/case) were selected to test the FROC observer study and 6 images with 8 signals were used during the training procedure.

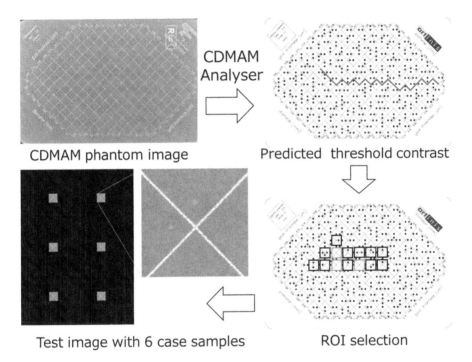

Fig. 2. Case sample preparation by using a CDMAM phantom. 126 case sample images without and with various number of signals (0–3 signals/case) were cropped along the threshold lines predicted by using a CDMAM Analyser and 20 test images (6 case samples per image) were produced.

To view the case sample images of the FROC observer study, a set of six case sample images were randomly selected and arranged on an image that had the same matrix size and standard DICOM header information as the original image (Fig. 2). Thus, 20 test images (6 case samples per image) were prepared for the FROC observer study.

2.2   Reading Session and True/False Positive Classification

The test image was displayed on a digital mammography LCD screen with high resolution (5 MP) and 10-bit grayscale (RadiForce GX540, EIZO Co. Ltd., Japan) and observed by using a publically available computer interface (ROC Viewer 2015 ver. 1.0 developed by the Japanese Society of Radiological Technology) [11]. By using this software, the observers determined the locations and the confidence ratings (ranging from 0.0 to 1.0) just by clicking on each of the 20 test images. The reading order of the 20 test images were determined in advance by using a random procedure. This was the same for all observers. There was no established reading order for the 6 case samples on the test image.

Six board-certified breast radiological technologists with experience ranging from 2 to 28 years (mean = 11.3 years) — all of whom were trained and certified for reading mammography by the Japan Central Organization on Quality Assurance of Breast Cancer Screening — participated in the FROC observer study. Because each observer interpreted 20 test images, in which case samples of three different imaging conditions were randomly mixed, we obtained confidence level ratings for 120 case samples with 153 signals (40 case samples with 51 signals per image condition) from one reading session. An input file of true positives, false positives, and true data with x-y locations and weight factors for the 153 signals was automatically produced by using a data management tool for calculating the figure of merit (FOM) values and testing statistically significant differences among the three different imaging conditions with the JAFROC software [9].

Our results obtained with the proposed FROC method were validated by comparison with those obtained from CDMAM Analyser version 1.55.

3   Results and Discussion

Although there was no statistically significant difference among the three conditions, the average FOM value and sensitivities of the 6 breast radiographers' performance improved with increasing dose level (Table 1). It is promising that the degrees of

Table 1. FOM and sensitivity (%) of 6 breast radiographers for each dose level compared with the inversed IQF obtained by CDMAM Analyser 1.55 and the total reading time for 120 case samples.

Reader	Dose level			Reading time (min)
	60 %	80 %	100 %	
1	0.56 (56.9 %)	0.58 (66.7 %)	0.59 (74.5 %)	19
2	0.57 (49.0 %)	0.58 (49.0 %)	0.58 (47.1 %)	12
3	0.57 (41.2 %)	0.59 (52.9 %)	0.60 (56.9 %)	26
4	0.60 (58.8 %)	0.61 (60.8 %)	0.61 (60.8 %)	37
5	0.57 (43.1 %)	0.57 (47.1 %)	0.59 (43.1 %)	9
6	0.60 (72.5 %)	0.61 (66.7 %)	0.62 (72.5 %)	29
Average	0.58 (53.6 %)	0.59 (57.2 %)	0.60 (59.2 %)	22.0
Inv. IQF	10.26	14.57	15.38	

difficulty of the case samples (sensitivity) were adequately selected by our proposed method. In addition, there was a high correlation between the average FOM and inverse image quality figure (inv. IQF) [12] in each dose level (r = 0.98). Furthermore, the average reading time for 20 test images (120 ROIs) was 22 min, which can be considered very short.

4   Conclusions

We propose a simplified method for performing an FROC observer study by using ROIs of CDMAM phantom images as case sample images. This new method would help researchers to plan and perform FROC observer studies in shorter time, with smaller errors and reduced complexity. In addition, by using a commercially available phantom employed for digital breast imaging systems, this method would provide reproducible results that can be utilized for comparing diagnostic accuracies of radiologic images obtained from two or more digital imaging system, various types of liquid crystal displays (LCDs), and/or imaging parameters.

Acknowledgments. The authors are grateful to the staff in the department of Radiology, Shizuoka Cancer Center. This work was supported by JSPS KAKENHI (Grant-in-Aid for Scientific Research) Grant Number 15K09898, and Pfizer Health Research Foundation.

References

1. Bijkerk, K.R., Thijssen, M.A.O., Arnoldussen, T.H.J.M.: Modification of the CDMAM contrast-detail phantom for image quality of Full Field Digital Mammography systems. In: Yaffe, M. (ed.) Proceedings of IWDM 2000, pp. 633–640. Medical Physics Publishing, Madison (2000)
2. Karssemeijer, N., Thijssen, M.A.O.: Determination of contrast-detail curves of mammography systems by automated image analysis. In: Proceedings of the 3rd International Workshop on Digital Mammography 1996, pp. 155–160 (1996)
3. Veldkamp, W.J., Thijssen, M.A., Karssemeijer, N.: The value of scatter removal by a grid in full field digital mammography. Med. Phys. **30**, 1712–1718 (2003)
4. Visser, R., Karssemeijer, N.: CDCOM Manual: software for automated readout of CDMAM 3.4 images. (note: CDCOM software, manual and sample images are posted at http://www.euref.org)
5. Young, K.C., Cook, J.J.H., Oduko, J.M., Bosmans, H.: Comparison of software and human observers in reading images of the CDMAM test object to assess digital mammography systems. In: Flynn, M.J., Hsieh, J. (eds.) Proceedings of SPIE Medical Imaging 2006, vol. 614206, pp. 1–13 (2006)
6. Young, K.C., Alsager, A., Oduko, J.M., Bosmans, H., Verbrugge, B., Geerste, T., et al.: Evaluation of software for reading images of the CDMAM test object to assess digital mammography systems. In: Proceedings of SPIE Medical Imaging 2008, vol. 69131C, pp. 1–10 (2008)

7. Figl, M., Hoffmann, R., Kaar, M., Semturs, F., Brasik, N., Birkfellner, W., et al.: Factors for conversion between human and automatic read-outs of CDMAM images. Med. Phys. **38**, 5090–5093 (2011)

8. Delakis, I., Wise, R., Morris, L., Kulama, E.: Performance evaluation of contrast-detail in full field digital mammography systems using ideal (Hotelling) observer vs. conventional automated analysis of CDMAM images for quality control of contrast-detail characteristics. Phys. Med. **31**, 741–746 (2015)

9. Chakraborty, D.P., Berbaum, K.S.: Observer studies involving detection and localization: modeling, analysis, and validation. Med. Phys. **31**, 2313–2330 (2004)

10. European Commission (EC): 2006 European Guidelines for Quality Assurance in Breast Cancer Screening and Diagnosis, 4th edn. Office for Official Publications of the European Communities, Luxembourg (2006)

11. Shiraishi, J., Fukuoka, D., Hara, T., Abe, H.: Basic concepts and development of an all-purpose computer interface for ROC/FROC observer study. Radiol. Phys. Technol. **6**(1), 35–41 (2013)

12. Oberhofer, N., Paruccini, N., Moroder, E.: Image quality assessment and equipment optimisation with automated phantom evaluation in Full Field Digital Mammography (FFDM). In: Krupinski, E.A. (ed.) IWDM 2008. LNCS, vol. 5116, pp. 235–242. Springer, Heidelberg (2008)

Equivocal Breast Findings Are Reduced with Digital Tomosynthesis

Maram Alakhras[1(✉)], Claudia Mello-Thoms[1], Roger Bourne[1],
Mary Rickard[2], and Patrick C. Brennan[1]

[1] Discipline of Medical Radiation Sciences,
Faculty of Health Sciences, University of Sydney, Sydney, Australia
{maram.alakhras, claudia.mello-thoms,
roger.bourne, patrick.brennan}@sydney.edu.au
[2] Sydney Breast Clinic, Sydney, Australia
mtr2006@bigpond.net.au

Abstract. The aim is to compare equivocal breast findings in digital breast tomosynthesis combined with digital mammography (DM+DBT) compared with DM alone for readers with different levels of DBT experience. Fifty cases (23 normal/benign, 27 cancer) were rated by 26 experienced breast radiologists (9, 9 and 8 individuals had no-, workshop- and clinical-DBT experience respectively) using a 5-point scoring scale (1 = normal, 5 = malignant). Ratings were compared between DM and DM+DBT for normal and cancer cases for all readers and for each sub-group of readers. Equivocal findings were 35 % of the total cancer-cases for DM compared with 24 % for DM+DBT for all readers grouped together with reductions also seen for each of the sub-groups. 31 % of normal cases were scored as equivocal in DM compared with 19 % in DM+DBT. Addition of DBT to DM reduces the number of equivocal breast findings regardless of the level of previous DBT experience.

Keywords: Digital breast tomosynthesis · Digital mammography · Equivocal

1 Introduction

The main limitation of mammography is the production of 2-dimensional (2D) breast images which may cause obscuring of breast abnormalities [1]. Missed cancer rates in mammography is relatively high (30 %) [1] with screening recall rates having a positive predictive value of 10 % [2]. In clinical breast imaging practice, a standard scoring system is usually used to report the likelihood of malignancy which is considered as a communication tool in mammography reports [3]. The use of a standardized reporting scale facilitates correct interpretation of breast findings and ensures accurate decisions about further management [4]. In Australia, a five-point scale (1 = Normal, 2 = Benign, 3 = Equivocal, 4 = Suspicious and 5 = Malignant) is used [5–9]. In this reporting scale, if the radiologist is uncertain about the correct diagnosis of the case, he/she will give it a score of 3 (equivocal) that indicates that the case will be recalled for further examinations to confirm the presence or absence of the disease. However, approximately 90 % of these cases will ultimately have a normal outcome [2]. Digital breast tomosynthesis is a recently introduced imaging tool which creates cross sectional

© Springer International Publishing Switzerland 2016
A. Tingberg et al. (Eds.): IWDM 2016, LNCS 9699, pp. 89–97, 2016.
DOI: 10.1007/978-3-319-41546-8_12

slices of the breast and may reduce tissue superimposition encountered in DM [10–12]. Therefore it results in higher number of detected cancers and lower number of false positive findings [8, 13]. In terms of image classifications, some previous studies have shown that the addition of DBT to DM may result in a higher number of 4–5 scores for cancer cases [7, 9] and more 1–2 scores for normal/benign cases [14, 15]. However, none of the previous studies has evaluated the impact of radiologists' level of DBT experience on the number of equivocal scorings, even though the impact of equivocal findings on the woman and screening services are significant.

The aim in the current study is to analyze equivocal breast scorings in DM and DM+DBT and assess the impact of adding two-view DBT to the standard two-view DM on the number of equivocal breast reporting for readers with different DBT experience.

2   Methods

2.1   Cases and Image Acquisition

This study was approved by our Institution Ethics Review Committee. A set of 50 cases from women who underwent DM and DBT were selected from a mix of screening and diagnostic patients by a state radiologist from Sydney Breast Clinic. Of these cases, 27 cases demonstrated cancer whilst 23 examinations had normal or benign findings. The majority of cancers were selected on the basis of difficulty where the lesions are not easily shown on DM images. All cases consisted of craniocaudal (CC) and mediolateral oblique (MLO) views for the right and left breasts except for two women who had a single breast removed. A summary of the types and sizes of each of the lesions is shown in Table 1.

Table 1. Sizes and the pathologic findings of the lesions that underwent biopsy

Lesion size	Number of lesions
≤ 10 mm	9
11–15 mm	12
16–20 mm	3
>20 mm	8
Total*	32
Pathologic findings	Number of lesions
Invasive ductal carcinoma	20
Invasive lobular carcinoma	3
Ductal carcinoma in situ (DCIS)	5
Medullary carcinoma	1
Mucinous carcinoma	1
Pleomorphic Lobular Carcinoma in Situ (LCIS)	1
Metastatic axillary lymph node	1

*: Some cases had more than one lesion

Selenia Dimensions digital system (Hologic, Inc. Bedford, MA, USA) which generates 15 low-dose projection images in a total scan angle of 15° was used for DM and DBT acquisitions. A combo imaging mode was applied for all cases, in which DM and DBT images are acquired during the same breast positioning and compression level, resulting in two datasets for each case available for review, one for DM and the other for DBT. After DBT acquisition, the data were used to reconstruct 1 mm thick slices, the number of slices for each case depending on the thickness of the compressed breast.

2.2 Image Interpretation

All images were interpreted by twenty-six experienced breast radiologists who read between 1000 and 5000 (median 4750) mammograms per year. Readers were categorized into three subgroups; readers with no DBT experience (n = 9); readers who had DBT workshop experience (n = 9); readers with clinical DBT experience (n = 8). Each radiologist read all cases in two sequential modes, DM followed by DM+DBT. For the first mode, DM images were displayed in two monitors and each radiologist reported his/her responses on a paper based report and gave each case a score based on a 5-point scale (1-Normal, 2-Benign, 3-Equivocal, 4-Suspicious, 5-Malignant) which has been developed by the Australian National Breast Cancer Centre (NBCC) in collaboration with the Royal Australian and New Zealand College of Radiologists (RANZCR) [16]. After reading DM images for each case, DBT images were made available on one monitor while the other monitor displayed DM images. The readers were asked to complete another report after the addition of DBT and give each case a score of 1–5. Images were displayed on a SecurView DX workstation (Hologic, Inc. Bedford, MA, USA) (CPU: High-end Dual Quad Processor, Memory: 16 GB High Speed RAM Minimum, Storage Space: 3.3 TB Minimum, Network Interface: 10/100/1000 Base T Ethernet) with 5-megapixel (MP) displays calibrated according to the Digital Imaging and Communications in Medicine (DICOM) part 14 standard [17]. Readers were able to use post-processing facilities including magnification, zooming and windowing while reviewing DM and DBT images.

2.3 Data Analysis

Based on radiologists' reports, equivocal responses on normal/benign and cancer cases were compared between the two modes (DM and DM+DBT) for all radiologists and for each sub-group of radiologists (according to the level of DBT experience). In addition, the number of equivocal breast findings on one mode and the change of their scores on the other mode were reported for normal/benign and cancer cases. Performance of each sub-group of readers was assessed using area under the receiver operating characteristic curve (ROC AUC).

3 Results

In this section, cancer and normal/benign cases with a score 3 in DM and/or DM+DBT will be discussed for all readers and for each sub-group of readers in terms of radiologists' DBT experience. Also, to demonstrate the performance of the individual radiologists' sub-groups, ROC AUC values will be included.

3.1 Cancer Cases

For all readers, the number of score 3 lesions was approximately 35 % (244/702) of the total number of cancer cases in DM compared with approximately 24 % (171/702) for DM+DBT as shown in Table 2. The percentage reduction of equivocal reportings after the addition of DBT was 40.6 % for readers with clinical experience compared with 22.2 % and 29.4 % for readers with no DBT and workshop DBT experience. Table 2 also shows ROC AUC values for each sub-group of readers.

Table 2. The difference in the number of equivocal findings of cancer cases between DM and DM+DBT, (ROC AUC is indicated within parentheses)*

Radiologists	DM	DM+DBT	Percentage decrease
No DBT	90 (0.682)	70 (0.775)	22.2 %
Workshop DBT	85 (0.680)	60 (0.790)	29.4 %
Clinical DBT	69 (0.681)	41 (0.789)	40.6 %
Total	244 (0.681)	171 (0.788)	30 %

*: ROC AUC values were reported in a previous publication [18]

Table 3 demonstrates that, for all radiologists, 33 % of cancer cases with score 3 in DM was assigned a RANZCR/NBCC categories 4–5 after the addition of DBT, Fig. 1 shows an example. The number and percentage of cases in each category in the second reading mode (DM+DBT) for cancer cases with score 3 in the first mode (DM) are shown in Table 3. These numbers are summarised for all readers and for each sub-group of readers.

Table 3. RANZCR/NBCC category in DM+DBT for lesions with RANZCR/NBCC category 3 in DM – Cancer cases

Radiologists	Score 3	Score 1–2	Score 4–5
No DBT	49 (54.44 %)	19 (21.11 %)	22 (24.44 %)
Workshop DBT	39 (45.9 %)	14 (16.5 %)	32 (37.6 %)
Clinical DBT	31 (44.9 %)	12 (17.4 %)	26 (37.7 %)
Total	119 (48.8 %)	45 (18.4 %)	80 (32.8 %)

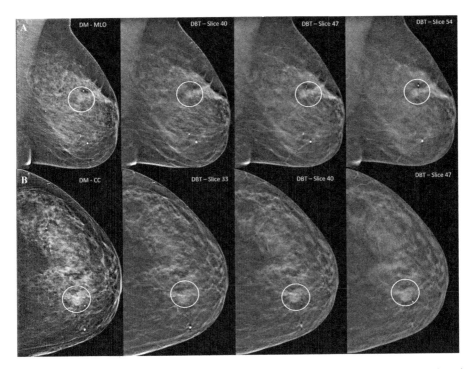

Fig. 1. Digital mammography and digital breast tomosynthesis mediolateral oblique (A) and craniocaudal (B) images for a stellate mass lesion. *This case was assigned a score 3 in DM and a score 4–5 in DM+DBT for 12 out of 26 radiologists.*

Table 4 shows that the majority of cases (~ 70 %), for all radiologists and for each subgroup of radiologists, with RANZCR/NBCC category 3 in DM+DBT were assigned a RANZCR/NBCC category 3 in the first mode (DM alone). Of these cases less than 7 % were assigned a score of 4 or 5 in DM.

Table 4. RANZCR/NBCC category in DM for lesions with RANZCR/NBCC category 3 in DM+DBT – Cancer cases

Radiologists	Score 3	Score 1–2	Score 4–5
No DBT	49 (70 %)	17 (24.3 %)	4 (5.7 %)
Workshop DBT	39 (65 %)	16 (26.7 %)	5 (8.3 %)
Clinical DBT	31 (75.6 %)	8 (19.5 %)	2 (4.9 %)
Total	119 (69.6 %)	41 (24 %)	11 (6.4 %)

3.2 Normal/Benign Cases

Table 5 shows that, for all radiologists, 31 % of the total number of normal/benign cases was given a RANZCR/NBCC category 3 in DM compared with 19 % in

DM+DBT. The percentage reduction of equivocal findings at DM after the addition of DBT is shown in Table 5.

Table 5. The difference in the number of equivocal findings of normal cases between DM and DM+DBT

Radiologists	DM	DM+DBT	Percentage decrease
No DBT	72	30	58 %
Workshop DBT	66	37	44 %
Clinical DBT	47	49	−4 %
Total	185	116	37 %

Table 6 shows that, for all radiologists, approximately half of normal/benign cases were downgraded to RANZCR/NBCC categories 1 and 2 after the addition of DBT, Fig. 2 shows an example. For no DBT and workshop DBT radiologists, more than 50 % of the normal cases with a RANZCR/NBCC category 3 in DM were scored as categories 1 or 2 after the addition of DBT to DM. However, for radiologists with clinical experience, the majority of these cases were scored as RANZCR/NBCC category 3 after adding DBT.

Table 6. RANZCR/NBCC category in DM+DBT for lesions with RANZCR/NBCC category 3 in DM – Normal/benign cases

Radiologists	Score 3	Score 1–2	Score 4–5
No DBT	20 (27.8 %)	46 (63.9 %)	6 (8.3 %)
Workshop DBT	25 (37.9 %)	37 (56 %)	4 (6.0 %)
Clinical DBT	29 (61.7 %)	17 (36.2 %)	1 (2.1 %)
Total	74 (40 %)	100 (54.1 %)	11 (5.9 %)

Table 7 shows the number of normal/benign cases that were assigned a score 3 in DM+DBT and their scores in DM. For normal/benign cases with category 3 in the second reading mode (DM+DBT), more than 50 % were scored as category 3 in the first mode (DM). The number of cases with different classifications in DM for all readers and each sub-group of readers is demonstrated in Table 7.

4 Discussion

In breast imaging, a scoring scale is usually used to facilitate the diagnosis and management of breast cancer. A 5-point scale is currently used in Australia and has been implemented in several research studies [5–8]. In this system, assigning a score 3 is considered an equivocal finding which means that the woman requires further tests to verify the diagnosis. Some previous studies have shown that some cancers were upgraded from score 3 to 4 or 5 using DBT [7], and that a higher number of cancer cases were assigned a score of 4 or 5 in DM+DBT compared with DM alone [9].

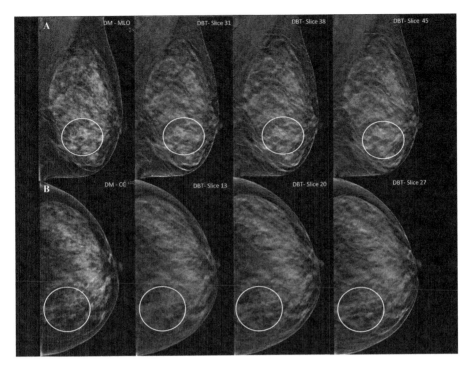

Fig. 2. Digital mammography and digital breast tomosynthesis mediolateral oblique (A) and craniocaudal (B) images for a benign case of architectural distortion and microcalcifications. *This case was assigned a score 3 in DM and a score 2 in DM+DBT for 9 out of 26 readers*

Table 7. RANZCR/NBCC category in DM for lesions with RANZCR/NBCC category 3 in DM+DBT – Normal/benign cases

Radiologists	Score 3	Score 1–2	Score 4–5
No DBT experience	20 (66.7 %)	9 (30 %)	1 (3.3 %)
Workshop DBT	25 (67.6 %)	11 (29.7 %)	1 (2.7 %)
Clinical DBT	29 (59.2 %)	18 (36.7 %)	2 (4.1 %)
Total	74 (63.8 %)	38 (32.8 %)	4 (3.4 %)

The current study however focused on the number of score 3 cases between DM and DM+DBT with particular consideration given to readers with different levels of DBT experience.

In the current study, we found that for all radiologists, the addition of DBT to the standard DM reduced the number of equivocal classifications by 11 % of the total number of cases (n = 50) (33 % for DM (429/1300) compared with 22 % (287/1300) for DM+DBT). Almost the same percentage reduction in score 3 cases was found for cancer (11 %) and normal/benign cases (12 %) after adding DBT to DM. Our work also demonstrated, for cases with category 3 in DM, that implementing DBT in addition to DM resulted in upgrading 33 % cancer cases to category 4 or 5 and downgrading 54 % normal/benign cases to category 1 or 2. These findings might be explained by the fact that DBT produces multiple slices of the breast which reduces tissue overlap facilitating more accurate reporting of breast images. If the radiologist is able to downgrade a normal/benign lesion from score 3 this may reduce the number of recalled women who undergo additional radiological and invasive examinations while they have no cancer which will also result in less stress, time and cost associated with recalling women with normal/benign findings. Also upgrading a malignant lesion from score 3 may decrease the need for performing additional examinations to ensure the presence or the absence of malignancy.

For cases with category 3 in the second mode, the majority of cancer and normal/benign cases for all readers were originally assigned a category 3 in the first reading mode (DM). For cancer cases, only ∼6 % of these equivocal finding in DM+DBT were assigned a score 4 or 5 in DM and only 3 % of normal cases was assigned a score 1 or 2 in DM.

In terms of radiologists' experience, our results demonstrated that, for equivocal findings in the first reading mode (DM), similar number of cancer cases was scored as equivocal in the second reading mode (DM+DBT) for the three subgroups of readers. However, it has to be acknowledged that for radiologists who had a clinical DBT experience the percentage reduction of category 3 cancer cases at DM+DBT compared with DM alone was more than that for readers who had no- or workshop-experience. It should be acknowledged however, that for normal/benign cases as readers get more experience and move from no DBT and DBT workshop experience to clinical DBT experience then the advantages of DBT with regard to equivocal findings might go down. The results showed that radiologists with clinical DBT reported more number of normal/benign cases as equivocal compared with the other two groups of readers. This might be partially explained by the abnormal prevalence (54 %) of cancer in our case set, which is not reflective of clinical practice. It is also important to acknowledge that all participant radiologists included in this study were experienced breast radiologists dedicated to DM reading. Also, DBT is considered as a new imaging modality so it can be argued that there is lack of extensive and prolonged DBT experience for all radiologists who participated in this study.

In conclusion, our results suggest that the use of DBT, as an adjunct to DM, may result in reducing the number of equivocal breast scorings for normal/benign and cancer cases. This reduction may be dependent on the radiologists DBT experience. Further studies including higher number of cases and higher number of readers in each experience subcategory should be performed. Future work should also consider the contribution of other factors on the number of category 3 cases such as breast density, lesion type and lesion size.

References

1. Pisano, E.D.: Diagnostic performance of digital versus film mammography for breast-cancer screening. N. Engl. J. Med. **355**(17), 1773–1783 (2006)
2. Yankaskas, B.C., et al.: Association of recall rates with sensitivity and positive predictive values of screening mammography. AJR **177**(3), 543–549 (2001)

3. Balleyguier, C., et al.: BIRADS™ classification in mammography. Eur. J. Radiol. **61**(2), 192–194 (2007)
4. Maxwell, A.J., et al.: The Royal College of Radiologists Breast Group breast imaging classification. Clin. Radiol. **64**(6), 624–627 (2009)
5. Poplack, S.P., et al.: Digital breast tomosynthesis: initial experience in 98 women with abnormal digital screening mammography. AJR **189**(3), 616–623 (2007)
6. Svane, G., et al.: Clinical experience of photon counting breast tomosynthesis: comparison with traditional mammography. Acta Radiol. **52**(2), 134–142 (2011)
7. Andersson, I., et al.: Breast tomosynthesis and digital mammography: a comparison of breast cancer visibility and BIRADS classification in a population of cancers with subtle mammographic findings. Eur. Radiol. **18**(12), 2817–2825 (2008)
8. Skaane, P., et al.: Comparison of digital mammography alone and digital mammography plus tomosynthesis in a population-based screening program. Radiology **267**(1), 47–56 (2013)
9. Tingberg, A., Andersson, I., Ikeda, D.M., Ruschin, M., Svahn, T., Timberg, P.: BIRADS classification in breast tomosynthesis compared to mammography and ultrasonography. In: Krupinski, E.A. (ed.) IWDM 2008. LNCS, vol. 5116, pp. 67–73. Springer, Heidelberg (2008)
10. Baker, J.A., Lo, J.Y.: Breast tomosynthesis: state-of-the-art and review of the literature. Acad. Radiol. **18**(10), 1298–1310 (2011)
11. David, G.: Tomosynthesis-based imaging of the breast. Acad. Radiol. **18**(10), 1203–1204 (2011)
12. Karellas, A., Vedantham, S.: Breast cancer imaging: a perspective for the next decade. Med. Phys. **35**(11), 4878–4897 (2008)
13. Ciatto, S., et al.: Integration of 3D digital mammography with tomosynthesis for population breast-cancer screening (STORM): a prospective comparison study. Lancet Oncol. **14**(7), 583–589 (2013)
14. Bernardi, D., et al.: Prospective study of breast tomosynthesis as a triage to assessment in screening. Breast Cancer Res. Treat. **133**(1), 267–271 (2012)
15. Gur, D., et al.: Digital breast tomosynthesis: observer performance study. AJR **193**(2), 586–591 (2009)
16. Breast Imaging: A Guide for Practice. National Breast Cancer Centre, Camperdown (2002)
17. Digital Imaging and Communication in Medicine (DICOM) Part 14: Grayscale Standard Display Function. National Electrical Manufacturer's Association (2011)
18. Alakhras, M.M., et al.: Effect of radiologists' experience on breast cancer detection and localization using digital breast tomosynthesis. Eur. Radiol. **25**(2), 402–409 (2015)

The Accuracy of an Estimating Method for the Mammary Gland Composition in the Mammography Using the CdTe-Series Photon Counting Detector

Ai Nakajima[1]([⊠]), Misa Kato[2], Chizuru Okamoto[1], Akiko Ihori[1],
Tsutomu Yamakawa[3], Shuichiro Yamamoto[3], Masahiro Okada[3],
and Yoshie Kodera[1]

[1] Department of Radiological Science, Graduate School of Medicine,
Nagoya University, Nagoya, Japan
nakajima.ai@e.mbox.nagoya-u.ac.jp
[2] School of Health Sciences, Nagoya University, Nagoya, Japan
[3] JOB Corporation, Yokohama, Japan

Abstract. We propose a method for estimating mammary gland composition and report the examined results to find the better conditions to improve the precision of the estimation. We use a cadmium telluride series (CdTe-series) detector as a photon-counting mammography detector in this study, since CdTe-series detectors detect photons in a wide energy range and provide highly accurate energy discrimination. An imaging system using a CdTe-series detector is simulated by MATLAB. We divide the spectrum of an X-ray, which is transmitted a phantom, into three energy bins and calculate the corresponding linear attenuation coefficients from the numbers of input and output photons. These linear attenuation coefficients are plotted in a three-dimensional (3D) scatter plot. Using this 3D scatter plot, we estimate the mammary gland composition and determine the optimal conditions to estimate.

Keywords: Photon counting · Digital mammography · Mammary gland composition

1 Introduction

Generally, breast cancer is difficult to be distinguished from mammary gland, using conventional mammography, because their linear attenuation coefficients are very close to each other. Moreover, it has been supposed that a risk of breast cancer is high when mammary gland content rate is high. Thus, mammary gland composition should be estimated to evaluate the risk of breast cancer. Many methods for estimating mammary gland composition has been reported. For example, Highnam proposed a method using standard mammogram form (SMF) [1]. We will propose a new method using photon-counting technology. Currently, a photon-counting mammography system that is one of digital mammography systems has been commercialized and used silicon semiconductor detectors. However, we use a cadmium telluride series (CdTe-series) detector as a

© Springer International Publishing Switzerland 2016
A. Tingberg et al. (Eds.): IWDM 2016, LNCS 9699, pp. 98–106, 2016.
DOI: 10.1007/978-3-319-41546-8_13

photon-counting detector in this study. Cadmium telluride series detector detect photons in a wide energy range, and their energy discrimination is highly accurate [2]. Thus, we could divide the spectrum of an X-ray into three energy bins and obtain not a two-dimensional (2D) scatter plot but a three-dimensional (3D) scatter plot. Three dimensional scatter plots are considered to have more information than 2D scatter plots. We are convinced that 3D scatter plot is superior to 2D scatter plot. Because high energy bin and low energy bin are apart from each other compare to 2D scatter plot and 3D scatter plot has high ability to visual express. Moreover, 3D scatter plot can render high dimension rather than 2D scatter plot. Therefore, a 3D scatter plot is appropriate for estimating mammary gland composition with high precision. We are going to compare and examine 3D scatter plot and 2D scatter plot in detail. Considering these properties, we propose a method for estimating mammary gland composition, using a MATLAB simulation. Moreover, we change the total photon number and the fraction of energy-binned photons to determine the optimal conditions giving the highest accuracy in this study.

2   Materials and Method

2.1   Simulation Geometry

We designed a CdTe-series detector using a MATLAB simulator and simulated a slit scan imaging system. Figure 1(a) shows the simulation geometry. The source-detector distance was 65 cm, the X-ray tube voltage was 50 kV, and the pixel size was 0.2 mm × 0.2 mm. Figure 1(b) schematically shows the phantom we designed.

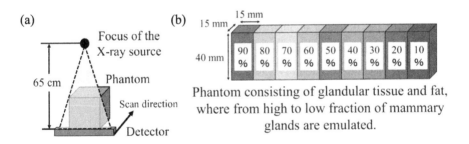

Phantom consisting of glandular tissue and fat, where from high to low fraction of mammary glands are emulated.

Fig. 1. (a) Simulation geometry (b) Phantom (Color figure online)

2.2   Method for Estimating Mammary Gland Composition

We divided the spectrum of an X-ray, which was transmitted through the phantom, into three energy bins and acquired the three images from one exposure corresponding to the three energy bins (Fig. 2). We denoted these bins as BIN1, BIN2 and BIN3 from a lower energy to a higher energy.

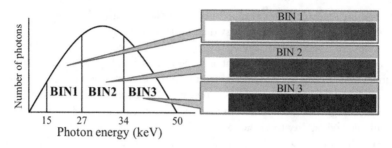

Fig. 2. Divided spectrum and the acquired three images.

The regions of interest (ROIs) are the background (BG) and the mammary gland areas (Fig. 3). The ROI size was 11 mm × 11 mm. In Fig. 3, the colors correspond to those of the phantom demonstrated in Fig. 1.

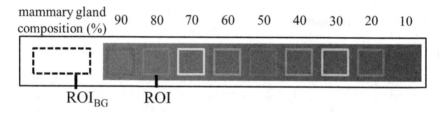

Fig. 3. Set ROIs (Color figure online)

The linear attenuation coefficients, μ_1, μ_2, and μ_3, for the three energy bins were calculated from the numbers of input and output photons. Then we calculated the normalized linear attenuation coefficients, which are symbolized as $\mu_1^\dagger$, $\mu_2^\dagger$, and $\mu_3^\dagger$ from BIN1 to BIN3. When expression (1) was used for $\mu_1^\dagger$, we did not need the information on the thickness (t). $\mu_2^\dagger$ and $\mu_3^\dagger$ were calculated in the same way.

$$\mu_1^\dagger = \frac{\mu_1 t}{t\sqrt{(\mu_1{}^2 + \mu_2{}^2 + \mu_3{}^2)}} \tag{1}$$

The 3D scatter plot was made from $\mu_1^\dagger$, $\mu_2^\dagger$, and $\mu_3^\dagger$. In Fig. 4, the colors correspond to those of the phantom depicted in Fig. 1. We denoted this 3D scatter plot as Xprism®. Xprism is the registered trademark of the JOB Corporation. The left figure shows the values of the individual pixels. The right figure shows the average values. Comparing the patient's data and 3D scatter plot, we estimated the mammary gland composition.

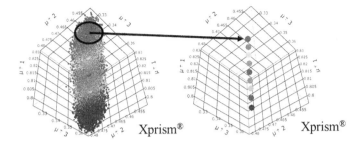

Fig. 4. Three-dimensional scatter plots at the same angle and scale. (Color figure online)

2.3 Optimal Condition Determination

To determine the optimal conditions to estimate the mammary gland composition, we changed some conditions to make the 3D scatter plot. We changed the total number of photons from 150 to 1000 counts/flame. One hundred fifty counts/flame is equal to 12360 photons/pixel. Hence, the total number of photons varied from 12360 to 82400. When the total numbers of photons was 82400, the average glandular dose was approximately 0.39 mGy. In addition, we changed the fraction of energy-binned photons as 1:1:1, 1:1:3, 1:3:1, and 3:1:1 by changing the binned energy threshold. Moreover, we corrected beam hardening in this study.

2.4 Evaluation Method

We prepared a new method to calculate the contrast-to-noise ratio (CNR). For this new CNR, the two scatter distributions should be calculated. In this report, we use the adjacent scatter distribution. Figure 5 shows an example. In expression (2), the numerator indicates the distance of adjacent average value, and the denominator indicates the average standard deviation (SD) value. Therefore, we use the distance of the adjacent average value as the contrast and the SD value as the noise.

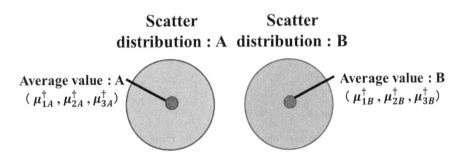

Fig. 5. Adjacent scatter distribution.

$$CNR = \frac{\sqrt{\left(\mu_{1A}^{\dagger} - \mu_{1B}^{\dagger}\right)^2 + \left(\mu_{2A}^{\dagger} - \mu_{2B}^{\dagger}\right)^2 + \left(\mu_{3A}^{\dagger} - \mu_{3B}^{\dagger}\right)^2}}{\sqrt{\frac{SD_A^2 + SD_B^2}{2}}} \tag{2}$$

3   Results

3.1   Total Number of Photons

Figure 6 is the 3D scatter plot obtained by the phantom simulation shown in Fig. 1. As the number of photons decreased, the points on the 3D distribution scattered widely. Conversely, as the number of photons increased, the points on the 3D distribution were densely convergent. As can be seen in Fig. 7, as the number of photons increased, the CNR value became large.

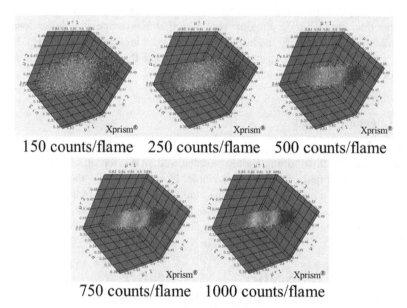

Fig. 6. Three-dimensional scatter plots. The number of photons was varied. The angle and scale are the same. (Color figure online)

3.2   Fraction of Photons

The shape of the distribution was changed, when the fraction of photons was varied (Fig. 8). In Figs. 9 and 10, when the fraction of photons for BIN2 increased like 1:3:1, the distance of the adjacent average points became long and the CNR value was large. Conversely, if the fraction of photons decreased like 1:1:3, the distance between the adjacent average points became short and the CNR value was small.

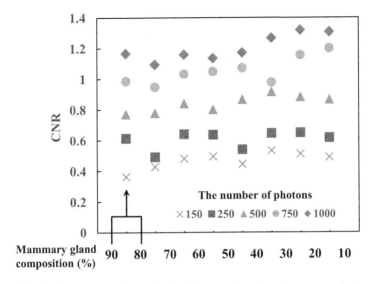

Fig. 7. Contrast-to-noise ratio plot. The number of photons was varied.

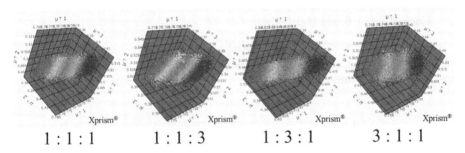

Fig. 8. Three-dimensional scatter plots. The fraction of photons was varied. The angle and scale are the same. (Color figure online)

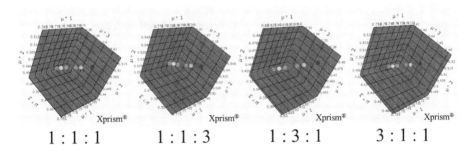

Fig. 9. Plots of the average points. The fraction of photons was varied. The angle and scale are the same. (Color figure online)

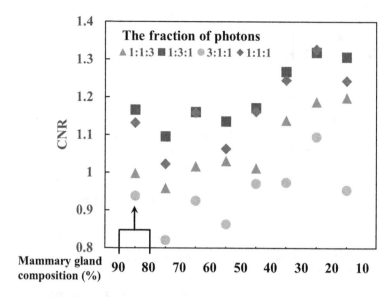

Fig. 10. Contrast-to-noise ratio plot. The fraction of photons was varied.

3.3 Correction of Beam Hardening

In Fig. 11, the CNR values were changed between the corrected CNR and non-corrected CNR. The CNR-corrected beam hardening was larger than CNR-non-corrected beam hardening.

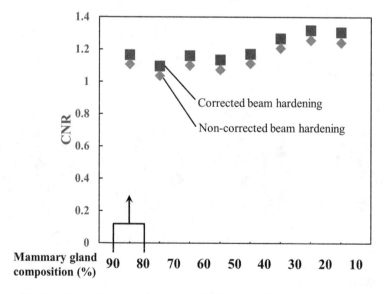

Fig. 11. Contrast-to-noise ratio plot. The fraction of photons was varied.

4   Discussion

As shown in Sect. 3.1, when the total number of photons was changed, the distribution of the individual pixel value and the CNR were also changed. A large CNR value indicates that the 3D scatter plot is appropriate for estimating the mammary gland composition. Thus, the precision of the estimation of the mammary gland composition is more accurate as the number of photons increase. In our calculation, the average glandular dose is very low. Hence, the estimation can be performed with high precision and low exposure dose.

When the fraction of photons was changed, the distribution of the average value and the CNR value were changed too. When the fraction of photons in BIN2 increased, we could well distinguish each average point. Moreover, the CNR value became large. Therefore, the distribution of the average points is appropriate for estimating the mammary gland composition. However, fraction 1:1:1 also had a high CNR value, but its distance of the adjacent average points was not so long. We assumed that this could be attributed to the method to calculate the CNR. In the CNR calculation, the shape of the scatter plots distribution is not considered. Thus, the CNR values were large, though they were not appropriate for the estimation. We need to improve the method for calculating the CNR.

The information on the thickness was not required for expression (1). Because of beam hardening, the normalized linear attenuation coefficient was not accurate. When beam hardening was corrected, the normalized linear attenuation coefficient approached an accurate value. Therefore, the CNR values became large when beam hardening was corrected, and the 3D scatter plot was appropriate for estimating the mammary gland composition. To make the precision of the estimation higher, further study should be conducted.

5   Conclusion

We could accurately estimate the mammary gland composition, using the method proposed in this study.

We examined the change in the number of photons and the fraction of photons, and we obtained the condition, under which the distribution of the values of the individual pixels were appropriate for estimating the mammary gland composition. The normalized linear attenuation coefficient was affected by beam hardening. Hence, when the beam hardening was corrected, its precision became accurate. In near future, we are going to find a condition, under which the exposure dose is lower and a higher precision is maintained. Additionally, we are going to make another factor affect the precision most severely. Moreover, we hope to develop a method for detecting the tumor tissue.

Acknowledgments. The authors thank Dr. Hiroaki HAYASHI and Ms. Natsumi KIMOTO from Tokushima University for their assistance on calculating the average glandular dose.

References

1. Highnam, R., Pan, X., Warren, R., et al.: Breast composition measurements using retrospective standard mammogram form (SMF). Phys. Med. Biol. **51**, 2695–2713 (2006)
2. Iwanczyk, J.S., Nygård, E., Meirav, O., et al.: Photon counting energy dispersive detector arrays for X-ray imaging. IEEE Trans. Nucl. Sci. **56**, 535–542 (2009)

Towards Optimization of Image Quality as a Function of Breast Thickness in Mammography: An Investigation of the Breast Thickness Compensation Schemes on Analogue and Digital Mammography Units

Lesley J. Grattan[✉] and Adam Workman

Northern Ireland Medical Physics Service, Belfast, UK
lesley.grattan@belfasttrust.hscni.net

Abstract. Historically, with film/screen mammography systems image quality as a function of breast thickness was constrained by the necessity to maintain constant dose to the film across all thicknesses. With digital units, no such constraint is placed upon the AEC system and different manufacturers have designed their own breast thickness compensation schemes. In this study, threshold contrast detail detectability measurements were made at three different simulated breast thicknesses using a CDMAM phantom on analogue and digital mammography units. The purpose was to understand how the design of the different AEC systems affected the image quality for thicker breasts in particular, when compared with that for a standard breast thickness on the same unit. The results showed that relative image quality for thicker breasts compared with standard breasts varies greatly with unit type, depending on the thickness compensation scheme implemented by the particular AEC system. The work highlights an urgent need for a more evidence based approach to determining optimal task-based image quality as a function of breast thickness.

Keywords: Digital mammography · Image quality · Breast thickness

1 Introduction

The determination of image quality adequate to fulfill a particular diagnostic task in medical imaging is extremely challenging; and particularly so in mammography given the subtleties of breast tissue and architecture which often characterize breast cancer. The resolution of the problem does not lend itself to a solely analytic interpretation due to the variety and complexity of clinical presentations. Therefore, pertinent information needs to be gathered from a range of sources such as clinical trials, task simulations and historical data. In the absence of conclusive evidence from the first two sources during the introduction of digital imaging in mammography, historical data on the performance of analogue imaging was relied upon to provide criteria for image quality measurements [1].

With analogue technology and the use of film, it was required to maintain a constant dose to the detector (film) across all thicknesses in order to produce usable images. The

© Springer International Publishing Switzerland 2016
A. Tingberg et al. (Eds.): IWDM 2016, LNCS 9699, pp. 107–115, 2016.
DOI: 10.1007/978-3-319-41546-8_14

need to limit dose to the breast necessitated the use of harder x-ray beams for thicker breasts which had the intrinsic effect of lowering the subject contrast due to a reduction in photoelectric absorption. In addition, the increased scatter volume of thicker breasts, exposed with harder x-ray beams, increased the amount of forward scattered radiation reaching the film (even with the grid in place) and meant that the image contrast to noise ratio was further reduced, with no option for recovery by post-processing.

With digital technology the requirement for constant detector dose no longer applies and there are currently several approaches adopted by manufacturers of digital mammography equipment. Some units are designed to still maintain a constant detector dose (i.e. pixel value) with thickness, while others are aiming for a constant measure of image quality (e.g. Signal difference to Noise Ratio (SDNR) or Contrast to Noise ratio (CNR) with breast thickness. Still others aim to maximize a figure of merit based on a combination of image quality and breast dose.

However, the question of what is the optimal image quality (and image quality metric) as a function of breast thickness remains unanswered. And secondary to this, what is the most appropriate design of automatic exposure control (AEC) system to achieve this within reasonable breast dose limits? In view of the changing breast tissue composition as a function of breast thickness - in general thicker breasts have a higher percentage of adipose tissue than thinner breasts [2]; it may not be necessary to maintain a constant level of image quality across all thicknesses. In their guidelines for quality assurance in mammography, EUREF has adopted a standard of a slowly decreasing SDNR as a function of increasing breast thickness, described by z factors, which was based partly on data from analogue units [1].

In this study we examine image quality measurements, namely threshold contrast detail detectability (TCDD), across a range of breast thicknesses using an analogue unit to obtain an understanding of the thickness-dependent image quality in use up until the introduction of digital mammography. TCDD measurements are a useful means of assessing image quality on analogue images where unlike digital systems the direct measurement of quantitative parameters such as CNR is not possible and the process of digitization of the films may introduce additional image noise or errors associated with quantization These results are compared with similar data from several digital mammography units in use in the UK Breast Screening Programme. Both calculated doses based on the CDMAM exposures, and clinical doses from a concurrent patient dose audit are presented alongside the image quality results. The differences shown between the units in their breast thickness compensation schemes highlight the need for a more evidence based approach in AEC design and testing standards.

2   Method

TCDD measurements were made using a CDMAM type 3.4 phantom (Artinis Medical Systems, Elst, NL, serial number 1148) on an analogue mammography x-ray system comprising a Hologic LoRad MIV unit and Fuji Fine AD film-screen system. This unit has a number of beam qualities available, giving the potential for optimization of image quality and breast dose as a function of breast thickness. The measurements were made at three different equivalent compressed breast thicknesses (CBT) of 32, 60 and 90 mm. These were simulated with PMMA and the 5 mm thick CDMAM phantom (which has an equivalent attenuation to about 10 mm PMMA) as shown in Table 1 below. The simulated compressed breast thickness values will be used throughout the paper.

Table 1. Simulation of compressed breast thickness using PMMA and a CDMAM phantom.

Compressed breast thickness (mm)	Equivalent PMMA thickness (mm)	PMMA thickness (mm) in addition to CDMAM phantom
32	30	20
60	50	40
90	70	60

In each case the height of the CDMAM phantom was maintained at 20 mm above the support platform to remove differences in magnification and geometric unsharpness between the three sets of measurements. A set of eight images was taken at each thickness using a range of cassettes selected from those in normal clinical use. All images were each read by two experienced observers. The readings were corrected according to the phantom manufacturer instructions, averaged and fitted with a smooth curve using Sigmaplot regression analysis (Sigmaplot v8.02, SSPS Inc., Chicago IL).

Similar sets of measurements were made on three digital mammography units: a Siemens Inspiration unit (using AEC high dose mode), a Hologic Selenia Dimensions unit (using auto-filter mode) and a GE Essential unit (using standard mode with the Profile Automatic Optimisation of Parameters (AOP) table). For the Inspiration and Dimensions units, the region of the detector used for AEC was set as static – for the Inspiration unit segmentation was turned off, and for the Dimensions unit the same AEC region was selected for each exposure. The Essential does not allow selection of a static AEC region; instead the exposure parameters were determined by the unit based on local dense regions in the main image area. (The mAs values for the CDMAM exposures on the Essential unit were within 10 % of those returned when imaging the corresponding thickness of PMMA). Since the purpose of the study was to examine the behaviour of the image quality metric as a function of breast thickness *within* each unit, these raw digital images were analysed using software to automatically read and score. The CDCOM v1.6 software [3] and the Matlab results analysis package from NCCPM in the UK were used for this purpose [4]. The analysis package includes a scaling factor to account for the human observer. All CDMAM results from one of the digital units were also manually read as a check between the two reading methods.

All the results were converted from threshold gold thickness (T_g) to threshold contrast (T_C) to take account of the different beam qualities used for different breast thicknesses using the method given in the EUREF guidelines [1]:

$$T_C = 1 - e^{-\mu T_g} \tag{1}$$

The average attenuation coefficient values for gold (μ) were calculated using mammography spectral models developed by Boone [5], with attenuation coefficients for the various filtering materials obtained from the NIST XCOM database

(Berger *et al.*) [6]. The attenuation of the beams was adjusted for the three different setups in Table 1.

Mean glandular doses (MGDs) were calculated with the Dance dose model [7, 8] using the parameters from the CDMAM exposures for each unit. Patient dose audits for the UK Breast Screening Programme were also carried out concurrently with the acquisition of the CDMAM data for the digital units. In brief, a sample of fifty women, aged between 50 and 70 years, were selected from each unit and their MGDs calculated using the Dance model. Fully clinical modes were used on each unit i.e. segmentation on the Inspiration unit and automatic selection of AEC region on the Dimensions and Essential units. The average dose was calculated at three CBT points: 31–33 mm, 60 mm and 89–91 mm. In order to improve the accuracy of the result, clinical data were included from other units of the same type which were found to have similar patient dose distributions to the unit on which the CDMAM exposures were taken. The Inspiration data came from 13 units and the Dimensions data from 3 units. Essential data were only obtained from a single unit.

3   Results

Results are shown from the manual reading of the films from the analogue unit both in terms of the initial threshold gold thickness results (Fig. 1) and threshold contrast (Fig. 2a) for the three simulated breast thicknesses. The threshold gold thickness results from the digital units read using the CDCOM software were fitted by the NCCPM analysis programme. The curve fits were within $\pm 2 \times$ SEM for all threshold gold thickness

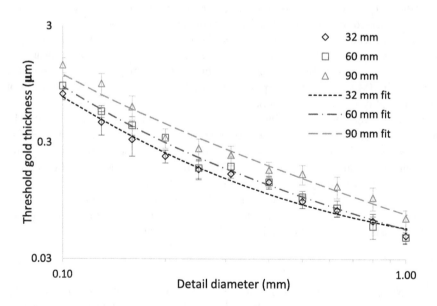

Fig. 1. Threshold gold thickness for film/screen system for three different simulated compressed breast thicknesses. Error bars show $2 \times$ sem.

data points. Threshold contrast values calculated from the fits using Eq. 1 are shown in Fig. 2b, c and d for the three digital units.

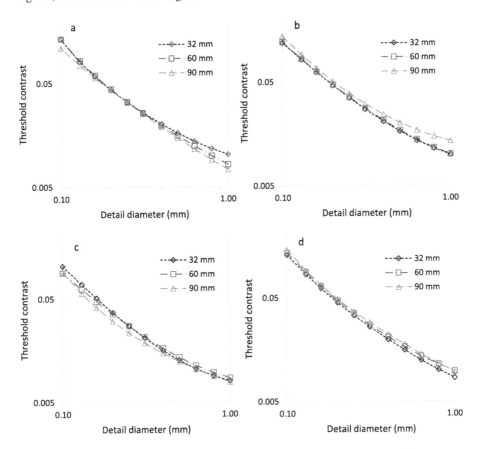

Fig. 2. Threshold contrast for three different simulated compressed breast thicknesses on (a) film/screen unit, (b) Inspiration unit, (c) Dimensions unit and (d) Essential unit.

To allow comparison of the thickness profiles from the different x-ray units, the threshold contrast measurements at the different CBTs (T_{C32}, T_{C90}) were normalized to the value obtained at 60 mm CBT (T_{C60}) for each of the CDMAM gold detail diameters between 0.1 and 1.0 mm. These ratios of T_{C60}/T_{C90} and T_{C60}/T_{C32} were then averaged over the detail diameter range. (The ratios determined for the purpose of checking agreement between the two reading methods agreed to within 4 % of each other). The results are plotted in Fig. 3 together with the z factors from Table 1.3 in the supplement to the EUREF guidelines [1]. A ratio greater than unity indicates a decrease in the threshold contrast detectability compared with the value at 60 mm CBT, i.e. an improvement in the image quality metric when compared with 60 mm CBT.

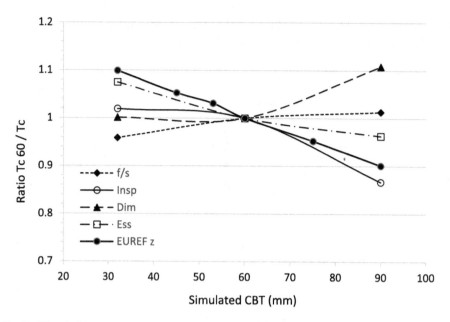

Fig. 3. Threshold contrast normalized to 60 mm compressed breast thickness for the film/screen system and three digital units. The lines are intended as a visual aid only; interpolated data is not implied. The z factors from the EUREF guidelines are also shown [1].

The doses calculated from the CDMAM exposures are shown in Fig. 4a for all units and from the clinical dose audit in Fig. 4b for the digital units. Reasonably good agreement of doses is seen between the two regimes which indicates that the CDMAM exposures are representative of the clinical operation of the units. Using the dose data from the CDMAM exposures, the ratios of the doses between 90 and 60 mm equivalent CBT are given in Table 2 for each of the units. These data combined with the T_{C60}/T_{C90} ratios give a measure of how effectively the increase in dose for the thicker breasts is used to improve image quality.

Table 2. Dose effectiveness for thicker breasts on each unit.

Unit	$Dose_{90}/Dose_{60}$	T_{C60}/T_{C90}	T_C ratio/Dose ratio
Film/Screen	1.53	1.01	0.66
Inspiration	1.78	0.87	0.49
Dimensions	1.47	1.11	0.76
Essential	2.06	0.96	0.47

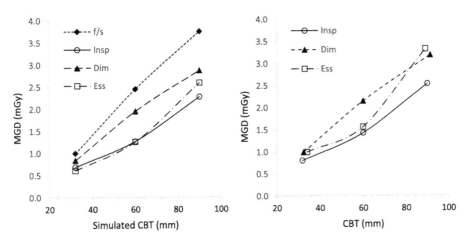

Fig. 4. Mean Glandular Dose calculated from (a) CDMAM exposures and (b) clinical dose audit data.

4   Discussion

The results presented here show that the current clinical situation may be quite varied, especially in the case of thicker breasts. The image quality and dose for thicker breasts is largely determined by the compensation scheme adopted by the manufacturer of a particular piece of equipment. The three digital units that we have tested demonstrate markedly different approaches to imaging thicker breasts. The Siemens Inspiration unit shows a 16 % reduction in measured image quality for 90 mm CBT compared with 60 mm CBT, whereas for the Hologic Dimensions unit the measured image quality *increases* by 10 % between 60 and 90 mm CBT. This may be a reflection of the increase in detector dose for increased thickness on this system. These units have different aims in the design of their breast thickness compensation schemes. The Inspiration unit aims for (and achieves) constant pixel value across the breast thickness range, whilst the Dimensions unit attempts to maintain a constant CNR with breast thickness [9]. The Essential unit using the Profile AOP aims to flatten out the image quality response as a function of CBT, and in particular aims to reduce the fall-off in image quality for thicker breasts. The result shown in Fig. 3 indicates a slight reduction of 4 % in image quality metric between 60 and 90 mm CBT for this unit.

The analogue unit ratios are unity and +5 %, indicating a threshold contrast which is largely independent of breast thickness. It should also be noted that the LoRad MIV unit employed a cellular grid and that the effect of this may be that the increase in scatter to primary ratio with increased breast thickness may have a smaller effect than with a conventional linear anti-scatter grid and therefore may explain the relatively small dependence of the ratio as a function of thickness [10].

The inclusion of the dose calculations in the analysis gives an indication of the dose penalty associated with the improvement in image quality metric for thicker breasts compared with standard breasts. The Dimensions unit shows the greatest increase in image quality per unit dose increase (Table 2). Out of the units tested here, for thicker breasts, the Dimensions uses the hardest beam of 34 kV, W/Ag. This finding suggests that the use of harder beams such as this, for thicker breasts may be advised.

One matter to consider in comparing the results of the threshold contrast of the units is that the actual limiting thickness of a material detectable in the breast will depend not only on the threshold contrast but also on the composition of the material and the quality of the beam used to image. In the situation where a more penetrating beam quality is used for imaging (as in the case with the Dimensions unit) the resulting lower subject contrast means that superior threshold contrast detectability for thicker breasts may be warranted. This may in turn mean a slightly different dose effectiveness for the Dimensions than that reported in Table 2. The interplay between the radiation quantity and quality of the harder beam and its effect on absorbed dose (when compared with a softer beam) is pertinent here.

The simulations described in this paper obviously differ from clinical practice in a number of ways. Even though exposure parameters and doses were well matched between the simulations and clinical exposures, there are still potential drawbacks in using phantoms to simulate breast tissue. Firstly, breast tissue adds structure to the images which is absent when using uniform PMMA and it may be the case that the detectability task when translated to clinical images with structured backgrounds is less dependent on breast thickness than is reported here with homogeneous materials [11]. Secondly, in using PMMA and CDMAM to simulate the attenuation of breast tissues we fail to match the scattering volume of breast tissue; and this disparity in scattering volume is greater for the simulation of thicker breasts – about 25 % less scattering volume is present in the experimental set-up compared with breast tissue. However, with gridded imaging the difference in forward scatter passing through the grid in each case will be small, and especially so, given that the 0.5 mm layer of aluminium included in the CDMAM phantom will produce proportionally more forward scatter than breast tissue.

The main conclusion to be drawn from the results is the large variation in the imaging of thicker breasts compared with a standard thickness. In particular, the difference in measured image quality for 90 mm breasts compared with 60 mm breasts was found to vary greatly with unit type with both an increase and decrease observed from digital units in clinical use. The question is of course what is the optimal compensation scheme? Was the image quality for thicker breasts from the film/screen systems satisfactory for the clinical task, or should we be looking to alter the thickness compensation scheme now that digital technology gives the opportunity to do so? Thicker breasts receive the highest radiation dose and therefore it would seem prudent that any move away from the historical analogue situation is evidence based. It may be that a clinical study and simulations with an emphasis on thickness dependence are required to establish the optimal thickness compensation scheme.

References

1. van Engen, R., Bosmans, H., Dance D., Heid, P., Lazzari, B., Marshall, N., Schopphoven, S., Thijssen, M., Young, K.: Digital mammography update: European protocol for the quality control of the physical and technical aspects of mammography screening. In: European Guidelines for Quality Assurance in Breast Cancer Screening and Diagnosis, 4th edn. – Supplements. European Commission, Luxembourg (2013)
2. Beckett, J.R., Kotre, C.J.: Dosimetric implications of age related glandular changes in screening mammography. Phys. Med. Biol. **45**, 801–813 (2000)
3. CDCOM v1.6. National Expert and Training Centre for Breast Cancer Screening and the Radboud University Nijmegen Medical Centre
4. CDMAM Analysis package v1.5.5. National Co-ordinating Centre for the Physics of Mammography, Guildford, UK; including Matlab 2012a. The Mathworks Inc., Natick (2012)
5. Boone, J.M., Fewell, T.R., Jennings, R.J.: Molybdenum, rhodium and tungsten anode spectral models using interpolating polynomials with application to mammography. Med. Phys. **24**, 1863–1874 (1997)
6. Berger, M.J., Hubbell, J.H., Seltzer, S.M., Chang, J., Coursey, J.S., Sukumar, R., Zucker, D.S., Olsen, K.: XCOM: Photon Cross Section Database, version 1.3. National Institute of Standards and Technology, Gaithersburg (2010). http://www.nist.gov/pml/data/xcom
7. Dance, D.R., Skinner, C.L., Young, K.C., Beckett, J.R., Kotre, C.J.: Additional factors for the estimation of mean glandular dose using the UK mammography dosimetry protocol. Phys. Med. Biol. **45**, 3225–3240 (2000)
8. Dance, D.R., Young, K.C., van Engen, R.E.: Further factors for the estimation of mean glandular dose using the United Kingdom, European and IAEA breast dosimetry protocols. Phys. Med. Biol. **54**, 4361–4372 (2009)
9. Smith, A.: Email communication to DXIMGMEDPHYS Mailbase. Hologic Inc., Bedford, December 2015
10. Smith, A.: Fundamentals of Digital Mammography: Physics, Technology and Practical Considerations, R-BI-016. Hologic Inc., Bedford, March 2005
11. Salvagnini, E., Bosmans, H., Monnin, P., Struelens, L., Verdun, F., Marshall, N.: The use of detectability indices as a means of automatic exposure control for a digital mammography system. In: Proceedings of SPIE, vol. 7961 (2011)

Lower Recall Rates Reduced Readers' Sensitivity in Screening Mammography

Norhashimah Mohd Norsuddin[1,2(✉)], Claudia Mello-Thoms[1], Warren Reed[1],
Patrick C. Brennan[1], and Sarah Lewis[1]

[1] Medical Imaging Optimisation and Perception Group (MIOPeG),
Discipline of Medical Radiation Sciences, Faculty of Health Science, The University of Sydney,
Cumberland Campus, East Street, Lidcombe, NSW 2141, Australia
nmoh5894@uni.sydney.edu.au, {claudia.mello-thoms,
warren.reed,patrick.brennan,sarah.lewis}@sydney.edu.au
[2] Diagnostic Imaging and Radiotherapy Programme, Faculty of Health Sciences,
The National University of Malaysia (UKM), 50300 Kuala Lumpur, Malaysia

Abstract. Higher recall rates have been related to increased false positive decisions, causing significant psychological and economical costs for both screened women and the mammography screening service respectively. This study compares breast readers' performance in a laboratory setting under varying levels of recall rates. Four experienced radiologists volunteered to read a single test set of 200 mammographic cases over three separate conditions. The test set contained of 180 normal and 20 abnormal cases and the participants were asked to identify each case that required to be recalled in line with three different target recall rates: control (unspecified or free recall (first read)), 15 % (second read) and 10 % (third read). Readers were required to mark the location of any malignancies using custom made detection software. The recall rates for the control condition ranged between 18.5 % and 34 %. Statistically significant differences were observed in sensitivity for control (median = 0.85) vs 15 % (median = 0.65, $z = -2.381$, $P = 0.017$), 15 % vs 10 % (median = 0.55, $z = -2.428$, $P = 0.015$) and control vs 10 % ($z = -2.381$, $P = 0.017$). ROC AUC was significantly different for control (median = 0.84) vs 15 % (median = 0.79, $z = -2.381$, $P = 0.017$) and 15 % vs 10 % (median = 0.75, $z = -2.381$, $P = 0.017$). Specificity significantly improved at lower recall rate of 10 % (median = 0.95) vs 15 % (median = 0.92, $z = -2.428$, $P = 0.017$). Setting specific target recall rates for readers significantly limited their performance in correctly identifying cancers. In this study, decreasing the number of recalled cases down to 10 %, significantly reduced cancer detection, with a significant improvement in specificity ($P \leq 0.05$).

Keywords: Recall rate · Sensitivity · Specificity · Screening mammography · Breast cancer

1 Introduction

Mammography is an effective imaging tool for detecting breast cancer at an early stage, however a relatively large number of screened women undergo unnecessary imaging

© Springer International Publishing Switzerland 2016
A. Tingberg et al. (Eds.): IWDM 2016, LNCS 9699, pp. 116–121, 2016.
DOI: 10.1007/978-3-319-41546-8_15

and invasive tests due to false positive findings. Such error may hamper the success of breast screening programs and reduce public confidence in medical screening programs [1, 2]. Some attention has been paid to variation in reader performance, particularly around recall rates using international comparisons of women attending breast screening programs. Overall, a large range of recall rates exists in screening practices, with recall rates quoted in the literature from below 1.4 % in the Netherlands up to 15 % in the United States [3] for initial screening. This variation was determined to some extent by factors including the mammographic technologies available at the point of screening, such as screen-film mammography (SFM) and full field digital mammography (FFDM) [4, 5]. Additionally, a woman's presentation can influence recall rate comparisons, especially when considering age, screening history, use of hormone therapy, breast density, possible previous invasive procedures and familial breast cancer history [6–9].

Considering that false positive results positively correlate with recall rates [10], some organizations have recommended specific recall policies as guidelines to evaluate the performance of readers in the screening population in their respective nations or states. In Australia, the National Accreditation Standards (NAS) has recommended a target recall rate of 10 % for the first screening and 5 % for subsequent screening across the population-based screening program. However it is known that some readers operate at considerably higher rates [11]. The intention of introducing recommended recall target rates is to optimize the trade-off between sensitivity and recall rate. However, extensive research has shown varying results around the question of an optimum recall rate [12–14]: a retrospective study by Schell et al. (2007) suggested that the best trade-off with sensitivity was at a 10 % recall rate for the first screen [14]; earlier work by Yankaskas et al. (2001) suggested that the effect of an increased recall rate on false positives can only be seen at the lower, limited range of recall rates between 4.9 % and 5.5 % [12, 13]; a Dutch study reported higher recall rates of more than 4 % are associated with an increase in false-positive decisions without an increase in the cancer detection rate [13].

Currently, there is a lack of evidence supporting the real effect of changing target recall rates upon readers' performance, particularly in relation to cancer detection rates. Other factors include the difficulty of altering embedded decision making practices and the advent of digital technologies. The purpose of this study is to further explore the relationship between recall rates and breast readers' performance in screening mammography to potentially improve the efficacy of breast screening programs.

2   Methods

Four experienced breast imaging radiologists who regularly report on screening mammograms for BreastScreen New South Wales (BSNSW) participated in this study. The mean number of years of experience was 16 and the mean case load read per year was 11,900 screening mammograms. Institutional ethical approval for this study was granted, informed consent was obtained from all participants and permission to use the images of patient materials was waived.

Each reader was asked to read a set of 200 de-identified digital mammographic examinations that were obtained from the BSNSW digital imaging library. The test set included 180 normal cases and 20 abnormal cases, with each abnormal case containing a single biopsy-proved malignancy. Each case consisted of a four-view digital mammogram, a cranio-caudal view (CC) and medio-lateral oblique (MLO) of both breasts and no prior images were provided. Cases were chosen by the BSNSW State Radiologist to represent a range of case difficulty, from subtle to obvious cancer presentation and a variety of normal mammographic appearances. The "truth" locations of all malignant cases were identified by an expert breast reader, who also had access to the prior images with biopsy confirmed malignancy. This expert radiologist did not participate as an observer in this experiment. The reading sequence order of cases was randomized separately for each reading session.

Each reader reviewed all images in the test set three times, each time with a different target recall rate. At the first reading session, no numerical percentage recall rate was imposed and readers were allowed to do a "free recall" when interpreting the cases. In the second read, the number of mammographic cases that readers could recall was reduced to 30 cases or 15 % and to 20 cases (10 %) in the third reading. The reading sessions were separated by a minimum of 2 months to reduce any memory effect, with the study running a total of 6 months for the three reads.

During the reading sessions, the readers identified and localized each mammographic case that they considered required recall in line with their target recall rates for conditions 2 and 3 (see below) and they were not permitted to exceed their target recall rate. The coordinates marked on each image of a case considered to have a malignant lesion by the readers (and hence "recalled"), were recorded on custom detection software. No time limit was set for the reporting session. No information was provided on the prevalence of abnormal cases or the number of lesions within each case. All images in the test set were displayed on two EIZO Radioforce GS510 medical-grade monitors (Ishikawa, Japan) driven by SECTRA (Linkonping, Sweden) workstations. Ambient lighting in this study was maintained at 20 to 40 lx.

Sensitivity, specificity and receiver operating characteristic (ROC) area under the curve (AUC) were calculated as measures of observer performance. The outcomes from the lesion marking were identified either as positive or negative by comparing markings with the truth table. A true positive (TP) score was recorded when a recall rating was correctly given to the side of the breast containing cancer.

A Kruskal-Wallis test was performed to determine significant differences across the 3 reading sessions. Post-hoc Mann-Whitney U test was performed to identify significant differences between pairs of sessions. Bonferroni adjustment was applied to the alpha values by dividing the alpha level of 0.05 by number of comparison made. Results therefore with the revised alpha level, a $P < 0.017$ were deemed to represent significant differences.

3   Results

Table 1 shows readers' scores for sensitivity, specificity and ROC AUC for the control, 15 % and 10 % recall rates respectively. The Kruskal-Wallis test showed significant differences in sensitivity ($P = 0.006$), specificity ($P = 0.007$) and ROC AUC ($P = 0.007$) across the three reading sessions (Table 1). The post-hoc Mann-Whitney U test shows significant changes in sensitivity, for control (free recall) versus (vs) 15 % ($z = -2.381$, $P = 0.017$) 15 % vs 10 % ($z = -2.428$, $P = 0.015$), and control vs 10 % $z = -2.381$, $P = 0.017$) respectively. Specificity was significantly different for 15 % v 10 % ($z = -2.397$, $P = 0.017$) and the ROC AUC was significantly different for control vs 15 % ($z = -2.381$, $P = 0.017$) and 15 % vs 10 % ($z = -2.381$, $P = 0.017$) (Table 2).

Table 1 Reader sensitivity, specificity, ROC AUC and median values at free call, 15% and 10% conditions

Reader	Sensitivity			Specificity			ROC AUC		
	Control (Free recall)	15%	10%	Control (Free recall)	15%	10%	Control (Free recall)	15%	10%
1	0.80	0.65	0.55	0.83	0.91	0.95	0.84	0.79	0.76
2	0.90	0.65	0.45	0.79	0.91	0.93	0.86	0.79	0.70
3	0.90	0.65	0.55	0.72	0.92	0.95	0.84	0.79	0.75
4	0.75	0.70	0.55	0.88	0.92	0.95	0.83	0.82	0.75
Median	0.85	0.65	0.55	0.81	0.92	0.95	0.84	0.79	0.75

Table 2 Kruskal-Wallis analysis and post hoc Mann-Whitney U test of sensitivity, specificity and ROC AUC

	Kruskal-Wallis Test	Post-hoc test (Mann-Whitney U test)		
		Control VS 15%	15% VS 10%	Control VS 10%
	P value ($P \leq 0.05$)	P value ($P \leq 0.017$)		
Sensitivity	**0.006**	**0.017**	**0.015**	**0.017**
Specificity	**0.007**	0.019	**0.017**	0.018
ROC AUC	**0.007**	**0.017**	**0.017**	0.019

4   Discussion

The results from this study demonstrate that readers operating in a free recall condition (mean recall rate of 25.6 %) detected more cancers when compared to a reduced specified recall rate (mean ROC of 0.84 and 0.75 respectively, $P = 0.006$). The largest reduction occurred when readers were tasked with reducing their recalled cases from free recall to 15 %. The sensitivity change observed in our study is in agreement with those reported by Gur et al. and Schell et al., suggesting that recalling more cases may result in a higher cancer detection rate [10, 14]. Our data does not concur with the Otten et al. study [13], as we did not observe a leveling off of cancer detection at the highest recall rate (free recall), however due to the enriched data set of 20 abnormal cases, we were unable to test the effect of reducing the recall rate further to 5 %, as studied by Yankaskas et al. and Otten et al. [12, 13].

Reading at a specific target recall rate also had a significant positive effect on specificity when considered across all 3 conditions ($P = 0.007$) and this change was most evident between the 15 % to 10 % recall conditions. The decreased specificity observed here concurs with previous findings by Otten et al. and Elmore et al., where higher recall rates correlate with an increase in false positive findings [13, 15]. To adhere to the specific reduced recall rate, the readers may have adopted a stricter reporting criterion compared to reading at the free recall condition and in turn increased their specificity, although there was also a significant decrease in sensitivity. Although our final specified target recall rate is similar to Australian clinical practice, such enforcement of a recall rate is not normally applied so rigorously. We speculate that the routine practice of double-reading in the Australian health care setting may have influenced decision making, as readers may be relying on their "double reading" partner to balance their recall rate.

In this study, the readers were not given access to any prior images nor were they provided with any clinical information, and there is some evidence to show the inclusion of prior images positively affects readers' performance [16, 17]. This experiment simulated recall conditions aligned to a first screen and therefore it is not unrealistic for readers to have limited clinical or past information about the cases. Equally, although the test set was enriched, this was necessary to gather meaningful observer performance within a laboratory setting. A study with a diversity of readers' number of years of practice and case load would allow for clarification of the importance of experience.

In conclusion, our data suggests that specific target recall rates reduce readers' performance in correctly identifying cancers at lower recall rates. Future research with this test set will include identifying the type of lesions/cancer characteristics that are most likely to be assigned a false negative finding as readers' target recall rates are reduced. Changes in established recall rates may have unintended consequences upon radiologists working in Australia who are accustomed to process of double. Anecdotally our participants stated they found it very difficult to alter their pre-set ideals of a target recall rate. Our work here has challenged the notion that lowering recall rates promotes increased accuracy within an Australian clinical setting.

References

1. Hofvind, S., et al.: False-positive results in mammographic screening for breast cancer in Europe: a literature review and survey of service screening programmes. J. Med. Screen. **19**(suppl 1), 57–66 (2012)
2. Brewer, N.T., Salz, T., Lillie, S.E.: Systematic review: the long-term effects of false-positive mammograms. Ann. Intern. Med. **146**(7), 502–510 (2007)
3. Yankaskas, B.C., et al.: International comparison of performance measures for screening mammography: can it be done? J. Med. Screen. **11**(4), 187–193 (2004)

4. Berns, E.A., Hendrick, R.E., Cutter, G.R.: Performance comparison of full-field digital mammography to screen-film mammography in clinical practice. Med. Phys. **29**(5), 830–834 (2002)
5. Lewin, J., et al.: Comparison of full-field digital mammography with screen-film mammography for cancer detection: results of 4,945 paired examinations. Radiology **218**(3), 873–880 (2001)
6. Castells, X., Molins, E., Macia, F.: Cumulative false positive recall rate and association with participant related factors in a population based breast cancer screening programme. J. Epidemiol. Community Health **60**(4), 316–321 (2006)
7. Carney, P.A., et al.: Individual and combined effects of age, breast density, and hormone replacement therapy use on the accuracy of screening mammography. Ann. Intern. Med. **138**(3), 168–175 (2003)
8. Lehman, C.D., et al.: Effect of age and breast density on screening mammograms with false-positive findings. Am. J. Roentgenol. **173**(6), 1651–1655 (1999)
9. Boyd, N.F., et al.: Mammographic density and the risk and detection of breast cancer. New Engl. J. Med. **356**(3), 227–236 (2007)
10. Gur, D., et al.: Recall and detection rates in screening mammography. Cancer **100**(8), 1590–1594 (2004)
11. BreastScreen Australia. National Accreditation Standards: BreastScreen Australia Quality (2008). http://www.cancerscreening.gov.au/internet/screening/publishing.nsf/Content/A03653118215815BCA257B41000409E9/$File/standards.pdf. Accessed 21 May 2014
12. Yankaskas, B.C., et al.: Association of recall rates with sensitivity and positive predictive values of screening mammography. Am. J. Roentgenol. **177**(3), 543–549 (2001)
13. Otten, J.D.M., et al.: Effect of recall rate on earlier screen detection of breast cancers based on the dutch performance indicators. J. Nat. Cancer Inst. **97**(10), 748–754 (2005)
14. Schell, M.J., et al.: Evidence-based target recall rates for screening mammography. Radiology **243**(3), 681–689 (2007)
15. Elmore, J.G., et al.: International variation in screening mammography interpretations in community-based programs. J. Nat. Cancer Inst. **95**(18), 1384–1393 (2003)
16. Soh, B.P., et al.: Mammography test sets: reading location and prior images do not affect group performance. Clin. Radiol. **69**(4), 397–402 (2014)
17. Soh, B.P., et al.: Screening mammography: test set data can reasonably describe actual clinical reporting. Radiology **268**(1), 46–53 (2013)

Simulation of Positron Emission Mammography Imaging with Pixelated CdTe.

Machiel Kolstein[✉] and Mokhtar Chmeissani

Institut de Física D'Altes Energies (IFAE),
The Barcelona Institute of Science and Technology,
Campus UAB, Bellaterra, 08193 Barcelona, Spain
mkolstein@ifae.es

Abstract. The Voxel Imaging PET (VIP) Pathfinder project presents a new approach for the design of nuclear medicine imaging diagnostic devices by using highly segmented pixel CdTe sensors. State-of-the-art PET devices are made from scintillator crystals which have an energy resolution of about 10 %. Because of their limited energy resolution, the scatter fraction is relatively large. Their limited spatial resolution will introduce a parallax error and deficiency in the depth of interaction (DOI) determination (> 5 mm FWHM) and therefore a wrong line of response (LOR). In this study, we present a design for a breast dedicated PET based on CdTe detectors which have an energy resolution of about 1 % and can be easily segmented into small voxels for optimal spatial resolution to provide a solution for these setbacks. This simulation study will assess the advantages of this design for breast imaging purposes.

1 Introduction

Current state-of-the art full body PET scanners have limited spatial resolution and, hence, their performance is limited when it comes to imaging cancerous tissue in the breast. To overcome this, dedicated PET scanners for breast imaging are developed. In this article, the nomenclature from [1] is used where Positron Emission Mammograph (PEM) systems refer to systems with two flat detectors on opposite sides of the breast and dedicated breast PET (DbPET) systems refer to a small ring of detectors within which the breast hangs pendant. Due to their restricted field of view (FOV), PEM and DbPET systems achieve higher cancer detection performance in terms of specificity than whole-body PET scanners. Additional benefits include lower cost and enhanced device portability.

Breast imaging devices currently in the market are based on arrays of scintillating crystal detectors. Such devices can provide an axial spatial resolution down to 2 mm FWHM [2] and high contrast images with 4 mm and 6 mm minimum detectable lesion size for 10:1 and 4:1 tumor to normal tissue ratio (TNR) respectively [3]. The typical thickness of a scintillator is 20 mm, which is a trade-off between good detection efficiency for 511 keV photons and maintaining good energy resolution. However, this causes a limitation to the precision of the depth

© Springer International Publishing Switzerland 2016
A. Tingberg et al. (Eds.): IWDM 2016, LNCS 9699, pp. 122–129, 2016.
DOI: 10.1007/978-3-319-41546-8_16

of interaction (DOI) estimation inside the scintillator ($> 5\,$mm FWHM [4]) which gives rise to the parallax error, introducing a lack of precision to the line of response (LOR) estimation. Moreover, scintillators have poor energy resolution (about 10 %), causing a large contamination of scatter events in the coincidence event sample. The two effects contribute to reduce the image quality and put a constraint on the minimum detectable tumor size and the correct assessment of the malignancy of small lesions. This article will evaluate a DbPET design with the aim to counteract the aforementioned limitations of state-of-the-art breast imaging devices.

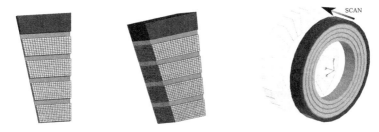

Fig. 1. From left to right: the basic VIP unit module, a ring section of 19 unit modules stacked together, and the complete DbPET scanner ring containing 28 sections, with an axial size of 40 mm, which can be moved axially to scan a longer range.

2   A Dedicated Breast PET Scanner with Pixelated CdTe

With the VIP design [5], one can achieve better image quality by using finely segmented CdTe which allows for a precise measurement of the gamma impact point and rejection of most of the scatter events because of the excellent energy resolution of about 1 % at 511 keV [6]. Figure 1 shows how the DbPET scanner is built up from the basic VIP unit module building block, consisting of 4 CdTe pixelated detectors, of 200 voxels each. Each voxel has a size of $1 \times 1 \times 2\,$mm^3 and is connected to its own independent readout channel for the energy, position, and arrival time of the incoming gamma. By traversing the VIP unit module, the incident radiation is facing 4 cm depth of interaction in CdTe to assure high detection efficiency. The unit module can be easily stacked to form large scale PET [5], PEM [7] or Compton camera [8] applications. For the DbPET device presented here, stacks of 19 basic unit modules are used. Because of the trapezoidal shape of the basic unit modules, a *gapless* ring can be made, consisting of 28 sections, where each section is a stack of 19 unit modules. The ring has an inner radius of 89 mm, an axial length of 40 mm and, in total, has 425600 data channels. The outer edges of the ring are shielded with a 10 mm thick tungsten layer. For our simulation studies, the 40 mm long ring is moved in small steps of 0.5 mm for a complete scan along the z-axis of the object under study. The design is made such that the patient will be in prone position with the breast hanging into the scanner FOV.

3 Method

For the simulation of particle generation and tracking, the Geant4-based Architecture for Medicine-Oriented Simulations (GAMOS) software [9] was used.

Electronics. The GAMOS output data are processed to account for electronics effects. Each voxel is treated as an independent detector measuring the deposited energy, position, and trigger time of any energy deposition above the trigger threshold. Energy depositions within the same voxel and during the same measuring time interval after the trigger are summed together. Energy depositions happening after the measuring interval and during the subsequential dead time are ignored.[1] During the data taking, hits are recorded in list-mode and sorted by their time stamps.

Coincidence Selection. The coincidence finding algorithm looks for hits that occur within the same time coincidence window. For 511 keV gammas it is possible to undergo a number of Compton scatterings in the scanner before their entire energy has been deposited. Therefore, hits that lie within a certain *Compton merging distance* are merged together, following the example of [5]. Additionally, when the sum of the enery deposits of two hits is 511 keV ± 8 keV, they are merged. After these steps, only events with two remaining hits are accepted, each with energy deposits of 511 keV ± 8 keV, within a coincidence time window of 20 ns. A measurement of the coincidence time resolution [10] has shown that for energies close to the trigger threshold of 20 keV, a coincidence window of 20 ns is necessary to detect at least 70 % of the photon pairs. LORs that lie outside the phantom radius are rejected. Table 1 shows a summary of all parameters.

Table 1. Electronics simulation and coincidence finding parameters used to simulate the VIP DbPET

Energy resolution	1.57 % FWHM @ 511 keV [6]
Trigger threshold	20 keV
Voxel measuring time	20 μs
Voxel dead time	130 μs
Coincidence time window	20 ns
Energy window	511 ± 8 keV
Compton merging distance (*see explanation in the text*)	10 mm

Image Reconstruction. For the image reconstruction, we used the List-Mode Ordered Subset Expectation Maximization (LM-OSEM) algorithm, as implemented by the VIP project [11], where attenuation correction is only applied in the case of the breast phantom.

---

[1] Note that this only affects the triggering pixel. All other pixels in the detector are still ready to measure new events.

4   Results

For all results, the 40 mm wide DbPET ring is moved in steps of 0.5 mm for a distance along the z-axis equal to the length of the object under study.

4.1   Sensitivity

To estimate the sensitivity of the VIP DbPET system, the NEMA NU 4-2008 protocol [12] for small animal PET is used, where the total sensitivity of the system is estimated by averaging over different axial positions of a ^{22}Na point source (a sphere with radius 0.15 mm) inside a 10^3 mm^3 acrylic cube. The protocol prescribes the use of ^{22}Na because of its long half-life, hence securing a constant value for the source activity. The additional 1274.5 keV gamma, emitted by ^{22}Na, can be neglected. The sensitivity for each slice i (i.e. axial source position z_i) is given by $S_i = \frac{R_i - B_i}{\text{Activity}}$, with R_i the counting rate and B_i the background rate set to 0 for simulation data. The total sensitivity is given by $S_{tot} = \frac{1}{N}\Sigma_i S_i$. The total absolute sensitivity is given by $S_{A,\text{tot}} = \frac{S_{tot}}{0.906}$, with 0.906 the branching ratio of β^+ emission of ^{22}Na [12]. Figure 2 shows the sensitivity for the ^{22}Na point source along 160 mm of the z-axis. The total absolute sensitivity of 3.6 cps/kBq is better than results for dual head PEM devices published previously by the VIP project [7] and by other groups [2].

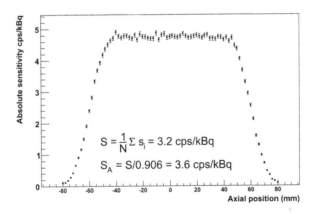

Fig. 2. Sensitivity for a single ^{22}Na point-like source along the z axis

4.2   Scatter and Random Fraction

To estimate the scatter fraction (SF) and the amount of random coincidence events as a function of source activity, we follow the NEMA NU 4-2008 guidelines [12] for small animal PET which specifies three different phantoms, corresponding to the size of a mouse, a rat or a monkey.[2] We used the monkey-like

---

[2] Note that the NEMA NU 4-2008 standard to measure the SF is different from the previously described standard to measure sensitivity.

phantom because it is closest in volume to the breast. The phantom consists of a line source of length 390 mm and 3.2 mm diameter filled with ^{18}F, placed at a radial distance of 30 mm from the center of a polyethylene tube of 100 mm diameter and 400 mm length. Figure 3 shows that the SF is negligible for all activities. The random coincidence rate is negligible until 10^6 Bq and gets dominant for activities higher than 10^8 Bq.

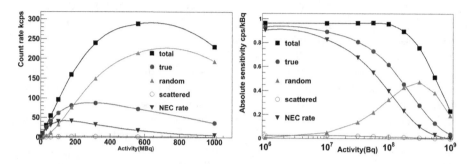

Fig. 3. Left: counting rates versus activity for the VIP DbPET with the monkey phantom. Right: the absolute efficiency versus activity

4.3   Derenzo Phantom

Figure 4 shows the results on a Derenzo phantom. Clearly, rods with diameter 1 mm and 2 mm center-to-center separation can be distinguished.

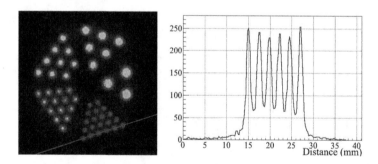

Fig. 4. Results with a Derenzo phantom. Shown are the transversal view along the XY plane and the line-profile through the 6 outer rods of smallest diameter (1 mm). A median linear filter is applied.

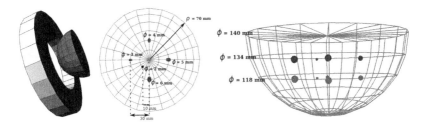

Fig. 5. Depiction of the simulated breast phantom. From left to right: A 3D view of the phantom and the DbPET ring, phantom front view and side view

4.4 Breast Phantom

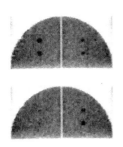

Fig. 6. Side view for the spheres of diameters 4 mm and 6 mm (*top*) and 3 mm and 5 mm (*bottom*).

Following the example of [13], we have simulated a breast phantom, as shown in Fig. 5. The phantom consists of a hemisphere filled with water. Spheres with diameters of 2, 3, 4, 5 and 6 mm are placed inside the phantom with a TNR of 4:1. For the image reconstruction with LM-OSEM, we used a basic attenuation correction procedure, where all pixels inside the phantom are assigned an attenuation correction factor of $0.0096\,\mathrm{mm}^{-1}$, and the weights of the LORs are normalized in proportion to how much of their length is traversing the phantom [14]. The results are shown in Figs. 6 and 7. For the line-profiles through the spheres with 3 mm and 5 mm diameters and with 4 mm and 6 mm diameters, the artificial high contents of the center bin is set to 0, to visualize the signal peaks more clearly. The spheres with diameters 3, 4, 5, and 6 mm can be clearly seen. The sphere with diameter 2 mm can be discerned even when it is on the level of the statistical fluctuations.

5 Conclusions

This article presents results of a simulation study of a dedicated breast PET (DbPET) design, using finely segmented CdTe as basic detector modules. The DbPET ring for breast imaging, as presented in this simulation study, showed an absolute sensitivity of 3.6 cps/kBq with the NEMA NU 4-2008 sensitivity test. The NEMA NU 4-2008 SF test shows that the DbPET device has negligible SF for all activities because of the excellent energy resolution of CdTe. The device has a negligible random fraction up to activities of 10^6 Bq. With a Derenzo phantom, rods with diameter 1 mm and center-to-center spacing 2 mm can be discerned in our simulations. With a breast shaped phantom filled with water and a TNR of 4:1, spheres with diameters down to 3 mm can be discerned.

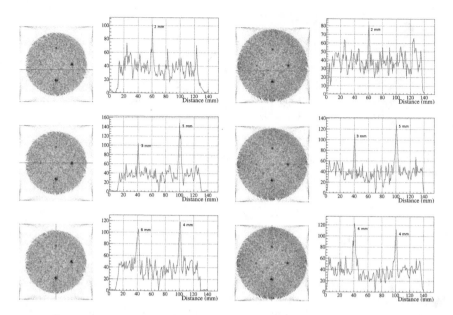

Fig. 7. Results with the breast phantom. *Top row:* the spheres with 2mm diameter. *Middle row:* the spheres with 3mm and 5mm diameters. *Bottom row:* the spheres with 4mm and 6mm diameters. *From left to right:* XY view at breast diameter 118mm and corresponding line profile, XY view at breast diameter 134mm and corresponding line profile.

Our conclusion is that the VIP design for a DbPET, as simulated in the study presented here, offers detection capabilities of small lesions that with current state of the art PEM are still not possible.

Acknowledgements. This work has received funding from the European Research Council under the European Union's Seventh Framework Programme (ERC Grant Agreement 250207, "VIP"). We also acknowledge the support from the Spanish MINECO under the Severo Ochoa excellence program (grant SO-2012-0234).

References

1. Hruska, C.B., O'Connor, M.K.: Nuclear imaging of the breast: translating achievements in instrumentation into clinical use. Med Phys. **40**(5), 050901 (2013)
2. Luo, W., et al.: Performance evaluation of a PEM scanner using the NEMA NU 4-2008 small animal PET standards. IEEE Trans. Nucl. Sci. **57**, 94–103 (2010)
3. MacDonald, L., et al.: Clinical imaging characteristics of the positron emission mammography camera: PEM Flex Solo II. J. Nucl. Med. **50**, 1666–1675 (2009)
4. Lerche, C.W., et al.: Dependency of energy-, position- and depth of interaction resolution on scintillation crystal coating and geometry. IEEE Trans. Nucl. Sci. **55**, 1344–1351 (2008)

5. Mikhaylova, E., et al.: Simulation of the expected performance of a seamless scanner for brain PET based on highly pixelated CdTe Detectors. IEEE Trans. Med. Imaging **33**, 332–339 (2014)
6. Ariño, G., et al.: Characterization of CdTe detector for use in PET. In: IEEE Conference Record on NSS & MIC, pp. 4598–4603 (2011)
7. De Lorenzo, G., et al.: Pixelated CdTe detectors to overcome intrinsic limitations of crystal based positron emission mammographs. J. Instrum. **8**, C01030 (2013)
8. Calderón, Y.: Design, Development, and Modeling of a Compton Camera Tomographer Based on Room Temperature Solid State Pixel Detector. Ph.D. Thesis, Universitat Autònoma de Barcelona (UAB) (2014)
9. Arce, P., et al.: Gamos: a framework to do Geant4 simulations in different physics fields with an user-friendly interface. Nucl. Instr. Meth. Phys. Res. A **735**, 304–313 (2014)
10. Ariño, G., et al.: Energy and coincidence time resolution measurements of CdTe detectors for PET. J. Instrum. **8**, C02015 (2013)
11. Kolstein, M., et al.: Evaluation of list-mode ordered subset expectation maximization image reconstruction for pixelated solid-state compton gamma camera with large number of channels. J. Instrum. **9**, C04034 (2014)
12. NEMA standards publication NU 4–2008: Performance measurements for small animal positron emission tomographs. National Electrical Manufacturers Association, Rosslyn, VA (2008)
13. Furuta, M., et al.: Basic evaluation of a C-shaped breast PET scanner. In: IEEE NSS & MIC Conference Record, pp. 2548–2552. IEEE (2009)
14. Ferreira, C.S., et al.: Scatter and attenuation corrections for a PEM detector using list-mode OSEM. In: IEEE Conference Record on NSS & MIC, pp. 1–4 (2013)

The International Use of PERFORMS
Mammographic Test Sets

Yan Chen[✉], Leng Dong, Hossein Nevisi, and Alastair Gale

Applied Vision Research Centre, Loughborough University, Loughborough, UK
y.chen@lboro.ac.uk

Abstract. To examine the utility of employing breast screening test sets internationally the data of 1,009 radiologists from the USA, UK and other European countries were examined as they inspected 20 carefully selected difficult recent screening cases. Some 720 UK radiologists, 247 American and 42 European radiologists took part. Whilst similar sensitivity scores between the three groups were found, the main difference was the lower specificity of the American radiologists reflecting their different recall clinical practice. It is argued that using test sets internationally provides participants with useful comparative performance information whilst also providing data on how the same cases are interpreted by radiologists from different countries.

Keywords: PERFORMS · Self-assessment · Performance

1 Introduction

There is international interest in using test sets to examine the performance of individual radiologists, and other screeners, from different countries when they examine and report the same set of cases. Such comparative examination can highlight particular training needs of groups or of indivdiual radiologists. Ideally any woman attending for screening, usually by full field digital mammography (FFDM), in any country should expect that their mammograms will be reported in a similar fashion so that any potential early signs of cancer are identified at the earliest treatable stage.

The use of such test sets has been nationally used in the UK for over 25 years. Here we report an initial investigation of how radiologists from different countries perform when they use such test sets.

In the UK all women aged 47–74 are invited for breast screening every three years. In England alone in 2014 some 2.2 million women were screened and 17,961 cancers detected [1]. Despite such figures, the actual daily presentation of a cancer case for an individual radiologist is actually quite rare and this very rarity, coupled with complexities of abnormality appearances can, and does, give rise to potential errors. To aid in screening error minimisation every individual who reads and reports screening mammograms in the UK must read at least 5,000 cases a year [2] which helps development of appropriate perceptual and cognitive skills concerning possible normal and abnormal appearances. They also have to take part in the PERFORMS scheme [3–5].

PERFORMS is the leading international breast screening self-assessment scheme and has been used nationally in the UK for over 27 years. It was established with the

© Springer International Publishing Switzerland 2016
A. Tingberg et al. (Eds.): IWDM 2016, LNCS 9699, pp. 130–135, 2016.
DOI: 10.1007/978-3-319-41546-8_17

NHS Breast Screening Programme and the Royal College of Radiologists. Each year every breast screening radiologist and advanced practitioner (trained technologist who also reads screening cases) reads two sets of carefully selected challenging de-identified FFDM cases. Difficult cases are selected for the PERFORMS scheme by an expert panel of breast radiologists and an overall panel decision about every case has been determined as well as known clinical and pathological outcome of the case.

Participants take part by downloading case sets to their PACS (Picture Archiving and Communication Systems) systems and report on these cases on their clinical workstations in breast screening centres whilst reporting on the cases using the PER-FORMS App which runs on any computing platform. For each case they identify key mammographic features and locate these on a graphic image of the case being examined and also rate various decisions about the features and the case. Finally, they also use a five point BIRADS-like scale to rate their overall decision about each breast.

Participants receive immediate feedback indicating how they have performed in terms of measures such as cancer detection, sensitivity, specificity and ROC measures. Subsequently individuals receive very detailed personal and confidential web based reports of how they have performed as compared anonymously to their peers. Currently over 850 breast screeners take part each year.

2   Methods

In order to determine how radiologists from different countries respond to the same set of challenging test cases the data of groups of radiologists were examined from three scenarios. First, a set of 20 FFDM cases were selected from the PERFORMS case database. These comprised difficult normal, benign and malignant examples and were drawn from recent screening cases from across the UK.

A PERFORMS mini-lab was run at a Breast Symposium in Orlando, in 2015, where 20 mammography workstations were provided for participants in a room with controlled light levels. Over the course of four days some 267 participants took part in this mini-lab, with 247 of them completing the whole test set, each reading the 20 cases within the allocated time slots.

In order to mimic the American screening situation, instead of using the UK five point decision rating scale per mammogram, the American three point screening BIRADS reporting scale was used [6]. To ensure the scale was employed appropriately, two American expert breast radiologists had previously first agreed the scale criteria and had also read the 20 cases and reported them using this reporting scale, thereby providing a standard radiological classification.

Later, in 2015, a similar mini-lab was run at a European breast screening confer-ence in London where four workstations were acquired and 42 European participants read the same 20 test cases over the course of the two day conference. Again the BIRADS scale was used. As before, the study took place in a room with appropriate controlled light levels.

For comparison purposes data from the UK PERFORMS scheme were extracted for these 20 cases. This gave 720 UK participants who had reported these cases. Additional data, including the number of years experience in breast screening and how many screening cases a year participants read were collected. This information will be reported elsewhere. Data from the three groups, American conference (US), European conference (EU) and the UK, were then examined for similarities and differences.

3 Results

Various data analyses were performed. Firstly, we examined the correct recall of abnormal cases (sensitivity) by the three groups of participants (Fig. 1) and the correct return to screen (specificity) decisions (Fig. 2) of the three groups. In terms of specificity the UK mean value was 78.94 %, US 66.78 % and EU 80.24 %. In terms of sensitivity the UK mean values was 83.46 %, US 82.18 % and EU 74.05 %.

One–way ANOVA showed that there was no significant difference in sensitivity among the three groups ($p = n.s.$). However, there was a significant difference in specificity among those groups. Post hoc showed that there was a significant difference between UK and US ($p < 0.001$) and a significant difference between UK and EU ($p < 0.05$). There was no significant difference between the US and EU groups ($p = n.s.$).

In addition, the percentage correct hits of the correct abnormality location (Fig. 3) was compared among the three groups. The area of interest was defined for each case which contained a key mammographic feature as the area around that feature using previously described criteria [7]: the UK mean value was 73.39 %, US 68.65 % and EU 66.77 %. ANOVA showed no significant difference among the three groups ($p = n.s.$).

The UK data here are based on a large group of individuals, many of whom have used the current version of our reporting APP several times before. This could potentialy give them an unfair advantage in this comparison. Therefore the UK data were re-examined but only concentrating on those individuals for whom examining these 20 cases was the first time they had taken part in the PERFORMS scheme. This is reported elsewhere.

4 Discussion

Firstly, the data show that is is perfectly feasible for radiologists from different nationalities to read and report the same test cases. The PERFORMS scheme offers this facility by making the clinical cases readily accessible to registered users who download the cases and then report on these using the PERFORMS on-line App. This App is available in multiple languages and has been designed to be transparent in use, requiring the minimum of user familiarisation using initial practice test cases before using the App to read any actual test cases.

When the same test cases are examined by radiologists from different countries then they achieve broadly similar sensitivity scores. This is reassuring and reinforces the globality of radiological education. The main difference between the three groups was found for the US specificity scores which we suggest reflects the different clinical management of potential assessment cases as compared to European countries.

It is proposed that this work demonstrates that the PERFORMS case sets and reporting App can be used successfully internationally to highlight group or individual performance

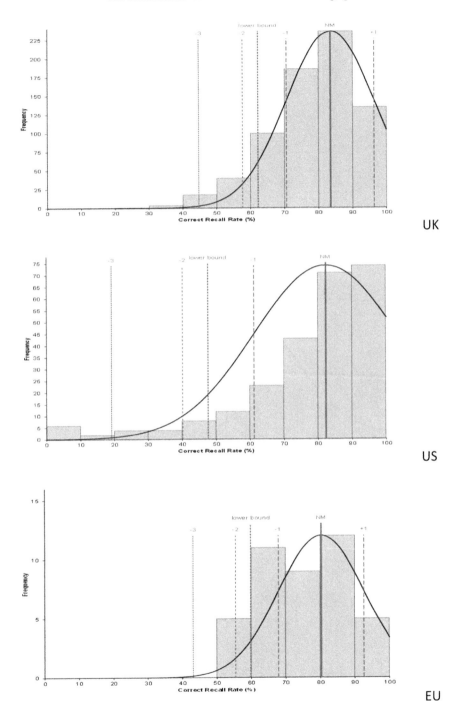

Fig. 1. Sensitivity of the three groups: UK, US, EU

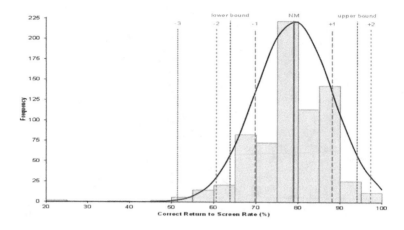

UK

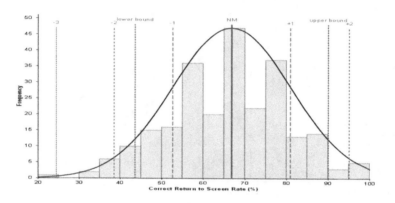

US

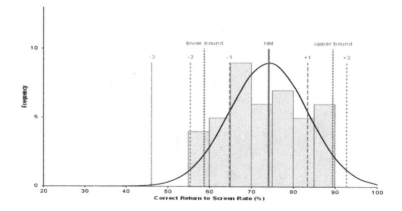

EU

Fig. 2. Specificity of the three groups: UK, US, EU

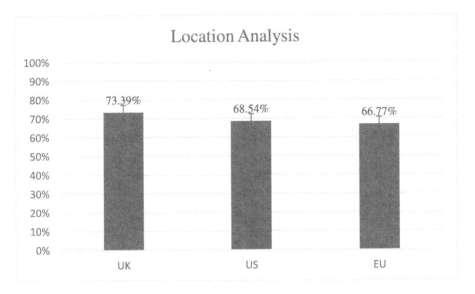

Fig. 3. Percentage of correct hits of Area of Interest (AOI)

difficulties and identify training needs for participants. This then can enhance their performance and help them target shortcomings as identified by the test sets.

Acknowledgements. We acknowledge the support of the NHSBSP and Public Health England.

References

1. Wilson, R.: Breast Screening Programme, England Statistics for 2013–14. Health and social care information centre, UK (2015)
2. Wilson, R., Liston, J.: Quality Assurance Guidelines for Breast Cancer Screening Radiology, vol. 59. NHSBSP publication, Sheffield (2011)
3. Gale, A.G.: PERFORMS – a self-assessment scheme for radiologists in breast screening. Semin. Breast Disease: Improv. Monit. Mammographic Interpretative skills **6**(3), 148–152 (2003)
4. Gale, A.G.: Maintaining quality in the UK breast screening program. In: Manning, D.J., Abbey, C. (eds.) Proceedings of SPIE Medical Imaging 2010: Image Perception, Observer Performance, and Technology Assessment, vol. 7627, pp. 1–11 (2010)
5. Gale, A.G., Scott, H.: Measuring radiology performance in breast screening. In: Michell, M. (ed.) Contemporary Issues in Cancer Imaging – Breast Cancer. Cambridge UP, Cambridge (2010)
6. D'Orsi, C.J., Sickles, E.A., Mendelson, E.B., Morris, E.A., et al.: ACR BI-RADS® Atlas, Breast Imaging Reporting and Data System. American College of Radiology, Reston (2013)
7. Dong, L., Chen, Y., Gale, A.G.: Breast screening: understanding case difficulty and the nature of errors. In: Abbey, C.K., Mello-Thoms, C.R. (eds.) Proceedings of SPIE Medical Imaging 2013: Image Perception, Observer Performance, and Technology Assessment (2013)

Dependence of Contrast-Enhanced Lesion Detection in Contrast-Enhanced Digital Breast Tomosynthesis on Imaging Chain Design

David A. Scaduto[1(✉)], Yue-Houng Hu[2], Yihuan Lu[3], Hailiang Huang[1], Jingxuan Liu[4], Kim Rinaldi[1], Gene Gindi[1], Paul R. Fisher[1], and Wei Zhao[1]

[1] Department of Radiology, Stony Brook Medicine, Stony Brook, NY 11794, USA
david.scaduto@stonybrookmedicine.edu
[2] Division of Medical Physics and Biophysics, Department of Radiation Oncology,
Dana-Farber Cancer Institute and Harvard Medical School, Boston, MA 02115, USA
[3] Departments of Radiology and Biomedical Engineering, Yale University, New Haven,
CT 06520, USA
[4] Department of Pathology, Stony Brook Medicine, Stony Brook, NY 11794, USA

Abstract. Contrast-enhanced digital breast tomosynthesis (CEDBT) may improve contrast-enhanced lesion conspicuity and relative contrast quantification by improving three-dimensional visualization of lesion morphology, and reducing the integration of attenuation information along the axial direction. Improved visualization of patterns of contrast-enhancement and improved iodine quantification may help differentiate between malignant and benign enhancing lesions. The dependence of dual-energy contrast-enhanced lesion detectability on imaging chain design is investigated. Lesion detectability and relative iodine quantification is comparable for subtraction in either reconstruction or projection domains for both phantom and patient images. SART generally produces greater SDNR than FBP, and scatter correcting projections further improves SDNR.

Keywords: Contrast-enhanced digital mammography · Contrast-enhanced digital breast tomosynthesis · Digital breast tomosynthesis · X-ray imaging · SDNR

1 Introduction

Contrast-enhanced digital mammography (CEDM) has been investigated recently to improve the conspicuity of mammographically occult breast pathologies. Similarly, contrast-enhanced digital breast tomosynthesis (CEDBT) has been proposed to improve breast cancer diagnosis by providing three-dimensional (3D) morphological information in addition to 3D physiological information through contrast-enhancement. A recent clinical study [1] showed superiority of CEDM, CEDBT and dynamic contrast-enhanced magnetic resonance imaging (DCE-MRI) over non-enhanced full-field digital mammography (FFDM) and non-enhanced DBT; however, none of the contrast-enhanced modalities was demonstrated to be superior to the others as assessed by the area under the receiver operating characteristic (ROC) curves.

© Springer International Publishing Switzerland 2016
A. Tingberg et al. (Eds.): IWDM 2016, LNCS 9699, pp. 136–144, 2016.
DOI: 10.1007/978-3-319-41546-8_18

While this result may suggest the addition of CEDBT to CEDM is unnecessary, this study did not report the specificity or false positive rate of any modality. Although numerous previous studies have reported sensitivities for CEDM ranging from 92 % −100 %, specificities are lower and more varied, ranging from 41 %−87 %, due to enhancement of benign pathologies [2–5].

The specificity of DCE-MRI similarly varies, however may be improved by the inclusion of additional factors to differentiate true and false positives. Differentiation of false positives from true positives in DCE-MRI is afforded by several characteristics; namely (1) accurate assessment of tumor margins, (2) observation of punctate or stippled enhancement of non-mass lesions, and (3) observation of contrast-kinetic curves [6].

Whereas planar mammography collapses all attenuation information to a single plane, DBT reduces this integrating effect by reconstructing projection images into a series of image slices, typically 1 mm thick, arranged parallel to the detector plane. This effectively reduces superposition of tissue structures, and provides improved localization of pathologies in 3D space. These results may provide CEDBT a technical advantage over CEDM in measuring all three benign/malignant differentiating characteristics.

First, the addition of 3D morphological information and reduction of superimposed structural noise provided by DBT has been shown to significantly improve tumor sizing and margin assessment. [7] Secondly, punctate or stippled enhancement patterns, generally indicative of benign fibrocystic changes, are characterized by multiple enhancing punctate foci 1−2 mm in diameter. [8] CEDBT may improve differentiation of these smaller individual foci from diffuse background parenchymal enhancement (BPE) by the addition of 3D information. Finally, while CEDM has been unable to reliably demonstrate contrast kinetic curves, initial results in CEDBT have shown promise. [9] By reducing the integration of signal from iodinated lesions along the axial direction, CEDBT may improve accurate quantification of iodinated lesions, and thus may improve observation of contrast kinetic information.

While the performance of DBT in identifying tumor margins has been investigated, further work remains in characterizing the performance of CEDBT in identifying small iodinated enhancements (stippled enhancement patterns) and accurately quantifying relative iodine concentration (kinetic curves).

We aim to investigate the ability of dual-energy CEDBT to identify small iodinated enhancements and accurately quantify relative iodine concentration, and the dependence of these tasks on imaging chain design. Specifically, lesion detectability, characterized by object signal-difference-to-noise-ratio (SDNR), is measured for dual-energy subtracted 3D CEDBT phantom images. Imaging chain design, including various image processing and reconstruction strategies, are investigated. We investigate iodine quantification by correlating iodine SDNR with known iodine concentration.

Additionally, SDNR for iodinated lesions is characterized for initial patients in an Institutional Review Board-approved clinical study. CEDBT datasets acquired for these patients are similarly processed and SDNR characterized with different imaging chain designs.

2   Methods

2.1   Image Acquisition

All image acquisitions were performed on a Siemens MAMMOMAT Inspiration Digital Breast Tomosynthesis prototype, modified for dual-energy contrast-enhanced imaging. The x-ray source is capable of producing 49 kVp x-ray beams and is equipped with a tungsten anode with a rhodium (Rh) filter and titanium (Ti) or copper (Cu) filters for low- and high-energy imaging, respectively. The amorphous selenium (*a*-Se) flat panel imager has also been designed for dual-energy imaging, wherein the photoconductor thickness has been increased from 200 μm to 300 μm to improve detective quantum efficiency at high energies.

2.2   Phantom Image Acquisition

Phantom imaging was performed using a CIRS (Norfolk, VA) model 020 BR3D breast simulating phantom with a custom solid iodine feature plate (see Fig. 1). This insert contains 16 cylindrical objects of four diameters (2, 3, 5 and 8 mm) and four concentrations of iodine (1, 2, 3 and 5 mg/ml). Four 1-cm tissue simulating slices were used, including the 1-cm solid iodine insert, for a total phantom thickness for 4 cm. Low- and high energy DBT scans of the phantom were acquired using W/Rh 28 kVp and W/Cu 49 kVp spectra, with approximately equal mean glandular doses (MGD) assigned to low- and high-energy scans, for a total MGD of 1.5 mGy. [10] The phantom was not moved and compression was maintained between scans.

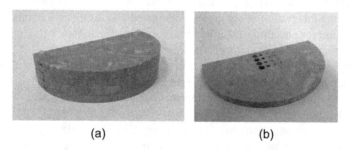

(a)   (b)

Fig. 1. (a) CIRS model 020 BR3D phantom and (b) custom solid iodine feature plate. Four 1-cm thick slices were used, including the solid iodine insert, for a total phantom thickness of 4 cm.

2.3   Patient Image Acquisition

Three patients with BI-RADS 4-5 suspicious findings were recruited as part of an Institutional Review Board-approved clinical study investigating CEDBT. After obtaining informed consent, each patient was injected with 1.5–2.0 ml of iodinated contrast medium per kilogram body weight at a rate of 2 ml/sec using a power-injector. After approximately 2 min, the affected breast was positioned and minimally compressed (<5 daN). A pair of dual-energy CEDM and CEDBT images were subsequently acquired, with approximately 33 % of the total dose allocated to the high-energy acquisitions. Each of the four acquisitions was separated by approximately 30 s, for a total study time of approximately 4.5 min post-injection.

2.4 Imaging Chain Design

Dual-energy subtracted reconstructions were produced from the low- and high-energy projections through six different imaging chain designs (see Fig. 1). Subtraction was performed in either the reconstruction or projection domain. While subtraction in the projection domain may remove the effect of reconstruction artifacts on subtracted images, system geometry instability may result in misregistered projections. Reconstruction was performed using either filtered back-projection (FBP) or an ordered-subset simultaneous algebraic reconstruction technique (OS-SART). [11] In the case of SART reconstructions, raw projections were either corrected for scatter radiation using a previously described scatter correction algorithm [12] or left uncorrected. Scatter radiation, manifest as a low-frequency drop in the modulation transfer function and additive quantum noise at all spatial frequencies, may obscure iodinated lesions and prevent accurate quantification of iodine. Since the filters applied in FBP typically remove the effect of scatter radiation, scatter correction was not applied to projections used in FBP reconstructions (Fig. 2).

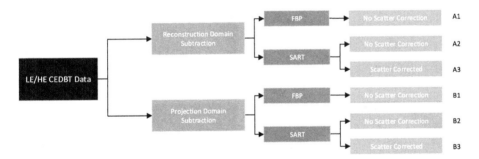

Fig. 2. Imaging chain design. Images were subtracted either in reconstruction or projection domains; reconstructed with either FBP or SART algorithms; and alternatively scatter corrected or uncorrected for SART reconstructions. A total of six imaging schemes were investigated.

2.5 SDNR Analysis

In-plane SDNR of the solid iodine objects was measured for each dual-energy subtracted reconstruction as

$$SDNR = \frac{q_O - q_B}{\sigma_B} \tag{1}$$

where q_O and q_B represent the signal intensity in an ROI of equal size in an area of uniform object and background respectively, and σ_B is the standard deviation of the pixel intensity in the ROI of background [13].

The dependence of object detectability on imaging chain design was investigated by measuring SDNR for iodine objects of every diameter; SDNR was similarly measured for iodinated lesions in patient images. Accuracy of relative iodine quantification was investigated by plotting phantom SDNR as a function of known iodine concentration and calculating the Pearson correlation coefficient r.

3   Results

3.1   Subtracted Reconstructions

Subtracted reconstructions were produced according to each of the six imaging strategies outlined for both phantom and patient datasets. Weighting factors w_s were derived analytically [11] and tuned to produce maximal tissue cancelation ($w_s \pm 0.1$). Example phantom and patient reconstruction slices are presented in Fig. 3.

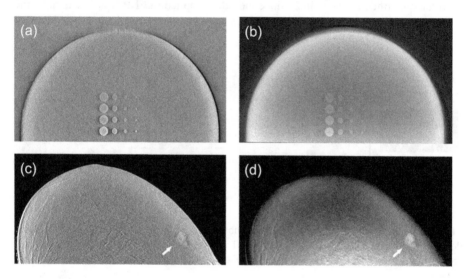

Fig. 3. Single slices from subtracted (top) phantom reconstructions and (bottom) patient reconstructions, subtracted in reconstruction domain with (a, c) FBP and (b, d) SART.

3.2   SDNR

SDNR was measured for each solid iodine insert in each dual-energy subtracted phantom reconstruction. As shown in Fig. 4, subtracting in the reconstruction domain produced SDNR comparable to subtracting in the projection domain. SART generally outperformed FBP, except for very low iodine concentration targets (<2 mg/ml), where FBP and SART results were comparable. The application of a ramp filter in FBP reduces contrast, thus degrading SDNR. Scatter correcting projections before SART reconstruction improved SDNR especially for low iodine concentrations (<3 mg/ml), though this is likely due to the placement of these low concentration objects at the center of the phantom, where scatter radiation is greatest. Iodinated lesion SDNR was similarly measured for each subtracted reconstruction for each of the three patients imaged (see Fig. 5); similar trends were observed, with no advantage of subtraction in one domain over the other.

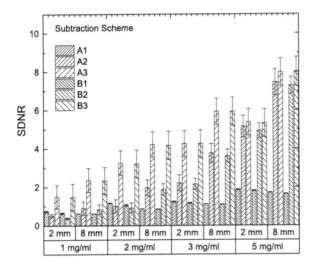

Fig. 4. SDNR of embedded iodine inserts in the phantom, measured for each subtraction scheme. Subtraction in reconstruction domain was essentially equivalent to subtraction in projection domain. SART (A2-A3/B2-B3) generally outperformed FBP when subtracting in either domain. Scatter correcting projections (A3/B3) before SART reconstruction improved SDNR in all cases.

Accuracy of relative iodine quantification was investigated by plotting SDNR as a function of iodine concentration; data were linearly fitted and Pearson's correlation coefficients r were calculated (see Fig. 6). Each algorithm performed nearly identically when comparing subtraction domains. Good correlation ($r > 0.98$) was seen for all imaging chain designs.

4   Discussion

Subtraction in the reconstruction domain was shown to produce essentially equivalent iodine SDNR when compared with subtraction in the projection domain for both phantom and patient images. While subtraction in either domain is thus feasible, subtraction in the reconstruction domain may allow for faster interleaved scans in which alternating low- and high-energy projections are acquired during a single scan, from which low- and high-energy reconstructions are generated and subsequently subtracted. [13] Further, patient motion did not result in low- and high-energy projection misregistration sufficient to impact SDNR.

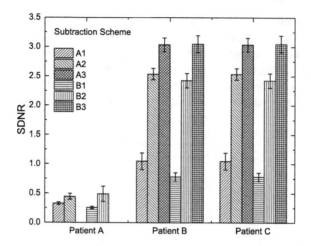

Fig. 5. SDNR of iodinated masses in each of three patients imaged with CEDBT. SART reconstruction outperformed FBP in all cases; scatter corrected projections increased SDNR in SART reconstructions. Subtraction in reconstruction domain was essentially equivalent to subtraction in projection domain. Data from Patient A could not be scatter corrected due to technical limitations of the correction algorithm.

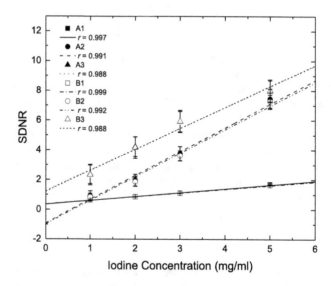

Fig. 6. Measured SDNR of 8 mm iodine objects for each subtraction scheme. Data were linearly fitted and Pearson correlation coefficients were calculated; $r > 0.98$ was demonstrated in all cases. Subtraction schemes in corresponding subtraction domains (e.g., A1/B1) produced virtually identical SDNR results, and thus appear to overlap in the plot.

SART was shown to generally outperform FBP, though judicious choice of reconstruction filters may improve FBP performance. Scatter correcting projections improves

SDNR for SART reconstructions, with the greatest improvement for iodine targets at the center of the phantom, where scatter radiation is greatest.

Strong correlation between iodine concentration and SDNR was observed for subtraction in either projection or reconstruction domain for FBP, suggesting that accurate relative iodine quantification may be achievable for dynamic CEDBT.

Finally, while these results describe the impact of subtraction scheme on contrast-enhanced lesion SDNR, the effect on residual noise remains to be studied. Future work will investigate the impact of subtraction domain, reconstruction algorithm, scatter presence and the impact of appropriate weighting factor on residual structural noise.

Acknowledgments. We gratefully acknowledge financial support from NIH (1 R01 CA148053 and 1 R01 EB002655), and Siemens Healthcare.

References

1. Chou, C.-P., Lewin, J.M., Chiang, C.-L., Hung, B.-H., Yang, T.-L., Huang, J.-S., Liao, J.-B., Pan, H.-B.: Clinical evaluation of contrast-enhanced digital mammography and contrast enhanced tomosynthesis – comparison to contrast-enhanced breast MRI. Eur. J. Radiol. **84**(12), 2501–2508 (2015)
2. Dromain, C., Thibault, F., Muller, S., Rimareix, F., Delaloge, S., Tardivon, A., Balleyguier, C.: Dual-energy contrast-enhanced digital mammography: initial clinical results. Eur. Radiol. **21**, 565–574 (2011)
3. Jochelson, M.S., Dershaw, D.D., Sung, J.S., Heerdt, A.S., Thornton, C., Moskowitz, C.S., Ferrara, J., Morris, E.A.: Bilateral contrast-enhanced dual-energy digital mammography: feasibility and comparison with conventional digital mammography and MR imaging in women with known breast carcinoma. Radiology **266**, 743–751 (2013)
4. Lobbes, M.B.I., Lalji, U., Houwers, J., Nijssen, E.C., Nelemans, P.J., Van Roozendaal, L., Smidt, M.L., Heuts, E., Wildberger, J.E.: Contrast-enhanced spectral mammography in patients referred from the breast cancer screening programme. Eur. Radiol. **24**, 1668–1676 (2014)
5. Luczyńska, E., Heinze-Paluchowska, S., Dyczek, S., Blecharz, P., Rys, J., Reinfuss, M.: Contrast-enhanced spectral mammography: comparison with conventional mammography and histopathology in 152 women. Korean J. Radiol. **15**, 689–696 (2014)
6. Baltzer, P.A.T., Benndorf, M., Dietzel, M., Gajda, M., Runnebaum, I.B., Kaiser, W.A.: False-positive findings at contrast-enhanced breast MRI: a BI-RADS descriptor study. Am. J. Roentgenol. **194**, 1658–1663 (2010)
7. Förnvik, D., Zackrisson, S., Ljungberg, O., Svahn, T., Timberg, P., Tingberg, A., Andersson, I.: Breast tomosynthesis: accuracy of tumor measurement compared with digital mammography and ultrasonography. Acta Radiol. **51**, 240–247 (2010)
8. Petralia, G., Bonello, L., Priolo, F., Summers, P., Bellomi, M.: Breast MR with special focus on DW-MRI and DCE-MRI. Cancer Imaging **11**, 76–90 (2011)
9. Froeling, V., Diekmann, F., Renz, D.M., Fallenberg, E.M., Steffen, I.G., Diekmann, S., Lawaczeck, R., Schmitzberger, F.F.: Correlation of contrast agent kinetics between iodinated contrast-enhanced spectral tomosynthesis and gadolinium-enhanced MRI of breast lesions. Eur. Radiol. **23**, 1528–1536 (2013)

10. Hu, Y.-H., Scaduto, D.A., Zhao, W.: Optimization of clinical protocols for contrast enhanced breast imaging. In: Nishikawa, R.M. Whiting, B.R. (eds.) SPIE Medical Imaging, p. 86680G. International Society for Optics and Photonics, Orlando, FL (2013)

11. Lu, Y., Peng, B., Scaduto, D.A., Zhao, W., Gindi, G.: Application of the ordered-subsets transmission reconstruction algorithm to contrast-enhanced dual-energy digital breast tomosynthesis. In: Proceedings of IEEE Nuclear Science Symposium and Medical Imaging Conference, IEEE NSS/MIC, Seattle, WA (2014)

12. Lu, Y., Peng, B., Lau, B.A., Hu, Y., Scaduto, D.A., Zhao, W., Gindi, G.: A scatter correction method for contrast-enhanced dual-energy digital breast tomosynthesis. Phys. Med. Biol. **60**, 6323–6354 (2015)

13. Hu, Y.-H., Zhao, W.: Experimental quantification of lesion detectability in contrast enhanced dual energy digital breast tomosynthesis, vol. 8313, pp. 83130A1–83130A10 (2012)

Evaluation of the *BreastSimulator* Software Platform for Breast Tomography: Preliminary Results

Giovanni Mettivier[1](✉), Kristina Bliznakova[2], Francesca Di Lillo[1],
Antonio Sarno[1], and Paolo Russo[1]

[1] Dipartimento di Fisica "Ettore Pancini", Università di Napoli Federico II,
and INFN Sezione di Napoli, Naples, Italy
(mettivier,dilillo,sarno,russo)@na.infn.it
[2] Department of Electronics, Technical University of Varna, Varna, Bulgaria
kristina.bliznakova@tu-varna.bg

Abstract. The aim of this work is the evaluation of the software *BreastSimulator*, as a tool for the creation of 3D uncompressed breast digital models and for the simulation and the optimization of Computed Tomography (CT) equipment. Three 3D digital breast phantoms were created, having different sizes and with realistic anatomical features. We calculated 2D X-ray CT projections simulating a breast tomogram with a dedicated cone-beam CT scanner. From the reconstructed CT slices, the power-law exponent, has been evaluated from the Noise Power Spectrum function $S(f) = \alpha/f^{\beta}$. The results were then verified by comparison against clinical CT and published data. The preliminary results of this study showed that the simulated model complexity may reproduce the real anatomical complexity of the breast tissues as described, in terms of β values, since the measured β coefficients are close to that of clinical CT data from a dedicated breast CT scanner.

Keywords: Breast computed tomography · Noise power spectrum · Breast software phantoms · X-ray simulations

1 Introduction

Digital Mammography (DM) is a fundamental technique in breast cancer diagnosis. DM returns a two-dimensional representation (2D) of a compressed three-dimensional object. Therefore, tissues belonging to different planes are all projected on the same X-ray image plane, making it difficult to detect possible abnormalities. In order to overcome this limitation, CT scanners dedicated to the breast have been developed using monochromatic [1, 2] or polychromatic [3, 4] X-ray beams, which return tomographic 3D images of the breast anatomy. However, these techniques need to be optimized before applying them clinically; thus, there is the need to develop X-ray imaging models for the compressed as well as uncompressed breast. Physical phantoms with realistic anatomical characteristics used for image quality assessment, have a high cost. On the other hand, the increasing use of powerful computers allows designing digital phantoms rather than physical phantoms.

© Springer International Publishing Switzerland 2016
A. Tingberg et al. (Eds.): IWDM 2016, LNCS 9699, pp. 145–151, 2016.
DOI: 10.1007/978-3-319-41546-8_19

Simple mathematical breast phantoms, usually in the form of a cylinder, a half-ellipsoid or slabs of homogeneous material with a given glandular to adipose breast tissue ratio, are widely used in simulations particularly for dosimetry and optimization of acquisition geometry [5, 6]. However, when it is necessary to investigate the detectability of lesions, the performance of image processing algorithms, the reconstruction algorithms, etc., the use of a homogeneous background is a limitation, since the anatomical noise is not reproduced.

BreastSimulator [7] is a software support tool for research in breast imaging. It allows the creation of realistic 3D uncompressed breast models. With this software, it is possible to simulate mammographic, tomosynthesis and tomographic breast imaging geometries with monochromatic and polychromatic beams.

This software was previously evaluated as a reliable tool for the simulation of DM systems [8] with good results. In this study, we evaluated *BreastSimulator*, as an appropriate X-ray simulator for dedicated breast CT. This investigation is based on the measure of anatomical noise, evaluated by calculating the β exponent deduced from the power spectral analysis of the CT simulated images.

2   Materials and Methods

2.1   Breast Simulator

The main components of Breast Simulator [7, 8] are the X-ray imaging module and the breast composition model. The first module contains information for the acquisition geometry, number of projections images, gantry angles and detector type. X-ray projections images are obtained with simulation of monochromatic X-ray photon transport starting from the X-ray source, passing through the breast model and reaching the detector (Fig. 1). The Siddon's algorithm for tracing the X-rays from the source to detector pixels is applied. Poisson quantum noise is also added to the original ideal images, using a Gaussian random number generator, with a variance set equal to the number of photons incident on each detector pixel. For simulating a poly-energetic beam, the images obtained at each monochromatic energy were averaged by weighting for the corresponding photon fluence in the spectrum.

The Breast module is used to generate breast models. The simulated features include breast shape, skin, the duct system (Fig. 2a) and terminal ductal lobular units, Cooper's ligaments (Fig. 2b), the pectoral muscle, the 3D mammographic background (glandular and adipose tissue) and breast abnormalities (masses, lesions, micro-calcifications).

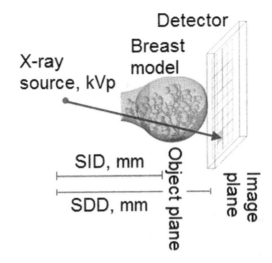

Fig. 1. Example of the simulated X-ray projection setup with the X-ray imaging module.

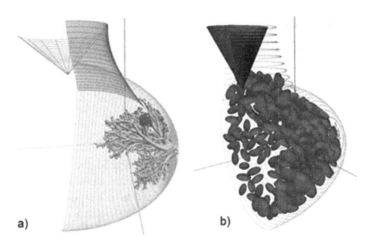

Fig. 2. Example of simulated breast elements (duct system (a) and Cooper's ligaments (b)) with the Breast module.

2.2   Setup Description

The simulated setup was a cone-beam irradiation geometry, with source to isocenter distance (SID) and source to detector distance (SDD) set to 458 mm and 866 mm, respectively. The detector was modeled with a size of 700×700 pixels, and a resolution of 3 pixels/mm, in order to match the resolution of the available clinical CT scan images. Scatter and detector responses have not been included in this simulation. Three realistic 3D uncompressed breast models were created with 64 bit Linux operating system on a

Intel Core 2 Quad Processor Q8200 2.33 GHz, with 8 GB RAM. Figure 3 shows the CT views for one of these models.

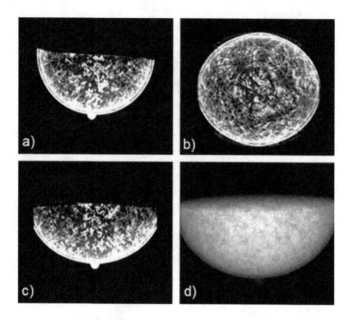

Fig. 3. Example of a sagittal (a), axial (b) and coronal (c) reconstructed CT slices and an X-ray projection (d) obtained with *BreastSimulator* software.

2.3   Assessment of the β Parameter

The projections of the simulated uncompressed breast (Fig. 3d) were reconstructed with a commercial software (Exxim COBRA) implementing the FDK algorithm, providing axial, coronal and sagittal views (Fig. 3a, b, c) in a virtual CT image of $(512)^3$ voxel of $(0.300 \text{ mm})^3$. From these reconstructed slices, the power-law exponent β derived from the Noise Power Spectrum (NPS) fitting function $S(f) = \alpha/(f^{\beta})$ has been evaluated [9], where f is the spatial frequency, evaluated in the range $0.05-0.5 \text{ mm}^{-1}$. To derive this value, 100 ROIs have been selected randomly inside a single coronal slice (Fig. 4a). Then, the 2D NPS was computed by means of the Fast Fourier Transform for each ROI and the mean 2D NPS was determined by averaging the NPS from the 100 ROIs. In order to obtain a 1D NPS, a radial profile was evaluated. Finally, we calculated the β coefficient, as the negative slope of the fitting line returned by computing a linear fit of $\log(\text{1D NPS})$ vs $\log(f)$ (Fig. 4c).

In order to make a comparison with measured clinical data the same procedure for the β evaluation was applied on clinical tomographic images kindly provided by the team at University of California Davis Medical Center (UCDMC) (1 patient) and Radboud University Medical Center (RUMC) (3 patients) which adopt two different clinical breast CT scanners (described in Refs. [9, 10], respectively) (Fig. 4c).

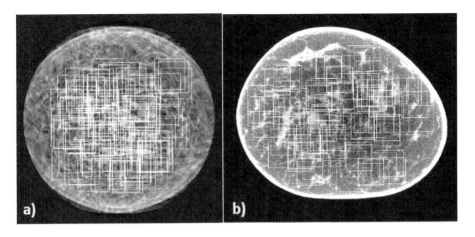

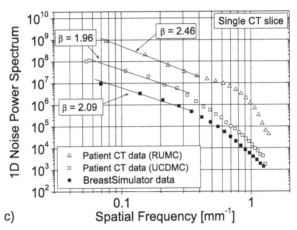

Fig. 4. (a) Example of the sampling carried out on an X-ray reconstructed axial slice obtained with BreastSimulator software and (b) on a real breast acquired with the RUMC scanner (@49 kV). (c) The NPS evaluated from these CT data and from a breast CT scan with the UCDMC scanner (@80 kVp).

3 Results

A number of 360 angular views were simulated, with a monochromatic (27 and 35 keV) and polychromatic X-ray beam (80 kVp). After CT reconstruction of such projections, from the resulting CT slices we evaluated the β coefficient; an example of NPS plots is shown in Fig. 4c, together with NPS data evaluated from two clinical breast CT slices.

We note that the trend of the NPS curves for simulated breasts is similar to that of the breast CT scan data, with a similar slope β of about 2 but with a different intercept ($\ln\alpha$). Hence, the simulated data show a lower power, at all frequencies, than patient data. In Table 1 are reported the measured β values for all the simulated and real breasts.

Table 1. Measured values on simulated and clinical CT scans

	Mono 27 keV	Mono 35 keV	Poly 80 kV	Poly 49 kV
Model breast 1	2.73	2.87	2.42	
Model breast 2	2.12	2.08	2.09	
Model breast 3	2.04	2.29	2.33	
RUMC scanner (3 patients)				1.86–2.46
UCDMC scanner (1 patient)			1.96	

4 Discussion

The results from the evaluation indicate that the parameter β (Table 1), calculated from the power spectral analysis on the simulated images, assumes values similar to those calculated on tomographic images from a dedicated breast CT scanner, with values of the exponent β close to 2. These values are in agreement also with published breast CT data for which the exponent was 1.86 on the average [11, 12].

5 Conclusions

In conclusion, we evaluated *BreastSimulator*, an X-ray simulation software for CT dedicated to the breast. Different breast models were simulated and the anatomical noise properties were evaluated by calculating the β exponent from the power spectral analysis of simulated images. The closeness between simulated values and values measured in a clinical scan indicates the potential of *BreastSimulator* in devising digital phantom for describing the complex anatomy of the female breast. We expect that by increasing the complexity of the present models for breast CT with *BreastSimulator* an even better description of the corresponding complexity of the anatomical structure will be obtained, in the uncompressed breast. This is related to the computing power evaluable for simulation. This would be particularly important for the description of dense breasts, for which the parameter β may be higher than in low-glandular composition breasts [12].

Future work is related to the design of more complex and realistic software breast phantoms via the implementation of a GPU based version of *BreastSimulator*, and to validation with a larger database of breast CT scans. Evaluation of the β values dependence on the thickness and the position of the slice will also be investigated.

Acknowledgments. Prof. J. Boone (UCDMC) and Prof. J. Sechopoulos (RUMC) kindly provided the sample CT images used for the validation of *BreastSimulator* with clinical data. This study was carried out in the framework of the European Commission Project MaXIMA (Three dimensional breast cancer models for X-ray Imaging research), Grant Agreement 692097 (H2020–TWINN – 2015) (Website: http://maxima-tuv.eu/).

References

1. Longo, R., et al.: Towards breast tomography with synchrotron radiation at Elettra: first images. Phys. Med. Biol. **61**, 1634–1649 (2016)
2. McKinley, R.L., et al.: Initial study of quasi-monochromatic X-ray beam performance for X-ray computed mammotomography. IEEE Trans. Nucl. Sci. **52**, 1243–1250 (2005)
3. Mettivier, G., et al.: Dedicated scanner for laboratory investigations on cone-beam CT/SPECT imaging of the breast. Nucl. Meth. A **629**, 350–356 (2011)
4. Sarno, A., Mettivier, G., Russo, P.: Dedicated breast computed tomography: basic aspects. Med. Phys. **42**, 2786–2804 (2015)
5. Mettivier, G., et al.: Glandular dose in breast computed tomography. Phys. Med. Biol. **61**, 569–587 (2016)
6. Lanconelli, N., et al.: Investigation of the dose distribution for a cone beam CT system dedicated to breast imaging. Physica Med. **29**, 379–387 (2013)
7. Bliznakova, K., et al.: A three-dimensional breast software phantom for mammography simulation. Phys. Med. Biol. **48**, 3699–3719 (2003)
8. Bliznakova, K., et al.: Evaluation of an improved algorithm for producing realistic 3D breast software phamtoms: application of mammography. Med. Phys. **37**, 5604–5617 (2010)
9. Lindfors, K.K., et al.: Dedicated breast CT: initial clinical experience. Radiology **246**, 725–733 (2008)
10. O'Connell, A., et al.: Cone-beam CT for breast imaging: radiation dose, breast coverage, and image quality. Am. J. Roentgenol. **195**, 496–509 (2010)
11. Metheani, K.G., et al.: Characterizing anatomical variability in breast CT images. Med. Phys. **35**, 4685–4694 (2008)
12. Chen, L., et al.: Association between power law coefficients of the anatomical noise power spectrum and lesion detectability in breast imaging modalities. Phys. Med. Biol. **58**, 1663–1681 (2013)

Effect of Dose on the Detection of Micro-Calcification Clusters for Planar and Tomosynthesis Imaging

Alistair Mackenzie[1(✉)], Andria Hadjipanteli[1], Premkumar Elangovan[2],
Padraig T. Looney[1], Rebecca Ealden[3], Lucy M. Warren[1], David R. Dance[1,4],
Kevin Wells[2], and Kenneth C. Young[1,4]

[1] National Coordinating Centre for the Physics of Mammography, Royal Surrey County Hospital,
Guildford, GU2 7XX, UK
`alistairmackenzie@nhs.net`
[2] Centre for Vision, Speech, and Signal Processing, Medical Imaging Group,
University of Surrey, Guildford, GU2 7XH, UK
[3] Medical Physics Department, Guy's and St Thomas' NHS Foundation Trust, London, UK
[4] Department of Physics, University of Surrey, Guildford, GU2 7XH, UK

Abstract. The aim of this study was to investigate the effect of dose on the detection of micro-calcification clusters in breast images using planar mammography and digital breast tomosynthesis (DBT). Planar and DBT images were created from mathematical models of breasts with and without inserted clusters of 5 identical calcifications. Regions of interest from the images were used in a series of 4-alternative forced choice human observer experiments using the clusters as targets. Three calcification diameters were used for each imaging condition. The threshold diameter required for micro-calcification detection was determined for a detection rate of 92.5 % at mean glandular doses of 1.25, 2.5, and 5 mGy. The measured threshold micro-calcification diameter was lower for planar mammography than for the DBT modality. The threshold micro-calcification diameter decreased with increasing dose for planar and DBT imaging. The image modality used had a larger effect on the threshold diameter than the dose change considered.

Keywords: DBT · Micro-calcifications · 4-alternative forced choice · Mean glandular dose

1 Introduction

There is evidence for improved cancer detection rates using digital breast tomosynthesis (DBT) compared to planar imaging for breast screening. DBT has some clear advantages over planar imaging due to the reduction of overlying and underlying tissue in the images which allows improved visualisation of suspicious regions in mammograms. However, there are a number of challenges in the introduction of DBT into a screening programme including practicalities such as transferring large amounts of data and increased time for reading the images. There are also challenges in the design of the DBT unit itself and it is not clear which of the many options are optimal for the image acquisition and presentation. It is important to investigate the effect that the magnitude of the dose may have

© Springer International Publishing Switzerland 2016
A. Tingberg et al. (Eds.): IWDM 2016, LNCS 9699, pp. 152–159, 2016.
DOI: 10.1007/978-3-319-41546-8_20

on cancer detection. The study presented here investigates the effect of dose on the threshold diameter of micro-calcifications in a cluster that can be detected in planar and DBT imaging using methods previously developed [1]. The study used simulated breast images and provided the opportunity to investigate the effects of increasing and decreasing the dose.

2   Method

2.1   Mathematical Model of Breast

A method of producing realistic breast models has been developed previously [2]. Using this method a skin outline was extracted from reconstructed DBT planes of the image of a real breast and a 3 mm thick skin layer added. To create the breast models features were extracted from reconstructed DBT planes of real breasts. The extracted features included glandular tissue, Cooper's ligaments, and blood vessels and these were de-noised. Each breast model was created by inserting the different structures into the breast volume. Each structure was rotated to change its appearance from the original images and to ensure a variety of models. By appropriate selection of structures, a simulated breast of a specific glandularity could be produced. The voxel size in the models was 100 µm × 100 µm × 100 µm.

In this study we created breast models with a compressed breast thickness (CBT) of 60 mm with a range of glandularity between 17 % and 19 %. Figure 1 shows examples of simulated planar and DBT images of the breast tissue phantoms calculated using the method described later (Sect. 2.3).

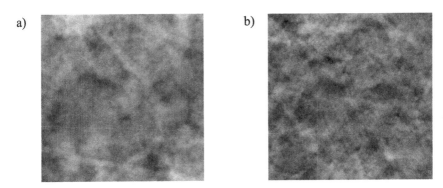

Fig. 1. Examples of simulated images (cropped to 27 mm × 27 mm) of a 3D breast phantom: (a) planar mammogram and (b) one DBT plane

2.2   Simulation of Micro-Calcification Clusters

The calcifications used for the simulation were chosen from a database of 400 calcifications acquired using microCT of breast biopsy samples [3]. It was decided to use a cluster of 5 micro-calcifications rather than a single calcification to create a more realistic target. For each cluster one calcification from the database was scaled to the required size. The calcification was inserted 5 times into a $2.5 \times 2.5 \times 2.5 \ mm^3$ cubic volume and with different rotations. The calcifications were placed randomly within the volume with a restriction that no calcifications could overlap in the planar projection. The voxel size of the cluster was between 15 and 30 μm. The process was repeated for different diameters of calcification (ranging from 110 to 245 μm). Sixty different clusters were produced for each diameter. Figure 2 shows examples of the planar projection of calcification clusters produced with two diameters.

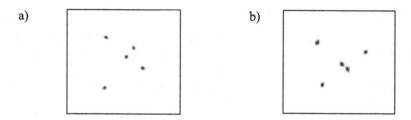

Fig. 2. Planar projection images of $(2.5 \times 2.5 \ mm^2$ area) clusters with two different microcalcification diameters before insertion: (a) 160 μm and (b) 245 μm.

2.3   Image Simulation

The process for simulating the imaging of the breast models with and without the inserted calcification cluster to create realistic 2D images and DBT image planes has been previously described [4]. Image acquisition using a Hologic Dimensions (Hologic Inc. Bedford, MA, USA) with an amorphous-selenium detector was simulated. The tube voltage and target/filter materials used in the x-ray simulation were: (i) planar: 30 kVp W/Rh, with anti-scatter grid (ii) DBT: 32 kVp W/Al, without anti-scatter grid. These are typical of the settings used clinically for imaging a breast of compressed thickness 6 mm. Fifteen projection images were acquired over a swing angle of $\pm$ 7.5° for DBT.

The breast models and calcification clusters were ray-traced separately to create planar and DBT projections. The calcification clusters were placed at a height of 30 mm above the breast support. The ray tracing process takes account of the grid transmission factor (for planar imaging), half value layer, tube movement, focal spot size, attenuation in the breast support and compression paddle. No movement of the breast was included in the simulation. The x-ray spectra were simulated using previously published data [5] and scaled so that the incident air kerma matched that required for a specified value of the mean glandular dose [6]. The mean glandular dose values were set at 1.25, 2.5 and 5 mGy for both planar and DBT. The resulting projected planar and DBT images were blurred to match the detector response and scatter was added. Noise was added with the correct magnitude and colour appropriate for the dose and beam quality using methods developed previously [7, 8].

Briona software (Real Time Tomography, LLC, Philadelphia, PA) was used to process the 2D planar images and to reconstruct the DBT planes from the projection images. After processing and reconstruction, for the observer studies the planar images were cropped into 30 mm × 30 mm regions of interest (ROIs) and the DBT planes were cropped to 30 mm × 30 mm ROIs in 11 planes with 1 mm spacing.

2.4   Observation and 4-Alternative Forced (AFC) Study

A 4-alternative forced choice (4AFC) study with human observers was used to determine the threshold diameter of calcifications that are detectable for the different doses and both planar and DBT modalities. In these studies each observer was shown groups of 4 cropped ROIs, only one of which contained a calcification cluster. The observer had to try and identify which of the ROIs had the cluster and was required to choose an ROI even if they could not see the cluster. Five physicists were used as observers. There were 6 sets of images, each set contained either planar or DBT images, three calcification diameters and was produced using one of three dose levels. Each set had 180 groups of four ROIs. Each observer was shown the images one set at a time.

The images were presented using an in-house graphical user interface (GUI) as shown in Fig. 3. A toto circle was used to indicate the possible location of the cluster in each image, as it has been shown to improve the selection of the correct ROI [9]. A 2D projection of only the calcification cluster was also shown to the observer as a signal cue. The observer could scroll through the 11 DBT planes and the central plane always contained the centre of the cluster volume. The DBT stack display wrapped around when the observer scrolled to the end of the stack. All experiments were undertaken using a 5 MP high-resolution monitor (Barco B-8500, 5 MP, Barco Inc., Belgium) at low lighting levels (< 10 lux) and no time limit was imposed.

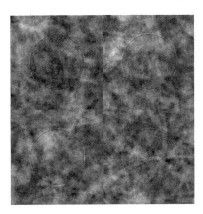

Fig. 3. Screenshot of the 4AFC GUI with signal cue for the planar images containing a 175 μm calcification cluster. In this case the cluster was present in the bottom left hand corner image (the cue was magnified only for this publication).

2.5   Data Analysis

The minimum detectable calcification size was defined as the value at which the observer makes 92.5 % correct decisions for a given experimental condition, which corresponds to a detectability index d' of 2.5 [10]. Diameters that resulted in a detection rate of 100 % or 25 % were not included in the results. A linear fit between d' and diameter was made for each modality, dose and observer, and the threshold diameter was determined for a d' of 2.5. The mean threshold diameter was then calculated for each of the three doses for DBT and 2D.

Analysis of variance (ANOVA) was performed on the results to identify any statistically significant differences between the minimum detectable calcification diameters of the three doses for planar and DBT.

3   Results

Figure 4 shows the threshold diameters of the calcifications for three different MGDs for planar and DBT imaging. A significant differences between the threshold diameters of the calcifications was found between the planar and DBT modes for each dose level ($p < 0.0001$). Differences between threshold diameters for images acquired at a dose of 1.25 mGy and 5 mGy compared to 2.5 mGy were also significant (maximum $p = 0.001$ for planar, maximum $p = 0.003$ for DBT).

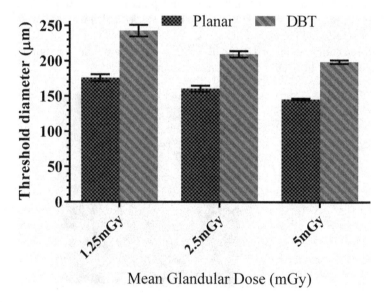

Fig. 4. Threshold calcification diameter for planar and DBT modalities for three MGDs (Error bars are 95 % confidence limits)

4   Discussion

The visibility of calcifications is affected by blurring processes during imaging. The DBT images were more blurred that the planar images as the images were acquired with a larger pixel pitch and there is some blurring from tube motion [11]. One advantage for DBT is the reduction in the background structure of the breast tissue. However, it has been shown that quantum noise affects the detection of calcifications more than background structure [12]. The threshold diameter of the planar images was between 50 and 70 μm smaller than for the DBT modality, depending on dose.

A dose of 2.5 mGy for 60 mm CBT is typical for the DBT system being simulated. The standard dose for planar imaging was raised to match the dose for DBT to provide a fair comparison between the imaging modalities. The effect of doubling the dose from 1.25 mGy or 2.5 mGy reduced the threshold diameter between 10 μm and 30 μm for planar imaging and DBT. Thus, the effect of dose on the threshold diameter was much smaller than that between imaging modalities at the same dose. It has been shown for planar imaging that the detection rate of calcification clusters will reduce if dose is lowered [13]. There must therefore be concerns that detection of calcification clusters will be lower in DBT and also the loss of the visibility of the smallest calcifications may affect the classification of clusters.

One of the advantages of using simulated clinical images is that we can investigate the effect of higher doses which is not possible using real clinical images. It indicates that is possible to see smaller calcifications at higher doses. Of course this does not definitely indicate that higher dose should be used. The benefits and detriments of detecting additional cancers would still need to be considered.

In this study we have assumed that the exposure time for each DBT projection is the same for the three dose levels and that the dose is changed by doubling or halving the tube current. This is the method for reducing dose on the Hologic system, but to increase the dose the exposure time for each projection is increased. This would mean that there should be more blurring included in this study for the high dose DBT mode as the tube travel is greater while the x-ray tube is on.

We used a 100 μm voxel size for the mathematical breast models. If a smaller voxel was used then the modelling may have been improved, but this would increase the simulation time to be impractically large. It was necessary to undertake finer sampling of the calcifications, where the voxel size was between 15 and 30 μm and so the ray tracing was undertaken separately for the breast and the cluster.

The DBT images were viewed in a stack rather than only showing the central plane. The number of images in the stack was chosen such that even for the largest calcifications there was no discernible shadow in the first and last image in the stack. The observer had control of the viewing of the images and could scroll through the stack or stop at individual planes. Typically the paradigm of an AFC test is object known and location known. Therefore, the observer was aware which image was the central plane. It was necessary to use a stack of images as the calcifications could be in focus in different planes and so the central plane may not be the best plane for viewing all of the calcifications. The ability to scroll through the planes also allowed the observer to identify calcifications which appeared and disappeared through the image stack.

5   Conclusions

This study measured the threshold diameter that micro-calcifications in a cluster can be reliably detected. It has been shown that the imaging modality and dose both have an effect on the threshold diameter.

Acknowledgements. This work is part of the OPTIMAM2 project and is supported by Cancer Research UK (grant, number: C30682/A17321). We thank Jack Miskell and Isobel Dodson for participating in this study. We are also grateful to the staff of Real Time Tomography for their help in using their software in this experiment.

References

1. Elangovan, P., Rashidnasab, A., Mackenzie, A., Dance, D.R., Young, K.C., Bosmans, H., Segars, W.P., Wells, K.: Performance comparison of breast imaging modalities using a 4AFC human observer study. In: Proceedings of SPIE Medical Imaging, vol. 9412, p. 94121T-1–7 (2015)
2. Elangovan, P., Dance, D.R., Young, K.C., Wells, K.: Simulation of 3D synthetic breast blocks. In: Proceedings of SPIE Medical Imaging, vol. 9783, p. 978308-1–8 (2016)
3. Shaheen, E., Van Ongeval, C., Zanca, F., Cockmartin, L., Marshall, N., Jacobs, J., Young, K.C., Dance, D.R., Bosmans, H.: The simulation of 3D microcalcification clusters in 2D digital mammography and breast tomosynthesis. Med. Phys. **38**, 6659 (2011)
4. Elangovan, P., Warren, L.M., Mackenzie, A., Rashidnasab, A., Diaz, O., Dance, D.R., Young, K.C., Bosmans, H., Strudley, C.J., Wells, K.: Development and validation of a modelling framework for simulating 2D-mammography and breast tomosynthesis images. Phys. Med. Biol. **59**, 4275–4293 (2014)
5. Boone, J.M., Fewell, T.R., Jennings, R.J.: Molybdenum, rhodium, and tungsten anode spectral models using interpolating polynomials with application to mammography. Med. Phys. **24**, 1863–1874 (1997)
6. Dance, D.R., Skinner, C.L., Young, K.C., Beckett, J.R., Kotre, C.J.: Additional factors for the estimation of mean glandular breast dose using the UK mammography dosimetry protocol. Phys. Med. Biol. **45**, 3225–3240 (2000)
7. Mackenzie, A., Dance, D.R., Workman, A., Yip, M., Wells, K., Young, K.C.: Conversion of mammographic images to appear with the noise and sharpness characteristics of a different detector and x-ray system. Med. Phys. **39**, 2721–2734 (2012)
8. Mackenzie, A., Dance, D.R., Diaz, O., Young, K.C.: Image simulation and a model of noise power spectra across a range of mammographic beam qualities. Med. Phys. **41**, 121901 (2014)
9. Kundel, H.L., Nodine, C.F., Toto, L.C., Lauver, S.C.: Circle cue enhances detection of simulated masses on mammogram backgrounds. Proc. SPIE Med. Imaging. **3036**, 81–84 (1997)
10. Burgess, A.: Image quality, the ideal observer, and human performance of radiologic decision tasks. Acad. Radiol. **2**, 522–526 (1995)
11. Mackenzie, A., Marshall, N.W., Dance, D.R., Bosmans, H., Young, K.C.: Characterisation of a breast tomosynthesis unit to simulate images. In: Proceedings of SPIE Medical Imaging, vol. 8668, 86684R-1–8 (2013)

12. Kotre, C.J.: The effect of background structure on the detection of low contrast objects in mammography. Br. J. Radiol. **71**, 1162–1167 (1998)
13. Warren, L.M., Mackenzie, A., Cooke, J., Given-Wilson, R.M., Wallis, M.G., Chakraborty, D.P., Dance, D.R., Bosmans, H., Young, K.C.: Effect of image quality on calcification detection in digital mammography. Med. Phys. **39**, 3202–3213 (2012)

Dosimetric Modeling of Mammography Using the Monte Carlo Code PENELOPE and Its Validation

Jason Tse[1,2(✉)], Roger Fulton[1], and Donald McLean[1,2]

[1] Faculty of Health Sciences, University of Sydney, Sydney, Australia
ttse4243@uni.sydney.edu.au
[2] Medical Physics and Radiation Engineering, Canberra Hospital, Canberra, Australia

Abstract. The Monte Carlo code PENELOPE (version 2014) and its software package PenEasy have been employed to closely simulate a commercial mammography system: Selenia Dimensions system (Hologic, Bedford, Mass) for dosimetric study. Normalized glandular dose (D_gN) was derived for specific filter combinations including tungsten/aluminum (W/Al), tungsten/rhodium (W/Rh) and tungsten/silver (W/Ag) for a range of clinically used voltages (kV). Breast models with thickness 2 cm, 4.5 cm and 8 cm and respective glandularity 100 %, 50 % and 0.1 % were included in the simulations. Derived D_gN values were in good agreement with well-accepted published values, with mean differences of 1.30 %, 2.17 % and 0.17 % for the W/Al, W/Rh and W/Ag anode/filter combinations, respectively. In the next phase of the study, this validated model will be modified to perform patient-specific dosimetry with an improved breast model and more realistic simulation of commercial mammography systems.

Keywords: Radiation dosimetry · Digital mammography · Tomosynthesis

1 Introduction

The mean radiation dose deposited in fibro-glandular tissues (known as mean glandular dose, D_g) is the common dose metric used to characterize the radiation risk from mammographic exposures. Direct determination of this dose quantity is currently impossible and medical physicists can only make estimates based on simplistic models. Thermoluminescence dosimetry (TLD) and Monte Carlo simulation methods have been employed to determine D_g and the latter is the generally preferred method nowadays owing to its flexibility.

To facilitate the determination of D_g in practice, a number of groups [1, 2] have published conversion factors to convert measurable incident air kerma to D_g. D_g normalized in this way to the incident air kerma at the entrance surface of the breast is termed normalized glandular dose (D_gN) in the USA. An equivalent set of factors, namely the g-, c- and s- factors, is commonly used in the UK and Europe and they share the same physical meaning as D_gN.

It is important to recognize that the derivation of D_g and D_gN is based upon a simplistic breast model which is a semi-circular cylinder consisting of a homogeneous mix of breast tissue (fibro-glandular and adipose tissue) enclosed by a layer of adipose

© Springer International Publishing Switzerland 2016
A. Tingberg et al. (Eds.): IWDM 2016, LNCS 9699, pp. 160–166, 2016.
DOI: 10.1007/978-3-319-41546-8_21

tissue (Fig. 1). Therefore, D_g does not provide a dose estimate for individual patients but rather a representative radiation dose estimate to a typical breast in the general population.

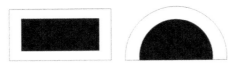

Fig. 1. The standard breast model in vertical cross-section (left) and top view (right). The black regions depict breast tissue, a homogeneous mixture of adipose and glandular tissue, and the white region refers to the adipose layer enclosing the breast tissue

In the present work, the Monte Carlo code PENELOPE (version 2014) [3, 4] and its software package PenEasy [5] have been employed to simulate a commercial mammography system for dosimetric study. Other simulation details have mirrored those used by Dance [1] to enable result comparison and method validation. We intend to use this model for subsequent investigations of patient-specific dosimetry in digital breast tomosynthesis. Here we present the details of the model, and its validation using published data.

2   Methods and Materials

2.1   Monte Carlo Simulation

The geometry of a commercial mammography unit (Selenia Dimensions Mammography System, Hologic, Bedford, MA, USA) was modeled as illustrated in Fig. 2. The breast support was made of carbon fiber of thickness 0.41 cm and the image receptor was a selenium slab of thickness 0.25 cm. Both slabs had the same dimensions of 29 cm by 24 cm which is the largest field-of-view for the mammography unit. An air gap of 2.5 cm was allowed between the breast support and image receptor as in the actual configuration. The anti-scatter grid was not explicitly modeled as the energy deposition in the image receptor was not of primary interest in this study.

Breast models of thickness 2 cm, 4.5 cm and 8 cm were included in the simulation. Breast glandularities of 100 %, 50 % and 0.1 % were respectively simulated in each of the three breast models. Glandularity, in this context, is defined as the weight proportion of the fibro-glandular tissues within the homogeneous breast tissue mixture. The radii of the models were fixed at 8 cm and the thickness of the adipose layer at 0.5 cm, identical to those used by Dance. The elemental composition and physical density of breast tissues were adopted from the work of Hammerstein [6].

The x-ray source was simulated as a perfect point source 70 cm from the image receptor. A series of simulations was performed with mono-energetic photon energies ranging from 6 keV to 40 keV (resolution of 1 keV) for each breast thickness. For each simulation run, 10 million mono-energetic photons were emitted from the source and collimated to irradiate the breast to achieve an uncertainty better than 0.5 % for energy

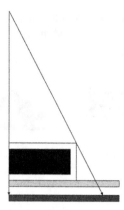

Fig. 2. A lateral view of the simulation geometry: a mono-energetic photon source located at 70 cm from the image receptor made of selenium (thickness: 0.25 cm), collimated to irradiate the simplistic breast model (Fig. 1) resting on the breast support made of carbon fiber (thickness: 0.41 cm). (Figure not to scale)

deposition. The interactions of every photon were traced until its energy fell below the 1 keV energy cut-off and the average energy depositions per photon in different materials were tallied. Photon interactions including Rayleigh scattering, photoelectric absorption and Compton scattering were accounted for in all simulations. Owing to the low tube voltage settings utilized in mammography (e.g. 25 kV - 45 kV), all electron transports were disabled, assuming that all secondary electrons would deposit their energy locally. Running on a personal computer with an Intel® Core™ Duo CPU of 2.00 GHz, each simulation took around five minutes which was considered acceptable and therefore no variance reduction technique was implemented.

2.2   Determination of DgN

D_gNs are derived by normalizing the glandular tissue dose by the incident air kerma at the breast entrance surface for different irradiation conditions. In the simulations above, the energies absorbed in the breast tissue were tallied for mono-energetic photon energies and the results were used to derive D_gN as proposed by Boone [7] i.e.

$$D_gN = \frac{D_g}{k_{in}} = \frac{\sum_{E_{min}}^{E_{max}} E_{ab,breast}(E) \, \Phi(E) \, G(E) \dfrac{A_{breast}}{m_{gland}}}{\sum_{E_{min}}^{E_{max}} E \, \Phi(E) \left(\dfrac{\mu_{en}}{\rho} \right)_{air}} \qquad (1)$$

where K_{in} is the incident air kerma at the entrance surface of the breast, $E_{ab,breast}$ (E) is the absorbed energy at photon energy E per incident photon, Φ (E) is the relative photon fluence at energy E of any arbitrary spectrum, A_{breast} is the entrance surface area of the breast model, m_{gland} is the mass of the fibro-glandular tissue, E is the mono-energetic photon energy and $(\mu_{en}/\rho)_{air}$ is the mass absorption coefficient of air at energy E.

G (E) is the scale factor relating the energy absorbed in breast tissue to that in fibro-glandular tissue and is the ratio between the mass absorption coefficient of fibro-glandular tissue and the weighted sum of coefficients of breast tissues by their proportions, i.e.

$$G(E) = \frac{\left(\frac{\mu_{en}}{\rho}\right)_g}{f_g\left(\frac{\mu_{en}}{\rho}\right)_g + (1-f_g)\left(\frac{\mu_{en}}{\rho}\right)_a} \tag{2}$$

where $(\mu_{en}/\rho)_g$ and $(\mu_{en}/\rho)_a$ are the mass absorption coefficients of fibro-glandular and adipose tissues, respectively, and f_g is the weight fraction of fibro-glandular tissue within the homogenous breast tissue mixture (1 for 100 %; 0.5 for 50 %; 0.01 for 0.1 %).

m_{gland}, the mass of the fibro-glandular tissue, is defined as

$$m_{gland} = 1/2\left(\pi R^2 T\right)\rho_g f_g \tag{3}$$

where R and T are the radius and thickness of the semi-circular cylindrical breast tissue of the simple breast model, ρ_g is the density of the glandular tissue; f_g is again the fraction of glandular tissue within the breast tissue mixture.

D_gNs were derived for the W/Al anode/filter combination (0.7 mm) with tube voltages ranging from 26 kV to 38 kV as used in the tomosynthesis image acquisition with the commercial mammography unit. Other combinations including W/Rh (0.05 mm) and W/Ag (0.05 mm), as utilized in two-dimensional image acquisitions, were simulated for a range of clinically used tube voltages: 25 kV to 31 kV and 30 kV to 32 kV, respectively. The energy spectra were generated using the method developed by Boone [8] with additional beryllium (Be) filtration of thickness 0.13 mm to match the actual thickness of 0.63 mm (Boone's spectra possess an inherent Be filtration of 0.5 mm) and a polycarbonate compression paddle of thickness 2.8 mm. The half value layers (HVL) for the different energy spectra were determined analytically and are summarized in Table 1.

Table 1. The three sets of x-ray beam qualities utilized in the present study.

Anode/Filter	Tube Voltages (kV)	Half-value layer (mm Al)
W/Al	26 – 38	0.452 – 0.718
W/Rh	25 – 31	0.488 – 0.563
W/Ag	30 – 32	0.590 – 0.616

2.3 Model Validation

The model was validated by comparing the derived D_gNs with the equivalent gcs- factors computed by Dance for identical irradiation conditions.

3   Results

D_gN values calculated in the present study were in good agreement with the published values, as illustrated in Figs. 3 and 4. The mean differences for the three anode/filter combinations: W/Al, W/Rh and W/Ag were respectively 1.30 %, 2.17 % and 0.17 % for all breast thicknesses of interest. The corresponding maximum differences were 2.75 %, 4.59 % and 0.39 %.

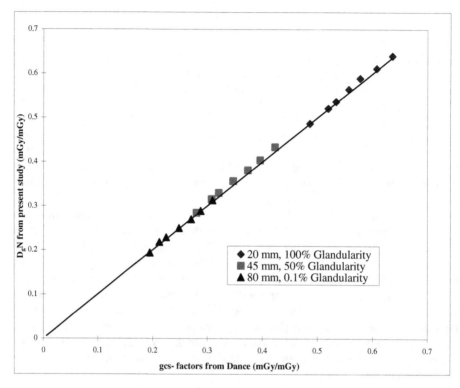

Fig. 3.   Comparison of the D_gN values derived for the tungsten/aluminum combination with the equivalent factors published by Dance for the breast thicknesses and compositions of interest. The solid black line is the line of identity.

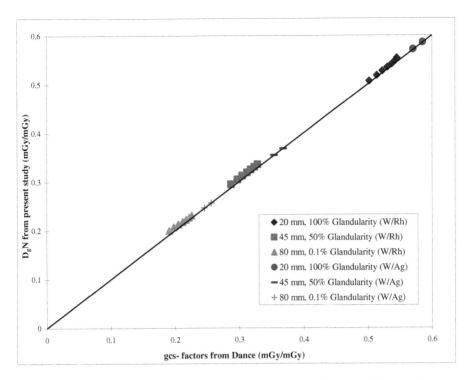

Fig. 4. Comparison of D_gN values drived for tungsten/rhodium and tungsten/silver combinations with the equivalent factors published by Dance for the breast thicknesses and compositions of interest. The solid black line is the line of identity.

4   Discussion and Conclusions

The dosimetric model developed by the code PENELOPE was successfully validated against that of Dance's which is the basis of the dosimetry methods for mammography in the UK and Europe. These results also confirmed the reliability of this Monte Carlo code to study dose deposition in the low energy range of diagnostic x-rays. The deviations from Dance's results are believed to be attributable to the different photon interaction cross-sections (maximum errors up to 10 %), the difference in the irradiation geometry (maximum errors up to 2.3 %) and the inaccurate scaling of G (E).

In this work, G (E) was retrospectively applied as opposed to the suggestions from Heggie and Wilkinson [9] that it should be applied on an interaction-by-interaction basis to accurately account for the energy depositions of the less energetic photons from Compton scattering events. Nonetheless, as reported by Boone, the associated systematic error would be less than 4 % for photon energies up to 50 keV for W/Al and in the range of 0.3 % for other anode/filter combinations as a result of the dominance of the photoelectric effect at low photon energies. Considering the low x-ray energies simulated, specific corrections were not implemented here. In future studies, however, interaction-by-interaction G (E) scaling may be crucial as the advanced mammography applications such as the contrast-enhanced and dual-energy mammography use higher tube potentials.

The next phase of the study is under way to investigate the possibility of patient-specific dosimetry. The present breast models will be refined based on the individual distribution of fibro-glandular tissue extracted from tomosynthesis images. The conditions of the simulation will also be improved to more closely mirror the actual settings of commercial mammography units with an aim to determine a more realistic and individualized breast dose estimation.

References

1. Dance, D.R.: Monte Carlo calculation of conversion factors for the estimation of mean glandular breast dose. Phys. Med. Biol. **35**, 1211–1219 (1990)
2. Wu, X., Barnes, G.T., Tucker, D.M.: Spectral dependence of glandular tissue dose in screen-film mammography. Radiology **179**, 143–148 (1991)
3. Baró, J., Sempau, J., Fernández-Varea, J.M., Salvat, F.: PENELOPE: An algorithm for Monte Carlo simulation of the penetration and energy loss of electrons and positrons in matter. Nucl. Instrum. Methods Phys. Res., Sect. B **100**, 31–46 (1995)
4. Sempau, J., Acosta, E., Baro, J., Fernández-Varea, J.M., Salvat, F.: An algorithm for Monte Carlo simulation of coupled electron-photon transport. Nucl. Instrum. Methods Phys. Res., Sect. B **132**, 377–390 (1997)
5. Sempau, J., Badal, A., Brualla, L.: A PENELOPE-based system for the automated Monte Carlo simulation of clinacs and voxelized geometries-application to far-from-axis fields. Med. Phys. **38**, 5887–5895 (2011)
6. Hammerstein, G.R., et al.: Absorbed radiation-dose in mammography. Radiology **130**, 485–491 (1979)
7. Boone, J.M.: Glandular breast dose for monoenergetic and high-energy X-ray beams: Monte Carlo assessment. Radiology **213**, 23–37 (1999)
8. Boone, J.M., Fewell, T.R., Jennings, R.J.: Molybdenum, rhodium, and tungsten anode spectral models using interpolating polynomials with application to mammography. Med. Phys. **24**, 1863–1874 (1997)
9. eLetters to the Editor - Glandular Breast Dose: Potential Errors. (2000)

Nonlinear Local Transformation Based Mammographic Image Enhancement

Cuiping Ding[1], Min Dong[1], Hongjuan Zhang[1], Yide Ma[1(✉)],
Yaping Yan[1], and Reyer Zwiggelaar[2]

[1] School of Information Science and Engineering,
Lanzhou University, Lanzhou, China
dingcpl4@lzu.edu.cn,
dm8800612dm@163.com
[2] Department of Computer Science,
Aberystwyth University, Aberystwyth, UK

Abstract. Mammography is one of the most effective techniques for early detection of breast cancer. The quality of the image may suffer from poor resolution or low contrast, which can effect the efficiency of radiologists. In order to improve the visual quality of mammograms, this paper introduces a new mammographic image enhancement algorithm. Firstly an intensity based nonlinear transformation is used for reducing the background tissue intensity, and secondly adaptive local contrast enhancement is realized based on local standard deviation and luminance information. The proposed method can obtain improved performance compared to alternative methods both covering objective and subjective aspects, based on 45 images. Experimental results demonstrate that the proposed algorithm can improve the contrast effectively and enhance lesion information (microcalcifications and/or masses).

Keywords: Mammography · Nonlinear transformation · Local contrast enhancement

1 Introduction

In recent years, the incidence rate of breast cancer has considerably increased. Mammography is one of the most commonly used and effective technologies to detect and diagnose breast cancer. Due to hardware limitations, a mammogram contains noise, which can impede the accuracy to early detection of different breast cancer abnormalities.

Image enhancement is an effective way to improve the visual quality of mammograms. In our work, we introduce a new mammographic image enhancement algorithm. Firstly, morphological opening is used to remove discrete noise. Then a nonlinear transfer function is utilized to reducing the background tissue intensity. Finally, adaptive local contrast enhancement is achieved using 2-D Gaussian convolution and local standard deviation. This algorithm can effectively suppress the background tissue intensity, and improve the image contrast.

© Springer International Publishing Switzerland 2016
A. Tingberg et al. (Eds.): IWDM 2016, LNCS 9699, pp. 167–173, 2016.
DOI: 10.1007/978-3-319-41546-8_22

2   The Proposed Algorithm

In this section, we propose a method based on nonlinear local enhancement exploiting their higher intensity and low contrast. This algorithm can effectively suppress the information of the tissue around the lesion, and improve the contrast.

2.1   Morphological Filter

A morphological opening operation is used as a processing tool to remove noise, which is important to image processing. The original image intensity $I(x, y)$ is normalized to $I_{n1}(x, y)$. The image intensity after the morphological opening is defined as $I_n(x, y)$. The structuring element is disk-shaped with a radius of two pixels.

2.2   Nonlinear Transfer Function

We use an exponential type nonlinear transfer function, whch is expressed as Eq. (1) to suppress the intensity of tissue around the lesion:

$$I_{e1} = I_n^{\lfloor 10\mu \rfloor} \tag{1}$$

where the operator $\lfloor \cdot \rfloor$ rounds its argument toward the nearest integer. I_n is the result of the morphological filtering. μ is the mean value of I_n. I_{e1} is the result after the nonlinear transfer function. As the value of $10\ \mu$ is expected to be smaller than unity, this transformation can be used to reduce the luminance of the image. Since the luminance of the lesions is generally higher than for normal tissue, the nonlinear transfer function can slightly reduce the intensity of lesion, and greatly reduce intensity of tissue around the lesion, resulting the highlight of lesion.

2.3   Gaussian Convolution and Local Standard Deviation

To get the average luminance information of the surrounding pixels, 2-D Gaussian convolution is carried out on I_{e1}. Suppose $G(x, y)$ denotes the 2-D Gaussian function. The convolution $I_{conv}(x, y)$ is defined as $I_{e1}(x, y) \otimes G(x, y)$. The mean and the standard deviation are estimated for a local window following the methodology described by Tao and Asari [9].

2.4   Adaptive Contrast Enhancement

The contrast enhancement is carried out using the following four equations [1]:

$$I_e(x, y) = 255 I_{e1}(x, y)^{E(x,y)} \tag{2}$$

$$E(x,y) = R(x,y)^P = \left[\frac{I_{conv}(x,y)}{I_{e1}(x,y)}\right]^P \tag{3}$$

$$P = 1 + \frac{3(Q - \min(Q))}{(\max(Q) - \min(Q))} \tag{4}$$

$$Q = \frac{1}{S} \tag{5}$$

$I_e(x,y)$ is the image intensity after contrast enhancement, $I_{conv}(x,y)$ is the average luminance information of the surrounding pixels with center at (x,y). $R(x,y)$ is the ratio between $I_{conv}(x,y)$ and $I_{e1}(x,y)$. The low contrast of some regions will be improved significantly, while the high contrast of other regions will only show limited improvement. A higher S reflects a higher contrast. So at region edges, the local standard deviation is relatively large, so the value of Q is quite small and vice versa. In order to get a better result, it is necessary to do certain restrictions on Q, that's why we use Eq. (4). Based on the experimental results, it is appropriate for Q to be normalized between 1 and 4, a range that can be data-adjusted. For example, if $I_{conv}(x,y)/I_{e1}(x,y)$ is greater than 1, then $E(x,y)$ is greater than 1. So $I_{e1}(x,y)^{E(x,y)}$ is less than $I_{e1}(x,y)$, which means the lower intensity of pixel will be lowered after the transformation and vice versa, leading the improvement of the contrast.

3 Results and Discussion

3.1 DataSet and Quantitative Measures

The mammograms used in this work are taken from the Mammography Image Analysis Society (MIAS) [2] and the Japanese Society of Medical Imaging Technology (JAMIT) [3]. The MIAS database contains 322 mammograms, which are 8 bits with a pixel size equal to 50×50 μm. The original screen-film mammograms of JAMIT are digitized with a pixel size of 100×100 μm and 10-bit gray-level resolution. The JAMIT database contains 40 mammograms and includes expert annotation of the lesion area. In general, the contrast of lesion area and the background is poor. Shape and size of the masses are irregular, and the borders can be ill-defined [4].

In order to quantify image enhancement, we use the Contrast Improvement Index (CII), the Peak Signal to Noise Ratio (PSNR), and the Distribution Separation Measure (DSM), and the Mean Opinion Score (MOS) as quantitative measure.

CII is defined as $C_{processed}/C_{original}$, where C is $(f - b)/(f + b)$, where f and b denote the mean gray level value of the target and the background, respectively. $C_{processed}$ and $C_{original}$ are the contrasts for the enhanced and original images.

PSNR is defined as $(p - b)/\sigma$, where p is the maximum gray level value and σ is the standard derivation of the background.

DSM is an evaluation method based on the probability distribution, which is defined as $\left(|D_2 - \mu_B^E| + |D_2 - \mu_T^E| - |D_1 - \mu_B^O| + |D_1 - \mu_T^O|\right)$, where $D_1 = (\mu_B^O \sigma_T^O + \mu_T^O \sigma_B^O)/(\sigma_B^O + \sigma_T^O)$, $D_2 = (\mu_B^E \sigma_T^E + \mu_T^E \sigma_B^E)/(\sigma_B^E + \sigma_T^E)$, where $\mu_B^O, \sigma_B^O, \mu_T^O, \sigma_T^O$ are respectively the mean and standard deviation of the grayscales comprising the background and target area, of the original image. And $\mu_B^E, \sigma_B^E, \mu_T^E, \sigma_T^E$ correspond to the mean and standard deviation of the grayscales of the enhanced image.

MOS is a subjective test and ten observers rank the performance of each original and corresponding enhanced images from 1 to 5, where a five score indicate the best visual quality.

3.2 Subjective Evaluation of Experimental Results

A dataset of 45 mammographic images was randomly selected from the JAMIT and MIAS databases, which included 30 abnormal and 15 normal images. All mammograms are cropped to contain a minimal amount of background. In order to show the effectiveness of the proposed method, it is compared with others: CLAHE [5], NUM [6], QUM [7], and RUM [8].

Table 1. Subjective evaluation for the enhanced results by differernt algorithms

Observers	Original	CLAHE	NUM	QUM	RUM	Our method
#1	1.83	3.48	3.07	1.71	2.15	**3.99**
#2	2.69	3.80	3.44	1.88	2.79	**4.02**
#3	1.66	3.14	3.25	1.41	2.53	**4.22**
#4	2.00	3.56	3.34	2.65	2.79	**4.68**
#5	2.14	3.48	3.07	1.50	2.24	**4.26**
#6	3.37	**3.93**	3.58	2.97	3.25	3.89
#7	3.28	3.32	3.37	3.19	3.11	**3.62**
#8	1.52	3.17	3.74	1.24	2.50	**4.21**
#9	1.47	3.26	3.65	1.56	2.31	**4.32**
#10	1.65	3.33	3.24	2.11	2.11	**4.11**
Average	2.16	3.45	3.38	2.02	2.58	**4.13**

The average subjective evaluation scores of each observer for all the test mammograms are shown in Table 1. The bottom row of Table 1 shows the average evaluation scores where our method gives the best overall visual quality with a score of 4.13, which is statistically significantly different from the other methods in Table 1.

We have selected 3 example enhancement results and display them in Figs. 1, 2 and 3. Mammograms from JAMIT database are negative films, so they are transformed to positive films at first, then input them to the various enhancement algorithms.

Figure 1 is a normal case and Figs. 2 and 3 are abnormal cases. Figures 1, 2 and 3 show that QUM and RUM are improved unsharp masking, which can enhance image details. However, we can observe from Figs. 2(e), (f) and 3(e), (f), that the lesions may

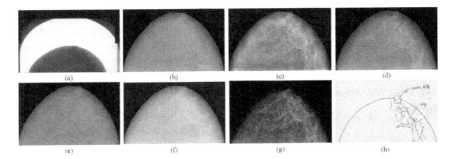

Fig. 1. Comparison of mammogram enhancement using different algorithms. (a) Original normal mammogram. (b) Positive film. (c) Enhanced result by CLAHE. (d) Enhanced result by NUM. (e) Enhanced result by QUM. (f) Enhanced result by RUM. (g) Enhanced result by our method. (h) Expert annotations.

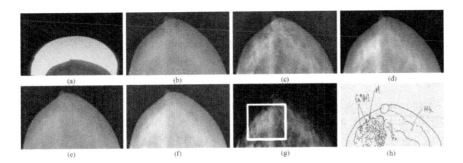

Fig. 2. Comparison of mammogram enhancement using different algorithms. (a) Original mammogram with mass and microcalcification. (b) Positive film. (c) Enhanced result by CLAHE. (d) Enhanced result by NUM. (e) Enhanced result by QUM. (f) Enhanced result by RUM. (g) Enhanced result by our method. (h) Expert annotations.

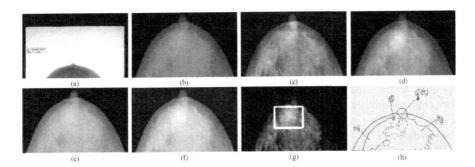

Fig. 3. Comparison of mammogram enhancement using different algorithms. (a) Original mammogram with mass and microcalcification. (b) Positive film. (c) Enhanced result by CLAHE. (d) Enhanced result by NUM. (e) Enhanced result by QUM. (f) Enhanced result by RUM. (g) Enhanced result by our method. (h) Expert annotations.

be still as difficult to detect as in the original images. From Figs. 2(d) and 3(d), although the NUM algorithm could suppress tissue information around the lesion, contrast is not clearly improved. CLAHE has better results than the above-mentioned, but it generates over enhancement in some regions, as shown in the Figs. 2(c) and 3(c). The proposed algorithm improves the contrast of mammograms and visual quality of the abnormal regions and removes the over-enhancement and background noise to a certain extent.

3.3   Objective Evaluation of Experimental Results

We used CII, PSNR, and DSM to measure the quality of the 30 abnormal mammograms. A higher score indicates better enhancement performance.

Table 2. Comparision average value of measure results based on different algorithms

	CLAHE	NUM	QUM	RUM	Our method
CII	0.94	1.25	0.95	0.95	**1.89**
PSNR	-0.01	0.01	0.04	-0.04	**0.21**
DSM	2.24	2.89	3.14	2.33	**4.43**

As shown in Table 2, the best results are boldfaced, our method produces higher values for CII, DSM, and PSNR, with the differences statistically significant.

4   Conclusion

We have proposed an adaptive mammographic image enhancement algorithm, which employs nonlinear transformation and neighborhood pixel information to enhance lesion. The luminance of the lesion region is generally higher than the normal tissue, the algorithm firstly reduces the luminance of the image and suppresses the background tissue information by using a nonlinear transfer function; then adaptive local contrast enhancement is achieved using a 2-D Gaussian convolution and image local standard deviation. We compared the proposed algorithm with several common enhancement algorithms both on objective and subjective performance. The experiment results show that our algorithm has better characteristics in most cases. The proposed algorithm can help improve the visualization of mammographic abnormalities, thereby it can be used in helping radiologists make accurate diagnosis.

Acknowledgment. This work is jointly supported by the National Natural Science Foundation of China (nos. 61175012 and 61201421), Natural Science Foundation of Gansu Province (nos. 145RJZA181), and the Fundamental Research Funds for the Central Universities of China (nos. lzujbky-2013-k06 and lzujbky-2015-196).

References

1. Tao, L., Asari, V.K.: Adaptive and integrated neighborhood-dependent approach for nonlinear enhancement of color images. J. Electron. Imaging **14**(4), 781–792 (2005)
2. Suckling, J., Parker, J., Dance, D.R., Astley, S., Hutt, I., Boggis, C., Ricketts, I., Stamatakis, E., Cerneaz, N., Kok, S.L., Taylor, P., Betal, D., Savage, J.: The mammographic image analysis society digital mammogram database. Excerpta Med. Int. Congr. Ser. **1069**, 375–378 (1994)
3. Japanese Society of Medical Imaging Technology. http://www.jamit.jp/cad-committe/caddbinfo. Accessed 11 Jan 2012
4. Guo, M., Dong, M., Wang, Z., Ma, Y.: A new method for mammographic mass segmentation based on parametric active contour model. In: Proceedings of IEEE Wavelet Analysis and Pattern Recognition Conference, pp. 27–33 (2015)
5. Pisano, E.D., Zong, S., Hemminger, B.M., Deluca, M., Johnston, R.E.: Contrast limited adaptive histogram equalization image processing to improve the detection of simulated spiculations in dense mammograms. J. Digit. Imaging **11**(4), 193–200 (1998)
6. Karen, P., Yicong, Z., Sos, A., Hongwei, J.: Nonlinear unsharp masking for mammogram enhancement. IEEE Trans. Inf Technol. Biomed. **15**(6), 918–928 (2011)
7. Hari, V.S., Gopikakumari, R.: Unsharp masking using quadratic filter for the enhancement of fingerprints in noisy background. Pattern Recogn. **46**(12), 3198–3207 (2013)
8. Ramponi, G., Polesel, A.: Rational unsharp masking technique. J. Electron. Imaging **7**(2), 333–338 (1998)
9. Tao, L., Asari, V.K.: Adaptive and integrated neighborhood-dependent approach for nonlinear enhancement of color images. J. Electron. Imaging **14**(4), 781–792 (2005)

A Hybrid Detection Scheme of Architectural Distortion in Mammograms Using Iris Filter and Gabor Filter

Mizuki Yamazaki[1], Atsushi Teramoto[1(✉)], and Hiroshi Fujita[2]

[1] Graduate School of Health Sciences, Fujita Health University, Aichi, Japan
82015309@fujita-hu.ac.jp
[2] Graduate School of Medicine, Gifu University, Gifu, Japan

Abstract. Architectural distortion in mammograms is the most frequently missed finding among breast cancer findings, the improvement of detection accuracy in existing commercial CAD software remains a challenge. In this study, in order to improve the detection accuracy of architectural distortion in mammography, we propose a hybrid automatic detection method that combines with the enhancement method of the concentration of line structure and massive pattern. In the method, the detection of the concentration of the line structure is conducted by the adaptive Gabor filter, and the enhancement of the massive pattern is performed by the iris filter. The concentration index is calculated from these filtered images; the lesion candidate regions are obtained. As for false positive (FP) reduction, 15 shape features are calculated from the candidate regions. Then, they are given to the support vector machine; the candidate regions are classified either as true positive or FP. In the experiment, we compared the results of the proposed method and physician interpretation report using 200 images (63 architectural distortions) from a digital database of screening mammography. Experimental results indicate that our method may be effective to improve the performance of computer aided detection in mammography.

Keywords: Computer-aided diagnosis · Mammography · Architectural distortion

1 Introduction

Breast cancer is the most common cancer in women around the world. Mammography screening has been recommended for breast cancer average-risk women over the age of 45 in the United States [1]. However, because most image data is generated in the image diagnosis, it is feared that the burden on the human reader is too high. Recently, computer-aided diagnosis (CAD) is expected to improve the diagnostic performance by reducing the burden on the human reader and preventing the oversight of lesions [2]. CAD for mammography has been used practically. Among the representative findings of breast cancer, it has reported that microcalcification and mass have detection accuracies of more than 90 %, whereas the detection accuracy of architectural distortion is low, approximately 60–80 % [3]. In order to improve the detection accuracy of architectural distortion, many studies have been conducted: Ichikawa et al. analyzed the

© Springer International Publishing Switzerland 2016
A. Tingberg et al. (Eds.): IWDM 2016, LNCS 9699, pp. 174–182, 2016.
DOI: 10.1007/978-3-319-41546-8_23

area of distortion in mammary glands using the mean curvature [4], Gou et al. developed the learning detection method by Fractal analysis and support vector machine, and compared their result with the results of neural networks [5]. Rangayyan et al. analyzed the mammary gland structure by using the Gabor filter [6]. In order to solve this problem, we developed a detection method as well that employed the Gabor filter [7]. However, it was difficult to detect distortion inside the highly concentrated mammary glands. Furthermore, the Gabor filter did not detect the distortion in case of plural findings at the same position in mammography.

In this study, we focus on the image feature of architectural distortion. Architectural distortion has been defined as the distortion and retraction of the breast structure [8]. Therefore, it seems that the obtained image characteristics tend to be massive patterns such as mass because the centers of retraction have low density in the image. In addition, both architectural distortion and mass are often observed in the invasive breast cancer in a mammogram. In order to improve the detection accuracy of architectural distortion in mammography, we propose a hybrid automatic detection method that combines with the enhancement method of the concentration of line structure and massive pattern. Further, we tried to improve the detection accuracy by a false positive (FP) reduction technique using the support vector machine (SVM).

2   Methods

Line structure enhancement processing and massive pattern enhancement processing are applied to the mammogram using the proposed method. After the candidate regions obtained from each processing are integrated, 15 shape features are calculated in each region. The shape features are input to SVM, the candidate regions are classified as true positive (TP) or FP. The procedure of the proposed method is described by the flowchart shown Fig. 1.

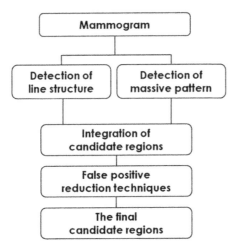

Fig. 1. Flowchart of the proposed method

2.1   Enhancement of Concentration of Line Structure

Normal mammary gland travels radially from the nipple; however, architectural distortion is a disturbance of this structure. In order to analyze the travelling of the mammary gland, the line structure is emphasized and detected using the adaptive Gabor filter that we have developed so far. In addition, architectural distortion often entails local retraction of the mammary gland, which is detected as the region of emphasis on the concentration of line structure. The processing procedure is described below.

(1) Preprocessing

By applying automatic binarization using the triangle method [9] and labeling to the original mammogram, unnecessary markers and noise are extracted from the breast region. The triangle method is for automatically calculating the threshold value using the density distribution curve $h(x)$ (x: density) that is obtained by density histogram. In the density distribution curve $h(x)$, the point where the end part of the low density side (the position of $h(x) > 0$) and the point where $h(x)$ is maximized are connected by a straight line. A perpendicular line is taken down to $h(x)$ from each position on the straight line. The position of the perpendicular line that maximizes the distance from both of the intersection until the straight line is searched. The intersection of the obtained perpendicular and $h(x)$ is found, and the corresponding value of the density x becomes threshold value.

(2) Detection of mammary gland

The mammary gland is detected by applying an adaptive Gabor filter. The Gabor filter is applied to detect the intensity and the direction of local line structure in the image [10, 11]. The operation expressions of the Gabor filter are shown in Eqs. (1)–(4).

$$g_\theta(x,y) = \exp\left(-\frac{x'^2 + \gamma^2 y'^2}{2\sigma^2}\right) \cos\left(2\pi\frac{x'}{\lambda}\right) \tag{1}$$

$$h_\theta(x,y) = f(x,y) \otimes g_\theta(x,y) \tag{2}$$

$$I(x,y) = \max_\theta[h_\theta(x,y)] \tag{3}$$

$$A(x,y) = \operatorname*{argmax}_\theta[h_\theta(x,y)] \tag{4}$$

In Eq. (1), the Gabor filter function has an anisotropic shape as shown in Fig. 2. σ is the standard deviation of the Gauss function, which is the parameter that determines the length of the long axis direction. γ represents the spatial aspect ratio of the Gabor function. λ is the wavelength; it is the parameter that adjusts the width of the short axis direction of the filter function. Further, we decide $x' = x\cos\theta + y\sin\theta$ and $y' = -x\sin\theta + y\cos\theta$, because the filter function $g_\theta(x, y)$ is rotated by an angle θ in the x-y plane.

As shown in Eq. (2), the Gabor filter performs a convolution of the original image $f(x, y)$ and the Gabor function $g_\theta(x, y)$ while θ is changed. The angle θ for which

$h_\theta(x, y)$ becomes maximum is calculated ($=\theta_{max}$). The angle θ_{max} becomes $A(x, y)$, $h_\theta(x, y)$ that is calculated using θ_{max} becomes $I(x, y)$. In Eqs. (3) and (4), the intensity output image $I(x, y)$ and the angle output image $A(x, y)$ are shown.

Further, mammary gland detection accuracy using the Gabor filter is significantly affected by the parameters of the Gabor function; therefore, it is not possible to set the parameters that detect all mammary gland patterns. Therefore, adaptive Gabor filter has plural Gabor filters that have different parameter sets, and the optimal filter (best fit filter) is selected for each pixel. This allows improvement in detection accuracy of line patterns compared to a single Gabor filter.

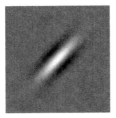

Fig. 2. Gabor filter function ($\sigma = 4.30$, $\gamma = 0.45$, $\lambda = 13.0$)

(3) Enhancement of the pattern of line concentration

To detect the concentration of the mammary gland structure, the primary mammary gland is detected by $I(x, y)$ and $A(x, y)$. Concentration of the mammary glands caused by retraction and spicula is detected using the concentration index [12].

(4) Extraction of candidate regions

The automatic binarization process is applied to the concentration index image. The number of candidate regions and pixel summation are changed by changing the binarization threshold. While changing the threshold for binarization, the number of candidate regions are counted. To increase the detection accuracy, the binarization is performed by the threshold value for which the largest number of candidate regions are detected, and the initial candidate regions of architectural distortion are obtained.

2.2 Enhancement of Massive Pattern

Regarding the detection of a massive pattern in a mammogram, the enhancement of the massive pattern and thresholding are conducted as follows. In a similar manner to the detection of concentration of line structure, processing is applied only to the breast area obtained in Sect. 2.1.

(1) Enhancement of massive pattern

The mass of breast cancer has massive structure, because there is the feature that the density in the image decreases toward the center from the edge of the mass, the gradient vector of changing density of each pixel in the mass is concentrated toward its center.

Architectural distortion is the finding of breast cancer that has distortion and retraction of the breast structure. Therefore, it seems that it has the massive pattern like mass and the gradient vector concentrates toward the center. In order to calculate the concentration index of the gradient vector, the iris filter [13] is used in this study. By using the iris filter, the concentration index is calculated from the angle information of the gradient vector of each pixel. As shown in Fig. 3, the pixels on the radial line of the N that are extended in any direction from the interest pixel are used. In each the radiation of the N, the range that maximizes the average of the cosine value of the angle formed by the direction from each pixel to the center point and the gradient vector at each pixel is searched. The concentration index c_j in that direction is the average of the cosine value in obtained range, as shown Eq. (5). The $\cos\theta_{ij}$ is the centrality evaluation value on the j-th of radiation and in radius vector i. R is the outer diameter of the filter and the r is the inner diameter when the pixel of interest is in the center. The iris filter output $C(x, y)$ is the average of the c_j obtained in all directions, as shown Eq. (6).

$$c_j = \max\left\{\sum_{i=0}^{n} \cos\theta_{ij}/i\right\}, R \leq n < r \tag{5}$$

$$C(x, y) = \frac{1}{N}\sum_{j=0}^{N} c_j \tag{6}$$

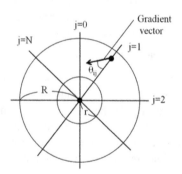

Fig. 3. Conceptual diagram of the iris filter

(2) Extraction of candidate regions

The concentration index image obtained from the iris filter is binarized; candidate regions of massive pattern enhancement process are extracted.

(3) Integration and FP reduction

The integrated candidate regions are obtained by taking the logical sum of the obtained candidate regions from each method.

Then, for FP reduction, shape features that reflect characteristics of architectural distortion and normal mammary gland structure are calculated for each candidate region. Shape features have 15 types: circularity, perimeter, average in the candidate region, contrast of the margin and center, etc. The calculated shape features are given to the SVM, which classifies FP and TP. The candidate regions that are not deleted as FPs are regarded as the final candidate regions.

3 Experiments

3.1 The Evaluation

In order to confirm the effectiveness of the proposed method, we conducted an evaluation using clinical images. We used 50 cases and 200 images provided by the Digital Database for Screening Mammography (DDSM) that has been published in the United States. This includes 20 normal cases and 30 abnormal cases with architectural distortion. The physician's report that has been attached to the data reveals that the 200 images have 63 architectural distortions. Further, there have been included cases that have architectural distortion only as well as cases with architectural distortion in mass. We evaluated the true-positive rate (TPR) of architectural distortion and FP in images, using physician's report and detection result. In addition, the previous method was applied in the same images, and we compared with TPR and FPs in the previous method and the proposed method. Furthermore, detection accuracy by performing FP reduction was also evaluated.

3.2 Results

In the initial detection without FP reduction, 54 architectural distortions were detected using by the proposed method, TPR was 85.7 %, and the FPs per image was 4.83. An example of a processing result is shown in Fig. 4. The examples of detected and undetected architectural distortion are shown in Figs. 5 and 6, respectively.

4 Discussion

From the result of evaluation by using clinical images, TPR of the initial detection by the proposed method was 85.7 %. That of our previous method was 82.45 %; The detection accuracy was improved over the previous method. The proposed method is added to the massive pattern enhancement process of the previous method, which could detect clearly massive shadow as mass. Moreover, it was possible to detect the massive pattern that secondarily occurred in the spicula and the around of retraction of the mammary gland structure. Therefore, it was shown from the evaluation result that the proposed method was effective to detect architectural distortion accompanied by mass. It is possible that the architectural distortion that could not be detected by the proposed method was excluded from the candidate regions by binarization, because the output value of each filter became small. Furthermore, due to the shape features, it is possible that the candidate regions are considered FPs by FP reduction processing.

After applying the FP reduction, FPs per image was 3.41 with the same TPR as initial detection. Using FP reduction method, 30 % of FPs were reduced; It became clear that the number of FP could be reduced by using SVM. Many FP regions that were not completely removed existed in locally high density in the image and high concentration of mammary glands in the entire breast. In the future, the shape features that focus on image characteristics will be calculated, and it will be necessary to consider more detailed FP reduction techniques.

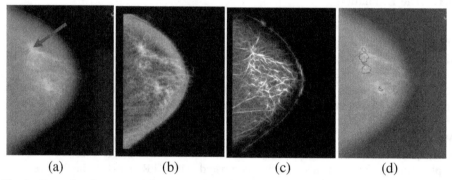

(a)   (b)   (c)   (d)

Fig. 4. Example of automated detection using clinical image. Arrow indicates the architectural distortion. (a) Original image, (b) Iris filtered image, (c) Intensity image by adaptive Gabor filter, (d) Detection result

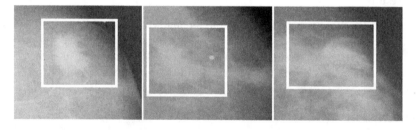

Fig. 5. Examples of detected architectural distortion

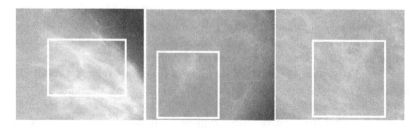

Fig. 6. Examples of undetected architectural distortion

5   Conclusion

In this study, in order to improve the detection accuracy of architectural distortion in mammography, we proposed a hybrid automatic detection method that combined with the enhancement method of the concentration of line structure and massive pattern. In the experiment using 50 cases (200 images) mammography, out of 63 architectural distortions, 54 regions were detected, and the TPR was 85.7 % It was possible to detect architectural distortion accompanied with mass and the massive pattern that secondarily occurred. Furthermore, at that time, FPs without FP reduction was 4.83 per image. However, FPs with FP reduction by using SVM was 3.41 per image. From this result, it is clear that FP reduction with SVM using the shape features is an effective technique. As future challenges, it will be necessary to further improve the detection accuracy and consider more detailed FP reduction methods.

Acknowledgment. This research was supported in part by a Grant-in-Aid for Scientific Research on Innovative Areas (#26108005), MEXT, Japan.

References

1. Oeffinger, K.C., et al.: Breast Cancer screening for women at average risk 2015 guideline update from the American Cancer Society. JAMA **314**(15), 1599–1614 (2015)
2. Fujita, H.: Present status of mammography CAD system. Med. Imaging Technol. **20**(1), 27–33 (2003)
3. Hatanaka, Y., Matdubara, T., Hara, T., et al.: A comparison between physicians' interpretation and a CAD system's Cancer detection by using a Mammogram database in a physicians' self-learning course. Radiol. Phys. Tech. **58**(3), 375–382 (2002). In Japanese
4. Ichikawa, T., Matsubara, T., Fujita, H., et al.: An automated extraction method for region of architectural distortion with concentration of mammary gland on mammograms. IEICE Trans. D-II **87**(1), 348–352 (2004)
5. Guo, Q., Shao, J., Ruiz, V.: Investigation of support vector machine for the detection of architectural distortion in mammographic images. Institute of Physics Publishing **15**, 88–94 (2005)
6. Rangayyan, R.M., Ayres, F.J.: Gabor filter and phase portraits for the detection of architectural distortion in mammograms. Med. Bio. Eng. Comput. **44**, 883–894 (2006)
7. Yoshikawa, R., Teramoto, A., Matsubara, T., Fujita, H.: Detection of architectural distortion and analysis of mammary gland structure in mammograms using multiple Gabor filters. Med. Imaging Technol. **30**(5), 287–292 (2012). In Japanese
8. The Japan Radiological Society and The Japan Society of Radiological Technology: Mammography Guidelines, 3rd edn. Igaku-Shoin Ltd., Tokyo (2014). In Japan
9. Zack, G.W., Rogers, W.E., Latt, S.A.: Automatic measurement of sister chromatid exchange frequency. J. Histochem. Cytochem. **25**(7), 741–753 (1977)
10. Grigorescu, S.E., Petkov, N., Kruizinga, P.: Comparison of texture feature based on Gabor filter. IEEE Trans. Image Process. **11**(10), 1160–1167 (2002)

11. Yoshikawa, R., Teramoto, A., Matsubara, T., Fujita, H.: Automated detection of architectural distortion using improved adaptive Gabor filter. In: Fujita, H., Hara, T., Muramatsu, C. (eds.) IWDM 2014. LNCS, vol. 8539, pp. 606–611. Springer, Heidelberg (2014)
12. Megata, Y., Oza, K., et al.: Features of local concentration patterns in line figures and their applications. IEICE Trans. D-II **77**, 1178–1179 (1994). In Japanese
13. Takeo, H., Shimura, K., Kobatake, H., Nawano, S.: Computer-aided diagnosis in CR mammography. Fujifilm Res. Dev. **43**, 47–54 (1997). In Japanese

Performance of Breast Cancer Screening Depends on Mammographic Compression

Katharina Holland[1]([⊠]), Ioannis Sechopoulos[1], Gerard den Heeten[2],
Ritse M. Mann[1], and Nico Karssemeijer[1]

[1] Radboud University Medical Center,
PO Box 9101, 6500 HB Nijmegen, The Netherlands
katharina.holland@radboudumc.nl
[2] Academic Medical Center Amsterdam,
PO Box 22660, 1100 DD Amsterdam, The Netherlands

Abstract. During mammographic acquisition, the breast is compressed between the breast support plate and the compression paddle to improve image quality and reduce dose, among other reasons. The applied force, which is measured by the imaging device, varies substantially, due to local guidelines, positioning, and breast size. Force measurements may not be very relevant though, because the amount of compression will be related to pressure rather than force. With modern image analysis techniques, the contact surface of the breast under compression can be determined and pressure can be computed retrospectively. In this study, we investigate if there is a relation between pressure applied to the breast during compression and screening performance.

In a series of 113,464 screening exams from the Dutch breast cancer screening program we computed the compression pressure applied in the MLO projections of the right and left breasts. The exams were binned into five groups of increasing applied pressure, in such a way that each group contains 20 % of the exams. Thresholds were 7.68, 9.18, 10.71 and 12.81 kPa. Screening performance measures were determined for each group. Differences across the groups were investigated with a Pearson's Chi Square test.

It was found that PPV and the cancer detection rate vary significantly within the five groups (p = 0.001 and p = 0.011 respectively). The PPV was 25.4, 31.2, 32.7, 25.8 and 22.0 for the five groups with increasing pressure. The recall rate, false positive rate and specificity were not statistically significant from the expectation (p-values: 0.858, 0.088 and 0.094 respectively). Even though differences are not significant, there is a trend that the groups with a moderate pressure have a better performance compared to the first and last category.

The results suggest that high pressure reduces detectability of breast cancer. The best screening results were found in the groups with a moderate pressure.

Keywords: Digital mammography · Screening · Performance · Pressure

© Springer International Publishing Switzerland 2016
A. Tingberg et al. (Eds.): IWDM 2016, LNCS 9699, pp. 183–189, 2016.
DOI: 10.1007/978-3-319-41546-8_24

1   Introduction

It is standard procedure to compress the breast during acquisition of a mammogram. The breast is compressed between the breast support plate and the compression paddle, causing a deformation of the breast into a more uniform thickness. Compression reduces the possibility of motion of the breast (and therefore motion artefacts), dose, tissue superposition and x-ray scatter [1–4]. A disadvantage of the compression is, that many women complain about discomfort and pain [5,6].

During the acquisition of the mammogram, the compression force is measured. There are however no clear guidelines about the applied force. The 'European guidelines for quality assurance in breast cancer screening and diagnosis' [7] for example say that: 'the compression of the breast tissue should be firm but tolerable', but no concrete values are given.

A better measurement for the compression might be the compression pressure. The pressure is defined as the force divided by the contact area. The contact area of the breast with the compression paddle depends strongly on the size of the breast. With the introduction of digital mammography, it is possible to save the applied force in the DICOM header and to estimate the contact area through image processing (e.g. with Volpara, Volpara Health Technologies, Wellington, New Zealand) or during the acquisition [8]. Therefore, it is possible to estimate the applied pressure. Previous studies have shown a considerable variation in pressure [9,10].

In the study by de Groot et al. [11] the force-standardized compression protocol was replaced by a pressure-standardized protocol. With the new protocol, the average pain score and the proportion of women experiencing severe pain was reduced by 10 % and 27 %, respectively, for medio lateral oblique (MLO) views, and 17 % and 32 %, respectively, in cranio caudal (CC) views, while for both protocols a similar average glandular dose and proportion of retakes was observed.

So far, it remains unknown how pressure affects screening performance. There might be an optimal pressure range, as too low or too high compression might reduce the ability to detect cancers. The aim of our study is to investigate screening program performance measures depending on the compression pressure applied during the acquisition of the mammogram. The results of this study might help to define better guidelines for the compression process during mammogram acquisition.

2   Methods

2.1   Data

In this study 'for processing' digital mammograms were used. The images are from the Dutch breast cancer screening program (Foundation of Population Screening Mid-West) in which women between 50–75 years of age are invited biennially to participate. Recall and breast cancer detection data was obtained from the screening registration system. All mammograms were acquired on Lorad Selenia systems (Hologic, Inc., Danbury, USA) between 2003–2011. A four month period in 2009 had to be excluded as no raw/'for processing' images were archived.

Institutional Review Board approval for this study was not required because the retrospective analysis of the anonymized mammograms does not fall within the remit of the Medical Research Involving Human Subject Act. However, a waiver to use the mammograms for research (in general) was obtained from the institutional review board.

In the screening program, MLO images and CC images were always acquired in the first screening round, while in subsequent screening rounds often only MLO images were taken. Additional CC images were taken in about 57 % of subsequent screening rounds, when an indication for an abnormality or high breast density was present. This number increased gradually and since 2014 it is obligatory to obtain two views in all rounds. In this study, only MLO images were used as MLO images were always acquired. In this way the systematic differences that exist in force and pressure between MLO and CC images are excluded from our results.

For the purposes of this study, the interval to determine the truth is defined as the interval up to the next screening round. Screen detected cancers (true positives (TP)) are defined as the cancers diagnosed after a recall of women for additional diagnostic tests. False positive (FP) examinations are exams of women recalled for additional tests in which no breast cancer was diagnosed. True negative (TN) examinations are examinations that did not lead to a recall and after which no breast cancer was diagnosed. Interval cancers are defined as the cancers that were found in the interval between the last examination and the next scheduled examinations. They are also called false negative (FN) examinations. All known FN examinations were excluded from the analysis. The remaining not recalled examinations are called negative examinations throughout this study, as it is unclear whether all examinations are TN examinations.

A research version of the software Volpara (version 1.5.0) was used to determine the pressure applied for the right and left MLO view. The algorithm determines the contact area between breast and compression paddle by image processing and reads the applied force measured by the acquisition system from the DICOM header. Volumetric percent density (PDV) was also determined with the software. Results of the left and right MLO views of each exam were averaged, resulting in a single score. In cases in which only one pressure estimate was available this estimate was used. The average pressure measurement was used to subdivide the exams in our study into five groups. Thresholds were chosen in such a way that each group contains 20 % of the exams.

2.2 Statistical Analysis

Many women in the data set had more than one screening examination. All examinations were used as independent samples, assuming that the applied compression depends on the technician and not on the indivudual women. Within the five groups the following performance measures with 95 % confidence intervals were determined: recall rate (number of women recalled among 1000 examinations), false positive rate (number of false positive results among 1000 examinations), screen detected breast cancer rate (number of screen detected breast cancers among 1000 women screened), specificity (number of negatives divided by the sum of the number of negatives and false positives), and positive predictive value (PPV - number of true positives divided by the number of recalls).

Differences across the different pressure groups were tested with the Pearson's Chi Square test. The way compression is applied to the breast might depend on the tissue composition of the breast. Therefore, the relationship between pressure and breast density was investigated and the coefficient of determination (R^2) was calculated.

3   Results

In total 113,956 examinations were available. Excluding examinations with unknown screening outcome, exams prior to an interval cancer (i.e. not detected in screening), and exams without available pressure measurement, 113,464 examinations of 54137 women were included in the analysis for this study. The pressure estimate was based on only one image in 3 exams with cancers, 15 false positive examinations, and 835 negative examinations.

To get the five groups, thresholds on the average pressure were applied at 7.68, 9.18, 10.71 and 12.81 kPa (group 1: 0 kPa < pressure ≤ 7.68 kPa, group 2: 7.68 kPa < pressure ≤ 9.18 kPa, group 3: 9.18 kPa < pressure ≤ 10.71 kPa, group 4: 10.71 kPa < pressure ≤ 12.81 kPa, group 5: pressure > 12.81 kPa).

Of the 113,464 examinations, 2,439 exams were recalled and 668 breast cancers were found. The number of false positives was 1,771 and 111,025 exams were negative. Table 1 gives an overview of the cancers, false positives and negatives across the five categories. The p-value of the associated Pearson's Chi Square test is 0.007. Next to the actual count, the expected count is displayed. In group three and four, more screen detected cancers and less false positive examinations were found than expected.

The overview of the screening performance measures is given in Table 2. Significant differences across the five groups are seen for the PPV and the cancer rate. Here the highest PPV is observed in group 3. No statistically significant differences were found in the recall rate and the false positive rate. Even though differences are not significant, there is a trend that the groups with a moderate pressure have lower false positive rate compared to the first and last groups. And that the highest pressure reduces the cancer detection rate.

The coefficient of determination (R^2) between breast density and pressure is 0.122. So, variation in percent breast density can account for only 12.2 % of the variation in applied pressure.

Table 1. Number of screen detected cancers, false positive examinations and negative examinations in the study population and in the five pressure classes, with in brackets the expected count and in gray the percentage of cases.

	total	group 1	group 2	group 3	group 4	group 5
N	113464	22739 20.0%	22816 20.1%	22598 19.9%	22636 19.9%	22675 20.0%
Screen detected cancer	668	126 18.9% (133.9)	149 22.3% (134.3)	161 24.1% (133.0)	122 18.3% (133.3)	110 16.5% (133.5)
False positive examinations	1771	371 20.9% (355.1)	328 18.5% (355.9)	331 18.7% (352.3)	351 19.8% (353.5)	390 22.0% (354.3)
Negative examinations	111025	22245 20.0% (22260.9)	22338 20.1% (22310.1)	22105 19.9% (22083.7)	22163 20.0% (22160.5)	22174 20.0% (22209.7)

Table 2. Screening performance measurements with 95% confidence intervals.

	Total	Group 1	Group 2	Group 3	Group 4	Group 5	Pearson's χ^2
Recall/1000	21.6 (20.7-22.3)	21.9 (20.0-23.8)	20.9 (19.0-22.8)	21.8 (19.9-23.7)	20.9 (19.0-22.8)	22.1 (20.1-24.0)	0.858
FP/1000	15.6 (14.9-16.3)	16.3 (14.7-18.0)	14.4 (12.8-15.9)	14.6 (13.1-16.2)	15.5 (13.9-17.1)	17.2 (15.5-18.9)	0.088
Cancers/1000	5.9 (5.4-6.3)	5.5 (4.6-6.5)	6.5 (5.5-7.6)	7.1 (6.0-8.2)	5.4 (4.4-6.3)	4.9 (3.9-5.8)	0.011
Specificity (%)	98.4 (98.4-98.5)	98.4 (98.2-98.5)	98.6 (98.4-98.7)	98.5 (98.4-98.7)	98.4 (98.3-98.6)	98.3 (98.1-98.4)	0.094
PPV (%)	27.4 (25.6-29.2)	25.4 (21.5-29.2)	31.2 (27.1-35.4)	32.7 (28.6-36.9)	25.8 (21.9-29.7)	22.0 (18.4-25.6)	0.001

4   Discussion and Conclusion

In this study, differences in performance measures were observed with respect to different pressure categories. Although only PPV is statistically significant different between the groups (also in case of applying Bonferroni correction for multiple testing), it can be observed that a better performance is observed for most measures for the groups with a moderate pressure (group $2 + 3$), compared to the other groups. These findings suggest, that a too low or too high compression may reduce screening program performance.

The results might be used to improve the compression process during the mammogram acquisition. Instead of controlling force, pressure could be used actively, for example with the setup explained in [8]. Furthermore, guidelines could be more specific in their recommendations, going from a descriptive recommendation ('firm but tolerable') to a quantitative recommendation in kPa.

So far, screening performance was measured with the true positives (screen detected breast cancers), false positives and negatives. Some cancers are however missed at screening and are detected in between screening rounds when they become symptomatic. It would be expected that the lower detection rate at high compression pressure would be reflected in an increase in the interval cancer rate in this group. Therefore, in future work we will look at the relation between interval cancer rate and pressure.

In this work we used a binning that created five groups, each containing 20 % of the exams. The bin width is however not the same for all groups. Especially the first and the last group cover a large range of values. An alternative binning, based on the compression pressure distribution, will be investigated.

Acknowledgements. The research leading to these results has received funding from the European Union's Seventh Framework Programme FP7 under grant agreement no 306088.

Special thanks to the Foundation of Population Screening Mid-West for providing the images and Ralph Highnam at Volpara for providing access to the Volpara Software.

References

1. Chen, B., Wang, Y., Sun, X., Guo, W., Zhao, M., Cui, G., Hu, L., Li, P., Ren, Y., Feng, J., Yu, J.: Analysis of patient dose in full field digital mammography. Eur. J. Radiol. **81**(5), 868–872 (2012)
2. Heine, J.J., Cao, K., Thomas, J.A.: Effective radiation attenuation calibration for breast density: compression thickness influences and correction. Biomed. Eng. Online **9**, 73 (2010)
3. Kopans, D.B.: Breast Imaging, 3rd edn. Lippincott Williams & Wilkins (2007)
4. Saunders Jr., R.S., Samei, E.: The effect of breast compression on mass conspicuity in digital mammography. Med. Phys. **35**(10), 4464–4473 (2008)
5. Dullum, J.R., Lewis, E.C., Mayer, J.A.: Rates and correlates of discomfort associated with mammography. Radiology **214**(2), 547–552 (2000)
6. Keefe, F.J., Hauck, E.R., Egert, J., Rimer, B., Kornguth, P.: Mammography pain and discomfort: a cognitive-behavioral perspective. Pain **56**(3), 247–260 (1994)

7. Perry, N., Broeders, M., de Wolf, C., Törnberg, S., Holland, R., Karsa, L.V.: European Guidelines for Quality Assurance in Breast Cancer Screeningand Diagnosis, 4 edn. (2008)

8. de Groot, J.E., Broeders, M.J.M., Branderhorst, W., den Heeten, G.J., Grimbergen, C.A.: A novel approach to mammographic breast compression: Improved standardization and reduced discomfort by controlling pressure instead of force. Med. Phys. 40(8), 081901 (2013)

9. Branderhorst, W., de Groot, J.E., Highnam, R., Chan, A., Böhm-Vélez, M., Broeders, M.J.M., den Heeten, G.J., Grimbergen, C.A.: Mammographic compression-a need for mechanical standardization. Eur. J. Radiol. 84(4), 596–602 (2015)

10. Mercer, C.E., Hogg, P., Lawson, R., Diffey, J., Denton, E.R.E.: Practitioner compression force variability in mammography: a preliminary study. Br. J. Radiol. 86(1022), 20110596 (2013)

11. de Groot, J.E., Branderhorst, W., Grimbergen, C.A., den Heeten, G.J., Broeders, M.J.M.: Towards personalized compression in mammography: a comparison study between pressure- and force-standardization. Eur. J. Radiol. 84(3), 384–391 (2015)

Monte Carlo Evaluation of Normalized Glandular Dose Coefficients in Mammography

Antonio Sarno[1,2(✉)], Giovanni Mettivier[1,2], Francesca Di Lillo[1,2], and Paolo Russo[1,2]

[1] Dipartimento di Fisica "Ettore Pancini", Università di Napoli "Federico II", Naples, Italy
[2] INFN Sezione di Napoli, Naples, Italy
{sarno,mettivier,dilillo,russo}@na.infn.it

Abstract. The mean glandular dose in mammography is evaluated via the normalized glandular dose coefficients (DgN), calculated via Monte Carlo simulations. The conversion from dose to the homogenous mixture to dose in the glandular tissue is made by considering an energy-dependent correction factor, G, which is the weighted mean of the energy absorption coefficients of adipose and glandular tissues. The authors implemented a GEANT4 code and evaluated, in the range 8–80 keV, the influence on the calculation of DgN values by (1) the method of G-weighting the dose, (2) the inclusion of bremsstrahlung radiation and (3) the energy threshold under which electrons are not tracked. The results for monochromatic DgN show that evaluating G retrospectively causes an underestimation up to 5 %, and that not considering bremsstrahlung or setting high electron energy cutoff may cause a bias up to 1 %, in the calculation of monochromatic DgN. These deviations may be negligible for polychromatic mammographic spectra.

Keywords: Breast cancer · Mammography · Breast dosimetry · Mean glandular dose · DgN

1 Introduction

In X-ray breast imaging, the mean dose to the glandular tissue (mean glandular dose – MGD), which is the radiosensitive part of the breast, is the reference dosimetric parameter. It is evaluated via Monte Carlo (MC) simulations, by computing the normalized glandular dose (DgN) factors that relate the MGD to the entrance surface air kerma (ESAK) at the entrance skin plane, as:

$$MGD = DgN \times ESAK \tag{1}$$

The MGD was proposed by Hammestein et al. in 1979 [1], and, today, coefficients provided by Wu et al. [2] in the USA and Dance et al. [3] in Europe represent the standard to compute the MGD.

In dose simulations, the breast is usually modeled as a homogeneous mixture of glandular and adipose tissue; then, in order to take into account exclusively the dose to the glandular tissue, the deposited energy is suitably weighted by a G factor, which depends on the photon energy E, evaluated as in Eq. (2)

© Springer International Publishing Switzerland 2016
A. Tingberg et al. (Eds.): IWDM 2016, LNCS 9699, pp. 190–196, 2016.
DOI: 10.1007/978-3-319-41546-8_25

$$G(E) = \frac{f_g \times \frac{\mu_{en}}{\rho}(E)_g}{f_g \times \frac{\mu_{en}}{\rho}(E)_g + (1 - f_g) \times \frac{\mu_{en}}{\rho}(E)_a} \quad (2)$$

where f_g is the breast glandular fraction by weight, μ_{en}/ρ is the mass energy absorption coefficient and the subscripts g and a indicate glandular and adipose tissue, respectively [4]. Boone et al. [4] in mammography, and Mittone et al. [5] in computed tomography dedicated to the breast, evaluated the G factor retrospectively, by weighting *a posteriori* the average dose to the breast tissue, on the G factor computed at the energy of primary incident radiation. On the other hand, Wilkinson and Heggie [6] claimed that, in the evaluation of the MGD, the G factor has to be evaluated "interaction-by-interaction", in other terms at the current energy of the photon during the transport process. Moreover, the DgN is usually evaluated in MC simulations by supposing that electrons release dose locally and do not produce bremsstrahlung radiation in tissue. In this work, the effects of including in the MC calculations the bremsstrahlung radiation produced by secondary electrons and its influence on the two G-evaluation approaches are evaluated, together with the influence of the electron tracking energy cutoff.

2   Methods

The MC simulations have been performed via the GEANT4 toolkit version 4.10.00. The code included the electromagnetic physics list – option 4, as suggested by the AAPM TG-195 [7]; this code was validated as suggested in the AAPM TG-195 [7]. In order to implement the different cases here investigated, the MC simulations were performed either by excluding the bremsstrahlung radiation or by including this process. Moreover, the MGD was evaluated either with default electron energy cutoff (by fixing the minimum range of tracked electrons to 1 mm corresponding to 342 keV energy cutoff in 20 % glandular breast tissue) or by setting the minimum electron range to 1 μm (corresponding to 990 eV energy cutoff in 20 % glandular breast tissue for GEANT4 toolkit). The ESAK was evaluated at the entrance skin plane, by scoring the photon flux on a 5-cm diameter circle at 2.5 cm from the chest wall and by computing the mono-chromatic air kerma as the photon energy fluence times the mass energy absorption coefficient of air. The DgN coefficients were then obtained by dividing the calculated MGD for the ESAK. At each energy, 10^8 photons were generated in order to achieve a coefficient of variation (the ratio between the standard deviation and the mean value of thesimulated quantity) of about 0.1 %. The statistical uncertainties were computed as suggested by Sempau et al. [8]. The breast was modeled as suggested in the AAPM TG-195 [7]. It is a 5-cm height semi-cylinder with diameter of 10 cm; the skin thickness is 2 mm; the patient body was modeled as a water box of volume $300 \times 300 \times 170$ mm^3; two PMMA compression plates (2 mm thick) were included. The isotropic X-ray source was at 595 mm from the upper surface of the breast skin and it was elec-tronically collimated in order to radiate exclusively a 140×260 mm^2 detector located at 15 mm from the bottom surface of the compressed breast. The breast material compo-sition was that suggested by Hammerstein et al. [1]. The G factor was computed via the mass energy absorption coefficients μ_{en}/ρ suggested by Fedon et al. [9] for the breast glandular and adipose tissues.

3 Results

Figure 1 shows in graphical form the validation of DgN data in this work against the data provided by Boone [10] with the SIERRA MC code. For this specific test (which shows an agreement of 0.2 % in terms of deviation from unity of the slope of the linear fitting function) the skin thickness of the breast was increased from 2 mm to 4 mm to match the geometry adopted in ref. [10]. Figure 2 shows the percentage deviation of the monochromatic DgN values (in the range 8-80 keV) among the cases under study. The deviation was calculated following Eq. 3:

$$\text{Percent deviation} = 100 \times \frac{\text{DgN}_r - \text{DgN}_x}{\text{DgN}_r} \tag{3}$$

where the subscription r indicates the reference value, and the subscript x indicates the generic case under study. Figure 2a is for 5-cm compressed breast thickness, while Fig. 2b is for 10-cm compressed breast thickness. At each energy, the reference value (i.e. deviation = 0 %) is that obtained by considering the bremsstrahlung processes in the simulations and by tracking electron with energy down to 990 eV in the breast. With reference to this condition, the deviation was evaluated either when bremsstrahlung production is excluded - both evaluating the G factor *a posteriori* (dashed line) or inter-action-by-interaction (cross symbols) - or when bremsstrahlung processes are included in the MC simulations and the default electron energy cutoff is set (continuous line). There is no significant difference if the G factor is evaluated interaction-by-interaction,

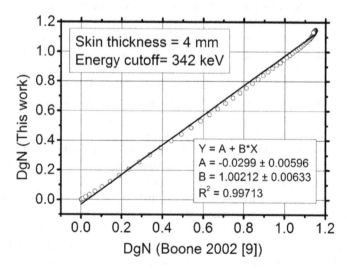

Fig. 1. DgN data validated with data in Ref. [9] by simulating a breast with 4-mm skin thickness and with a default cutoff for electron tracking; a linear fit shows an agreement within 0.2 %.

whether the bremsstrahlung process is excluded or it is included, but the default electron energy cutoff is set. These two cases present a maximum percentage deviation of 1 %, and determine an overestimation of DgN of about 1 % at 50 keV, both for a compressed breast thickness of 5 cm (Fig. 2a) or 10 cm (Fig. 2b). The process of G-weighting *a posteriori* the deposited dose leads to a DgN underestimation of 1 % at 40 keV, up to 5 % at 80 keV for a compressed breast thickness of 10 cm.

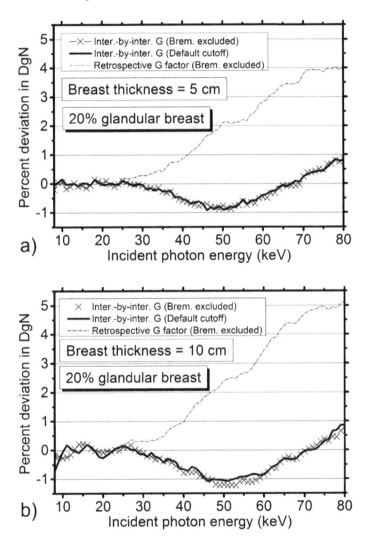

Fig. 2. Percentage deviation of DgN from the low energy electron cutoff simulation in the cases of bremsstrahlung processes exclusion, with retrospective G factor weighting (dashed line) and with interaction-by-interaction weighting (crossed line) and in the case of simulation with default electron energy cutoff and interaction-by-interaction weighting (crossed symbol).

Figure 3 shows DgN values, in the various simulated cases, for two polychromatic mammographic spectra: Mo/Mo 32 kV (filter thickness = 30 μm; mean energy = 17.3 keV) and W/Rh 40 kV (filter thickness = 50 μm; mean energy = 21.5 keV). The uncertainty reported is due exclusively to the statistical precision of the simulations. For the former spectrum there are no significant differences in polychromatic DgN values between the examined cases. Differences up to 0.5 % can be observed with the W/Rh spectrum at 40 kV.

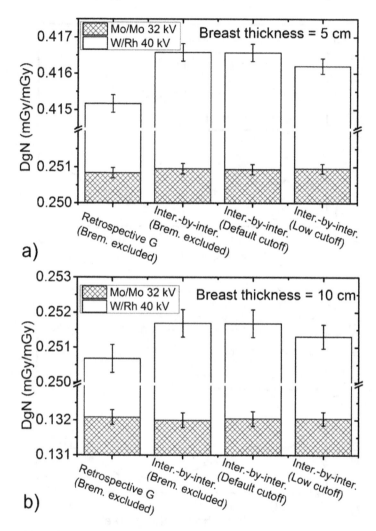

Fig. 3. DgN for polychromatic spectra (Mo/Mo 32 kV and W/Rh 40 kV) for a compressed breast thickness of 5 cm (a) and 10 cm (b).

4   Conclusions

In principle, breamsstrahlung photons (produced by slowing down electrons generated by interaction of a primary or secondary photon in breast tissue) should be taken into account (e.g. via a suitably defined G factor) when calculating the DgN values for mammography with MC simulations. To the authors' knowledge, this does not occur for published DgN data with various MC codes. This work, performed using a GEANT4 MC code validated against TG 195 data [7], shows that the exclusion of bremsstrahlung processes produces an overestimation in monochromatic DgN up to 1 % at about 50 keV primary photon energy. Moreover, it confirmed the occurrence of an underestimation caused by the retrospective G-weighting of the dose deposited in the breast, of 1 % at 40 keV and 5 % at 80 keV, for 20 % glandular fraction and 10-cm thick breast. However, differences in polychromatic DgN may be negligible in the case of mammographic spectra, up to 0.5 % for a W/Rh spectrum at 40 kV.

In recent works [11, 12], the homogeneous breast assumption in MC simulations has been shown to overestimate the dose to the breast of about 30 % compared to the dose estimated via an anthropomorphic breast phantom with a real glandular tissue distribution. Moreover, *in vivo* evaluation via computed tomography dedicated to the breast [13] demonstrated that breast skin thickness is about 1.45 mm on the average instead of the 5 mm (of adipose shielding) supposed in the EU quality assurance protocol. Simulating a breast skin thickness of 1.45 mm instead of 4 mm might overestimate the DgN by about 15 % for a Mo/Mo mammographic spectrum [13]. Compared to these results, the bias showed in this work, related to the electron energy cutoff, results much lower. Further improved determinations via MC simulations will be performed by the authors' group, aiming at revisiting models adopted for the DgN calculation in mammography.

References

1. Hammerstein, G.R., et al.: Adsorbed radiation dose in mammography 1. Radiology **130**(2), 485–491 (1979)
2. Wu, X., et al.: Spectral dependence of glandular tissue dose in screen-film mammography. Radiology **179**(1), 143–148 (1991)
3. Dance, D.R.: Monte Carlo calculation of conversion factors for the estimation of mean glandular breast dose. Phys. Med. Biol. **35**(9), 1211–1219 (1990)
4. Boone, J.M.: Glandular breast dose for monoenergetic and high-energy X-ray beams: Monte Carlo assessment. Radiology **213**(1), 23–37 (1999)
5. Mittone, A., et al.: Radiation dose in breast CT imaging with monochromatic x-rays: simulation study of the influence of energy, composition and thickness. Phys. Med. Biol. **59**(9), 2199–2217 (2014)
6. Wilkinson, L., Heggie, C.P.: Glandular breast dose: potential errors. Radiology **213**, 1 (2001)
7. Sechopoulos, I., et al.: Monte Carlo reference data sets for imaging research: executive summary of the report of AAPM research committee task group 195. Med. Phys. **42**(10), 5679–5691 (2015)
8. Sempau, J., et al.: Monte Carlo simulation of electron beams from an accelerator head using PENELOPE. Phys. Med. Biol. **46**(4), 1163–1180 (2001)

9. Fedon, C., et al.: GEANT4 for breast dosimetry: parameters optimization study. Phys. Med. Biol. **60**(16), N311–N323 (2015)
10. Boone, J.M.: Normalized glandular dose (DgN) coefficients for arbitrary x-ray spectra in mammography: computer-fit values of Monte Carlo derived data. Med. Phys. **29**(5), 869–875 (2002)
11. Sechopoulos, I., et al.: Characterization of the homogeneous tissue mixture approximation in breast imaging dosimetry. Med. Phys. **39**(8), 5050–5059 (2012)
12. Hernandez, A.M., et al.: Breast dose in mammography is about 30 % lower when realistic heterogeneous glandular distributions are considered. Med. Phys. **42**(11), 6337–6348 (2015)
13. Huang, S.-Y., et al.: The effect of skin thickness determined using breast CT on mammographic dosimetry. Med. Phys. **35**(4), 1199–1206 (2008)

Breast Density Assessment Using Breast Tomosynthesis Images

Pontus Timberg[1](✉), Andreas Fieselmann[2], Magnus Dustler[1], Hannie Petersson[1], Hanna Sartor[3], Kristina Lång[4], Daniel Förnvik[1], and Sophia Zackrisson[3]

[1] Medical Radiation Physics, Department of Translational Medicine, Lund University, Skåne University Hospital, 205 02 Malmö, Sweden
pontus.timberg@med.lu.se
[2] Siemens Healthineers, Erlangen, Germany
[3] Medical Radiology, Department of Translational Medicine, Lund University, Skåne University Hospital, 205 02 Malmö, Sweden
[4] Unilabs AB, 205 02 Malmö, Sweden

Abstract. In this work we evaluate an approach for breast density assessment of digital breast tomosynthesis (DBT) data using the central projection image. A total of 348 random cases (both FFDM CC and MLO views and DBT MLO views) were collected using a Siemens Mammomat Inspiration tomosynthesis unit at Unilabs, Malmö. The cases underwent both BI-RADS 5th Edition labeling by radiologists and automated volumetric breast density analysis (VBDA) by an algorithm. Preliminary results showed an observed agreement of 70 % (weighted Kappa, $\kappa = 0.73$) between radiologists and VBDA using FFDM images and 63 % ($\kappa = 0.62$) for radiologists and VBDA using DBT images. Comparison between densities for FFDM and DBT resulted in high correlation ($r = 0.94$) and an observed agreement of 72 % ($\kappa = 0.76$). The automated analysis is a promising approach using low dose central projection DBT images in order to get radiologist-like density ratings similar to results obtained from FFDM.

Keywords: Breast density · BI-RADS · Mammography · Breast tomosynthesis

1 Introduction

Breast density is an independent risk factor for developing breast cancer [1–3]. In common practice radiologists visually evaluate breast density in mammograms. However, the visual evaluations have shown to be associated with some drawbacks such as being subjective and inconsistent and could be misleading if directly related to risk [4]. Hence, an increasing demand for robust and objective breast density assessment has arisen and software has been shown to produce both reliable and valid result using full-field digital mammography (FFDM) images [5]. There is also a request to be able to estimate glandular content in digital breast tomosynthesis (DBT) images and to obtain comparable results with that of FFDM. Another possible way, rather than only quantifying the content of dense tissue, is to take into account the dense tissue distribution and the masking effect on tumors. This has now been acknowledged in the revised breast

© Springer International Publishing Switzerland 2016
A. Tingberg et al. (Eds.): IWDM 2016, LNCS 9699, pp. 197–202, 2016.
DOI: 10.1007/978-3-319-41546-8_26

imaging-reporting and data system (BI-RADS) criteria in the 5th Edition [6]. For DBT, the existing approaches (whether automatic or semiautomatic) deal with the central projection image, which resembles more or less a low dose mammogram [7, 8].

The purpose of this study was to investigate the automated volumetric breast density analysis (VBDA) by comparing volumetric breast density (VBD) obtained for DBT images and FFDM images and conventional BI-RADS assessment by radiologists. The implementation in clinical practice and risk assessment of available methods, whether evaluated by radiologists or software methods, is out of the scope of this paper.

2   Materials and Methods

The automatic VBDA method computes volumetric breast density based on a physical model of the image acquisition process [9]. It assumes that the breast consists of fatty and glandular tissue. From a reference value of fat in the image, the known compressed breast thickness and the attenuation values of these two components the height of glandular tissue above each detector pixel can be estimated. The VBDA method also provides an alternative set of percent densities taking into account the effect of masking. This so called masking risk analysis is used to find local accumulated dense tissue regions that have a high probability of masking tumors. The outcome is a masking risk score that is computed by first determining connectivity of dense tissue in a density map using different thresholds and then finding the area of enclosed dense regions using morphological processing that utilizes a linear classifier and a non-linear mapping function [9]. The masking risk score is implemented in a certain percent VBD (%VBD) interval between categories (b) and (c) to mimic the BI-RADS 5th Edition criteria. BI-RADS 5th Edition is divided into breast composition categories: (a) entirely fatty breast; (b) scattered areas of fibroglandular density; (c) heterogeneously dense which may obscure small masses; and (d) extremely dense breast, which lowers the sensitivity of mammography.

The VBDA method was tested on 348 random cases (mean age of 57 ± 4 years, mean compressed breast thickness of 52 ± 13 mm) from the Malmö breast tomosynthesis screening trial (MBTST). The current study was approved by the Regional Ethical Review Board at Lund University (Dnr 2009/770). The MBTST is a population-based screening trial design to compare the screening efficacy of one-view DBT to two-view DM, described in more detail elsewhere [10]. All images were acquired on a single Mammomat Inspiration tomosynthesis unit (Siemens Healthcare GmbH, Erlangen, Germany) set to yield an average glandular dose of 1.2 mGy for a 53 mm standard breast comprised of 50 % glandularity in FFDM mode and 1.6 mGy in DBT mode [11]. All DBT images were acquired without an x-ray scatter grid. Four FFDM images (bilateral craniocaudals (CC) and mediolateral obliques (MLO) views) and two DBT projection image sets (bilateral MLOs) from each woman were available, allowing the average %VBD percentages to be determined for each breast. The %VBDs were converted to BI-RADS 5th Edition values using fixed %VBD thresholds. In cases where there was a discrepancy between the BI-RADS values of the left and right breast of a subject, the maximum value was chosen to avoid underestimation of density.

All FFDM cases were reviewed by four radiologists according to the BI-RADS 5th Edition criteria. The outcome, using a panel majority vote (PMV) per case, was compared with the VBDA method (using both FFDM CC and MLO images and DBT MLO images only). The MLO projections for both modalities were also compared using VBDA in terms of %VBD. Statistical analysis was performed using weighted Kappa (κ) and Pearson's correlation coefficient (r) to investigate agreement and correlation, respectively.

3 Results

The median breast volume of the DBT cases as estimated by VBDA was 698 cm^3 (range from 78 to 2450 cm^3) and the median %VBD was 5.0 % (range from 1.5 to 42.0 %). The result for the comparison of %VBD using DBT and FFDM MLO data from the VBDA method is presented in Fig. 1. The correlation coefficient and the observed agreement in density categories was r = 0.94 and 72 % (κ = 0.76), respectively. For the radiologists' BI-RADS labeling (using FFDM CC and MLO images) versus VBDA (DBT MLO) images the observed agreement was 63 % (κ = 0.62). For the radiologist's BI-RADS labeling versus VBDA FFDM images the observed agreement was 70 % (κ = 0.73). A confusion matrix for radiologists versus VBDA DBT is presented in Table 1, which shows the distribution of cases along each BI-RADS criterion.

Table 1. Confusion matrix of BI-RADS categories from radiologists' PMVs and VBDA using DBT images.

		BI-RADS (PMV)	BI-RADS (PMV)	BI-RADS (PMV)	BI-RADS (PMV)	
		a	b	c	d	*sum*
BI-RADS (VBDA)	a	**17**	17	0	0	*34*
BI-RADS (VBDA)	b	25	**136**	43	0	*204*
BI-RADS (VBDA)	c	0	19	**69**	1	*89*
BI-RADS (VBDA)	d	0	0	17	**4**	*21*
	sum	*42*	*172*	*129*	*5*	*348*

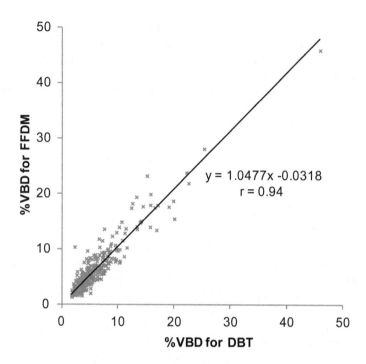

Fig. 1. Correlation of the DBT and FFDM %VBD data (includes a linear fit, equation and Pearson's correlation coefficient). The outlier at 50 % VBD was an extremely dense thin breast.

4   Discussion

The VBDA method provided a reasonably reliable way to automatically assess breast density, with an agreement in line with other published studies [8]. A moderate agreement ($\kappa = 0.55$) between radiologists and software determined scores in a large study population (using BI-RADS 4th Edition) was shown in a recent publication by Sartor et al. [12]. In another study by Lau et al. [13], automatic assessment of breast density was used on 315 cases acquired in combo mode to compare VBD from DBT projections and FFDM achieving a high agreement (κ of 0.79) and strong correlation ($r = 0.95$). It should be noted that their approach did not take into account the masking effect related to BI-RADS 5th Edition. Tagliafico et al. used a semiautomatic method comparing FFDM, DBT and magnetic resonance imaging (MRI) on 48 patients [7]. They found a high correlation ($r = 0.97$) with MRI for both DBT and FFDM. The results for FFDM did overestimate density by roughly 15 % compared to MRI and DBT which yielded similar density values.

The VBDA method assigned more cases to BI-RADS category (d) than the radiologists, and less to BI-RADS category (a). However, it is not clear if this represents an overestimation of the density and masking by the software, or an underestimation by the radiologists. The VBDA method calculates a relative density value, which is then assigned to a category based on certain pre-set thresholds, while the radiologists assign cases according to BI-RADS 5th Edition which is not entirely linear to the amount of density. Optimization of the thresholds separating the various categories could increase agreement between software and radiologists. Only in one single case (in the comparison of radiologists and VBDA BI-RADS ratings on FFDM images) was there a discrepancy of more than one category between radiologists' PMV and the VBDA score, which indicates that the differences between the software and the radiologists is likely to be minor.

One limitation in this study was that the evaluation by radiologists in FFDM images used both CC and MLO views, while the DBT images were only available in the MLO view. The software could hence not handle the contributing effect of the CC view which in turn may result in a changed BI-RADS rating and as a consequence lower agreement was observed. Also, using only the central projection rather than the whole projection set or the whole reconstructed DBT image volume for density assessment is a compromise. More image data is likely to improve breast density assessment and might be included in future releases. The cases were randomly selected with the drawback that rather few dense cases were included. An alternative approach would be to use equal amounts in each BI-RADS category.

In conclusion, the VBDA software may be a promising method of evaluating breast density. More validation studies are required, and reliable ways to match BI-RADS and VBD, as they cope with different approaches. It might be preferable that any association between risk, both of cancer and of masking, and volumetric density is studied directly without adding BI-RADS as a confounding factor.

Acknowledgdements. The authors would like to thank all participating radiologists at Unilabs Malmö. This work was financially supported by Siemens Healthcare GmbH (Erlangen, Germany) who also provided the breast tomosynthesis unit.

Disclaimer. The concepts and information presented in this paper are based on research and are not commercially available.

References

1. McCormack, V.A., dos Santos Silva, I.: Breast density and parenchymal patterns as markers of breast cancer risk: a meta-analysis. Cancer Epidemiol. Biomark. Prev. **15**, 1159–1169 (2006)
2. Boyd, N.F., Guo, H., Martin, L.J., Sun, L., Stone, J., Fishell, E., Jong, R.A., Hislop, G., Chiarelli, A., Minkin, S.: Mammographic density and the risk and detection of breast cancer. N. Engl. J. Med. **356**, 227–236 (2007)
3. Boyd, N.F., Martin, L.J., Yaffe, M.J., Minkin, S.: Mammographic density and breast cancer risk: current understanding and future prospects. Breast Cancer Res. **13**, 223 (2011)
4. Yaffe, M.J.: Mammographic density. Measurement of mammographic density. Breast Cancer Res. **10**, 1–10 (2008)
5. Alonzo-Proulx, O., Mawdsley, G.E., Patrie, J.T., Yaffe, M.J., Harvey, J.A.: Reliability of automated breast density measurements. Radiology **275**, 366–376 (2015)
6. D'Orsi, C.J., Sickles, E.A., Mendelson, E.B., Morris, E.A., et al.: ACR BI-RADS® Mammography. ACR BI-RADS Atlas, Breast Imaging Reporting and Data System, pp. 141–167 (2013)

7. Tagliafico, A., Tagliafico, G., Astengo, D., Airaldi, S., Calabrese, M., Houssami, N.: Comparative estimation of percentage breast tissue density for digital mammography, digital breast tomosynthesis, and magnetic resonance imaging. Breast Cancer Res. Treat. **138**, 311–317 (2013)

8. Highnam, R., Brady, S.M., Yaffe, M.J., Karssemeijer, N., Harvey, J.: Robust breast composition measurement - VolparaTM. In: Martí, J., Oliver, A., Freixenet, J., Martí, R. (eds.) IWDM 2010. LNCS, vol. 6136, pp. 342–349. Springer, Heidelberg (2010)

9. Fieselmann, A.: Volumetric breast density combined with masking risk: enhanced characterization of breast density from mammography images. In: IWDM Proceedings (2016)

10. Lång, K., Andersson, I., Rosso, A., Tingberg, A., Timberg, P., Zackrisson, S.: Performance of one-view breast tomosynthesis as a stand-alone breast cancer screening modality: results from the Malmö Breast Tomosynthesis Screening Trial, a population-based study. Eur. Radiol. **26**, 184–190 (2016)

11. Van Engen, R., Bouwman, R., Dance, D., Heid, P., Lazzari, B., Marshall, N., Schopphoven, S., Strudley, C., Thjissen, M., Young, K.: Protocol for the quality control of the physical and technical aspects of digital breast tomosynthesis system. EUREF, European Guidelines for Quality Assurance in Breast Cancer Screening and Diagnosis (2013)

12. Sartor, H., Lång, K., Rosso, A., Borgquist, S., Zackrisson, S., Timberg, P.: Measuring mammographic density: comparing a fully automated volumetric assessment versus European radiologists' qualitative classification. Eur. Radiol. 1–7 (2016)

13. Lau, S.K.H.N., Aziz, F.A., Highnam, R., Chan, A.: Volumetric breast density and mean glandular dose estimated from digital breast tomosynthesis projections and digital mammograms. World Congress on Medical Physics and Biomedical engineering, BR261-SD-WEB2 (2015)

Detailed Analysis of Scatter Contribution from Different Simulated Geometries of X-ray Detectors

Elena Marimon[1,2(✉)], Hammadi Nait-Charif[1], Asmar Khan[2],
Philip A. Marsden[3], and Oliver Diaz[4]

[1] Centre for Digital Entertainment, University of Bournemouth, Bournemouth, UK
{Elena.MarimonMunoz,hncharif}@bournemouth.ac.uk
[2] Dexela Ltd, PerkinElmer, London, UK
{Elena.Munoz,Asmar.khan}@perkinelmer.com
[3] Unitive Design, London, UK
phil@unitivedesign.co.uk
[4] ViCOROB Research Institute, University of Girona, Girona, Spain
oliver.diaz@udg.edu

Abstract. Scattering is one of the main issues left in planar mammography examinations, as it degrades the quality of the image and complicates the diagnostic process. Although widely used, anti-scatter grids have been found to be inefficient, increasing the dose delivered, the equipment price and not eliminating all the scattered radiation. Alternative scattering reduction methods, based on post-processing algorithms using Monte Carlo (MC) simulations, are being developed to substitute anti-scatter grids. Idealized detectors are commonly used in the simulations for the purpose of simplification. In this study, the scatter distribution of three detector geometries is analyzed and compared: Case 1 makes use of idealized detector geometry, Case 2 uses a scintillator plate and Case 3 uses a more realistic detector simulation, based on the structure of an indirect mammography X-ray detector. This paper demonstrates that common configuration simplifications may introduce up to 14 % of underestimation of the scatter in simulation results.

Keywords: Digital mammography · Scatter · Post-processing · Monte carlo · X-ray detector

1   Introduction

Scattered radiation remains one of the main challenges in digital mammography [1], limiting the quantitative usefulness of radiographic images. It reduces the quality of the image, degrades the contrast and the signal to noise ratio, reduces the dynamic range and therefore affects the diagnosis of low contrast lesions and small microcalcifications [2, 3].

At present, the most widespread technique to reduce the scattered radiation in mammography, makes use of anti-scatter grids. However, anti-scatter grids are an incomplete solution, adding complexity and cost to the mammography system manufacturing. Although they help to improve image quality, they also attenuate primary

© Springer International Publishing Switzerland 2016
A. Tingberg et al. (Eds.): IWDM 2016, LNCS 9699, pp. 203–210, 2016.
DOI: 10.1007/978-3-319-41546-8_27

radiation, leading to an increase in the patient dose delivered (up to a factor of 3) to maintain a constant Detector Air Kerma (DAK) [1, 4, 5].

The limitations of the anti-scatter grids have contributed to the emergence of new scatter reduction methods, based on image post-processing. Although scatter can be estimated using Monte Carlo (MC) simulations, faster and more flexible methods, such as the convolution-based scatter estimation method, have lately become more attractive [4, 6, 7]. This method is based on the idea that the scatter in the system is spatially diffuse, thus it can be approximated by a two-dimensional low-pass convolution filter of the primary image [3]. In this paper, we study the scatter contribution of different detector geometries and their influence on the simulated filters, i.e. point spread function (PSF) kernels, in order to study possible simplifications in future scatter modelling.

2   Methodology

The image recorded in a digital mammography detector is the combination of energy deposited by primary and scattered X-ray photons. In this work, the contribution of the detector geometry to the final scatter PSF (SPSF) kernels will be analyzed.

2.1   Software Used

MC simulations, based on the GEANT4 toolkit (version 10.01.p02), were used to study the production of scattered radiation in the simulated mammography geometry. GEANT4 is a widely used toolkit for simulating physical processes, including those occurring in mammography [8–10].

2.2   Scatter Point Spread Function

SPSF kernels are obtained from the MC simulation using a narrow X-ray beam which is represented by a normally-incident two-dimensional spatial delta function, i.e. the X-ray beam is simulated following the narrow pencil beam method [2, 7, 10]. Energy from scattered radiation (S) was binned into 1 mm radius (r) concentric annuli (up to 100 mm). These were then normalized to the primary image $P(0)$ to create SPSFs. These SPSFs were also normalized by the area of the annuli, $A(r)$, as described in [11].

$$SPSF(r) = \frac{s(r)}{P(0)A(r)} \left[mm^{-2} \right] \tag{1}$$

2.3   Validation Geometries

Before the simulations were performed, the scatter PSF code was validated using, as a benchmark, the values given in the report of the American Association of Physicists in medicine (AAPM) task group 195, case 3 – Mammography and breast tomosynthesis [12, 13].

The geometry used for the validation included breast compression and support paddles, both made of PMMA and 2 mm thick, a semi-circular cylinder as breast phantom - 46 mm thick, composed by 80/20 % of adipose/glandular tissue and surrounded by a 2 mm thick skin layer - and a 13 mm air gap between the support paddle and an idealized detector surface. The Source to Image Distance (SID) was 660 mm. A patient body made of water was also included, adjacent to the breast phantom's chest wall side and centered in the vertical direction with the breast phantom. Figure 1-A shows a diagram of the geometry [12, 13].

A combination of two X-ray beams (cone and pencil beam) and two X-ray spectra (monoenergetic and polyenergetic) were used for the validation, see Table 1. The spectrum values were obtained from [12]. For each of them, the primary radiation, Compton scattering, Rayleigh scattering and multiple scattering were measured in 7 different regions of interest (ROIs), as described by [12]. Enough particles to produce Standard Error of the Mean (SEM) values equal or lower than 1 % were run. The maximum discrepancies were obtained when recording the multiple scattering values.

Table 1. The table shows the four X-ray source/spectrum combinations used for the validation of the scatter PSF code. The last column shows the maximum discrepancy found when comparing the results with the AAPM report – group 195- Case 3 data [12].

Validation	Source type	Spectrum	AAPM comparison (%) Average (Maximum)
V1	Cone Beam	Mono energetic (16.8 keV)	0.82 (4.0)
V2	Cone Beam	30 kVp Mo/Mo (HVL = 0.3431 mmAl)	0.48 (3.6)
V3	Pencil Beam	Mono energetic (16.8 keV)	0.37 (1.6)
V4	Pencil Beam	30 kVp Mo/Mo (HVL = 0.3431 mmAl)	0.29 (1.9)

2.4 Geometry Used in This Study

The mammography geometry used was slightly modified from the one suggested in the AAPM-group 195 report, [12], to adjust it to the needs of this study. Firstly the patient body was not included in the simulation, as we were only interested in studying the scattering produced in the center of the breast, and secondly the D-shaped phantom was changed to a cylinder-shaped phantom, Fig. 1-B shows an example of this geometry.

In this report, the SPSF kernels are simulated using a narrow pencil beam and spectrum of 30 kVp Mo/Mo (HVL = 0.3431 mmAl). The photon cross-section "Electromagnetic physics option 4 package" was used both for the validation and the experiment. 20 to 60 runs, of 10^9 X-ray photons each, were simulated, ensuring uncertainties lower than 1.5 %. All presented values are represented as:

$$q \pm 3s \tag{2}$$

where, $\bar{q}$ is the mean of the value under study and s represents the uncertainty. s were calculated following Eq. (3), as suggested by Sempau et al. [14]:

$$s = \sqrt{\frac{1}{N}\left(\frac{\sum_i q_i^2}{N} - q^{-2}\right)} \tag{3}$$

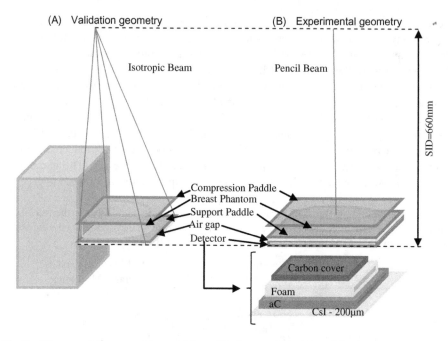

Fig. 1. Diagram of the geometries used for validation purposes (A) and for the experiments (B). Figure A shows an example using a cone beam aligned with the chest wall of the breast phantom. Figure B shows the pencil beam example and a detector added after the air gap.

where, N is the number of runs and q_i is the value under study for run N = i.

2.5 Experiment and Analysis

To evaluate the contribution of the detector geometry to the simulated PSF, three different detector setups were compared:

1. Case 1 - Ideal detector geometry: The detector is assumed to be an ideal X-ray sensitive surface. The energy stored comes from all X-ray photons that reach the detector surface.
2. Case 2 - Simplified detector geometry: The detector is assumed to be only the scintillator plate (200 μm CsI on a 1.5 mm of amorphous Carbon (aC) substrate [15]), placed right after an air gap of 13 mm.
3. Case 3 - Realistic detector geometry: The different layers of the detector down to the scintillator surface are considered and their contribution studied. A carbon cover was placed after the 13 mm air gap. Then, a second air gap was added between the cover and the Case 2 scintillator plane. The second air gap is an approximation used to simulate a piece of foam, see Fig. 2. The data was obtained via private communication with PerkinElmer Inc.

Case 2 simplification is often found in the literature, in cases where the detector structure is unknown. To evaluate how effective this simplification is, Case 3 simulates

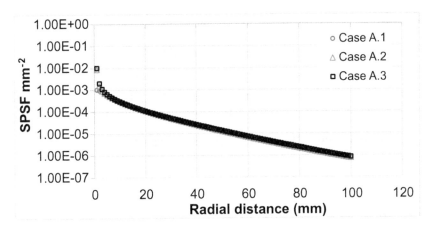

Fig. 2. The plot shows the SPSF(r) curves obtained when using an ideal detector (Case A.1), a scintillator plate (Case A.2) and a realistic detector geometry (Case A.3). (Color figure online)

a more realistic detector structure. The interactions occurring after the X-rays are scintillated were not taken into account.

For the three detector geometries described above, three breast thicknesses and three breast glandularity percentages - material composition obtained from Hammerstein et al. [16] - were analyzed. Table 2 shows all of the combinations under study. Data from experiment A are taken as the reference values. Radial symmetry was assumed in this study, since the pencil beam hits a location far from the edges of the simulated phantom.

Table 2. The table shows the characteristics of the different experiments that have been studied. It specifies the breast thickness and glandularity of the phantom

Exp.	Breast Thickness (mm)	Glandularity (%)	Detector geometry: Cases 1,2,3
A	50	20	A.1, A.2, A.3
B	30	20	B.1, B.2, B.3
C	80	20	C.1, C.2, C.3
D	50	35	D.1, D.2, D.3
E	50	50	E.1, E.2, E.3

The figure of merit used for the analysis of the result was the total SPR, SPR_T, see (4), which corresponds to the area under the SPSF' curve and represents the amount of total scatter.

$$SPR_T = \int_{r=0}^{r=r\max} SPSF'(r)dr \tag{4}$$

$$SPSF'(r) = SPSF(r)A(r) \tag{5}$$

3   Results

3.1   Comparison of the Scatter Kernels Obtained for Each Geometry

Figure 2 shows the SPSF(r) for cases A.1, A.2 and A.3. The figure shows the spatial distribution of the scatter as a function of radial distance. The plot on top of Fig. 2 is used to highlight the differences between the cases, using results from A.1 as reference.

3.2   Comparison of the SPR$_T$ Obtained for Each Experiment

The area under the SPSF(r) curve, i.e. SPR$_T$, allows the comparison of the total scatter contribution of the different experiments, see Table 3. The table also shows the ratio between cases 1 and 3 and cases 2 and 3, giving an estimation of the change in the scattering between cases and experiments. The values were calculated for a radial distance of 100 mm.

Table 3. The table shows the average SPR$_T$ values and their uncertainty (3 s, %) for the three detector geometries and five experiments run (A-E) and the ratios between C1-C3 and C2-C3.

	Total SPR (Error in %)				
Exp.	Case 1	Case 2	Case 3	C1/C3	C2/C3
A	0.60 (0.04)	0.64 (0.04)	0.67 (0.04)	0.90	0.95
B	0.40 (0.04)	0.43 (0.04)	0.46 (0.04)	0.86	0.94
C	0.92 (0.13)	0.97 (0.14)	0.10 (0.14)	0.92	0.97
D	0.61 (0.07)	0.65 (0.08)	0.68 (0.08)	0.90	0.95
E	0.62 (0.08)	0.66 (0.08)	0.69 (0.08)	0.90	0.95

Looking at the last two columns of Table 3, the ratio of C1 or C2 with respect C3 can be seen in Fig. 3 (expressed in %).

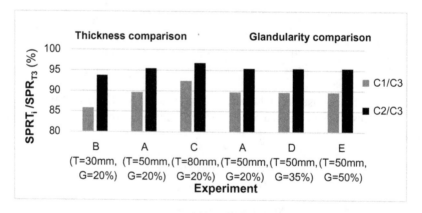

Fig. 3. The plot shows the ratio between the ideal detector geometry C1 (and the scintillator plate geometry C2) and the more realistic geometry (C3) for different breast thickness (T) and glandularity (G) combinations.

4   Discussion and Conclusions

Convolution-based scattering removal methods have been suggested in the literature for scattering reduction in mammography as an alternative to the anti-scatter grids [3, 6, 7]. This method makes use of simplified MC simulations for kernel (PSF) calculations, which are used to post-process acquired images.

A realistic mammography geometry is required for the PSF simulations, to account for scatter from elements such as compression paddles and breast support which can have a large contribution in the final image [10, 17]. This work focuses on the contribution of the detector geometry to the SPRs. To that end, three geometries have been studied for three different glandularities and thicknesses: an ideal case where the detector does not contribute to the scatter (Case 1), an intermediate case where the detector is approximated by a scintillator plate (Case 2) and a more realistic detector structure (Case 3).

Figure 2 shows a plot of the SPSF as a function of the radial distance. In the graph, it is possible to see that cases 2 and 3 show a peak at shorter radial distances, up to 4 mm, that is not present in Case 1. This is in line with previous observation of Diaz [11].

Considering the overall scatter contribution (see Table 3), the total amount of scatter increases with additional layers of material. As expected, a more complex detector geometry presents higher scatter to primary ratio values. If Case 1 and Case 3 are compared, a discrepancy between 10–14 % is found for the different experiments, while a discrepancy between 3–6 % can be seen when comparing cases 2 and 3. These results show that it is important to add the detector information into the simulations. If the dimensions and component materials are unknown, simply adding the scintillator (substrate and CsI:Tl) to the geometry can improve the scatter simulation by 5–8 %, when compared with the detailed detector geometry, Case3.

The changes in the ratio between the cases, as a function of variations in the glandularity or the thickness of the breast, can be seen in Fig. 3. The figure shows the percentage discrepancy from the reference experiment. The results show that Case 1 is more affected by the phantom changes than Case 2.

For thinner breasts (experiment B), the variation with Case 3 is higher, so the importance of including the detector details in the simulation increases. As thicker breast phantoms have greater contribution to the total SPR, we believe that the relative contribution from the detector geometry to the total SPR is decreased.

Glandularity variations do not seem to have a considerable effect on the ratio between the cases. This is in line with the literature, [10, 18].

Acknowledgements.   This work has been done in collaboration with PerkinElmer. The authors would like to thank FilmLight Ltd for their donation of computer resources.

Oliver Díaz is supported by the European Union within the Marie Sklodowska-Curie Innovative Training Networks (H2020-MSCA-IF-2014 SCARtool project, reference 657875) and the Ministry of Economy Competitiveness of Spain, under project reference DPI2015- and 68442-R.

References

1. Wang, A. et al.: Asymmetric scatter kernels for software-based scatter correction of grid-less mammography. SPIE Medical Imaging, vol. 94121, pp.1–7 (2015)
2. Boone, J.M., Cooper, V.N.: Scatter/primary in mammography: Monte Carlo validation. Med. Phys. **27**(8), 1818–1831 (2000)
3. Ducote, J.L., Molloi, S.: Scatter correction in digital mammography based on image deconvolution. IOP – Phys. Med. Biol. **55**, 1295–1309 (2010)
4. J. Binst et al.: Evaluation of automated CDMAM readings for non-standard CDMAM imaging conditions: Grid-less acquisitions and scatter correction. Oxford University Press – Radiation Protection Dosimetry, pp. 1–4 (2015)
5. Krol, A., et al.: Scatter reduction in mammography with air gap. Med. Phys. **23**(7), 1263–1270 (1996)
6. O. Diaz., et al.: A fast scatter field estimation for digital breast tomosynthesis. In: Proceedings of SPIE Medical Imaging, vol. 8313 (2012)
7. Diaz, O., et al.: Estimation of scattered radiation in digital breast tomosynthesis. IOP Phys. Med. Biol. **59**, 4375–4390 (2014)
8. Allison, J., et al.: GEANT4 developments and applications. IEEE Trans. Nucl. Sci. **33**(1), 270–278 (2006)
9. Feijó, P.V., Hoff, G.: GEANT4 validation on mammography applications. In: IEEE Nuclear Science Symposium (2008)
10. Sechopoulos, I., et al.: Scatter radiation in digital tomosynthesis of the breast. Med. Phys. **34**(2), 564–576 (2007)
11. Diaz, O.: Scattered radiation in projection X-ray mammography and digital breast tomosynthesis. Ph.D. Thesis, University of Surrey (2013)
12. Sechopoulos, I., et al.: The report of AAPM Task Group 195: Monte Carlo Reference Data Sets for Imaging Research. AAPM (2015)
13. Sechopoulos, I., et al.: Monte Carlo reference data sets for imaging research: executive summary of the report of AAPM research committee task group 195. Med. Phys. **42**, 5679 (2015)
14. Sempau, J., Sánchez-Reyes, A., Salvat, F., et al.: Monte Carlo simulation of electron beams from an accelerator head using PENELOPE. Phys. Med. Biol. **46**(4), 1163–1186 (2001)
15. Hamamatsu photonics: Scintillator plates – Hamamatsu photonics. Hamamatsu photonics. http://www.hamamatsu.com/jp/en/product/category/3100/3010/index.html. Accessed 23 Mar 2016
16. Hammerstein, G.R., Miller, D.W., White, D.R., Masterson, M.E., Woodard, Q.J., Laughlin, J.S.: Absorbed radiation dose in mammography. Radiology **130**, 485–491 (1979)
17. Dance, D.R., Day, G.J.: The computation of scatter in mammography by Monte Carlo methods. Phys. Med. Biol. **29**, 237–247 (1984)
18. Boone, J., et al.: Scatter/primary in mammography: comprehensive results. Med. Phys. **27**(10), 2408–2416 (2000)

Calibration Procedure of Three Component Mammographic Breast Imaging

Serghei Malkov[1(✉)], Jesus Avila[1], Bo Fan[1], Bonnie Joe[1],
Karla Kerlikowske[2], Maryellen Giger[3], Karen Drukker[3],
Jennifer Drukteinis[4], Leila Kazemi[1], Malesa Pereira[4],
and John Shepherd[1]

[1] Department of Radiology and Biomedical Imaging,
University of California, San Francisco, USA
{Serghei.Malkov,jesus.avila,BO.FAN,Bonnie.Joe,
John.Shepherd}@ucsf.edu
[2] Departments of Medicine and Epidemiology and Biostatistics,
University of California, San Francisco, USA
Karla.Kerlikowske@ucsf.edu
[3] University of Chicago, Chicago, IL, USA
{m-giger,kdrukker}@uchicago.edu
[4] Moffitt Cancer Center, Tampa, FL, USA
{jennifer.drukteinis,Malesa.Pereira}@moffitt.org

Abstract. Our purpose was to investigate the influence of phantom and biological materials on a 3-component decomposition using dual-energy mammography protocol (3CB).

Materials and Methods: A novel dual-energy 3CB mammography technique concludes in quantifying of the lipid, protein, and water thicknesses. The protocol was designed to be used on full-field digital mammography system by including an additional high-energy image with the clinical image. We study influence of calibration phantom and regression techniques on three component outputs. Two types of phantoms were used: solid water/wax/Delrin phantom and bovine phantom consisted of fat and lean muscle compartments. The linear and quadratic model equations were analyzed using linear and ridge regressions. The elaborated calibration protocol was applied to breast images with different compositions and sizes. In addition, the protocol was validated using cadaver breasts of known compositions.

Results: We found that there were many negative values of protein components when we applied our solid water/wax/Delrin calibrations using 51 ROIs for clinical dual energy mammogram analysis. This behavior could be explained by potential over fitting and not exact correspondence of biological and phantom material. Creating a calibration related to bovine tissue provided higher accuracy and realizable thicknesses for clinical breast composition components, and achieved satisfactory results for cadaver breast compositions.

Conclusion: Using a bovine calibration, the 3CB technique provides higher accuracy for lipid, water and protein compositional breast measurements than using plastic tissue equivalents alone.

Keywords: Breast composition · Dual energy digital mammography · Ridge regression

© Springer International Publishing Switzerland 2016
A. Tingberg et al. (Eds.): IWDM 2016, LNCS 9699, pp. 211–218, 2016.
DOI: 10.1007/978-3-319-41546-8_28

1   Introduction

Cancerous lesions have been found to differ in composition from benign tissue [1]. Invasive cancer is supposed to be highly angiogenic and presents with substantially more water than healthy tissue [2, 3]. Moreover, collagen protein has been found to be significantly higher in invasive tumors in both mouse and human tissues [4]. Raman spectroscopic measurements of ex-vivo breast tissues demonstrate the existence of unique signature of lesion water, lipid and protein content sufficient to discriminate lesion types [5]. A novel in-vivo imaging technique is designed to quantify the lesion and background tissue compositions in terms of protein, water and lipid content by combining a dual-energy digital mammography protocol with highly accurate thickness measurements from an in-place calibration phantom [6]. The purpose of this technique is to create a more accurate model of probability of cancer whose primary impact will be to reduce the number of negative biopsies while maintaining high specificity in breast imaging. However, the application of this technique in clinical study faced some problems related to negative values mostly in the protein component during decomposition step. It should be noted that the similar problem was reported for three component breast tissue decomposition of breast computed tomography [7]. Our calibration approach has been to create a stable phantom of biologically equivalent materials at different thicknesses and image this phantom at different kVp setting. However, the relationship of phantom materials can be unique to kVp in dual energy imaging. That is, the phantom materials may represent on fraction of lipid/water/protein at one X-ray technique but a completely different fraction at another technique. Since accuracy is considered against the biological materials, this can cause unrealistic solutions when looking at actual breast tissue. The purpose of this paper is to investigate how calibration using our phantom materials differed from bovine tissue calibration under a broad range of clinical mammographic techniques. We then investigated how to apply this difference to improving the phantom calibration. Finally, we tested our improved calibration model using both clinical mammograms and cadaveric mastectomy specimens.

2   Methods

We imaged our standard 3CB and bovine phantoms with known lipid/water/protein amounts using a range of X-ray exposure conditions. We then created two calibration models for these phantoms. We applied these two calibrations to screening mammograms and to cadaveric mastectomy samples, compared 3CB compositional outputs, and reported the improvements of our estimates.

2.1   Datasets

Participants undergoing breast biopsy (BIRADS 4 or 5 lesions) were recruited before their biopsies in terms of an ongoing prospective multi-center study. We use the following exclusion criteria: prior breast cancer, prior breast interventions such as biopsy, breast alterations, and mammographically occult findings. Breast biopsies were reviewed by a clinical pathologist. The lesions were delineated by the study radiologist on CC and MLO views, and the compositional measures of the whole breasts, local areas within lesions and their peripheries were derived. In addition, two individual frozen cadaver breasts (one each from two donors) were used in this study. Tissue samples from the cadaver breasts have been sent for chemical analysis and homogenization (Anresco Laboratories, San Francisco, CA).

2.2   3CB Imaging

The 3CB imaging technique concludes in quantifying of the lipid, protein, and water thicknesses for each pixel in a mammogram. The protocol was designed to be performed on standard full-field digital mammography systems by acquiring the standard clinical mammogram and an additional high-energy image. The 3CB method combines the dual-energy X-ray mammography attenuations and breast thickness map to solve for the three unknowns water, lipid, and protein content. Breast thickness was measured using the SXA phantom as previously described [8]. Then compositional thickness maps are extracted by calibrating to known thicknesses and compositions in a 3CB phantom. In this report, we used a single Hologic Selenia full-field digital mammography system (Hologic, Inc.). The second mammogram was acquired at a 39 kVp/Rh filter combination. An additional 3-mm thick X-ray filter was placed in the beam. The total dose of this procedure is estimated to be approximately 10 % more than that of the screening mammogram alone. The lesion water, lipid, and protein compositions were reported as the pixel component thicknesses of the delineated region. Two types of calibration phantoms were used: a solid water/wax/Delrin (CP51) phantom, and a bovine phantom consisting of fat and lean muscle compartments. A picture of these phantoms is shown in Fig. 1. The CP51 phantom had 51 ROIs with 2, 4 and 6-cm thicknesses, solid water/wax volumetric compartments of 0, 0.25/0.75, 0.5/0.5, 0.75/0.25 and 1 fractions. In addition, Delrin was added to each fraction to create 0, 10 %, 20 % and 30 % thickness of Delrin. The bovine phantoms had 15 ROIs with thicknesses of 2, 4 and 6 cm and pure lean muscle, pure fat trimmings and other three compartments closed to 0.25/0.75, 0.5/0.5, 0.75/0.25 muscle/fat fractions. We used water/lipid/protein volumetric fractions estimates of 0.81/0.012/0.178 for lean muscle and 0.13/0.855/0.015 for fat samples in the bovine phantom calibration [9]. The linear and quadratic model equations were analyzed using multiple linear and ridge regressions. The ridge regression analysis has been tuned by varying λ coefficient. It is equal to 0 for linear regression [10]. The elaborated calibration protocol was applied for a selected set of breast images with different compositions and sizes. In addition, the protocol was validated using cadaver breasts of known compositions. The homogenized tissues were also undergone a dual-energy X-ray scan, from which average water, lipid, and protein content was calculated. A flat field correction procedure for low and high energy images using 4 cm CIRS 50/50 slab was applied to all images. In addition, all images were corrected for the incident beam intensity during their negative log transformation. Breast thicknesses were measuring using an in-image SXA phantom. The thickness validation procedure concluded in a weekly scanning of specially

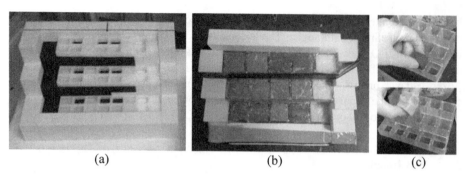

Fig. 1. The pictures of the calibration phantoms: (a) calibration phantom of solid water/wax/protein components, 51 ROIs, wax – blue, solid water – yellow, Delrin - white; (b) bovine calibration phantom consisted of solid water, lean muscle, pure fat trimmings, fat and lean muscle combinations; (c) insertion procedure of lean muscle and fat components into the phantom frame. (Color figure online)

designed quality assurance phantom [11]. Quality assurance thickness scans demonstrated thickness error below 0.2 mm.

3   Results

At this time point, the 3CB images of 226 patients have been collected and processed. This set of 226 dual energy mammograms excluding a few outliers has been processed using the CP51 phantom calibration tables created from 51 ROIs solid water/wax/Delrin for each kVp. The calibration coefficients have been estimated using a linear regression model of quadratic equations. We found that there were many negative values of protein components when we applied the CP51 calibration. We consider that such deviation errors could be explained by potential over fitting and not exact correspondence of biological and phantom materials. To investigate this behavior we tried the following calibration procedure modifications: (a) creating the biological material calibration model based on the bovine phantom consisted of 15 lean muscle and fat combinations; (b) downgrading from quadratic to linear model equations; (c) the ridge regression with a variation of λ parameter. Application of linear equation model decreased a magnitude of negative protein values or removed them but at the expense of increasing the calibration error in comparison with quadratic model, and the results tend to be biased. The λ parameter helps to some extent but gives rise into error calibration increase, either. The positive contribution of introduction of λ concluded in decreasing the noise after decomposition transformation. Eventually, all the analysis was done using quadratic equation model, and a small λ coefficient equal to 0.01 was used for the regularization term in case of the ridge regression. An example of the analysis results of the lesion ROI and the whole breast using the CP51 and the bovine phantoms is shown in the Table 1. As one can see, using the bovine phantom calibration we can get rid of negative protein values for both lesion ROI and whole breast mean estimates. The values of relative calibration errors for both phantoms have approximately the same amplitudes.

Table 1. Three component decomposition of the lesion area delineated in the patient dual-energy mammograms. Water, lipid and protein rows are related the breast component thicknesses of 3CB analysis. CP water, lipid and protein errors represent relative component decomposition errors of the CP51 and bovine phantom ROIs.

Region type	Lesion ROI		Whole breast	
Phantom type	Bovine phantom	CP51 phantom	Bovine phantom	CP51 phantom
Water, cm	1.69	3.93	1.86	3.30
Lipid, cm	1.67	1.21	1.07	0.65
Protein, cm	0.52	−1.26	0.61	−0.41
CP water error, %	1.62	2.11	1.62	2.11
CP lipid error, %	1.90	0.62	1.90	0.62
CP protein error, %	2.04	7.63	2.04	7.63

Figure 2. represents clinical mammogram, water, lipid, and protein thickness maps. The 3CB imaging decomposition maps were derived using the bovine phantom calibration. The lesion areas were delineated by the radiologist and shown by green lines. As expected, the water and lipid maps are inverse to each other, and the protein map follows the water gray scale trend.

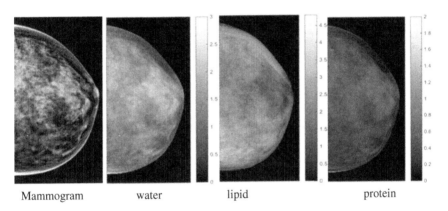

Mammogram   water   lipid   protein

Fig. 2. 3CB imaging technique decomposition (water, lipid, and protein thickness) maps and clinical mammogram. The bovine phantom calibrations were used for decomposition. The lesion area is delineated by radiologist. The composition thickness maps are presented in cm scale. (Color figure online)

The protein distributions representing the lesion ROI and the whole breast that processed for 15 patients using both the CP51 and bovine phantom calibrations are shown in the Fig. 3. As one can see there are no negative protein thicknesses for both lesion ROI and whole breast mean values obtained using bovine phantom calibrations. In case of the CP51 phantom calibration the protein thickness distributions are wider and mostly spread into negative thickness direction. The testing of these calibration procedure modifications using the whole patient set available is presently under way.

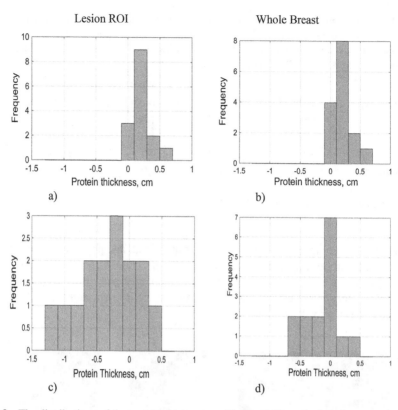

Fig. 3. The distributions of the protein thicknesses of lesion ROIs and whole breasts calculated using the bovine (a, b) and CP51 (c, d) phantom calibrations.

The results of comparison of Anresco Laboratories and 3CB measurements of cadaver breast fractional compositions are presented in the Table 2. Application of elaborated calibration procedure for two cadaver breast samples (dense and not dense tissues) demonstrated satisfactory correspondence with measured compositions in case

Table 2. Comparison of Anresco Laboratories and 3CB measurements of cadaver breast compositions (in fractional %). MAE is a mean absolute error of component fraction.

Variable	Anresco measurements		3CB, Bovine phantom		3CB, CP51 phantom		Bovine phantom MAE	CP51 phantom MAE
Sample name	MT1	6337R	MT1	6337R	MT1	6337R	Combined	Combined
Water, %	73.49	8.81	45.99	3.24	85.71	59.75	8.27	17.18
Lipid, %	13.53	90.79	39.29	98.67	26.66	81.76	8.41	7.51
Protein, %	12.1	0.29	14.73	−1.91	−12.36	−41.51	1.21	16.02
Ash, %	0.88	0.11	–	–	–	–	–	–

of the bovine phantom calibration. These two sample measurements demonstrated mean absolute errors of 8.2 %, 8.4 %, and 1.2 % for water, lipid, and protein component fractions. This is a significant improvement in comparison with the CP51 phantom calibration especially for the protein fraction.

4 Conclusions

Thus, we found a set of calibration conditions using bovine tissue as breast equivalent material that generated realizable clinical breast composition components and achieved satisfactory results for cadaver breast compositions. We expect to continue further improving the calibration procedure in order to decrease composition breast measurement errors for a variety of breast compositions, sizes, and X-ray characteristics. Future studies include redoing these proof of concept scans with bovine samples that have a calibration chemical composition of lipid, water, and protein.

Acknowledgements.   The authors would like to acknowledge the following funding sources: National Cancer Institute No. R01 CA166945, R21CA157254, and the California Breast Cancer Research Program No. 18IB-0042.

References

1. Weind, K.L., Maier, C.F., Rutt, B.K., Moussa, M.: Invasive carcinomas and fibroadenomas of the breast: comparison of microvessel distributions–implications for imaging modalities. Radiology **208**(2), 477–483 (1998)
2. Cerussi, A., Shah, N., Hsiang, D., Durkin, A., Butler, J., Tromberg, B.J.: In vivo absorption, scattering, and physiologic properties of 58 malignant breast tumors determined by broadband diffuse optical spectroscopy. J. Biomed. Opt. **11**(4), 044005–044016 (2006)
3. Sha, L., Ward, ER., Stroy, B.: A review of dielectric properties of normal and malignant breast tissue. In: Proceedings of IEEE SoutheastCon. IEEE, pp. 457–462 (2002)
4. Provenzano, P.P., Inman, D.R., Eliceiri, K.W., et al.: Collagen density promotes mammary tumor initiation and progression. BMC Med. **6**(1), 11 (2008)
5. Zhu, C., Breslin, T.: Diagnosing breast cancer by using Raman spectroscopy. Breast Dis. Year Book Q. **17**(1), 34 (2006)
6. Laidevant, A.D., Malkov, S., Flowers, C.I., Kerlikowske, K., Shepherd, J.A.: Compositional breast imaging using a dual-energy mammography protocol. Med. Phys. **37**(1), 164–174 (2010)
7. Ding, H., Zhao, B., Baturin, P., Behroozi, F., Molloi, S.: Breast tissue decomposition with spectral distortion correction: a postmortem study. Med. Phys. **41**(10), 101901 (2014)
8. Malkov, S., Wang, J., Kerlikowske, K., Cummings, S.R., Shepherd, J.A.: Single X-ray absorptiometry method for the quantitative mammographic measure of fibroglandular tissue volume. Med. Phys. **36**(12), 5525–5536 (2009)
9. Ding, H., Ducote, J.L., Molloi, S.: Breast composition measurement with a cadmium-zinc-telluride based spectral computed tomography system. Med. Phys. **39**(3), 1289–1297 (2012)

10. Hoerl, A.E., Kennard, R.W.: Ridge regression: biased estimation for nonorthogonal problems. Technometrics **12**(1), 55–67 (1970)
11. Malkov, Serghei, Wang, Jeff, Duewer, Fred, Shepherd, John A.: A calibration approach for single-energy x-ray absorptiometry method to provide absolute breast tissue composition accuracy for the long term. In: Maidment, Andrew D.A., Bakic, Predrag R., Gavenonis, Sara (eds.) IWDM 2012. LNCS, vol. 7361, pp. 769–774. Springer, Heidelberg (2012)

Local Detectability Maps as a Tool for Predicting Masking Probability and Mammographic Performance

Olivier Alonzo-Proulx[1(✉)], James Mainprize[1], Heba Hussein[2],
Roberta Jong[2], and Martin Yaffe[1,3]

[1] Physical Sciences, Sunnybrook Research Institute,
2075 Bayview Avenue, Toronto, ON M4N 3M5, Canada
{oliviera,james.mainprize,
martin.yaffe}@sri.utoronto.ca
[2] Department of Medical Imaging, Sunnybrook Health Sciences Centre,
2075 Bayview Avenue, Toronto, ON M4N 3M5, Canada
{hebamostafa.hussein,roberta.jong}@sunnybrook.ca
[3] Department of Medical Biophysics, University of Toronto,
2075 Bayview Avenue, Toronto, ON M4N 3M5, Canada

Abstract. High mammographic density is associated with reduced sensitivity of mammography. Recent changes in the BI-RADS density assessment address the potential for dense tissue to mask lesions, but the assessment remains qualitative and achieves only moderate agreement between radiologists. We have developed an automated, quantitative algorithm that generates a local detectability (d_L) map, which estimates the likelihood that a simulated lesion would be missed if present. The d_L map is computed by tessellating the mammogram into overlapping regions of interest, for which the detectability of a simulated lesion by a non-prewhitening model observer is calculated using local estimates of the noise power spectrum and volumetric breast density. The algorithm considers both the effects of loss of contrast due to density and the distracting appearance of density on lesion conspicuity.

In previous work, it has been shown that the mean d_L from the maps are strongly correlated to detection performance by computerized and human readers in a controlled reader study. Here, we investigate how various statistical features of the d_L maps (gray-level histogram and co-occurrence features) are related to the diagnostic performance of mammography in a set of images comprised of 8 cancer cases that were mammographically occult and 40 cancer that were detected in screening mammography.

Keywords: Breast density · Breast cancer · Parenchymal tissue patterns · Mammography screening · Sensitivity · Masking · Diagnostic performance

1 Introduction

Elevated levels of breast density cause a reduction in the sensitivity of mammography. It has been shown that the sensitivity drops from 86 %–95 % in the lower density mammograms to 59 %–89 % for the densest mammograms [1–3]. Due to this

© Springer International Publishing Switzerland 2016
A. Tingberg et al. (Eds.): IWDM 2016, LNCS 9699, pp. 219–225, 2016.
DOI: 10.1007/978-3-319-41546-8_29

limitation, several jurisdictions have implemented a mandatory reporting of density to mammography screening clients. In the US and Canada, density is commonly assessed with the BI-RADS categorization scale, which is a good indicator of the potential of density to mask lesions [4]. However, inter-rater agreement between radiologists is only moderate, with reported Cohen's kappa scores of 0.44–0.54 [5, 6].

We have developed an automatic, quantitative algorithm that generates a local detectability map, which estimates the likelihood that a lesion of a specific size and shape would be detected within any area of the mammogram. The metric incorporates the effects of the texture, spatial distribution and amount of dense tissue on lesion conspicuity. In this preliminary study, we investigate how various features of the detectability maps differ between mammograms where cancer was occult and mammograms where cancer was detected.

2 Methods

2.1 Local Detectability Calculation

The method used to compute the d_L maps has been described elsewhere [7, 8]. In short, the map is created by dividing the breast into an overlapping grid of small (12.8×12.8 mm) regions of interests (ROIs) and calculating the detectability d' of a signal-known exactly non-prewhitening model observer [9] in each ROI:

$$d'^2 = \frac{\left[C \iint MTF^2(u,v)W^2(u,v)dudv \right]^2}{\iint S(u,v)MTF^2(u,v)W^2(u,v)dudv},$$ (1)

where C is the peak lesion signal difference, u and v the spatial frequency on the x and y directions, respectively, $MTF(u, v)$ is the modulation transfer function for the mammography imaging system, $S(u, v)$ is the normalized noise power spectrum (NNPS), and $W(u, v)$ is the Fourier transform of the simulated lesion, in this case a 5 mm full-with half maximum Gaussian profile. The MTF was directly measured for the imaging system using in this study, a Senographe Essential (GE Healthcare). The NPS was computed from the multi-taper approach of Wu et al. [10] and fitted to a surface to further reduce the variance. The contrast, C, is computed by comparing the difference in attenuation of a Gaussian-shaped lesion of invasive ductal carcinoma [11] and a corresponding attenuation from an equivalent thickness of breast tissue whose level of glandularity has been set to match the local estimate of the volumetric breast density (VBD) for that ROI. See Fig. 1 for examples of d_L maps.

2.2 Clinical Image Dataset

Research Ethics Board approval was obtained to analyse VBD and d_L on de-identified mammograms acquired at the Sunnybrook Health Sciences Centre, and to review the clinical records of cancer patients. We conducted a search in the Breast Cancer Research Biomatrix database to identify (1) mammographically-occult cancers and (2) cancers

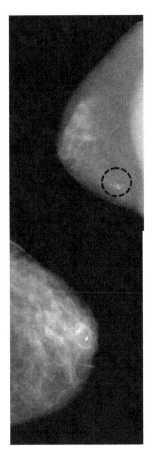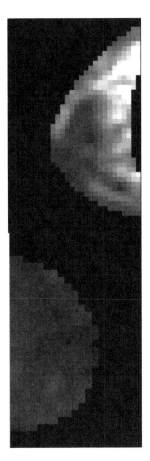

Fig. 1. Examples local detectability maps (top and bottom right) with the corresponding mammograms (top and bottom left). The maps are scaled from 0 to 10 where dark pixels represent low detectability. The top and bottom images are from the found and missed cancer sets, with an average d_L of 5.0 and 1.6, respectively. The found lesion is outlined with a dashed circle.

found via mammography screening. The occult or "missed" cancers were those that had (a) a pathology-confirmed cancer diagnosis, (b) a MRI or ultrasound guided biopsy procedure or a lumpectomy and (c) a negative digital mammogram (i.e. with a BIRADS of 1, 2 or 3) within 18 months prior to the diagnosis. The "found" cancers detected by screening were those that had (a) a pathology-proven cancer diagnosis and (b) a non-negative digital mammogram (i.e. with a BIRADS of 0, 4, 5 or 6) within 2 months prior to the diagnosis. We further restricted the found cases to invasive cancers, since the d_L maps correspond to the detectability of masses, and to those for which we had data available in the contralateral (unaffected) breast, to avoid the potential masking effect of the mass itself. There were 8 missed and 40 found cancers, from women with mean ages of 47.9 and 62.4 years, respectively. There were 6 invasive and 2 *in situ* cancers in the missed cancer set, and the average time difference between the mammograms and the diagnosis was 3.7 months. There were two cases in the missed cancer set for which the contralateral breast data was unavailable; we then used the ipsilateral breast data.

2.3   Feature Analysis

We computed a series of statistical features on the d_L maps, as shown in Table 1. The gray-level histogram features are computed directly from the d_L values, while the co-occurrence features are computed from the gray-level co-occurrence matrix (GLCM), using the `graycomatrix` and `graycoprops` functions in MATLAB R2013a. The GLCM were computed using 64 histogram bins, for values ranging between 0 and 14 (the 98th percentile in this dataset), and for the 0° direction to the nearest neighbor (*e.g.* for the offset [0 1]). The features were calculated for each image, and were averaged per patient and per breast side.

Table 1. List of statistical features computed on the d_L maps.

Feature type	Feature name
Gray-level histogram	Mean, 95th percentile, 5th percentile, std. deviation, sum, entropy, kurtosis, skewness
Co-occurrence	Contrast, correlation, energy, homogeneity

2.4   ROC Performance of Detectability Features

We first investigated the performance of each feature in discriminating between missed and found cancers by computing the area under the curve (AUC) of the receiver-operator characteristics (ROC) curve. The 95 % confidence interval (95 CI) was calculated using 5000 bootstrap replicas. The `perfcurve` function in Matlab R2013a was used for the computation.

3   Results

3.1   ROC Performance of Detectability Features

The ROC performance of the d_L features is shown in Table 2. Figure 2 shows the ROC curves for the 2 features (Mean and GLCM Contrast) which had the largest significant AUCs. We also computed the AUC of the ROC curve using VBD as the discrimination threshold. The AUC = 0.67 [95CI 0.40–0.84] was not statistically significant. The mean (standard deviation) of the VBD in the missed and found groups were respectively 21.9 % (12.5) and 16.4 % (8.7). Figure 3 shows the ROC curve for the VBD.

Table 2. AUC of the ROC curve of the d_L features in discriminating between missed and found cancers. The non-significant AUCs are highlighted with an asterix. The features which are inversely correlated to the missed status are shown in italic. Also shown is the Pearson correlation r of each feature vs. the mean d_L.

Feature	AUC	r	Feature	AUC	r
Mean	*0.74*	1.0	5th percentile	*0.68**	0.84
Std. deviation	*0.70*	0.81	95th percentile	*0.73*	0.95
Sum	*0.73**	0.72	Contrast 0°	*0.77*	0.92
Entropy	0.63*	−0.52	Correlation 0°	0.51*	0.00
Kurtosis	0.55*	−0.44	Energy 0°	0.73	−0.76
Skewness	0.57*	−0.47	Homogeneity 0°	0.72	−0.91

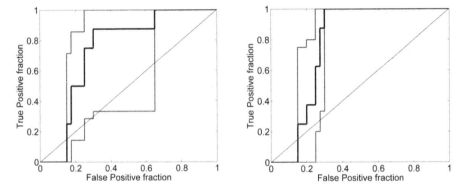

Fig. 2. ROC curves of the mean and GLCM contrast d_L features in discriminating between missed and found cancers. The lighter lines represent the 95 CI on the true positive fraction.

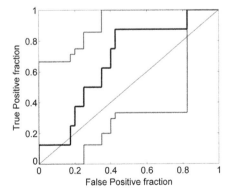

Fig. 3. ROC curve of the VBD in discriminating between missed and found cancers. The ligher lines represent the 95 CI on the true positive fraction.

4 Discussion

The results presented in this paper demonstrate the potential for the d_L maps to predict clinical diagnostic accuracy. In Sect. 2.1 we show that there are 6 features of the detectability maps which can significantly discriminate between missed and found cancers, with AUCs ranging between 0.70 and 0.77. In contrast, the VBD was not a statistically significant discriminator, despite the fact that the d_L maps are partially derived from the density maps. However, we note that there are strong similarities in those statistically significant features: most of them are strongly correlated to the mean d_L.

There are several limitations in this study. First, the sample size of missed cancers in this study is very small. Second, the results may be biased by the patient selection. The patients with occult cancers were younger than those with found cancers, and thus may have different breast tissue texture. Furthermore, due to sample size constraints, we included bilateral cancers in the missed set, which may induce a bias in the d_L values due to the mass itself. In the future, we plan to conduct a similar study with a larger number of missed and found cancers, which will enable us to construct a predictive model (using multivariate binomial logistic regression) of the missed cancer status using a selection of d_L features as predictors.

Acknowledgements. This project has been supported financially by research grants from The Ontario Institute for Cancer Research.

References

1. Kerlikowske, K., Hubbard, R.A., Miglioretti, D.L., Geller, B.M., Yankaskas, B.C., Lehman, C.D., Taplin, S.H., Sickles, E.A.: Comparative effectiveness of digital versus film-screen mammography in community practice in the United States: a cohort study. Ann. Intern. Med. **155**, 493–502 (2011)
2. Pisano, E.D., Gatsonis, C., Hendrick, E., Yaffe, M., Baum, J.K., Acharyya, S., Conant, E.F., Fajardo, L.L., Bassett, L., D'Orsi, C., Jong, R., Rebner, M.: Diagnostic performance of digital versus film mammography for breast-cancer screening. N. Engl. J. Med. **353**, 1773–1783 (2005)
3. Pisano, E.D., Hendrick, R.E., Yaffe, M.J., Baum, J.K., Cormack, J.B., Hanna, L.A., Conant, E.F., Fajardo, L.L., Bassett, L.W., Orsi, C.J.D., Jong, R.A., Rebner, M., Tosteson, A.N.A., Gatsonis, C.A.: Diagnostic accuracy of digital versus film mammography: exploratory analysis of selected population subgroups in DMIST. Radiology **246**, 376–383 (2008)
4. Mandelson, M.T., Oestreicher, N., Porter, P.L., White, D., Finder, C.A., Taplin, S.H., White, E.: Breast density as a predictor of mammographic detection: comparison of interval- and screen-detected cancers. J. Natl. Cancer Inst. **92**, 1081–1087 (2000)
5. Ciatto, S., Houssami, N., Apruzzese, A., Bassetti, E., Brancato, B., Carozzi, F., Catarzi, S., Lamberini, M.P., Marcelli, G., Pellizzoni, R., Pesce, B., Risso, G., Russo, F., Scorsolini, A.: Categorizing breast mammographic density: intra- and interobserver reproducibility of BI-RADS density categories. Breast **14**, 269–275 (2005)

6. Redondo, A., Comas, M., Macià, F., Ferrer, F., Murta-Nascimento, C., Maristany, M.T., Molins, E., Sala, M., Castells, X.: Inter- and intraradiologist variability in the BI-RADS assessment and breast density categories for screening mammograms. Br. J. Radiol. **85**, 1465–1470 (2012)

7. Mainprize, J.G., Wang, X., Ge, M., Yaffe, M.J.: Towards a quantitative measure of radiographic masking by dense tissue in mammography. In: Fujita, H., Hara, T., Muramatsu, C. (eds.) IWDM 2014. LNCS, vol. 8539, pp. 181–186. Springer, Heidelberg (2014)

8. Mainprize, J.G.: Olivier Alonzo-Proulx, R.A.J., Yaffe, M.J.: Quantifying masking in clinical mammograms via local detectability of simulated lesions. Med. Phys. **43**, 1249–1258 (2016)

9. Burgess, A.E.: Statistically defined backgrounds: performance of a modified nonprewhitening observer model. J. Opt. Soc. Am. A: **11**, 1237–1242 (1994)

10. Wu, G., Mainprize, J.G., Yaffe, M.J.: Spectral analysis of mammographic images using a multitaper method. Med. Phys. **39**, 801–810 (2012)

11. Johns, P.C., Yaffe, M.J.: X-ray characterisation of normal and neoplastic breast tissues. Phys. Med. Biol. **32**, 675–695 (1987)

The Effect of Breast Composition on a No-reference Anisotropic Quality Index for Digital Mammography

Bruno Barufaldi[1,2(✉)], Lucas R. Borges[1,2], Marcelo A.C. Vieira[1],
Salvador Gabarda[3], Andrew D.A. Maidment[2], Predrag R. Bakic[2],
David D. Pokrajac[4], and Homero Schiabel[1]

[1] Department of Electrical and Computer Engineering,
University of São Paulo, São Carlos, Brazil
Bruno.Barufaldi@uphs.upenn.edu
[2] Department of Radiology, University of Pennsylvania, Philadelphia, USA
[3] Spanish Council for Scientific Research, Institute of Optics, Madrid, Spain
[4] Department of Information and Computer Sciences,
Delaware State University, Dover, USA

Abstract. There are several methods to evaluate objectively the quality of a digital image. For digital mammography, objective quality assessment must be performed without references. In a previous study, the authors investigated the use of a normalized anisotropic quality index (NAQI) to assess mammography images blindly in terms of noise and spatial resolution. Since the NAQI is used as a quality metric, it must not be highly dependent on the breast anatomy. Thus, in this work, we analyze the NAQI behavior with different breast anatomies. A computerized system was used to synthesize 2,880 anthropomorphic breast phantom images with a realistic range of anatomical variations. The results show that NAQI is only marginally dependent on breast anatomy when images are acquired without degradation (<12 %). However, for realizations that simulate the acquisition process in digital mammography, the NAQI is more sensitive (33 %) to variations arising from quantum noise. Thus, NAQI can be used in clinical practice to assess mammographic image quality.

Keywords: Breast anatomy · Image quality index · Anisotropy · Digital mammography

1 Introduction

The evaluation of mammography image quality is important in clinical practice to assure optimal performance of the radiologists. To execute this task, a large dataset of clinical mammograms must be assessed by a group of radiologists through standardized subjective methods [1]. These approaches are expensive, time-consuming and influenced by inter-observer subjectivity. An alternative is the use of objective image quality assessment, where the goal is to provide computational models that can automatically predict perceptual image quality [2].

© Springer International Publishing Switzerland 2016
A. Tingberg et al. (Eds.): IWDM 2016, LNCS 9699, pp. 226–233, 2016.
DOI: 10.1007/978-3-319-41546-8_30

There are several methods to evaluate the quality of a digital image objectively. Generally, such methods calculate the similarity between the degraded image and a reference image, which is assumed to have perfect quality (ground-truth) [2]. However, these methods cannot be applied to digital mammography because the ideal image without degradation is not available in clinical practice. Thus, for digital mammography, objective quality assessment must be performed without any reference. No-reference or "blind" image quality assessment is an extremely difficult task, as they have to predict the perceptual quality of distorted images with no information about the reference images [2].

In a previous paper [3], we investigated a no-reference image quality index to assess mammographic images acquired within a range of radiation doses (noise) and detector sizes (blur). The results reported by this index, the normalized anisotropic quality index (NAQI), followed the same behavior as other well-established full-reference indexes, such as the *peak signal-to-noise ratio* (PSNR) and *structural similarity index* (SSIM), when evaluating digital mammograms acquired with anthropomorphic breast phantoms.

However, the NAQI is normalized by the entropy of the image. The anatomical features of the breast exert some influence on this normalization. Since the anatomy varies among patients, it would be an undesirable feature if the NAQI were more sensitive to the variations on breast anatomy then to image quality. The purpose of the current study is to analyze the sensitivity of the NAQI to a range of breast anatomies and image qualities, using a large set of synthetic mammograms generated by an anthropomorphic breast software phantom [4, 5] with a realistic range of anatomical variations.

2   Method

The anisotropic quality index [6] is calculated using the generalized Rényi entropy (R_α) and the normalized pseudo-Wigner distribution (W_z)

$$R_\alpha = \frac{1}{1-\alpha} \log_2 \left(\sum_n \sum_k P^\alpha[n,k] \right) \qquad (1)$$

$$W_z[n',k'] = 2 \sum_{m=-N/2}^{(N/2)-1} Z[n'+m]Z^*[n'-m]e^{-2i(2\pi m/N)k'} \qquad (2)$$

where $P[n,k]$ is the discrete space-frequency distribution, n and k are spatial and frequency components, and α is a constant for the space-frequency distributions; n' and k' represent the spatial and frequency discrete variables, m is a parameter used for shifting and z^* is the complex conjugate of z. To consider the entropy directions, $z[n']$ is a 1D sequence of N gray values of pixels.

Based on Eqs. 1 and 2, the Rényi entropy for a pixel located at the position n, described at the pseudo-Wigner domain, is given by

$$R_3[n] = -\frac{1}{2}\log_2\left(\sum_{k=1}^{N} \breve{P}_n^3[k]\right); \tag{3}$$

where the probability distribution P_n has been obtained from the normalization of coefficients W_z.

In considering the statistical dispersion of entropy, spatial resolution and noise have an inverse correlation with anisotropy. To overcome this problem, the proposed metric uses the anisotropy with directional dependency, since this measurement decreases in accordance with the amount of degradation.

The proposed metric, based on result of Eq. 3, is given by:

$$\bar{R}[\theta_s] = \sum_{n} R_3[n, \theta_s] \Big/ M; \tag{4}$$

where M is the image size and $\theta_s \in [\theta_1, \theta_2, \ldots, \theta_S]$ represents the S different orientations that are considered to measure the entropy.

3 Materials

All images used in this work were generated using an anthropomorphic breast software phantom developed by the University of Pennsylvania [4, 5]. The tissue simulation is controlled by user-selected parameters, that can cover anatomical variations seen clinically. All phantoms had a voxel size of $(0.1 \text{ mm})^3$, a simulated breast volume of 1500 mL, and a compressed breast thickness of 6.4 cm. To test the robustness of the image quality measure, in this study we specifically varied:

- Thickness of Cooper's ligaments: 0.04 mm and 0.06 mm;
- Number of tissue compartments: 167, 333, 500, and 1,000;
- Percent of compartments labeled dense: 0 %, 5 %, and 10 %, corresponding to overall glandularity of 15 %, 21 %, and 26 %, respectively;
- Size and shape of compartments: three sets of parameters selected;
- Skin thickness: 1.2 mm and 1.5 mm.

The combination of the anatomical features mentioned above generated 144 different phantoms, which were then simulated 10 times using different position seeds, resulting in the equivalent of 1,440 patients.

Mammographic projections were synthesized based upon the simulation of a clinical mammography Selenia Dimensions system (Hologic Inc., Bedford, MA), with 70 μm pixel size. The x-ray acquisition parameters were chosen assuming automatic exposure control (AEC) and also half of the recommended mAs to simulate 50 % dose reduction on the radiation dose. Therefore, a total of 2,880 FFDM were generated. Figure 1 shows examples of simulated images.

A subset of the anatomical configurations was chosen, fixing the skin thickness to 1.2 mm and the size and shape of compartments to just one value. A total of 240 images were then generated considering an ideal acquisition system with no noise. This image set was used to study the impact of breast anatomy individually, without any influence of the image quality.

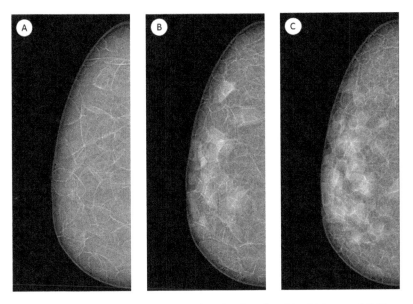

Fig. 1. Examples of three digital phantoms that simulate the skin thickness of 0.12 mm and 0.04 mm of Copper's ligaments. (A) Breast density overall of 15 % and number of compartments of 167; (B) 21 % and 500; and (C) 26 % and 1,000.

All experiments were performed using a ROI size of 2,791 × 709 pixels, containing as much of the inner breast tissue as possible to avoid background bias. The window size (w) and number of directions of the NAQI algorithm were set to 16 pixels and 5 angles ($\Theta = [0°, 45°, 90°, 135°, 180°]$), respectively.

4 Results

First, the NAQI was evaluated over a dataset of 240 ground-truth images, generated considering an ideal acquisition system with no noise. Second, all the 144 different breast anatomies, with 10 random realizations were evaluated at two different radiation dose levels: the one given by the AEC and 50 % of it. The total number of images considered in the second subsection is 2,880.

4.1 Impact of Breast Anatomy

Table 1 presents the NAQI reported for the phantom simulations, arranged by four classes of compartments (167, 333, 500 and 1000) and two groups of ligament thickness (0.04 mm and 0.06 mm).

Note that the NAQI is reduced as the number of compartments and the percent of compartment's density are increased. On the other hand, NAQI increases with the thickness of Cooper's ligaments.

Table 1. Proposed blind index (NAQI) calculated for 10 synthetic images of each type, without any degradation, categorized by number of compartments, Cooper's ligament thickness and breast skin thickness.

Average of NAQI				
No. Compartments	Overall percentage density (PD)			Total NAQI reduction
	15 %	21 %	26 %	
167	0.348	0.344	0.336	−4 %
333	0.333	0.326	0.318	−2 %
500	0.325	0.322	0.315	−3 %
1,000	0.318	0.315	0.310	−4 %
Total NAQI reduction	−9 %	−8 %	−8 %	
Ligament thickness				
0.06 (mm)	0.352	0.347	0.339	−4 %
0.04 (mm)	0.310	0.306	0.301	−4 %
Total NAQI reduction	−12 %	−12 %	−11 %	
Skin thickness				
1.2 (mm)	0.331	0.327	0.320	−3 %

4.2   Impact of Dose Reduction

The next set of experiments was performed using the set of 2,880 images simulated with 100 % and 50 % dose. In this experiment we investigated if variations on breast anatomy are more relevant then the changes on image quality.

Figure 2 shows the reported values of NAQI for different breast densities, number of compartments, and radiation dose. Figures 3 and 4 show the equivalent results for variations in the thickness of the Cooper's ligament and skin thickness, respectively.

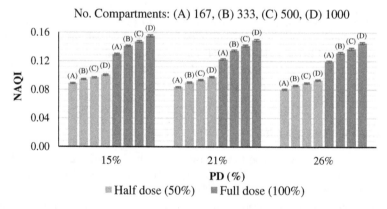

Fig. 2. Reported NAQI for each breast density and number of compartments. (Color figure online)

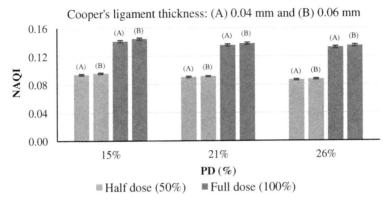

Fig. 3. Reported NAQI for each breast density and thickness of Cooper's ligament. (Color figure online)

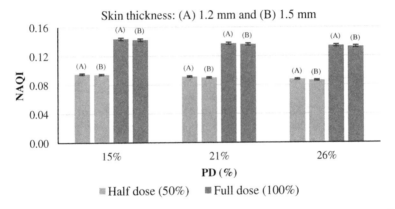

Fig. 4. Reported NAQI for each breast density and skin thickness. (Color figure online)

As a final experiment, we compared the distributions reported by the NAQI values at both radiation levels, as shown by Fig. 5. Using both distributions, we calculated the ROC curve that illustrates the performance of a binary classifier that would apply the NAQI to discriminate images at different doses. The reported AUC was 0.994.

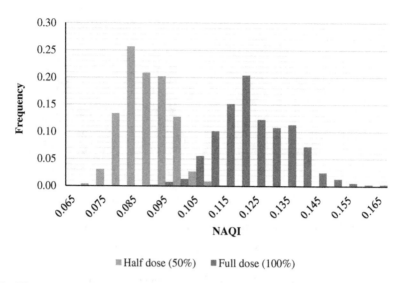

Fig. 5. Histogram distribution of NAQI showing the variation in accordance with the breast anatomy and radiation dose (half and full dose). (Color figure online)

5 Discussion and Conclusions

In this work, we evaluated the dependency of the NAQI to breast anatomy and radiation dose. To assess the image quality properly, the proposed index must report a stronger dependency to image quality than to breast anatomy.

The first experiment used noiseless images with a range of anatomies to assess how the breast composition individually influences the NAQI. The results of this experiment, presented in Table 1, showed that the NAQI decreases at most 12 % when only the anatomy changes.

In the second experiment, the images were simulated with quantum noise in accordance with the AEC in digital mammography, corresponding to the standard radiation dose (full dose) and 50 % dose of a clinical mammographic projection. The variation on image quality due to dose reduction yielded a decrease of 33 % in the NAQI. Figures 2 and 3 show how each anatomic feature affects the metric on image quality. It is evident that changes on image quality (between blue and red columns) cause greater variation in the metric than do variations in breast anatomy (within red and blue columns).

Moreover, in a detailed analysis, the NAQI trend is inverted in terms of the number of compartments, i.e., the anisotropic index tends to be higher because of the increased complexity arising from the larger number of compartments (from 167 to 1,000). This inverse relationship proves that the index is highly sensitive to quantum noise. Thus, although the AEC adjusts the exposure factors to different breast profiles, denser phantoms tend to achieve lower NAQI.

The discrete histogram distribution based upon the NAQI values differentiates with high accuracy (AUC = 0.994) good quality images (full dose) and low quality (half dose).

For future work, the authors will analyze a large institutional clinical data set to provide a more complete statistic.

Acknowledgments. The authors would like to thank São Paulo Research Foundation (FAPESP grant #2013/18915-5) and the Brazilian Foundation for the Coordination of Improvement of Higher Education Personnel (CAPES grant #99999.014175/2013-04 and grant #88881.030443/ 2013-01) for the financial support given to this project. The authors would also like to acknowledge the support of the National Institutes of Health/National Cancer Institute grant 1R01-CA154444 and the U.S. National Institute of General Medical Sciences (P20 GM103446) from the National Institutes of Health. The content of this paper is solely the responsibility of the authors and does not necessarily represent the official views of the funding agencies. We thank Real Time Tomography (RTT) for providing assistance with image processing. We also acknowledge Abdullah-Al-Zubaer Imran, Niara Medley, Rick Emory, and Vernita Adkins for their assistance generating software breast phantoms and projections. ADAM is a member of the scientific advisory board and shareholder of RTT.

References

1. Li, Y., Poulos, A., Mclean, D., Rickard, M.: A review of methods of clinical image quality evaluation in mammography. Eur. J. Radiol. **74**, e122–e131 (2010). doi:10.1016/j.ejrad.2009.04.069
2. Wang, Z., Bovik, A.C.: Modern image quality assessment. Synth. Lect. Image Video Multimed. Process. (2006). doi:10.2200/S00010ED1V01Y200508IVM003
3. Oliveira, H.C.R., Barufaldi, B., Borges, L.R., Gabarda, S., Bakic, P.R., Maidment, A.D.A., Schiabel, H., Vieira, M.A.C.: Validation of no-reference image quality index for the assessment of digital mammographic images. In: SPIE Med Imaging, San Diego, CA, p. 978713-2 (2016). doi:10.1117/12.2217229
4. Bakic, P.R., Pokrajac, D.D., De Caro, R., Maidment, A.D.: Realistic simulation of breast tissue microstructure in software anthropomorphic phantoms. In: Fujita, H., Hara, T., Muramatsu, C. (eds.) IWDM 2014. LNCS, vol. 8539, pp. 348–355. Springer, Heidelberg (2014). doi:10.1007/978-3-319-07887-8_49
5. Bakic, P.R., Zhang, C., Maidment, A.D.A.: Development and characterization of an anthropomorphic breast software phantom based upon region-growing algorithm. Med. Phys. **38**, 3165–3176 (2011). doi:10.1118/1.3590357
6. Gabarda, S., Cristóbal, G.: Blind image quality assessment through anisotropy. J. Opt. Soc. Am. Opt. Image Sci. Vis. **24**, B42–B51 (2007). doi:10.1364/JOSAA.24.000B42

Grid-Less Imaging with Anti-scatter Correction Software in 2D Mammography: A JAFROC Study Using Simulated Lesions

Frédéric Bemelmans[1]([⊠]), Nelis Van Peteghem[1],
Xenia Bramaje Adversalo[1], Elena Salvagnini[1],
Chantal Van Ongeval[1,2], and Hilde Bosmans[1,2]

[1] Department of Imaging and Pathology, KU Leuven,
Herestraat 49, 3000 Leuven, Belgium
frederic.bemelmans@outlook.com
[2] Department of Radiology, UZ Leuven,
Herestraat 49, 3000 Leuven, Belgium

Abstract. *Purpose:* To perform a virtual clinical trial study to assess the justification of the grid-less mammography acquisition mode with scatter correction software, as developed by Siemens Healthcare (PRIME mode). *Materials and methods:* The study was performed on a Siemens mammography unit using the conventional acquisition mode (system 1) and a second system used PRIME. Mean glandular doses (MGD) were compared from data of 5981 images. A paired t-test for all thickness groups (<29 mm, 30–49 mm, 50–70 mm, >69 mm) separately and combined had shown a significantly higher average MGD for system 1 (NON-PRIME) when compared to system 2 (PRIME), with an overall decrease of 11.7 %. The next phase in justification focused on detectability performance, in particular for screening applications. A dataset mimicking an enriched screened population was created by simulating previously developed anthropomorphic mass models and microcalcification clusters in 60 out of 100 normal mammograms of system 1 (NON-PRIME). The same physical lesions were then simulated into 60 out of 100 PRIME, normal mammograms. Care was taken to simulate each lesion model in matched mammograms PRIME-NON PRIME in terms of BI-RADS score, in a region with the same background glandularity (obtained after analysis with Volpara) and in a breast of the same thickness group. All images were visualized with ViewDEX software and four radiologists performed the free search detectability study. A JAFROC analysis was executed and detectability was quantified by means of the AUC. *Results:* Present approach allowed the realization of paired virtual clinical data sets starting from 200 normal mammograms. The results of all readers separately as well as combined showed approximately the same AUC for PRIME and NON-PRIME (0.57 vs 0.60), and the ANOVA analysis showed no statistical significant difference in detectability of the lesions between PRIME and NON-PRIME (p-value 0.36). The same result was found if the dataset was subdivided for both types of lesions: masses (p-value 0.88) and microcalcification clusters (p-value 0.33). *Conclusion:* Results state that the MGD is significantly lower in PRIME mode than with the conventional acquisition while lesion detectability remained constant for all four radiologists.

© Springer International Publishing Switzerland 2016
A. Tingberg et al. (Eds.): IWDM 2016, LNCS 9699, pp. 234–242, 2016.
DOI: 10.1007/978-3-319-41546-8_31

Keywords: Simulated lesions · Virtual clinical trials · Grid-less imaging · 2D mammography · PRIME · JAFROC · MGD

1 Introduction

Full field digital mammography is the modality of choice for breast cancer detection. Today, new digital mammography technologies are still being developed for an even better performance by optimizing the systems at different stages of acquisition, processing and display. Present work tests the effect of the grid-less acquisition mode with scatter correction software as developed by Siemens Healthcare (PRIME mode) in terms of Mean Glandular Dose (MGD) and lesion detectability. We have focused on the screened population as performance is most critical for this application. The MGD was studied first from a large patient dose survey performed on a system with and without PRIME. Rather than running a large and time consuming clinical trial, patient images of these systems were used for the partially virtual clinical trial. It started from real mammograms into which lesions were simulated corresponding to 3D models that had been validated for realism in earlier work [1, 2]. The study also used scatter fractions with and without grid for the Siemens Inspiration system [3]. The partially virtual clinical trial approach allows to simulate lesions in matched pairs of images, namely in images with the same glandularity, the same thickness and the same local glandularity estimation, yet acquired with or without PRIME. Visibility of the lesions was also tuned by their size and choice of attenuation coefficient. Additionally, the same physical lesions were simulated into regions of interest (ROIs) with the same local glandularity estimation in the matched mammogram, allowing paired processing that could not be performed in real clinical trials. A free search study was conducted to evaluate lesion detectability in both conditions.

2 Method and Materials

2.1 Mean Glandular Dose

The study was performed on a SIEMENS mammography unit (Mammomat Inspiration, Erlangen, Germany) using the conventional acquisition mode (system 1) and a second SIEMENS Mammomat Inspiration system using PRIME. The dose was clinically investigated by performing a patient dose survey on these systems with the TQM software package (qaelum NV, Belgium). In total, 5981 2D digital mammograms were extracted from the PACS system, collected in a time period of three months: 2931 mediolateral oblique images and 3050 cranio-caudal images. These images were further subdivided into seven different thickness groups (10–19 mm, 20–29 mm, 30–39 mm, 40–49 mm, 50–59 mm, 60–69 mm, >69 mm). The largest thickness group was discarded, because the system uses the anti-scatter grid again from 70 mm. Thus a comparison between PRIME and NON-PRIME is not possible above 69 mm. The Mean Glandular Dose (MGD) was extracted from the image headers and a paired t-test was executed to compare the patient doses of the two systems for all thickness groups, combined and separately.

2.2   Partially Virtual Clinical Trial

A dataset mimicking an enriched screened population was set up by simulating previously developed 3D lesion models into normal 2D cranio-caudal mammograms obtained from routine screening activities. It started from 350 mammograms, 100 NON-PRIME and 250 PRIME images, judged to be normal by an expert radiologist. The simulation started with the 100 NON-PRIME images. Three-dimensional mass models and microcalcification clusters were simulated into 60 out of these 100 normal mammograms of both groups [1, 2]. A validated software framework was used to create projection templates of the 3D lesions that can then be added to base line images of patients. These base images were for processing images that have been linearized in terms of detector air kerma and after subtraction of the estimated scatter fraction at the place of insertion. After adding the lesion template, the theoretical scatter fraction is added again. This framework accounts for system geometry, the x-ray spectra (kV, T/F combination), the local glandularity of the ROI, Modulation Transfer Function (MTF) and the scatter fraction [3]. The main difference between conventional acquisitions and PRIME is the scatter fraction. The local glandularity score is used to define the attenuation coefficient of the tissue that is theoretically being replaced by a mass lesion. The hybrid images were then processed using the software tool provided by the vendor. Firstly, the lesions were simulated into the normal, NON-PRIME mammograms. We created 10 'easy to find' lesions (5 microcalcs, 5 masses), 10 difficult lesions and 40 lesions were made subtle. As a result, 30 images contained microcalcification clusters and 30 images contained masses, while 40 2D mammograms were lesion-free. The same physical lesions with the same size and attenuation coefficient, were then simulated in 100 normal PRIME mammograms. 100 out of 250 PRIME mammograms were carefully selected to create the right match with the NON-PRIME images. Care was taken to simulate each lesion model in matched mammograms PRIME-NON PRIME in terms of BI-RADS score, in a region with the same background glandularity (obtained after analysis with Volpara [4]) and in a breast of the same thickness group.

The 200 mammograms were randomly subdivided into 4 sets of 50 images. The four image datasets of the partially virtual clinical trial were read by four radiologists using a free search paradigm to detect lesions and to subsequently classify them with the VIEWDEX viewing software [5]. The software allows the user to pan, zoom, window/level and put marks in an image. After the reader selected a region, three questions needed to be answered: (1) Confidence with the presence of the lesion on a 5 point scale (from suggestive for a lesion to definitely a lesion); (2) Which type of lesion is observed (mass or microcalcification cluster); (3) BI-RADS score of the lesion.

The output of the VIEWDEX software was used to calculate the fraction of true positive (TP) and false positive (FP) cases, both of them necessary input parameters for the FROC (free response receiver operating characteristic). In contradiction to the ROC method, the FROC method takes into account the suspicious locations marked by the reader to verify the TP or FP character of the case, which resembles more the clinical practice [6]. The JAFROC software (JAFROC, version 4.2.1) [7] was used for a jackknife-alternative free-response receiver operating characteristic (JAFROC) analysis. Detectability was quantified by means of the AUC of an Alternative FROC study (lesion localization fraction as a function of false positive fraction). The larger the AUC, the higher the detectability of the lesions. One-way ANOVA statistics was performed for the statistical comparison between conventional mammography and PRIME, and for all further subdivisions of the dataset.

3 Results and Discussion

Table 1 shows the average Mean Glandular dose with its standard deviation for both systems and each thickness group. The smallest thickness group (10-19 mm) was left out of the study: our radiographers insist on using the Mo/Mo target/filter combination for thin breasts (this mode brings the anti-scatter grid in place). This choice is considered justified too (next to the use of W/Rh) based on an older study in our department [8]. The largest thickness group (>69 mm) was also excluded because the system automatically switches off the PRIME mode for breasts thicker than 69 mm. The average MGD is lower for each thickness category for the PRIME system. The highest dose reduction (27.3 %) was found for the smaller breasts (20–29 mm); a decreasing dose reduction is noticeable for increasing breast thickness. The average dose reduction for all breast thicknesses combined (20–69 mm) was found to be 11.7 %. This dose reduction was found to be statistically significant (p-value 1.53E-45). The study reflect how the system is pre-programmed.

Table 1. Average MGD, SD and p-values for both systems for different breast thickness categories (20–29 mm; 30–39 mm; 40–49 mm; 50–59 mm; 60–69 mm) and for all breast thickness categories combined

Breast thickness (mm)	SYSTEM 1 (NON-PRIME)		SYSTEM 2 (PRIME)		SYSTEM 1 vs SYSTEM 2	
	Nr. of images	MGD ± SD (mGy)	Nr. of images	MGD ± SD (mGy)	Dose reduction	p-value
20–29	321	1.01 ± 0.20	186	0.73 ± 0.14	27.3 %	5.48E-49
30–39	684	1.12 ± 0.30	342	0.85 ± 0.18	23.8 %	1.75E-46
40–49	1073	1.22 ± 0.34	506	1.03 ± 0.25	15.9 %	2.96E-29
50–59	1056	1.37 ± 0.36	680	1.26 ± 0.36	8.4 %	9.27E-11
60–69	637	1.62 ± 0.44	496	1.46 ± 0.41	9.9 %	3.25E-10
20–29	3771	1.29 ± 0.40	2210	1.14 ± 0.40	11.7 %	1.53E-45

Table 2 indicates the figure of merit (FoM) for the full dataset from the JAFROC analysis for all four radiologists separately and combined. The full dataset denoted an average Area Under the Curve (AUC) for the NON-PRIME mode of 0.57 with 95 % CI of 0.52–0.61. The AUC for the PRIME mode was slightly larger with 0.60 and 95 % CI of 0.56–0.64. The results of the one-way ANOVA demonstrated that there was no statistically significant difference between both modes. This was also confirmed for each of the readers separately (p-values ranging from 0.17 to 0.94). These results justify the use of grid-less imaging with anti-scatter correction software for detectability of lesions. The AUC of both systems are a bit low, indicating that the datasets are quite difficult. This is a result of simulating more lesions in a subtle way and some even in a non-obvious way. The AUC of the systems are still acceptable to evaluate the performance of the radiologists and to compare PRIME and NON-PRIME.

Table 2. AUC and the 95 % CI for the JAFROC analysis for the full dataset

ALL LESIONS					
	NON-PRIME		PRIME		
Observer	AUC	95 % CI	AUC	95 % CI	P-VALUE
1	0.59	0.54–0.65	0.59	0.53–0.65	0.9461
2	0.57	0.52–0.61	0.61	0.56–0.65	0.2437
3	0.56	0.51–0.62	0.60	0.54–0.65	0.4328
4	0.54	0.48–0.60	0.61	0.55–0.67	0.1739
AVERAGE	0.57	0.52–0.61	0.60	0.56–0.64	0.3626

Figure 1 FoM curves plot lesion localization fraction (LLF) as a function of the false positive fraction (FPF). The AUC of the PRIME function seems slightly higher than the NON-PRIME function. As indicated previously (Table 2), this effect was not found to be significant.

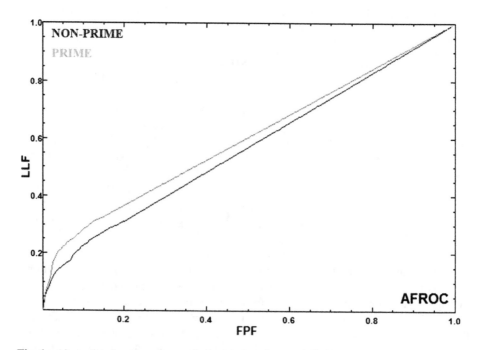

Fig. 1. Alternative free-response receiver operating characteristic (AFROC) curve for all lesions and for all readers combined with: red = NON-PRIME and green = PRIME (Color figure online)

In a next step, the dataset was subdivided for the two different lesion types: masses and microcalcification clusters. The aim of this subdivision was to evaluate whether there was a significant difference in detectability of either masses or the microcalcification clusters for conventional acquisition mode versus PRIME.

Table 3 shows the FoM for detectability of masses only for all four radiologists separately and combined. The mass dataset denoted an average AUC for the conventional mode of 0.54 with 95 % CI of 0.50–0.58. The AUC for the PRIME mode was found to be approximately the same, namely 0.54 and 95 % CI of 0.51–0.58. The results of the one-way ANOVA demonstrated that there was no statistically significant difference between both modes. This was also confirmed for each of the readers separately (p-values ranging from 0.60 to 0.93). These results demonstrate that grid-less imaging with anti-scatter correction software is a good candidate for the task of mass detectability. The AUC of both systems are quite low, indicating that the datasets are more difficult, but the scores are still acceptable to compare both modalities.

Table 3. AUC and the 95 % CI for the JAFROC analysis for the mass images

MASSES					
	NON-PRIME		PRIME		
Observer	AUC	95 % CI	AUC	95 % CI	P-VALUE
1	0.55	0.50–0.60	0.54	0.49–0.59	0.7642
2	0.55	0.51–0.59	0.55	0.51–0.59	0.9258
3	0.53	0.48–0.57	0.54	0.49–0.59	0.7844
4	0.52	0.46–0.58	0.55	0.49–0.61	0.6026
AVERAGE	0.54	0.50–0.58	0.54	0.51–0.58	0.8763

This result is also demonstrated in Fig. 2 which shows the FoM curve, namely Lesions localization fraction as a function of the false positive fraction. The AUC of both curves are approximately overlapping, indicating that there is no difference in detectability of the masses between conventional imaging and PRIME.

Table 4 shows the FoM for the microcalcification clusters for all four radiologists separately and combined. The microcalcification cluster dataset denoted an average AUC for the NON-PRIME mode of 0.59 with 95 % CI of 0.54–0.63. The AUC for the PRIME mode was found to be slightly higher with an average AUC of 0.62 and 95 % CI of 0.58–0.67. The one-way ANOVA concluded that the values of PRIME and NON-PRIME were not statistically significantly different (p-value 0.33). This result was also confirmed for all radiologists separately (p-values ranging from 0.23 to 0.75). Again, these results indicate that there is no statistically significant difference in microcalcification detectability between PRIME and NON-PRIME mode.

Figure 3 shows the lesion localization fraction as a function of the false positive fraction for the microcalcification clusters. The graph suggests that the AUC of the PRIME is different from the AUC of the NON-PRIME. As already addressed, this difference was not found to be significant. From these results it can be stated that,

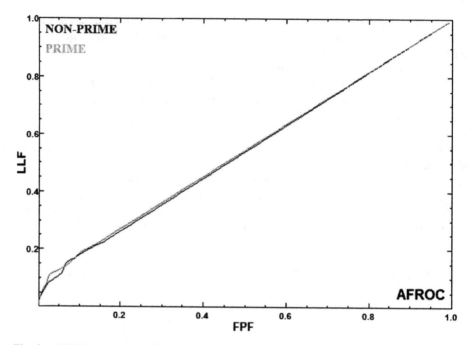

Fig. 2. AFROC curve for all mass images and for all readers combined with: red = NON-PRIME and green = PRIME (Color figure online)

Table 4. AUC and 95 % CI from JAFROC analysis (AFROC area) of microcalcification clusters readings

μCALC CLUSTERS					
	NON-PRIME		PRIME		
Observer	AUC	95 % CI	AUC	95 % CI	P-VALUE
1	0.61	0.59–0.67	0.54	0.49–0.59	0.7642
2	0.56	0.51–0.60	0.55	0.51–0.59	0.9258
3	0.59	0.48–0.57	0.54	0.49–0.59	0.7844
4	0.58	0.46–0.58	0.55	0.49–0.61	0.6026
AVERAGE	0.59	0.50–0.58	0.54	0.51–0.58	0.8763

for present collection of microcalcification clusters and base line images, detection is not significantly different conventional and PRIME imaging.

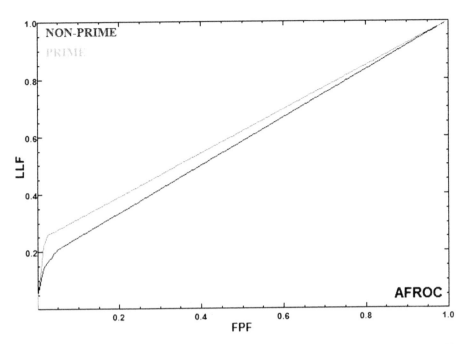

Fig. 3. AFROC curve for all microcalcification clusters and for all readers combined with: red = NON-PRIME and green = PRIME (Color figure online)

4   Conclusion

This study aimed to evaluate grid-less acquisition mode with scatter correction software as developed by Siemens Healthcare (PRIME mode) in a comparative study with conventional acquisitions. Next to a classical patient dose survey, a partially virtual clinical trial was used to assess detectability: radiologists had to search for (simulated) masses and clusters of microcalcifications in otherwise normal mammograms, mimicking an enriched screening data set.

A paired t-test analysis indicated a significantly lower MGD for PRIME versus the conventional acquisition mode for breasts with a thickness of 20 mm to 69 mm. The same results was found when the breasts were subdivided into different thickness groups (20–29 mm, 30–39 mm, 40–49 mm, 50–59 mm and 60–69 mm).

The AUC of the JAFROC study was approximately the same for PRIME and NON-PRIME, which was supported by the ANOVA analysis for all radiologists separately as well as combined. We did not find any statistically significant difference in detectability between PRIME and NON-PRIME. These results were also found if the dataset was separated into the two types of lesions: the masses and microcalcification clusters.

There are obvious limitations to this study: we used a type of virtual clinical trial, termed 'partially virtual', as we started from real mammograms rather than simulating the complete imaging chain. This has the advantage that a lot of hidden or obvious characteristics are included in the base line images. The software correction software will also perform as in clinical practice as even after insertion of the (subtle) lesions, the mammograms cannot be distinguished from real mammograms. Compared to a real clinical trial, present approach can be fast. A limitation is linked to the number of cases, the number and the type of the masses and the fact that a trial is never truly representative for the reality as there is no consequence for the patient from the readings.

Our results indicate that the system with PRIME is preprogrammed to operate at a lower MGD level, overall 11.7 %, while detectability assessed from a dataset mimicking an enriched screened population was not statistically significantly different. This makes the system with PRIME a suitable alternative for 2D mammography with grid for thicknesses <70 mm.

References

1. Shaheen, E., Van Ongeval, C., Zanca, F., Cockmartin, L., Marshall, N., Jacobs, J., Young, K. C., Dance, D.R., Bosmans, H.: The simulation of 3D microcalcification clusters in 2D digital mammography and breast tomosynthesis. Med. Phys. **38**(12), 6659–6671 (2011)
2. Shaheen, E., De Keyzer, F., Bosmans, H., Dance, D.R., Young, K.C., Van Ongeval, C.: The simulation of 3D mass models in 2D digital mammography and breast tomosynthesis. Med. Phys. **41**(8), 081913 (2014)
3. Salvagnini, E., Bosmans, H., Struelens, L., Marshall, N.W.: Quantification of scattered radiation in projection mammography: four practical methods compared. Med. Phys. **39**(6), 3167–3180 (2012)
4. Highnam, R., Brady, S.M., Yaffe, M.J., Karssemeijer, N., Harvey, J.: Robust Breast Composition Measurement - Volpara. In: Martí, J., Oliver, A., Freixenet, J., Martí, R. (eds.) IWDM 2010. LNCS, vol. 6136, pp. 342–349. Springer, Heidelberg (2010)
5. Håkansson, M., Svensson, S., Zachrisson, S., Svalkvist, A., Båth, M., Månsson, L.G.: VIEWDEX: an efficient and easy-to-use software for observer performance studies. Rad Prot Dosimetry **139**(1–3), 42–51 (2010)
6. Chakraborty, D.P.: Recent advances in observer performance methodology: jackknife free response ROC (JAFROC). Radiat. Prot. Dosim. **114**(1-3), 26–31 (2005)
7. Chakraborty, D.P., Berbaum, K.S.: Observer studies involving detection and localization: modeling, analysis, and validation. Med. Phys. **31**(8), 2313–2330 (2004)
8. Toroi, P., Zanca, F., Young, K.C., Van Ongeval, C., Marchal, G., Bosmans, H.: Experimental investigation on the choice of the tungsten/rhodium anode/filter combination for an amorphous selenium-based digital mammography system. Eur. Radiol. **17**(9), 2368–2375 (2007)

Towards a Phantom for Multimodality Performance Evaluation of Breast Imaging: A 3D Structured Phantom with Simulated Lesions Tested for 2D Digital Mammography

Kristina Tri Wigati[1,2], Lesley Cockmartin[3], Nicholas Marshall[1,3], Djarwani S. Soejoko[2], and Hilde Bosmans[1,3(✉)]

[1] Department of Imaging and Pathology, Medical Imaging Research Center, KU Leuven, Leuven, Belgium
`kristinatri.wigati@student.kuleuven.be,`
[2] Department of Physics, Faculty of Mathematics and Natural Sciences, University of Indonesia, Depok, Indonesia
`djarwani@fisika.ui.ac.id`
[3] Department of Radiology, University Hospitals Leuven, Leuven, Belgium
`{lesley.cockmartin,nicholas.marshall,`
`hilde.bosmans}@uzleuven.be`

Abstract. The aim of this work is to test whether a 3D structured phantom with simulated lesions can be used for performance evaluation of 2D digital mammography, as a step towards a multimodality phantom. A phantom, developed for breast tomosynthesis was therefore applied on 23 digital mammography systems. Ten images were acquired at the clinically used dose and for 11 systems also at half and double dose. The images were read in a four-alternative forced choice (4-AFC) paradigm by 5 readers. CDMAM phantom acquisitions were also performed. It was possible to calculate diameter thresholds of the simulated masses and microcalcifications that guarantee 62.5 % correct response. The results showed the expected sensitivity with mean glandular dose: detectability of microcalcifications improved with dose, whereas the detectability of masses was not affected. Systems of the same manufacturer and operated at similar doses had very similar detectability scores. Percentage correctly detected microcalcifications with average diameter 119 μm correlated with CDMAM based gold thickness thresholds. Present phantom, developed and tested for tomosynthesis, is also a good candidate for 2D mammography, suggesting its use for (future) benchmarking of at least two types of imaging systems.

Keywords: 3D structured phantom · Spiculated masses · Non-spiculated masses · Microcalcifications · Image quality

1 Introduction

With new imaging modalities being introduced for radiological imaging of the breast, a generally accepted phantom for performance testing would be of great use. Current new generation mammography devices include breast tomosynthesis, contrast

© Springer International Publishing Switzerland 2016
A. Tingberg et al. (Eds.): IWDM 2016, LNCS 9699, pp. 243–253, 2016.
DOI: 10.1007/978-3-319-41546-8_32

enhanced spectral mammography and breast CT. Their (future) role has to be explored and justified. All new modalities aim to enhance particular features of lesions or breast tissue, yet at this point, 2D digital mammography remains the standard in breast cancer screening. Justification of new modalities may therefore be helped from a comparison with 2D mammography.

Test objects that have been used extensively in full field digital mammography (FFDM) are not well suited to judge the advantages of new modalities if the elements of potential benefits are not included in the test. As an example: tomosynthesis is being developed for its ability to reduce overlapping tissue. This aspect cannot be tested with a test object that lacks any 3D structure around a detectability target.

The challenge of testing digital breast tomosynthesis (DBT) had made us develop a new phantom with a 3D structure and simulated lesions for task based performance evaluation in terms of lesion detectability. The choices of number and types of lesions allowed a four-alternative forced choice (4-AFC) evaluation mode. The aim of present study is to test whether the same 3D structured phantom with simulated lesions can be used for performance evaluation of 2D digital mammography, making it a second modality that can be tested with the same phantom and providing basically the same metric as in DBT, namely detectability of lesions. This approach may help in justification cases or for benchmarking of systems.

Present study includes three main phases. First, establish the performance scores that 2D digital mammography obtains with the new phantom when being used under clinical exposure conditions, by calculating diameter thresholds and number of detected targets. This will then automatically lead to minimal scores that a 2D digital mammography unit should reach. Second, study the sensitivity of the 3D structured phantom in response to dose variation. Third, compare the applicability of the new phantom for performance testing with the experience of a routinely used phantom with the same purpose, namely the CDMAM phantom.

2   Materials and Methods

2.1   The 3D Structured Phantom

Figure 1 and Table 1 show the 3D structured phantom and its inserted lesions [1]. The 3D structured background was created with acrylic spheres of 6 different diameters (15.88, 12.70, 9.52, 6.35, 3.18, and 1.58 mm) (United States Plastic Corp., Ohio, USA) that were submersed in a cylindrical container that was otherwise filled with water [2–4]. The container has a semi-circular shape with a thickness of 48 mm and diameter of 200 mm, equivalent with a compressed breast thickness of 60 mm. Five spiculated and 5 non-spiculated 3D printed masses, and 5 microcalcification groups with various sizes, aimed for covering a clinically relevant range, were inserted in the phantom. Spiculated and non-spiculated masses were created from a database of 3D voxel models by Shaheen *et al.* [5]. Two lesions that, after insertion in DBT, had received a high realism and high malignancy score by the radiologists, were selected for 3D printing. The masses were made of the material NEXT (Materialize, Leuven) in order to approximate the linear attenuation coefficient of cancerous tissue in real breast [1].

The microcalcifications are formed from calcium carbonate ($CaCO_3$) (Leeds Test Objects, Leeds, UK) and available in 5 size groups. The spheres are not fixed in their position, while the lesions have been glued on a little support in PMMA. This approach generates always new 3D structured backgrounds after a simple shaking of the phantom. This variability was introduced in the phantom on purpose: it is a straightforward way for the application of model observer based evaluations in digital breast tomosynthesis (DBT) and 2D digital mammography. Present study will be followed by more studies developing automated reading, most probably using the model observer approach.

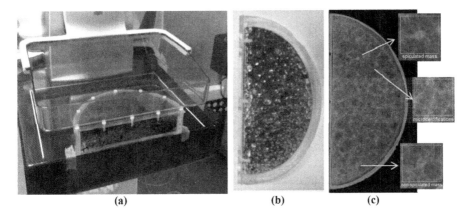

(a)   (b)   (c)

Fig. 1. (a) A semi-circular phantom with structured background filled with spheres of 6 different diameters and inserted target objects representing spiculated masses, non-spiculated masses and microcalcifications [1], (b) Photograph of the phantom from the top, and (c) "For presentation" 2D mammogram of the phantom

Table 1. Diameter of the inserted target object.

Spiculated masses				Non-spiculated masses				Microcalcifications	
X (mm)	Y (mm)	Z (mm)	Average (mm)	X(mm)	Y(mm)	Z(mm)	Average (mm)	Diameter range (μm)	Average (μm)
4.4	4.4	1.6	3.8	1.6	1.4	1.9	1.8	90-100	95
6.1	6.1	2.3	4.8	2.2	2.0	2.7	2.3	112-125	119
8.8	8.8	3.2	6.9	3.2	2.8	3.8	3.3	140-160	150
12.2	12.2	4.5	9.7	4.5	4.0	5.3	4.6	180-200	190
16.6	16.6	6.1	13.1	6.1	5.4	7.2	6.2	224-250	237

2.2   Image Acquisitions

Twenty three digital mammography systems that are used on routine basis in the Belgian breast cancer screening were included in the study. All the systems and their exposure factors are shown in Table 2. Eleven systems were assessed with the 3D structured phantom and the CDMAM phantom at three dose levels: the clinically used dose (also called AEC dose, as this is the setting controlled by the automatic exposure control (AEC) of the system for the phantom), half this dose (also called half AEC dose), and double AEC dose. Twelve systems were only assessed with the 3D structured phantom at AEC dose level. For each dose level, 10 "for presentation" images of the 3D structured phantom and at least eight "for processing" images of the CDMAM phantom were acquired on each system.

Table 2. Digital mammography systems in the present study and their exposure factors.

No	System	A/F	kV	mAs manual		
				Half AEC	AEC	Double AEC
1	Agfa DX-M + CR HM 5.0 (1)	Mo/Rh (25μm)	30	32.0	63.0	125.0
2	Agfa DX-M + CR HM 5.0 (2)	Mo/Rh (25μm)	28		80.0	
3	Fuji Profect CS + CR HR-BD	Mo/Rh (25μm)	28	50.0	100.0	200.0
4	Fuji Amulet S	W/Rh (50μm)	30	45.0	90.0	180.0
5	Fuji Amulet Innovality	W/Rh (50μm)	30	36.0	71.0	138.0
6	GE Senographe Essential (1)	Rh/Rh (25μm)	29	28.0	56.0	110.0
7	GE Senographe Essential (2)	Rh/Rh (25μm)	29	36.0	71.0	140.0
8	GE Senographe Essential (3)	Rh/Rh (25μm)	29		71.0	
9	GE Senographe Essential (4)	Rh/Rh (25μm)	29		63.0	
10	GE Senographe Essential (5)	Rh/Rh (25μm)	29		71.0	
11	GE Senographe Essential (6)	Rh/Rh (25μm)	29		56.0	
12	Hologic Selenia Dimensions	W/Rh (50μm)	31	70.0	140.0	280.0
13	IMS Giotto Image 3DL	W/Rh (50μm)	31	99.0	198.0	300.0
14	Philips MicroDose L50	W/Al (50μm)	35	6.5	12.5	23.5
15	Philips MicroDose L30 (1)	W/Al (50μm)	38		12.0	
16	Philips MicroDose L30 (2)	W/Al (50μm)	32		16.0	
17	Siemens Mammomat Inspiration (1)	W/Rh (50μm)	30	50.0	100.0	200.0
18	Siemens Mammomat Inspiration (2)	W/Rh (50μm)	30		90.0	
19	Siemens Mammomat Inspiration (3)	W/Rh (50μm)	30		100.0	
20	Siemens Mammomat Inspiration (4)	W/Rh (50μm)	30		90.0	
21	Siemens Mammomat Inspiration (5)	W/Rh (50μm)	30		90.0	
22	Siemens Mammomat Inspiration (6)	W/Rh (50μm)	31		80.0	
23	Siemens Mammomat Inspiration PRIME	W/Rh (50μm)	30	45.0	90.0	180.0

2.3   Image Analysis

The 3D structured phantom images were read in a 4 AFC paradigm: a segment with lesion (signal) was shown next to 3 signal free images. These image compositions were shown in random order to 5 human readers using our in house developed visualisation program [6]. Since there were 15 inserted target objects (5 spiculated masses, 5 non-spiculated masses, and 5 groups of microcalcifications) in ten "for presentation" images, 150 images of signal and 450 selected images of background had to be prepared for every system. In this study, each image segment of signal and background had a dimension of 20 mm × 20 mm. Two hundred sets of image segments of background were used out which 450 segments have been randomly chosen, some of them obviously several times. The observers were allowed to adjust contrast, brightness and zoom level to reach the optimum condition for observation. Ultimately, the percentage correctly detected signals (PC) was calculated.

The PC value was then fitted as a function of diameter. As the psychometric curve had shown high correlation coefficients, this function was applied and subsequently a diameter threshold was defined, namely the diameter corresponding to a PC of 62.5 %:

$$PC = 0.25 + \frac{0.75}{1 + \left(\frac{d}{dtr}\right)^{-f}} \tag{1}$$

where d is diameter, dtr is diameter threshold, and f is a parameter of the psychometric curve that is obtained after fitting [1, 7].

The CDMAM phantom acquisitions were analyzed with CDCOM software following the procedure in the European Guidelines, a common practice in our quality control activities [8, 9].

2.4   Mean Glandular Dose Calculation

Mean glandular dose (MGD) was calculated according to the work of Dance *et al.* and copied in the European guidelines [8, 9].

$$MGD = K\,g\,c\,s \tag{2}$$

where K is the incident air kerma (without backscatter, filtered by the compression paddle) at the top surface of the breast. The g-factor transforms the incident air kerma into absorbed dose to the glandular tissue, assuming a glandularity of 50 %. The c-factor is a correction factor that accounts for the glandularity if that is different from 50 %. The s-factor is related with the choice of beam quality used.

3   Results

3.1   The Diameter Threshold

In present study, 14 types of objects were analyzed (4 spiculated masses, 5 non-spiculated masses, and 5 microcalcifications). The phantom contained 5 spiculated masses but one mass was not used for the analysis due to its anomalous characteristics [1]. Figure 2 shows diameter threshold values of spiculated masses (a), non-spiculated

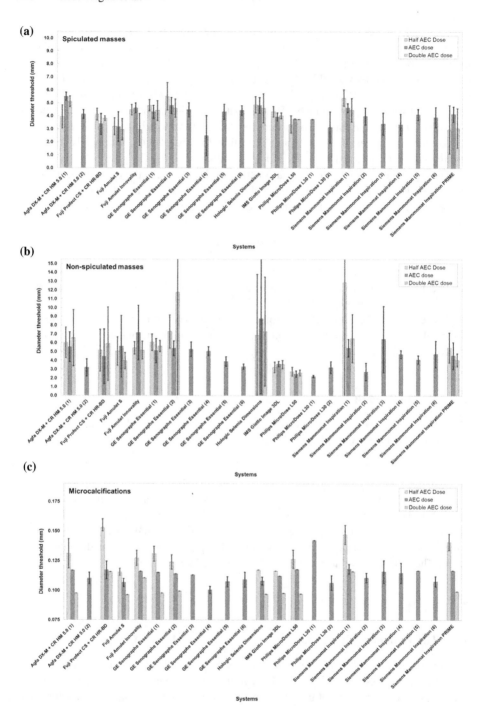

Fig. 2. Diameter thresholds of spiculated masses (a), non-spiculated masses (b) and microcalcifications (c). (Color figure online)

masses (b), and microcalcifications (c) that were obtained from the psychometric curve fits. We could derive such a curve for all systems operating at their clinical working condition. In a next phase, we calculated also the values for the half and double dose conditions.

At AEC dose level, the following system averaged diameter threshold values were obtained: 4.02 mm [range 3.73–4.32 mm] for spiculated masses, 4.64 mm [range 3.98–5.31 mm] for non-spiculated masses and 0.114 mm [range 0.110–0.117 mm] for microcalcifications. According to these values, 3[range 3–4] spiculated masses, 1[range 1–2] non-spiculated mass and 4 groups of microcalcifications were correctly detected for this range of systems.

3.2   Mean Glandular Dose

The MGD at AEC dose level of the 23 systems ranged from 0.75 mGy to 3.32 mGy (Table 3).

Table 3. Mean glandular dose of 23 systems acquired at half AEC dose, AEC dose, and double AEC dose, calculated with the method described by Dance.

No	System	MGD (mGy)		
		Half AEC dose	AEC dose	Double AEC dose
1	Agfa DX-M + CR HM 5.0 (1)	0.96	1.90	3.76
2	Agfa DX-M + CR HM 5.0 (2)		1.68	
3	Fuji Profect CS + CR HR-BD	1.02	2.05	4.10
4	Fuji Amulet S	0.69	1.38	2.76
5	Fuji Amulet Innovality	0.54	1.07	2.08
6	GE Senographe Essential (1)	0.58	1.17	2.30
7	GE Senographe Essential (2)	0.81	1.60	3.16
8	GE Senographe Essential (3)		1.43	
9	GE Senographe Essential (4)		1.39	
10	GE Senographe Essential (5)		1.47	
11	GE Senographe Essential (6)		1.16	
12	Hologic Selenia Dimensions	0.79	1.58	3.16
13	IMS Giotto Image 3DL	1.66	3.32	5.03
14	Philips MicroDose L50	0.41	0.80	1.50
15	Philips MicroDose L30 (1)		0.92	
16	Philips MicroDose L30 (2)		0.75	
17	Siemens Mammomat Inspiration (1)	0.60	1.19	2.38
18	Siemens Mammomat Inspiration (2)		1.08	
19	Siemens Mammomat Inspiration (3)		1.24	
20	Siemens Mammomat Inspiration (4)		1.14	
21	Siemens Mammomat Inspiration (5)		1.14	
22	Siemens Mammomat Inspiration (6)		1.09	
23	Siemens Mammomat Inspiration PRIME	0.54	1.07	2.15

3.3   Dose Sensitivity

Diameter thresholds as a function of MGD are shown for all lesions (spiculated masses, non-spiculated masses, and microcalcifications from 11 systems) in Fig. 3.

The diameter thresholds of spiculated masses and non-spiculated masses are not affected by the dose, although a decreasing trend with dose was observed. On the other hand, diameter thresholds of microcalcifications decreased significantly as dose was increased. Therefore, the change of dose significantly affects the microcalcification detection task performance, but not mass detection. This finding confirms the observations in many other and earlier studies [10–13]. A possible explanation for the difference in the effect of dose on masses versus the effect of dose on microcalcifications must be related with the different effects of anatomical structure noise at the one hand and system (quantum) noise at the other hand. In the study by Burgess et al., it was observed that mammographic backgrounds are dominated by a high magnitude of low spatial frequency components. Lowering dose has a relatively small effect on these low frequency components compared to the higher frequencies in which system noise is known to dominate. Therefore, a variation in dose leads to a smaller effect on the detection of (lower frequency) masses when compared to the detection of microcalcifications that are tiny objects with high frequencies that have to be discriminated from the high (dose affected) frequencies of the small region around the microcalcifications [13].

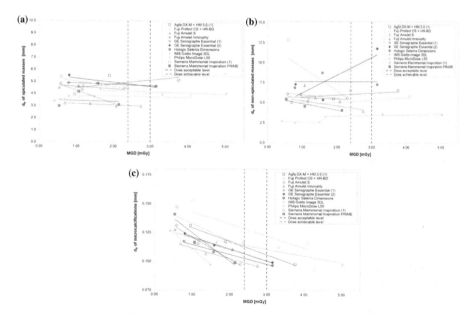

Fig. 3. Correlation between MGD and diameter threshold for spiculated masses (a), non-spiculated masses (b) and microcalcifications (c) from 11 systems tested at three dose levels. (Color figure online)

3.4   Comparison Between the 3D Structured Phantom and the CDMAM Phantom

Correlating the results of the 3D structured phantom and the CDMAM phantom is relevant and interesting for microcalcifications in the 3D structured phantom at the one hand and the smallest gold disks in the CDMAM phantom at the other hand. Figure 4 shows the correlation of the PC values of the group of microcalcifications with average diameter of 119 µm in the 3D structured phantom and the thickness thresholds of the gold disk with diameter 100 µm and present in the CDMAM phantom for all the systems in our study.

Pooled data analysis of all the systems showed that if a digital mammography system would be working at 62.5 % PC for the particular group of microcalcifications with diameter 119 µm, then the CDMAM analysis would show a thickness threshold of 1.50 µm for the 0.1 mm gold disk. This value is very close to the acceptable gold thickness threshold of 1.68 µm in the EUREF guidelines. PC values above 62.5 % for that group of microcalcifications may guarantee compliance with the EUREF criteria.

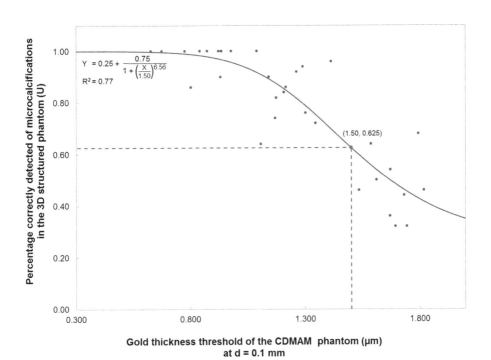

Fig. 4. Correlation between the percentage correctly detected microcalcifications of the group with average size 119 µm of the 3D structured phantom and gold thickness thresholds as obtained from CDMAM analysis of the same systems.

4   Discussions and Conclusions

The performance of each system to display the spiculated masses, non-spiculated masses, and microcalcifications is known to be multifactorial, and depending on the type of image detector, beam quality, dose setting and image processing, as these factors play a role in limiting spatial resolution, contrast, latitude or dynamic range, noise and artifacts. The modulation transfer function has a great impact on the spatial resolution. The X-ray energy spectrum, which is determined by the target material, kVp, and filtration (either inherent in the tube or added), is known to strongly affect the contrast resolution. System performance tests have a role as they allow to summarize all these aspects with a single measure [14]. From the results of present study, it is not clear which of all factors has the largest effect on the performance as tested here but a single performance test phantom will never explain all possible reasons of higher or lower scores. There remains a role for more detailed physics testing.

Detection of microcalcifications is mainly limited by spatial resolution and the effect of quantum and/or detector system noise. The use of fewer quanta (dose reduction) could increase the random noise or quantum mottle (for fixed signal) and therefore decrease SNR and reduce the ability to discern subtle differences in contrast. The visibility of masses is governed more by contrast resolution. The effect of tissue superimposition in 2D projection imaging is thought to merely limit the detection of mass lesions [10, 11, 14]. These characteristics have been confirmed in the dose response curve that was performed with the new phantom.

Present phantom allowed to list threshold diameters for spiculated lesions, non spiculated lesions and microcalcifications, with dose and size having a predictable impact on lesion detectability. These factors, next to the correlation with CDMAM readings, make it a candidate phantom for 2D digital mammography. Obviously, our data base is still limited and we do not have validated explanations for some of the lower or higher scores in our analysis. This could be further explored in the future.

The 3D structured phantom had been successfully applied on DBT. The same phantom being useful for 2D mammography has obvious practical advantages. More importantly, expressing performance in the same way between 2D mammography and DBT triggers comparative studies or bench marking. A next modality to test is breast CT. This must be feasible with similar background material and the same targets, brought together in a different container. Testing contrast enhanced spectral mammography may be possible with iodine including targets. Including breast MRI in this analysis is an ultimate challenge.

Acknowledgements. We would like to acknowledge the 4-AFC readers: Andreas Stratis, Frédéric Bemelmans, Michiel Dehairs, and Xochitl Lopez Rendon.

References

1. Cockmartin, L., Marshall, N.W., Zhang, G., Lemmens, K., Shaheen, E., Van Ongeval, C., Fredenberg, E., Dance, D.R., Salvagnini, E., Michielsen, K., Bosmans, H.: A structured phantom for detection performance comparison between breast tomosynthesis and digital mammography, Ph.D. thesis (2015)

2. Cockmartin, L., Marshall, N.W., Bosmans, H.: Design and evaluation of a phantom with structured background for digital mammography and breast tomosynthesis. In: Maidment, A.D., Bakic, P.R., Gavenonis, S. (eds.) IWDM 2012. LNCS, vol. 7361, pp. 642–649. Springer, Heidelberg (2012)
3. Cockmartin, L., Bosmans, H., Marshall, N.W.: Comparative power law analysis of structured breast phantom and patient images in digital mammography and breast tomosynthesis. Med. Phys. **40**(081920), 1–17 (2013)
4. Gang, G.J., Tward, D.J., Lee, J., Siewerdsen, J.H.: Anatomical background and generalized detectability in tomosynthesis and cone-beam CT. Med. Phys. **37**, 1948–1965 (2010)
5. Shaheen, E., De Keyzer, F., Bosmans, H., Dance, D.R., Young, K.C., van Ongeval, C.: The simulation of 3D mass models in 2D digital mammography and breast tomosynthesis. Med. Phys. **41**(081913), 1–17 (2014)
6. Zhang, G., Cockmartin, L., Bosmans, H.: A four-alternative forced choice (4AFC) software for observer performance evaluation in radiology. Poster presentation at the SPIE Conference, San Diego (2016)
7. Figl, M., Hoffmann, R., Kaar, M., Semturs, F., Brasik, N., Birkfellner, W., Homolka, P., Hummel, J.: Factors for conversion between human and automatic read-outs of CDMAM images. Med. Phys. **38**, 5090–5093 (2011)
8. European Commission: European guidelines for quality assurance in breast cancer screening and diagnosis, 4th ed. Europe against Cancer, Office for Official Publications of the European Communities, Luxembourg (2006)
9. van Engen, R., Bosmans, H., Heid, P., Lazzari, B., Schopphoven, S., Thijssen, M., Young, K., Dance, D., Marshall, N.W.: Supplement to the European Guidelines, 4th edn. Health and Consumer Protection - European Communities (2011)
10. Warren, L.M., Mackenzie, A., Cooke, J., Given-Wilson, R.M., Wallis, M.G., Chakraborty, D.P., Dance, D.R., Bosmans, H., Young, K.C.: Effect of image quality on calcification detection in digital mammography. Med. Phys. **39**, 3202–3213 (2012)
11. Timberg, P., Bàth, M., Andersson, I., Mattsson, S., Tingberg, A.: Visibility of microcalcification clusters and masses in breast tomosynthesis image volumes and digital mammography: a 4AFC human observer study. Med. Phys. **39**, 2431–2437 (2012)
12. Ruschin, M., Timberg, P., Båth, M., Hemdal, B., Svahn, T., Saunders, R., Samei, E., Andersson, I., Mattsson, S., Chakraborty, D.P., Tingberg, A.: Dose dependence of mass and microcalcification detection in digital mammography: free response human observer studies. Med. Phys. **34**, 400–407 (2007)
13. Burgess, A.E., Jacobson, F.L., Judy, P.F.: Human observer detection experiments with mammograms and power-law noise. Med. Phys. **28**, 419–437 (2001)
14. Kanal, K.M., Krupinski, E., Berns, E.A., Geiser, W.R., Karellas, A., Mainiero, M.B., Martin, M.C., Patel, S.B., Rubin, D.L., Shepard, J.D., Siegel, E.L., Wolfman, J.A., Mian, T.A., Mahoney, M.C., Wyatt, M.: ACR-AAPM-SIIM practice guideline for determinants of image quality in digital mammography. J. Digit. Imaging **26**, 10–25 (2013)

Novel Technology

Simulation and Visualization to Support Breast Surgery Planning

Joachim Georgii[1(✉)], Torben Paetz[1], Markus Harz[1], Christina Stoecker[1],
Michael Rothgang[1], Joseph Colletta[2], Kathy Schilling[2],
Margrethe Schlooz-Vries[3], Ritse M. Mann[3], and Horst K. Hahn[1]

[1] Institute for Medical Image Computing, Fraunhofer MEVIS, Bremen, Germany
joachim.georgii@mevis.fraunhofer.de
[2] Boca Raton Regional Hospital, Boca Raton, FL, USA
[3] Radboud University Medical Centre, Nijmegen, The Netherlands

Abstract. Today, breast surgeons plan their procedures using pre-operatively placed metal clips or radioactive seeds and radiological images. These images show the breast in a positioning different from the one during surgery. We show a research prototype that eases the surgeon's planning task by providing 3D visualizations based on the radiological images. With a FEM-based deformation simulation, we mimic the real surgical scenario. In particular, we have developed a ligament model that increases the robustness of a fully automatic prone-supine deformation simulation, and we have developed specific visualization methods to aid intra-operative breast lesion localization.

1 Introduction

For their planning in breast surgery, surgeons use the pre-operatively acquired radiological images showing the anatomy as well as the lesion. Surgeons mentally transform the three-dimensional information from breast MRI or the projection information from mammograms to the actual 3D surgical scenario, including all involved deformations. This also encompasses the spatial linking of landmarks from one modality to the other, and the correlation of size and shape of structures. Most importantly, breast presentation during surgery (supine positioning) usually differs substantially from breast presentation in radiological images (compressed view in mammography, prone positioning in MRI). Since surgeons often sketch the surgical plan on the patients skin, e.g. indicating the closest point to the tumor or the necessary cuts to access the lesion, we hypothesize that a meaningful 3D representation of the required information might

- improve the surgical outcome,
- reduce the time needed for the intervention,
- bring added confidence for less experienced surgeons.

For many patients facing surgery, contrast-enhanced breast MRI images are available. Breast MRI is in many parts of the world the acknowledged reference

A. Tingberg et al. (Eds.): IWDM 2016, LNCS 9699, pp. 257–264, 2016.
DOI: 10.1007/978-3-319-41546-8_33

standard to assess a patient with biopsy-proven cancer for contralateral and additional ipsilateral disease prior to therapy. We hence aim to improve and facilitate surgery planning based on breast MRI images. We visualize landmarks, the lesion extent including margins, and respective distances to anatomical structures for a simulated breast shape that mimics the actual surgical positioning. This lets the surgeon comprehend the relevant information intuitively. The 3D visualizations of the tumor localization and tumor extent might potentially reduce re-excision rates and allow more reliable planning of the access path and the excision extent. The absolute size of the surgical target volume influences the treatment decision and determines the cosmetic outcome and resection strategy (segmentectomy, quadrantectomy, mastectomy). Decisions on systemic treatment before or after surgery are again mainly based on tumor grade and size.

To the best of our knowledge, only little research on breast surgery planning has been documented to date. There have been advances in the simulation of cosmetic outcomes of breast lumpectomies (see www.vph-picture.eu). Attempts of surgical support have been made based on supine breast MR images and mapping out sketches of the structures onto the patient skin [14]. Other work describes how to support interventions directly, assuming knowledge on the intended surgical approach and extent [11]. Specifically, to simulate the supine positioning from prone MR data additional supine MR images have been used in combination with FE modelling [1,2,4,6]. Besides the breast specific related work our planning approach draws inspiration from surgery planning software designed for other organs, like the lung [3,12,17,19,21,22] or the liver [5,7,9,10,18].

2   Methods

This paper describes a novel modeling approach for realistic prone-to-supine deformation simulation that is the basis of a research prototype for breast surgery planning. In particular, it presents a novel ligament model for the deformation simulation, as well as recent fundamental advancements of the applied visualization methods. The advanced method for simulating supine positioning from prone position MRI images provides increased robustness. The 3D visualizations illustrate the relevant structures more clearly and allow for improved perception of the patient situation and tumor localization.

2.1   Visualization of Target Volume

We propose to present the patient anatomy using spatial visualizations designed to give surgeons an intuitive understanding of the surgical scenario. Thus, we reduce the need to mentally transform radiological data (slice information) to the real 3D world and facilitate the assessment of the patient-specific situation. A preparatory data processing step segments the relevant anatomical structures automatically or with minimal user interactions. This comprises segmentation of the breast-skin boundary [24], the breast-chest wall boundary [23], the nipples [8], the breast parenchyma [16], and breast tumors [13]. The tumor segmentation requires a single mouse click onto the lesion.

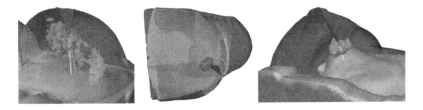

Fig. 1. Visualization of the lesion, the parenchyma and the breast quadrants as well as the distances of the lesion to nipple (blue), closest point on the skin (red) and chest wall (white). (Color figure online)

Orientation guides. Interpreting the information from radiological images, surgeons pre-operatively draw a marker on the patient's skin indicating the closest point on the skin to the tumor. This task is supported by the software by calculating the closest distance between the lesion and the skin. To increase depth perception, besides the distances from the lesion to the nipple and the closest point on the skin, a surface patch in between the connecting lines is drawn. Thereby, the surgeon also gets information about the on-surface distance between the nipple and the closest point on the skin. We furthermore included a visualization of the breast quadrants for more orientation aid. To visualize the risk structures in the vicinity of the tumor, all risk structures (nipple, skin, or chest wall) within a user-chosen distance are highlighted. See Figs. 1 and 2 for examples of the provided orientation guides.

Quantitative parameters to decide on resection strategy and planning of intervention. Among other factors, the decision on the adequate resection strategy (segmentectomy, quadrantectomy, mastectomy) depends on the volume of the resected area in relation to the breast volume. Segmentectomy, in general, is feasible if the volume to be resected does not exceed 20% of the breast volume. In the demonstrator, the relative volume of the planned area to be resected is computed and visualized. Further quantification parameters for the decision on the resection strategy and for planning the surgical intervention are the closest distance of the tumor to the skin, the distance of the tumor to the nipple, and the closest distance of the tumor to the chest wall. The demonstrator computes and visualizes these distances.

The demonstrator supports the visualization and the computation of the quantification parameters both for the original MRI data (prone position) as well as for a simulated supine positioning. The next section describes the model building and computations to estimate a supine positioning of the patient from the prone breast MRI.

2.2   A Ligament Model for Prone-Supine Deformation Simulation

We aim to present the breast shape in the positioning of the patient during surgery. This requires the computation of the breast shape change, since MRI

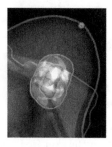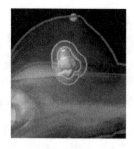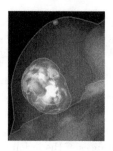

Fig. 2. Visualization of safety margins for different lesions. Note that the structures at risk are shown in red. (Color figure online)

data is acquired in prone position (face down), but the patient is positioned in supine position during surgery (face up). Our simulation approach is based on the work of Pätz et al. [15]. They use a patient-specific finite element model, which is automatically generated from acquired MR images. The breast is modeled with linear elasticity in combination with sliding contact conditions on the chest wall. To increase the robustness of the mentioned approach, we have developed a ligament model that is incorporated into the sliding approach. Since Cooper ligaments are not easily visible on breast MR images, and a patient-specific segmentation would be time-consuming, we have developed a simplified generic model based on two assumptions:

1. The Cooper ligaments are fully stretched in the prone MR images used for model generation.
2. The Cooper ligaments are directed from the chest wall towards the nipple.

Based on these assumptions, we build a spring-mass system along the finite element (FE) model, which is initialized in the prone positioning. For each point of the FE model that is located at the chest wall, we establish a spring to the nipple position, and the distance between these points in the prone position is set as rest length. During each step of the deformation simulation, the current spring length and orientation is computed and used in the sliding update process, which is an update of the positions (Dirichlet boundary conditions) of the sliding vertices based on the internal stresses of the breast. Given the intended update of the sliding vertex $\hat{u}$ (which is derived from the internal stress, see [15]) and the spring to the nipple l with rest state l_0, we compute a scalar factor α as follows:

α	$\frac{\|l\|}{\|l_0\|} \leq 1$	$\frac{\|l\|}{\|l_0\|} > 1$
$\hat{u} \cdot l < 0$	$1 - \frac{\|l\|^2}{\|l_0\|^2}$	0
$\hat{u} \cdot l \geq 0$	1	$1 + \left(\frac{1}{\|l_0\|} - \frac{1}{\|l\|} \right) \frac{\hat{u} \cdot l}{\|\hat{u}\|}$

Note that the upper row handles the case where the sliding will increase the ligament length, while the lower row handles the cases where the sliding will decrease the ligament length. Similar, the left column handles under-stretched ligaments, whereas the right column handles over-stretched ligaments. The new position update of the sliding vertex in single step is then $\alpha\,\hat{u}$. Note that the ligament model only affects the position update of the sliding vertices and effectively and efficiently serves as a stopping criterion for the amount of sliding. By means of the ligament model, the sliding in the prone-to-supine simulation is less sensible to the elastic modulus, and thus the robustness of the prone-to-supine simulation is significantly increased.

3   Results and Discussion

Figure 3 shows simulation results for stiffness values from 1000 to 3500 N/m^2. Including the ligament model into the FE model brings about several advantages over previous approaches. The novel ligament model increases the robustness of the prone-supine simulation with respect to the input parameters. Furthermore, the embedding of the ligament model only marginally increases the computational costs per simulation step by less than 1ms. More importantly, the number of steps required until convergence is noticeably reduced by the ligament model as can be seen in Table 1. This is due to the increased robustness that allows adaptive displacement updates of the sliding vertices. It is worth mentioning that in contrast to the approach by Pätz et al. [15] we can simulate smaller elastic moduli robustly, and thus we can mimic more sliding and increased deformability in the simulation, addressing the common fact that breast cancer is more frequent in obese and elderly women with fatty-replaced breasts that deform gravely.

Summarizing, we can state that the prone-to-supine simulation using the ligament model is advantageous in the computation of the breast shape in supine positioning for breast surgery planning. Parameters such as the direction of gravity (i.e. the angulation in patient positioning) and the stiffness can be adjusted

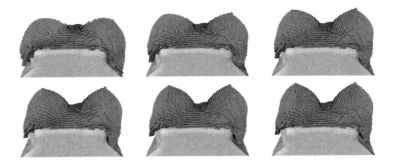

Fig. 3. Simulated supine positioning for the same model using stiffness values from 1000 (upper left) to 3500 (lower right). Due to the ligament model, convergence is achieved within 30 to 50 simulation steps, yielding simulation times of 13 to 21 s for the model consisting of 33,156 hexahedral elements with 117,378 degrees of freedom.

Table 1. Prone-to-supine simulation statistics. Elastic modulus: 1500 N/m^2. We show the number of hexahedral elements, the computation time for one iteration step, the number of steps to convergence without and with ligament model (w/o LM, w/LM).

ID	#hexahedra	time/step (ms)	#steps (w/o LM)	#steps (w/LM)
case0	19375	123	81	67
case1	12981	95	87	81
case2	18252	119	98	35
case3	20614	134	82	69
case4	18385	121	85	72
case5	43064	296	71	32
case6	33156	220	78	58
case7	37831	245	61	38
case8	21502	152	90	76
case9	35380	230	76	57

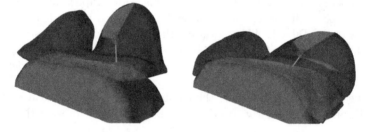

Fig. 4. Comparison of the surgery planning visualizations in prone (left) and simulated supine (right) positioning. Note the significant shape change.

interactively by the surgeon, and the adapted visualizations can already be shown after very few iteration steps, since the iteration starts from a reasonable initial solution.

Figure 4 shows the visualizations both in original prone and simulated supine positioning. The closest point of the tumor on the skin is shown to the surgeon, as well as the on-surface distance to the nipple position. The visualizations have been developed in close collaboration with two clinical sites in the U.S. and the Netherlands. Surgeons expect an improved, faster, and more intuitive understanding of the tumor localization using the novel 3D visualizations in the simulated supine positioning. Therefore, planning the surgical access path to the tumor is expected to be simplified compared to a planning based on radiological data alone. Showing the patients breast in the surgery positioning has been described to be highly valuable for the surgeon's pre-surgical preparation. First, the position of the tumor in relation to the nipple and the point on the skin closest to the tumor as well as information on the distance of the tumor to the skin can be derived from the planning software. Second, as an outlook surgeons expect the visualizations also to be used in pre-treatment discussions with breast cancer patients.

4   Conclusion and Future Work

We have accomplished important basic steps towards a functional breast surgery support software. At its core are a robust and automatic prone-supine deformation simulation as well as intuitive 3D visualization methods. Nevertheless, the field of breast surgery support is still at its beginning. Consequently, the future work will mainly focus on quantitative evaluation and practical exploration.

One of the visions is the usage of the 3D visualizations intra-operatively, which has already been briefly presented [20]. Particularly, it provides an illustration of an augmented reality component integrated on an iPad which is designed to be used by surgeons directly in the OR.

Acknowledgments. The presented work has partially been funded under the European Union FP7 Virtual Physiological Human grant number 601040, VPH-PRISM.

References

1. Behrenbruch, C., Marias, K., Armitage, P., Moore, N., Clarke, J., Brady, M.: Prone-supine breast MRI registration for surgical visualisation. In: Proceedings of Medical Image Understanding and Analysis, pp. 109–112 (2001)
2. Carter, T.J., Tanner, C., Crum, W.R., Beechey-Newman, N., Hawkes, D.J.: A framework for image-guided breast surgery. In: Yang, G.Z., Jiang, T.-Z., Shen, D., Gu, L., Yang, J. (eds.) MIAR 2006. LNCS, vol. 4091, pp. 203–210. Springer, Heidelberg (2006)
3. Eguchi, T., Takasuna, K., Kitazawa, A., Fukuzawa, Y., Sakaue, Y., Yoshida, K., Matsubara, M.: Three-dimensional imaging navigation during a lung segmentectomy using an iPad. Eur. J. Cardio-Thorac. Surg. Official J. Eur. Assoc. Cardiothorac. Surg. **41**(4), 893–897 (2012)
4. Eiben, B., Vavourakis, V., Hipwell, J., Kabus, S., Buelow, T., Lorenz, C., Mertzanidou, T., Reis, S., Williams, N., Keshtgar, M., Hawkes, D.: Symmetric biomechanically guided prone-to-supine breast image registration. Ann. Biomed. Eng. **44**(1), 154–173 (2016)
5. Gavaghan, K.A., Peterhans, M., Oliveira-Santos, T., Weber, S.: A portable image overlay projection device for computer-aided open liver surgery. IEEE Trans. Bio-Med. Eng. **58**(6), 1855–1864 (2011)
6. Han, L., Hipwell, J., Eiben, B., Barratt, D., Modat, M., Ourselin, S., Hawkes, D.: A nonlinear biomechanical model based registration method for aligning prone and supine mr breast images. IEEE Trans. Med. Imaging **33**(3), 682–694 (2014)
7. Hansen, C., Zidowitz, S., Ritter, F., Lange, C., Oldhafer, K., Hahn, H.: Risk maps for liver surgery. Int. J. Comp. Ass. Radiol. Surg. **8**, 419–428 (2013)
8. Harz, M.T.: Complexity Reduction in Image-Based Breast Cancer Care. Ph.D. thesis, University of Bremen (2014). http://elib.suub.uni-bremen.de/edocs/00104007-1.pdf
9. Koehn, A., Matsuyama, R., Endo, I., Schenk, A.: Liver surgery data and augmented reality in the operation room: experiences using a tablet device. Int. J. Comput. Assist. Radiol. Surg. Surg./Interv. Navig. S111 (2014)

10. Lang, H., Radtke, A., Hindennach, M., Schroeder, T., Fruehauf, N., Malago, M., Bourquain, H., Peitgen, H., Oldhafer, K., Broelsch, C.: Impact of virtual tumor resection and computer-assisted risk analysis on operation planning and intraoperative strategy in major hepatic resection. Arch. Surg. **140**, 629–638 (2005)
11. Liao, H., Inomata, T., Sakuma, I., Dohi, T.: 3-D augmented reality for MRI-guided surgery using integral videography autostereoscopic image overlay. IEEE Trans. Bio-Med. Eng. **57**(6), 1476–1486 (2010)
12. Limmer, S., Stoecker, C., Dicken, V., Krass, S., Wolken, H., Kujath, P.: Computer-assisted visualization of central lung tumours based on 3-dimensional reconstruction. In: CT Scanning Techniques and Applications, pp. 205–228 (2011)
13. Moltz, J., Bornemann, L., Kuhnigk, J.M., Dicken, V., Peitgen, E., Meier, S., Peitgen, H.O.: Advanced segmentation techniques for lung nodules, liver metastases, and enlarged lymph nodes in CT scans. IEEE J. Select. Topics Sig. Process. **3**, 122–134 (2009)
14. Nakamura, R., Nagashima, T., Sakakibara, M., Sangai, T., Fujimoto, H., Arai, M., Shida, T., Kaneoya, K., Ueda, T., Nakatani, Y., Hashimoto, H., Miyazaki, M.: Breast-conserving surgery using supine magnetic resonance imaging in breast cancer patients receiving neoadjuvant chemotherapy. Breast **17**(3), 245–251 (2008)
15. Pätz, T., Harz, M., Wang, L., Stöcker, C., Schilling, K., Colletta, J., Schlooz-Vries, M., Hahn, H., Georgii, J.: Sliding motion in breast deformation modeling. In: 3rd MICCAI Workshop on Breast Image Analysis (2015)
16. Razavi, M., Wang, L., Gubern-Merida, A., Ivanovska, T., Laue, H., Karssemeijer, N., Hahn, H.K.: Towards accurate segmentation of fibroglandular tissue in breast mri using fuzzy c-means and skin-folds removal. In: 18th International Conference on Image Analysis and Processing (2015)
17. Saji, H., Inoue, T., Kato, Y., Shimada, Y., Hagiwara, M., Kudo, Y., Akata, S., Ikeda, N.: Virtual segmentectomy based on high-quality three-dimensional lung modelling from computed tomography images. Interact. CardioVasc. Thorac. Surg. **17**, 227–232 (2013)
18. Schenk, A., Haemmerich, D., Preusser, T.: Planning of image-guided interventions in the liver. IEEE Pulse **2**, 48–55 (2011)
19. Stoecker, C., Bornemann, L., Dicken, V., Krass, S., Kuhnigk, J., Zidowitz, S., Peitgen, H.: CT-based patient individual anatomical modeling of the lung and its impact on thoracic surgery. In: World Congress on Medical Physics 2009, IFMBE Proceedings, vol. 25. pp. 1592–1595 (2010)
20. Stoecker, C., Harz, M., Schlooz-Vries, M., Mann, R., Schilling, K., Colletta, J., Georgii, J., Paetz, T., Hahn, H.K.: MRI-based visualization and augmented reality for breast surgery planning and guidance. In: Proceedings of CURAC (2015)
21. Stoecker, C., Welter, S., Klemm, W., Beckers, F., Witte, B., Krass, S.: Computer assistance in lung surgery for segment resections and minimally invasive surgery. In: Proceedings of CURAC, pp. 299–304 (2015)
22. Volonte, F., Robert, J., Ratib, O., Triponez, F.: A lung segmentectomy performed with 3D reconstruction images available on the operating table with an iPad. Interact. CardioVasc. Thorac. Surg. **12**, 1066–1068 (2011)
23. Wang, L., Filippatos, K., Friman, O., Hahn, H.K.: Fully automated segmentation of the pectoralis muscle boundary in breast MR images (2011)
24. Wang, L., Platel, B., Ivanovskaya, T., Harz, M., Hahn, H.: Fully automatic breast segmentation in 3d breast MRI. In: 2012 9th IEEE International Symposium on Biomedical Imaging (ISBI), pp. 1024–1027 (2012)

Single Section Biomarker Measurement and Colocalization via a Novel Multiplexing Staining Technology

Tyna Hope[1(✉)], Dan Wang[1], Sharon Nofech-Mozes[2], Kela Liu[1],
Sireesha Kaanumalle[4], Yousef Al-Kohafi[4], Kashan Shaikh[4],
Robert Filkins[4], and Martin Yaffe[1,3]

[1] Physical Sciences, Sunnybrook Research Institute, Toronto, Canada
thope@sri.utoronto.ca
[2] Department of Anatomic Pathology,
Sunnybrook Health Science Centre, Toronto, Canada
[3] Department of Medical Biophysics, University of Toronto, Toronto, Canada
[4] GE Global Research Center, Niskayuna, USA

Abstract. Measuring colocalization of multiple biomarkers may contribute to understanding tumor growth and progression. Traditionally, multiple biomarkers colocalization has been performed by processing multiple serial tissue sections. To provide true colocalization measures, we are investigating single section multiplexing techniques. Utilizing a fluorescent-based sequential stain and bleach system (SSB) we investigated multiplexing 8 markers in breast cancer tissue microarray sections. The experiments consisted of a 4 predictive biomarker panel (ER, PR, HER2, and Ki67) and markers to assist in the image processing. The goals included comparing the immunofluorescent signal with bright field single chromogen IHC scores, the measurements of tumor heterogeneity, and to discover technical challenges. Early results suggest that SSB signals correspond to traditional IHC staining. Additionally, our work has highlighted improvements to workflow and the staining process. We present a review of our progress and expectations for this technology.

Keywords: Biomarker multiplexing · Quantitative image analysis · Pathology

1 Background

The disruption of normal cell signal transduction and cell signal pathways are the hallmark of cancer development and progression [1]. Protein expression and receptor presence (biomarkers) in cells are indicators of the state of these pathways. Conversely, endocrine and HER2/neu targeted therapies are unlikely to have an effect in tumors not expressing hormone receptors or HER2/neu respectively [2].

However, subsets of patients do not respond to these treatments, even in the presence of their targets or develop resistance after initial response [3, 4]. Since the threshold for labelling breast tumors as positive for hormone receptors is set at 1 % and that for HER2 at 10 %, it is not surprising that tumors labelled positive for certain markers may have a variable proportion of positive cells. When ER, PR, HER2, Ki67

© Springer International Publishing Switzerland 2016
A. Tingberg et al. (Eds.): IWDM 2016, LNCS 9699, pp. 265–273, 2016.
DOI: 10.1007/978-3-319-41546-8_34

biomarkers are assessed it is expected to find subsets of tumors with different profiles. The significance of intratumoral heterogeneity on disease biology and its possible role in treatment failure is not yet understood and requires more investigation [5].

The most common practice is to access biomarkers at the protein expression level by individual immunohistochemical (IHC) study on sequential tissue sections, although multigene prognostic and predictive assay are emerging, in particular for hormone positive breast cancer [6–8]. But this approach tests different group of cells in every level. In comparison, multiplexing allows to test multiple markers in the same cells. In addition, by using multiplexing, several steps in a given signal transduction cascade can be studied at once rather than focusing on any single molecule or could allow characterization of the immune microenvironment.

Multiplexing through concurrent IHC chromogens has the limitation that when the same sub-cellular compartment is targeted multiple times, quantitative analysis becomes difficult (if not impossible). Multiplexing with concurrent immunofluorescent tags often involves signal overlap and autofluorescence [9] which confounds the attribution of the signal to the correct biomarker. This technique is also limited by the availability of proper fluorescent tags.

To accomplish the goal of obtaining quantitative measures of multiple biomarkers for individual cells, the Biomarker Imaging Research Laboratory (BIRL) has been working with a prototype device from GE Global Research Center (GEGRC). This technology is capable of sequentially staining and bleaching (SSB) a single section multiple times, allowing the measurement of multiple biomarkers on a cell by cell basis. In the following sections, the technology will be described, the lessons learned shared and the new opportunities for discovery discussed.

2   Objectives and Data

GE Global Research Center has developed a novel technology with an automated staining system for immunofluorescence-labeling, multiplexing, imaging and analysis of onco-proteins in fixed tissues [10]. This multiplexing platform enables studying multiple biomarker expressions on the same tissue section at subcellular level (nuclear, membrane, and cytoplasmic).[1] The Biomarker Imaging Research laboratory is interested in assessing the technology to determine if there is an association between the output signal and traditional single chromogen IHC scores, its repeatability, and tumor heterogeneity. The first breast panel under investigation is ER, PR, HER2, and Ki67. Additional markers such as epithelial marker cytokeratin (CK), and nuclear and membrane markers, are used for the registration and segmentation algorithms. Figure 1 shows the multiple SSB signals that can be viewed simultaneously.

We are reporting on the calibration and validation experiments, utilizing 3 invasive breast cancer tissue microarray sections (TMAs), AS2000, AS3000, and AS4000 (Table 1). AS2000 and AS3000 are used for calibration of the system, to determine if

---

[1] GEGRC provided support to the Biomarker Imaging Research Laboratory (BIRL) in the form of the equipment and the reagents.

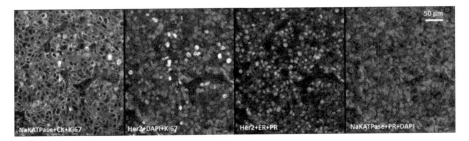

Fig. 1. Biomarker multiplexed images from a triple positive breast cancer patient using SSB technique. From Left to Right: NaKATPase + CK + Ki67; Her2 + DAPI + Ki67; Her2 + ER + PR; NaKATPase + PR + DAPI. NaKATPase (purple); CK (cyan); Ki67 (white); Her2 (red); DAPI (yellow); ER (green); PR (blue). Scale on all images is as shown in the right image. (Color figure online)

Table 1. TMAs used in the calibration and validation experiments. Omitted cores are due to missing tissue.

TMA	Patients, cores	Cores included	Biomarkers for calibration & validation
AS2000	55,3	144	ER and PR
AS3000	50,3	136	Ki67 and Her2
AS4000	50,2	99	ER, PR, Ki67, HER2

there is agreement between the signal obtained from multiplexing and signals obtained from the traditional single stained serial sections. The AS4000 TMA is used to validate the analysis on an independent set of tumors using the calibration methods.

3 Methods

3.1 Staining Methods

A description of the equipment and the staining methods used, has been published previously [11]. During the course of the experiments, we found that we had to make one adjustment. In order to avoid false positive signals caused by antibody species cross-reaction, an additional staining round with normal serum was performed following the HER2 and ER staining round [12].

3.2 Image Acquisition, Processing and Signal Measurement

User-selected areas were acquired in TIFF format at 20× magnification, equivalent to 0.37 μm/pixel resolution with a field-of-view of 764 μm × 764 μm per image. To correct for variable illumination over the field-of-view, a blank slide image was acquired and pixel wise division performed prior to analysis of the biomarker images.

The DAPI images in each step were registered to the reference step, and then images of all other channels were adjusted. The bleached and stained images are normalized with respect to their exposure times and the dark pixel value (pixel intensity value at zero exposure time). Autofluorescence, typically present in FFPE tissues, was then separated from target fluorophore signals by subtracting bleaching images from the corresponding normalized stained image. For sub-cellular quantitation, GE developed segmentation algorithms to identify membrane, cytoplasm, and nuclei using NaKATPase, cytokeratin, and DAPI images respectively. Finally, the pixel intensity statistics (e.g. median) were recorded for each compartment and cell shape metrics.

4 Results and Observations

Currently we are focusing on reliability and association of single stains to scoring performed by pathologists using conventional IHC methods.

Two pathologists at our institution performed the scoring of the IHC DAB stained samples, a practicing breast pathologist and a researcher. Scoring ER, PR, and Ki67 is performed by estimating the percentage of invasive cancer cells that have nuclear stain and then assigning the label positive for those patients that have more than 1 % positive cells, with the pathologists' scores averaged. HER2 IHC is scored according to the 2013 ASCO/CAP guidelines as 0/1+ (negative), 2+ (equivocal), 3+ (positive) per image. Scoring HER2 is based upon the pattern of membranous staining, evaluating intensity and circumferential pattern to obtain the percentage of cells with the aforementioned labelling. Prior to analysis, the data were cleaned to remove cores without invasive carcinoma or to remove poorly segmented cells.

Multiple analyses were performed using the pathologists' scores and the image processing data. The first method was subcellular compartment threshold derivation to determine if it is possible to obtain a grade comparable to the pathologist with the SSB intensity data. Since we do not have prior knowledge as to the correct threshold, multiple thresholds were applied until the best fit to the data was reached (Fig. 2) for the nuclear markers. The goal was to try to match the pathologists' continuous score, however this technique was not pursued because clinical decision is made on dichotomized values. For the HER2 signal we made a comparison between the membrane and another cell compartments which is more in line with the traditional scoring method (Fig. 3). The agreement between the two pathologists (Spearman correlation) was 0.84 ($p < 0.001$) for ER and 0.99 ($p < 0.001$) for PR. For HER2, measured by Cohen's Kappa, Kappa = 0.99 ($p < 0.001$).

Next, we applied more advanced models as we suspected their results could more closely match the pathologists' scores. For the ER model, we used the median intensity statistics from the nuclear region of each cell and then for the entire image extracted scale-insensitive population statistics for the group of cells in the image. For instance, the kurtosis of the median nuclear intensities of all cells is one of 10 image features. After applying exclusion criteria, 25 negative cores and 115 positive cores in the calibration set were used to create a model using the random forest classifier within Cran R [13, 14]. The random forest classifier has a built in error metric, similar to cross-validation, called the out-of-bag (OOB) error rate. The resulting OOB error rate was 5.7 % (94.3 % accuracy) with a 95 % confidence interval of (0.8905, 0.975).

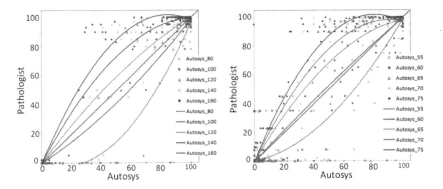

Fig. 2. Multiple thresholds applied to nuclear intensity data. For each threshold the percentage of positive cells was compared to pathologists' score to determine best fit. Left: ER, Right: PR. (Color figure online)

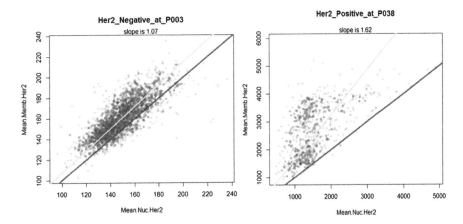

Fig. 3. Comparison of membrane mean intensity vs. nuclear mean intensity for HER2. Positve and negative HER2 cores showed different relationships between membrane and nuclear signal. The red line is a reference, with slope = 1, wheras the yellow line is the best fit line to the data. (Color figure online)

For the HER2 model, we generated features by comparing the median intensity of the membrane to nuclear or cytoplasmic cellular compartments for each cell and then, once every cell comparison was generated, extracted scale-insensitive population statistics for the group of cells in the image. For instance the standard deviation of the contrast between each membrane to cytoplasm intensity for all cells is one of the five image features. Since there is no clinical difference in 0+ and 1 + HER2 scores, we chose to combine them, as negative, to create a three class model. After application of exclusion criteria, 107 negative, 6 equivocal, and 18 tumours positive for HER2 in the calibration set were used for random forest model development within Cran R. The resulting OOB error rate was 4.6 % (95.4 % accuracy) with class error rates of 3.7 %, 33 % and 0 % on negative, equivocal and strong positive respectively.

We have yet to independently validate the ER and HER2 models however we are encouraged by the results. We are working with pathologists at our institution on scoring protocols for the Ki67 signal as a clinical protocol is still under development [15, 16]. The PR staining was adjusted for AS4000 to prevent cross reacting with ER, similar to the reported Ki67 and HER2 interaction, so PR analysis will be limited to AS4000. We have yet to address the issue of sensitivity to noise, such as the impact of DCIS cells included in the image analysis pipeline and imperfect segmentation.

5   Future

While there still are technical challenges, such as cross-reactivity, the impact of multiple bleaching steps, limitation of commercial antibodies available for this technique, lack of context that is available with IHC and validation of signals, this technology has the potential to provide novel insights. This technology may provide the ability to assess new biomarker panels and to quantify biomarker heterogeneity.

With many options to combine multiple biomarkers, the first step may be to view per cell measures of the various signals within the relevant cell compartment. By preserving the cell context information, we can visualize the cell phenotypes that are within a sample, such as with scatter plots (Fig. 4) (Cran R package scatterplot3d [17]). We may also reveal sub-populations by using cluster analysis with an evaluation method such as Calinski-Harabasz [18] (Cran R package vegan [19]) (Fig. 5).

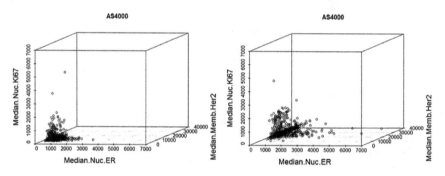

Fig. 4. Scatter plots of per cell Ki67, ER and HER2 signal. Left: ER, PR, HER2 negative Right: ER, PR, HER2 positive

While cell context information is interesting, it does require accurate segmentation and registration algorithms. If it is possible to gain insights through analysis of common relationships on population assessment only (Fig. 6), this requirement could be relaxed. This information may allow clinicians to identify those patients that could benefit from drug treatments geared to particular cell signaling pathways or to address microenvironment modifications induced by cancer cells [5].

These methods not only allow investigation of invasive cancer cells, but also DCIS which is timely given treatment options are now under closer scrutiny [20]. Through

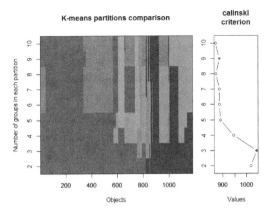

Fig. 5. Cluster assessment of a triple negative case using ER, Her2 and Ki67 median cell compartment intensities as features. The Calinski criteria applied to K-means suggests 3 clusters. (Color figure online)

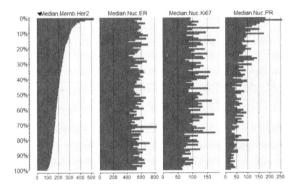

Fig. 6. Simultaneous plots of HER2, ER, PR, and Ki67 for one patient. The data are sorted on the maximum HER2 signal with each row containing 8 cells and showing the average cells.

quantitative assessment of existing biomarkers and the investigation of new panels, such as ER, PR, HER2, Ki67, cox-2, P16, P53 [21], greater insight may be gained to identify clinically significant cases with risk to recur as invasive cancer, or markers of indolent tumors that could be managed with breast conserving therapy or observation.

While biomarker quantification through image analysis can reduce subjectivity and improve quantitative accuracy, enhancing the technique with multiplexing opens new opportunity to study interaction between biomarkers, test predefined panels such as "IHC4" [22] and enable analysis of fluorescent DNA in situ hybridization and RNA ISH. Moreover, as molecular techniques are improving, there is potential for future studies of protein colocalization integrated with genomic and transcriptomic profiling.

References

1. Hanahan, D., Weinberg, R.A.: Hallmarks of cancer: the next generation. Cell **144**, 646–674 (2011)
2. Kelloff, G.J., Sigman, C.C.: Cancer biomarkers: selecting the right drug for the right patient. Nat. Rev. Drug Discov. **11**, 201–214 (2012)
3. Nielsen, D.L., et al.: Efficacy of HER2-targeted therapy in metastatic breast cancer. Monoclonal antibodies and tyrosine kinase inhibitors. The Breast **22**, 1–12 (2013)
4. Gong, I.Y., et al.: Determination of clinically therapeutic endoxifen concentrations based on efficacy from human MCF7 breast cancer xenografts. Breast Cancer Res. Treat. **139**, 61–69 (2013)
5. Marusyk, A., Almendro, V., Polyak, K.: Intra-tumour heterogeneity: a looking glass for cancer? Nat. Rev. Cancer **12**, 323–334 (2012)
6. Cronin, M., et al.: Analytical validation of the oncotype DX genomic diagnostic test for recurrence prognosis and therapeutic response prediction in node-negative, estrogen receptor–positive breast cancer. Clin. Chem. **53**(6), 1084–1091 (2007)
7. Gnant, M., et al.: Identifying clinically relevant prognostic subgroups of postmenopausal women with node-positive hormone receptor-positive early-stage breast cancer treated with endocrine therapy: a combined analysis of ABCSG-8 and ATAC using the PAM50 risk of recurrence score and intrinsic subtype. Ann. Oncol. **26**, 1685–1691 (2015)
8. Delahaye, L.J.M., et al.: Performance characteristics of the MammaPrint® breast cancer diagnostic gene signature. Personalized Med. **10**(8), 801–811 (2013)
9. Monici, M.: Cell and tissue autofluorescence research and diagnostic applications. Biotechnol. Annu. Rev. **11**, 227–256 (2005)
10. Gerdes, M.J., et al.: Highly multiplexed single-cell analysis of formalin-fixed, paraffin-embedded cancer tissue. Proc. Natl. Acad. Sci. U. S. A. **110**(29), 11982–11987 (2013)
11. Clarke, G.M., et al.: A novel, automated technology for multiplex biomarker imaging and application to breast cancer. Histopathology **64**, 242–255 (2014)
12. Wang, D., et al.: Ki-67 membranous staining: biologically relevant or an artifact of multiplexed immunofluorescent staining. AIMM (2015)
13. R Core Team: A language and environment for statistical computing. R Foundation for Statistical Computing, Vienna, Austria (2014)
14. Liaw, A., Wiener, M.: Classification and regression by randomForest. R News **2**(3), 18–22 (2002)
15. Dowsett, M.: Assessment of Ki67 in breast cancer: recommendations from the international Ki67 in breast cancer working group. JNCI **103**(22), 1656–1664 (2011)
16. Polley, M.-Y.C., et al.: An international study to increase concordance in Ki67 scoring. Mod. Pathol. **28**, 778–786 (2015)
17. Ligges, U., Mächler, M.: Scatterplot3d - an R package for visualizing multivariate data. J. Stat. Softw. **8**(11), 1–20 (2003)
18. Calinski, T., Harabasz, J.: A dendrite method for cluster analysis. Commun. Stat. **3**(1), 1–27 (1974)
19. Oksanen J.J., et al. Vegan: Community Ecology Package. R package version 2.3-2 (2015)
20. O'Connor, S.: Why doctors are rethinking breast-cancer treatment. TIME **186**(14), 30–36 (2015)

21. Bartlett, J.M., et al.: Ductal carcinoma in situ of the breast: can biomarkers improve current management? Clin. Chem. **60**(1), 60–67 (2014)
22. Bartlett, J.M.S., et al.: Validation of the IHC4 breast cancer prognostic algorithm using multiple approaches on the multinational team clinical trial. Arch. Pathol. Lab. Med. **140**, 66–74 (2016)

Breast Conserving Surgery Outcome Prediction: A Patient-Specific, Integrated Multi-modal Imaging and Mechano-Biological Modelling Framework

Björn Eiben[1]([⊠]), Rene Lacher[1], Vasileios Vavourakis[1], John H. Hipwell[1],
Danail Stoyanov[1], Norman R. Williams[2], Jörg Sabczynski[3], Thomas Bülow[3],
Dominik Kutra[3], Kirsten Meetz[3], Stewart Young[3], Hans Barschdorf[3],
Hélder P. Oliveira[4], Jaime S. Cardoso[4], João P. Monteiro[4],
Hooshiar Zolfagharnasab[4], Ralph Sinkus[5], Pedro Gouveia[6],
Gerrit-Jan Liefers[7], Barbara Molenkamp[7], Cornelis J.H. van de Velde[7],
David J. Hawkes[1], Maria João Cardoso[6], and Mohammed Keshtgar[8]

[1] Centre for Medical Image Computing, University College London, London, UK
bjoern.eiben.10@ucl.ac.uk
[2] Surgical and Interventional Trials Unit, University College London, London, UK
[3] Philips Technologie GmbH Innovative Technologies, Hamburg, Germany
[4] INESC TEC, Porto, Portugal
[5] Imaging Sciences and Biomedical Engineering, King's College London, London, UK
[6] Champalimaud Foundation, Lisbon, Portugal
[7] Leiden University Medical Center, Leiden, Netherlands
[8] Royal Free Hospital, London, UK

Abstract. Patient-specific surgical predictions of Breast Conserving Therapy, through mechano-biological simulations, could inform the shared decision making process between clinicians and patients by enabling the impact of different surgical options to be visualised. We present an overview of our processing workflow that integrates MR images and three dimensional optical surface scans into a personalised model. Utilising an interactively generated surgical plan, a multi-scale open source finite element solver is employed to simulate breast deformity based on interrelated physiological and biomechanical processes that occur post surgery. Our outcome predictions, based on the pre-surgical imaging, were validated by comparing the simulated outcome with follow-up surface scans of four patients acquired 6 to 12 months post-surgery. A mean absolute surface distance of 3.3 mm between the follow-up scan and the simulation was obtained.

Keywords: Breast imaging · Oncoplastic breast surgery · Surgical planning · Image registration · Surface reconstruction · Finite element · Mathematical modelling

© Springer International Publishing Switzerland 2016
A. Tingberg et al. (Eds.): IWDM 2016, LNCS 9699, pp. 274–281, 2016.
DOI: 10.1007/978-3-319-41546-8_35

1   Introduction

Breast cancer today is the most common cancer for women in the developed world with 464,000 new cases reported in Europe in 2012 alone [1]. Early diagnosis and improved treatment fortunately make breast cancer an increasingly treatable disease and, as a result, the patients' *quality of life* is a significant issue following the completion of primary cancer care. Breast Conserving Therapy (BCT) was shown to lead to an improved body image and a higher level of satisfaction with the overall treatment result [2], however up to 30 % of BCT procedures have been reported to produce cosmetically suboptimal outcomes [3].

Providing tools that enable predictions of the outcome of proposed BCT procedures to be made, could inform a shared decision making process between patient and clinician, and manage patient expectations regarding their expected cosmetic outcome. Specifically, such tools could be used at various points in the patient consultation process to develop an appropriate surgical option, given the constraints of tissue excision and safe surgical margins etc., which is aesthetically acceptable to the patient.

In this work we present an overview of a processing workflow that was developed in the PICTURE project[1]. The workflow facilitates such patient-specific, surgical outcome predictions on the basis of clinical Magnetic Resonance Imaging (MRI) and optical surface scans. Development of surface reconstruction methodologies that are designed to work with low-cost RGBD (abbreviation for red, green blue, and depth) cameras, i.e. Microsoft Kinect, could make the system easier to adopt by removing the need for high-cost dedicated acquisition systems. To quantify the accuracy of the outcome predictions, we use follow-up surface scans of four clinical cases. Figure 1 shows an overview of the implemented processing workflow, where each component is represented by a coloured box.

2   Input Data and Pre-processing

2.1   Surface Reconstruction

A 3D surface model of the patient's torso is an important prerequisite to produce a realistic visualisation of the personalised aesthetic outcome simulation. The patient's upper body as well as the skin texture information is digitally represented as a coloured, triangle-based mesh. This can be achieved by using a dedicated scanning system provided by the company 3dMD that instantaneously captures surface data and reconstructs three-dimensional models with sub-millimetre accuracy while utilising active multi-view stereo-photogrammetry. As an alternative, low-cost source of surface data, we also make use of recent depth-sensing technology employing RGBD cameras of the Microsoft Kinect series. With both Kinect sensors working with light in the near-infrared range, the first Kinect device is a structured-light scanner while the second generation uses time-of-flight technology for depth estimation. In order to produce a single consistent

---

[1] www.vph-picture.eu.

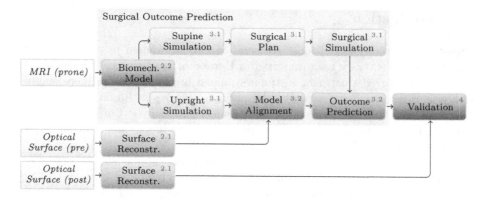

Fig. 1. Data processing and analysis work-flow. From the input MRI and surface data a personalised mechano-biological model is generated that, together with a surgical plan, facilitates simulation of the surgical outcome. The prediction is validated using follow-up surface reconstructions. The numbers inside the boxes correspond to the sections where more detail is provided (Color figure online)

dense surface profile, Kinect data acquisition follows a predefined protocol in which a sequence of images from a number of viewpoints, taken along a circular path around the patient, is recorded. The data from these multiple, consecutive Kinect images needs to be fused into a unified model of the patient. Prior to this fusion, the subsurface visible in each individual image is aligned with a reference coordinate system (the SLAM problem). To that end, a processing pipeline based on the KinectFusion framework is used [4]. To improve results in our clinical data acquisition setting, the pipeline is extended via a pre-processing step to discard unreliable data points and via global pose optimization step to mitigate pose errors [5]. Also, colour from the RGB images is integrated and mapped onto the surface. Having redundant systems for surface acquisition in place, we aim to show that portable consumer-level depth sensors are capable of creating surface data of sufficient quality for this application, and hence have the potential to reduce imaging costs and complexity in a clinical scenario. While the highly-accurate 3dMD surface is generally superior to the Kinect-based surface, the latter provides a realistic geometry of good quality, able to resolve minor details reliably. Figure 2 shows the estimated Kinect camera trajectory that was recovered during surface reconstruction alongside a side-by-side comparison of the surface reconstruction results of the three different systems.

2.2 Biomechanical Model Generation

A patient-specific biomechanical model is generated from routine clinical T1- or T2-weighted structural MRI scans. A binary region of interest mask is first segmented from these images, and discretised to create a three-dimensional mesh using a number of open-source libraries and tools, i.e. *VTK*, *Gmsh* and *Netgen*. Each tetrahedral finite element of the resulting mesh is then labelled as adipose

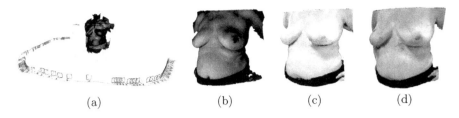

(a)   (b)   (c)   (d)

Fig. 2. Surface reconstruction and side-by-side comparison for one exemplary patient (a) Reconstruction volume, estimated Kinect camera trajectory and overlaid reconstructed surface (b) 3dMD result (c) Kinect V2 coloured surface (d) Kinect V1 coloured surface (Color figure online)

or fibroglandular tissue, according to segmentation of these classes from the input MR volume, and assigned the appropriate constitutive material relation according to published population based statistics. The breast skin surface is modelled using triangular membrane elements and is assumed traction-free in the biomechanical model. Finally, the lateral planar boundaries are defined as traction-free, the superior and inferior planes are constrained to 2D in-plane motion, and the chest surface is fixed.

3 BCT Modelling Framework

3.1 Surgical Simulation Tool

We have developed a surgical simulation tool to model BCT interventions performed on breast cancer patients. The integrated tool is a three-dimensional, multiscale, finite element (FE) numerical framework, capable of simulating breast tissue deformations and the physiological tissue recovery process following surgery. The modelling framework encompasses breast tissue biology and solid mechanics in a multiscale manner. At the macroscopic level, tissue biomechanics is described using a standard continuum mechanics approach, with breast tissues being modelled as a neo-Hookean material [6] and the skin as a hyperelastic membrane [7]. At the microscopic level, cell (i.e. fibroblasts and epithelial cells etc.) concentration, proliferation and cell-cycle in the operated-breast region is explicitly described via an established diffusion transport equation [8]. Following Moreo et al. [9], fibroblasts are also considered to actively contribute to the contraction of the wound in the model. Additionally, tissue recovery and angiogenesis is modelled using a simplified non-linear mathematical model. Hence, in the operated region of the patient-specific breast model, the transport of chemical agents (i.e. macrophage-derived growth factor, vascular endothelial growth factor) regulating inflammation, cell proliferation and angiogenesis is explicitly specified using a pair of Kolmogorov-Petrovsky-Piskounov equations [10,11]. In common with the early work of Maggelakis [12], neo-vascularisation in the recovering tissue, and oxygen-level and nutrient transport is described mathematically

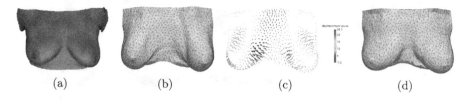

Fig. 3. Surface alignment procedure in the upright position. The optical surface scan (a) acts as a target to which the upright simulation (b) is adapted. A material parameter optimisation step followed by a non-linear surface warping (c) is used to update the biomechanical simulation (d) so that it fits the target surface (a). (Color figure online)

as a diffusion process. The present computational framework has been implemented into our open-source finite element project *FEB3*,[2] which incorporates several high-performance numerical libraries, i.e. *libmesh*, *PETSc*, and *MPICH*.

In the grey shaded rectangle of Fig. 1, the workflow of the BCT modelling framework is illustrated, where the core modules of the surgical simulation tool are depicted in boxes. Starting from the FE model (c.f. Sect. 2.2) an inverse deformation analysis [13] is carried out to predict tissue pre-stressing due to the effect of gravity. Then, conventional forward deformation analysis, to predict the breast shape in the supine and upright position, is performed. Subsequently, surgical planning takes place in which the virtual patient (i.e. the predicted breast shape in the supine setting) is visualised through a graphical user interface by the surgeon. At this point, annotations of the surgical plan on the virtual patient-specific model are specified, namely the skin incisions, the resected breast tissue volume (including the lesion and margins) and optional tissue mobilisation. The finite element model is then updated accordingly and is fed back to the surgical simulation tool, where the wound-healing simulation during a 3-month period of the patient's recovery is carried out. The final prediction of the patient-specific breast is then transformed into the upright configuration and, subsequently, compared with the corresponding pre-operative breast shape.

3.2 Model-to-Surface Alignment and Outcome Prediction

The FE methodology described in Sect. 3.1 facilitates the transformation of the prone MRI based model to another configuration such as upright. Despite the use of a rigorous simulation framework, inaccuracies in the model persist and, as a result, the upright simulation does not completely match the optical upright surface. Such inaccuracies are for instance caused by (i) an uncertainty about the patient-specific material parameters and (ii) deformations of the breast in the prone MRI acquisition configuration due to contact between the breast and the scanner. Figure 3 shows an example case where the upright simulation (Fig. 3(b)) differs from the upright scan (Fig. 3(a)) especially due to medial indentation of the breast during MRI acquisition. Correction of such deformations based on a

---

[2] https://bitbucket.org/vasvav/feb3-finite-element-bioengineering-in-3d/wiki/Home.

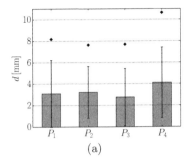
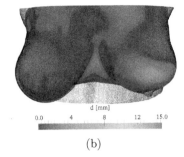

(a)   (b)

Fig. 4. Validation results. (a) Absolute surface distance d between the simulated surgical outcome predictions for patients P_1 to P_4 and the corresponding optical follow-up surface scans. The grey bars represent the mean values, the whiskers the standard deviations and the diamonds the 95th percentile of the measured distances. (b) The simulated surgical outcome for case P_1 with the colour coded surface distances, as well as the post-surgical surface scan as a wire-frame. (Color figure online)

pure mechanical simulation is difficult. Hence we make use of the optical upright surface in order to address both issues above in a two-step procedure [14].

In a first step the global alignment between the upright simulation and the target surface is improved by optimising the material parameters of the biomechanical model. After this global alignment, local refinements are carried out by the means of a surface warping step. In this step the skin nodes are driven towards the target surface, while the deformation is regularised by a smoothness term and an area-change penalising term. The deformation vector field and the final alignment result for an example case are shown in Fig. 3(c) and (d) respectively.

The alignment procedure results in an updated biomechanical model which then can be further transformed according to the displacements calculated by the surgical simulation (Sect. 3.1). In combination with a texture transfer from the reconstructed optical surface to the biomechanical model, a photo-realistic visualisation of the surgical outcome prediction becomes possible.

4 Validation

In order to validate the BCT modelling framework, we compared the generated surgical outcome predictions with follow-up surface scans (c.f. bottom most input in Fig. 1). The follow-up scans were acquired 6–12 months after surgery, and registered to the simulated outcome using a rigid Iterative Closest Point algorithm [15].

The results in terms of the mean absolute surface distance for the first four patients with complete data sets are shown in Fig. 4(a). The mean distance in all four cases is computed to be 3.3 mm. Figure 4(b) shows the surgical outcome simulation as a coloured surface, together with the follow-up acquisition as a wire-frame. The colours represent the evaluated distance between follow-up and prediction. It can be observed that the mechano-biological simulation predicts the overall deformity of the breast very well and within clinically useful accuracy. However, due to the relatively large time gap between baseline and follow-up scans, the breast shape might change due to effects unrelated to surgery – such as weight loss or gain. Such effects, presently not considered by the surgical outcome prediction, will increase the surface distance measure.

5   Conclusion

This paper presents an overview of our simulation methodology which enables breast shape changes due to breast conserving surgery to be predicted. The patient-specific mechano-biological models are derived from magnetic resonance images acquired in the prone configuration. In addition, optical surface scans are used to improve model predictions in the upright configuration. Breast surface acquisition is carried out using a 3dMD system alongside Microsoft Kinect v1 or v2 devices, with the aim of investigating and developing methodologies that allow reliable and high-fidelity surface reconstruction. We have developed a novel surgical simulation tool that incorporates a multiscale mechano-biological finite element solver. The modelling framework can facilitate simulations of large deformations of the breast due to gravity, but can also predict breast tissue deformities and scarring caused by the physiological wound healing process.

The modelling framework was evaluated by performing surgical simulations using imaging data acquired from four patients. This data included pre-operative MRIs, surface scans and the corresponding surgical plans specified by the surgeon who performed the procedure. The numerical predictions were compared and validated against clinical follow-up surface scans acquired 6–12 months after BCT. This resulted in a mean absolute surface error, over all four cases, of 3.3 mm. The PICTURE project also investigated the use of biomechanical models that do not require a pre-surgical MRI. However, these results will be presented in future work.

In this contribution, we demonstrate that efficient integration of different input modalities and detailed mechano-biological modelling tools can achieve accurate predictions of complex surgical interventions, such as BCT. In the future such predictions could promote improved and visually enriched communication between clinicians and patients. Personalised information about planned procedures could facilitate a shared decision making process in which decisions are made with more confidence.

Acknowledgements. The authors would like to acknowledge the financial support of the European FP7 project *VPH-PICTURE* (FP7-ICT-2011-9, 600948) and the Marie Curie Fellowship project *iBeSuP* (FP7-PEOPLE-2013-IEF, 627025). The authors are also indebted to members of the Royal Free Hospital NHS Foundation Trust for their support of this research; in particular Dominic Baxter for patient recruitment, Georgina Bartl for data administration and David Bishop, Emily Appleby, Imogen Ashby and Susan Smart for medical photography.

References

1. Ferlay, J., Steliarova-Foucher, E., Lortet-Tieulent, J., Rosso, S., Coebergh, J.W.W., Comber, H., Forman, D., Bray, F.: Cancer incidence and mortality patterns in Europe: estimates for 40 countries in 2012. Eur. J. Cancer **49**(6), 1374–1403 (2013)
2. Curran, D., van Dongen, J., Aaronson, N., Kiebert, G., Fentiman, I., Mignolet, F., Bartelink, H.: Quality of life of early-stage breast cancer patients treated with radical mastectomy or breast-conserving procedures: results of EORTC trial 10801. Eur. J. Cancer **34**(3), 307–314 (1998)
3. Hill-Kayser, C.E., Vachani, C., Hampshire, M.K., Lullo, G.A.D., Metz, J.M.: Cosmetic outcomes and complications reported by patients having undergone breast-conserving treatment. Int. J. Radiat. Oncol. Biol. Phys. **83**(3), 839–844 (2012)
4. Newcombe, R.A., Izadi, S., Hilliges, O., Molyneaux, D., Kim, D., Davison, A.J., Kohi, P., Shotton, J., Hodges, S., Fitzgibbon, A.: Kinectfusion: real-time dense surface mapping and tracking. In: 2011 10th IEEE International Symposium on Mixed and Augmented Reality (ISMAR), pp. 127–136 (2011)
5. Lacher, R., Hipwell, J., Williams, N., Keshtgar, M., Hawkes, D., Stoyanov, D.: Low-cost surface reconstruction for aesthetic results assessment and prediction in breast cancer surgery. In: 2015 37th Annual International Conference of the IEEE Engineering in Medicine and Biology Society (EMBC), pp. 5871–5874 (2015)
6. Samani, A., Plewes, D.: A method to measure the hyperelastic parameters of ex vivo breast tissue samples. Phys. Med. Biol. **49**(18), 4395–4405 (2004)
7. Veronda, D., Westmann, R.: Mechanical characterization of skin - finite deformations. J. Biomech. **3**(1), 111–124 (1970)
8. Murray, J.: Mathematical Biology I: An Introduction. Interdisciplinary Applied Mathematics, 3rd edn. Springer, New York (2011)
9. Moreo, P., García-Aznar, J., Doblaré, M.: Modeling mechanosensing and its effect on the migration and proliferation of adherent cells. Acta Biomater. **4**(3), 613–621 (2008)
10. Sherratt, J., Murray, J.: Mathematical analysis of a basic model for epidermal wound healing. J. Math. Biol. **29**(5), 389–404 (1991)
11. Olsen, L., Sherratt, J., Maini, P.: A mechanochemical model for adult dermal wound contraction and the permanence of the contracted tissue displacement profile. J. Theor. Biol. **177**(2), 113–128 (1995)
12. Maggelakis, S.: A mathematical model of tissue replacement during epidermal wound healing. Appl. Math. Model. **27**(3), 189–196 (2003)
13. Vavourakis, V., Hipwell, J., Hawkes, D.: An inverse finite element u/p-formulation to predict the unloaded state of in vivo biological soft tissues. Ann. Biomed. Eng. **44**(1), 187–201 (2016)
14. Eiben, B., Vavourakis, V., Hipwell, J.H., Kabus, S., Lorenz, C., Buelow, T., Williams, N.R., Keshtgar, M., Hawkes, D.J.: Surface driven biomechanical breast image registration. In: Webster, R.J., Yaniv, Z.R. (eds.) Medical Imaging 2016: Image-Guided Procedures, Robotic Interventions, and Modeling. Proceedings SPIE, vol. 9786, 97860W–97860W-10 (2016)
15. Besl, P., McKay, N.: A method for registration of 3-D shapes. IEEE Trans. Pattern Anal. Mach. Intell. **14**(2), 239–256 (1992)

The Characteristics of Malignant Breast Tumors Imaged Using a Prototype Mechanical Imaging System as an Adjunct to Mammography

Magnus Dustler[1]([✉]), Daniel Förnvik[1], Pontus Timberg[1], Hannie Petersson[1], Anders Tingberg[1], and Sophia Zackrisson[2]

[1] Medical Radiation Physics, Department of Translational Medicine, Faculty of Medicine, Lund University, Skåne University Hospital, Malmö, Sweden
magnus.dustler@med.lu.se
[2] Department of Imaging and Functional Medicine, Skåne University Hospital, Malmö, Sweden

Abstract. Breast cancer is diagnosed by a combination of modalities. Measuring the elasto-mechanical properties of suspicious lesions, by e.g. ultrasound elastography, can help differentiate malignant from benign findings. Using a prototype Mechanical Imaging (MI) system as an adjunct to mammography, the aim of this study was to characterize tumors using MI and compare the readings to those from the contralateral breast. Thirteen bilateral MI sets from women with malignant breast lesions were included in this study, drawn from a larger set of 155 women recalled from screening. The results showed that mean lesion pressure was significantly greater than the mean pressure of the corresponding breast, 7.5 ± 7.0 kPa compared to 2.5 ± 1.6 kPa ($P = 0.01$). There was no evidence for a difference in mean pressure or standard deviation of the MI image between symptomatic and contralateral asymptomatic breasts ($P = 0.24$ and 0.68). The results support that it is possible to use MI to distinguish malignant cancers from normal breast tissue. Still, further investigations of the characteristics of benign lesions are necessary to ascertain the usefulness of the system.

Keywords: Mammography · Mechanical imaging · Elastography · Screening

1 Introduction

Breast tumors, because of their different tissue composition and density, can be distinguished from normal breast tissue in a number of ways. The premier method of breast cancer detection, mammography, employs differences in x-ray absorption, MRI uses differences in water and/or fat content and ultrasound images display variations in the acoustical impedance of tissue [1]. Often a combination of modalities is needed to properly diagnose a lesion as malignant or benign.

Another way of detecting and differentiating malignant lesions is through the use of elastography, i.e. through measuring elasto-mechanical properties. Though markedly different in many respects, ultrasound [2, 3], MRI [4, 5] and other [6] forms of elastography all rely on measuring the relationship between deformation (strain) and applied

© Springer International Publishing Switzerland 2016
A. Tingberg et al. (Eds.): IWDM 2016, LNCS 9699, pp. 282–288, 2016.
DOI: 10.1007/978-3-319-41546-8_36

force (stress) of different kinds of tissue – the elastic modulus – and thereby differentiating them.

Manual examination of the breast, i.e. palpation, is essentially a form of unaided elastography. Whether performed as self-examination or by a physician or other medical professional, it relies on applying a force to the breast and sensing the resistance to deformation [7]. During screening mammography it is standard practice to ask women whether they have felt any new lumps in their breast, and for the radiographer to mark such areas on the mammogram for later review [8]. Such areas of increased resistance may later be associated with malignant lesions. Similarly, interval breast cancers, and breast cancer among women who do not participate in the screening program, often present as self-detected lumps which are further palpated by a medical professional before further referral to the breast clinic. Studies on excised lesions show that there are marked difference in elastic modulus between various lesions and normal breast tissue (fat and fibroglandular tissue) [9, 10]. The elastic modulus of malignant lesions appears to be greater than that of benign lesions, indicating that they are stiffer and can thus be distinguished by measuring there response to deformation.

So-called mechanical imaging (MI) systems which apply a set level of force to an area of the breast and measure the resulting pressures (stresses) arising due to essentially even deformations in breast tissue have been described and discussed in the literature, providing a way of quantifying the results of breast palpation [10–12]. Our group has used a prototype MI-system to investigate breast compression procedures in several earlier studies, including the compression of breast with malignant lesions [13–15]. We are currently working on a project which analyzes whether the addition of MI to screening mammography can be used to reduce false positives and improve sensitivity.

The aim of the current study was to characterize and categorize mechanical imaging of malignant lesions using our prototype system, and compare readings with the contralateral breast, using the material from the larger project.

2   Materials and Methods

2.1   Mechanical Imaging System

The prototype MI-system employs the Iscan 9801 FSR (force sensing resistor) pressure sensor (Tekscan Inc, South Boston, MA, USA). The sensor matrices consist of 16×6 sensor elements each, with a resolution of 12.7 mm and were consistently re-calibrated during the study to take into account sensor wear. The sensor is designed to work optimally with pressures up to 34 kPa, with a 256-channel resolution. A single sensor matrix is shown in Fig. 1.

Two sensor matrices of were attached to the bottom of the compression paddle of a mammography system, MAMMOMAT Inspiration (Siemens Healthcare, Erlangen, Germany), as shown in Fig. 2. The setup allows a 2D distribution of pressure on the breast to be acquired along with a minimal-dose (5 mAs) mammogram to be able to match sensor readings with breast structures in a full-dose diagnostic mammogram. Using the prototype system, the sensor would be too prominent on a full-dose mammogram for the image to be used diagnostically.

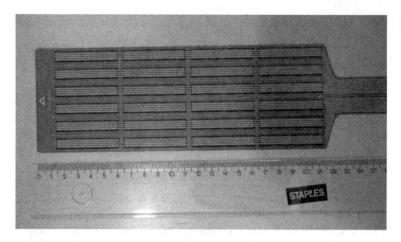

Fig. 1. Iscan 9801 sensor. Each strip contains four equally sized sensor elements. The sensor is approximately 0.16 mm thick.

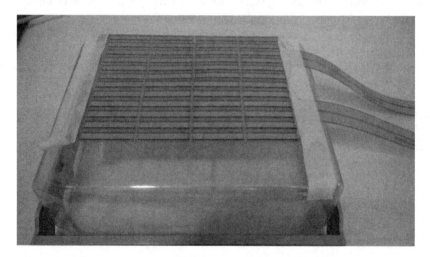

Fig. 2. Two Iscan 9801 sensors attached to the bottom of a MAMMOMAT compression paddle.

2.2   Study Population

The study population used for this institutional review board approved study (dnr 2013/620) consists of 19 cancer cases drawn from 155 women recalled from primary screening with suspicion of breast cancer. This sub-study includes all biopsy proven cancers from the main study, except for two cases of (very-rare) non-hodgkins lymphoma. Six cases had to be excluded from the later analysis due to the location of the lesion not being pressurized (three cases), the lesion not being present on the image in the employed projection (one case) and technical malfunction (two cases). This left 13 cancer cases for the analysis.

2.3   Data Acquisition and Analysis

All women had contralateral MI-examination of the breasts acquired alongside normally indicated clinical mammography, breast ultrasound and biopsies. MI-readings were acquired in either the cranio-caudal or medio-lateral oblique projection, depending on which projections was deemed to be most beneficial for including the suspicious lesion in the central part of the breast. A suspicious area of the breast was marked on the mammogram and matched with corresponding pressure readings from the MI-system, using the low-dose mammogram as a guide. The pressure on the sensor element deemed to match the center of the lesion and the mean lesion pressure (the mean pressure of 3 × 3 elements centered over the lesion) was compared to the mean pressure of the breast (excluding the innermost row of sensor elements, closest to the chest wall, as pressures in that are very high compared to the rest of the breast and frequently exceed the systems saturation pressure). The mean and standard deviation of the pressure readings of the symptomatic breast was compared with equivalent values of the contralateral breast. Pathology results were drawn from the hospital reporting system.

Table 1. Pressure data for the 13 included cancer cases. (ILC: Invasive Lobular Carcinoma, IDC: Invasive Ductal Carcinoma, DCIS: Ductal Carcinoma in situ, Tubular: Tubular Carcinoma)

	Lesion type, grade, laterality and size	Central lesion, kPa	Mean lesion, kPa	Mean R, kPa	Mean L, kPa	SD R, kPa	SD L, kPa
1	ILC 2, L, 7 mm	12.6	7.6	2.4	1.8	3.7	2.8
2	IDC 3, R, 19 mm	2.4	2.3	1.4	1.4	1.4	2.2
3	ILC 2, R, 35 mm	8.0	4.0	1.0	1.7	2.4	1.4
4	Tubular 1, L, 10 mm	8.1	12.7	2.2	4.7	2.7	4.4
5	IDC 2, R, 13 mm	0.8	4.8	0.9	0.7	1.6	1.0
6	ILC 2, L, 10 mm	20.3	17.5	4.7	4.5	5.0	6.0
7	DCIS 3, R, 25 mm	1.6	1.1	1.7	1.0	1.8	1.2
8	IDC 2, R, 18 mm	3.0	4.3	1.2	0.8	1.6	1.5
9	IDC 1, R, 22 mm	3.4	1.4	1.0	1.4	1.5	1.6
10	IDC 2, L, 15 mm	12.2	9.7	1.4	5.4	1.6	6.8
11	IDC 1, L, 16 mm	47.4	24.5	3.4	4.1	4.5	9.5
12	IDC 3, R, 30 mm	9.6	5.5	2.4	4.4	2.9	4.2
13	DCIS 2, R, 4 mm	1.5	1.6	2.0	2.6	2.1	2.3

3   Results

The paired Student's t-test showed no statistical difference between the normalized standard deviations or mean pressures (P = 0.24 and 0.68, respectively) of the symptomatic and asymptomatic breasts. The mean and central lesion pressure were both significantly greater (7.5 ± 7.0 kPa and 10.1 ± 12.6 kPa, respectively) than the mean pressure (2.5 ± 1.6 kPa) of the corresponding breast (P = 0.01 and 0.04, respectively). A total of 11 (84 %) cases had a mean lesion pressure greater than the breast mean pressure; the remaining two cases were both DCIS. Figure 3 shows an example of a combined mammography and MI set (subject 1) (Table 1).

There was no correlation between tumor size and mean or central lesion pressure, (R = 0.14 and −0.08, respectively).

4   Discussion

The results show the possibility of using MI in conjunction with mammography to differentiate tumors from normal tissue, as both the central pressure over the tumor and the mean pressure in its vicinity are significantly greater than the mean pressure of the symptomatic breast. Central pressure over the lesion in is likely to suffer from uncertainties, because of the difficulty of exactly matching pressure readings with the mammogram due both to the masking effect of the pressure sensors and the differences in positioning between the low and full dose images, making mean pressure over the 3 × 3

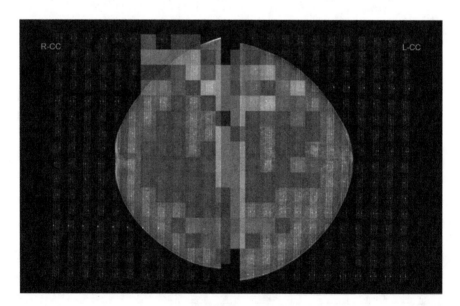

Fig. 3. Bilateral MI-image of symptomatic woman (7 mm ILC grade 2). The malignant lesion is located in the upper quadrant of the left breast. Please refer to inset for a full-dose mammographic image of the lesion. Note that the innermost rows of values are excluded from the analysis.

elements closest to the lesion a more reliable measure. The fact that there was no observed correlation between tumor size and pressure is interesting, and suggests that it is not only the size of the tumor itself, but also its composition and its effect on surrounding tissue which affects its apparent stiffness, though it should be stressed that the number of included tumors was relatively small.

It is notable that the two cases of DCIS had central and mean lesion pressure lower than the surrounding breast, indicating that there was no tissue reaction in these cases. A larger investigation of DCIS (in isolation, i.e. with no other associated mass) is warranted in order to check if this is always the case. If so, possible future clinical users of the MI-system would have to take this into account when evaluating DCIS.

It could be expected that there would be some asymmetry in the breasts, but it could not be quantified by either mean pressure readings or standard deviation. Differences in compression force, breast size and breast positioning likely influence such results, and in the future have to be compensated for if the influence of a possible tumor is to be detected in isolation.

In conclusion, the study shows promising results using a prototype Mechanical Imaging system in conjunction to aid in the detection of malignant lesions. In order to investigate this further, a more sophisticated method needs to be employed, which also takes into account benign lesions and asymptomatic breasts.

Acknowledgements. The authors would like to acknowledge the contributions of Dr. Ingvar Andersson. We would also like to acknowledge the Unilabs staff at the Malmö Breast Centre for their contribution to the acquisition of the data. This study was supported by a grant from Stiftelsen för cancerforskning vid onkologiska kliniken vid Universitetssjukhuset MAS.

References

1. Zhi, H., Ou, B., Luo, B.M., Feng, X., Wen, Y.L., Yang, H.Y.: Comparison of ultrasound elastography, mammography, and sonography in the diagnosis of solid breast lesions. J. Ultrasound Med. **26**, 807–815 (2007)
2. Cespedes, I., Ophir, J., Ponnekanti, H., Maklad, N.: Elastography - elasticity imaging using ultrasound with application to muscle and breast in-vivo. Ultrason. Imaging **15**, 73–88 (1993)
3. Itoh, A., Ueno, E., Tohno, E., Kamma, H., Takahashi, H., Shiina, T., Yamakawa, M., Matsumura, T.: Breast disease: clinical application of US elastography for diagnosis. Radiology **239**, 341–350 (2006)
4. Sinkus, R., Lorenzen, J., Schrader, D., Lorenzen, M., Dargatz, M., Holz, D.: High-resolution tensor MR elastography for breast tumour detection. Phys. Med. Biol. **45**, 1649–1664 (2000)
5. Sinkus, R., Tanter, M., Xydeas, T., Catheline, S., Bercoff, J., Fink, M.: Viscoelastic shear properties of in vivo breast lesions measured by MR elastography. Magn. Reson. Imaging **23**, 159–165 (2005)
6. Engelken, F.J., Sack, I., Klatt, D., Fischer, T., Fallenberg, E.M., Bick, U., Diekmann, F.: Evaluation of tomosynthesis elastography in a breast-mimicking phantom. Eur. J. Radiol. **81**, 2169–2173 (2012)
7. Mahoney, L., Csima, A.: Efficiency of palpation in clinical detection of breast-cancer. Can. Med. Assoc. J. **127**, 729–730 (1982)

8. Mathis, K.L., Hoskin, T.L., Boughey, J.C., Crownhart, B.S., Brandt, K.R., Vachon, C.M., Grant, C.S., Degnim, A.C.: Palpable presentation of breast cancer persists in the era of screening mammography. J. Am. Coll. Surg. **210**, 314–318 (2010)

9. Krouskop, T.A., Wheeler, T.M., Kallel, F., Garra, B.S., Hall, T.: Elastic moduli of breast and prostate tissues under compression. Ultrason. Imaging **20**, 260–274 (1998)

10. Wellman, P.S., Dalton, E.P., Krag, D., Kern, K.A., Howe, R.D.: Tactile imaging of breast masses: first clinical report. Arch. Surg. **136**, 204–208 (2001)

11. Sarvazyan, A.: Mechanical imaging: a new technology for medical diagnostics. Int. J. Med. Inform. **49**, 195–216 (1998)

12. Egorov, V., Kearney, T., Pollak, S.B., Rohatgi, C., Sarvazyan, N., Airapetian, S., Browning, S., Sarvazyan, A.: Differentiation of benign and malignant breast lesions by mechanical imaging. Breast Cancer Res. Treat. **118**, 67–80 (2009)

13. Fornvik, D., Andersson, I., Dustler, M., Ehrnstrom, R., Ryden, L., Tingberg, A., Zackrisson, S., Aaltonen, K.: No evidence for shedding of circulating tumor cells to the peripheral venous blood as a result of mammographic breast compression. Breast Cancer Res. Treat. **141**, 187–195 (2013)

14. Dustler, M., Andersson, I., Brorson, H., Frojd, P., Mattsson, S., Tingberg, A., Zackrisson, S., Fornvik, D.: Breast compression in mammography: pressure distribution patterns. Acta Radiol. **53**, 973–980 (2012)

15. Fornvik, D., Dustler, M., Andersson, I., Brorson, H., Timberg, P., Zackrisson, S., Tingberg, A.: Pressure distribution in mammography: compression of breasts with malignant tumor masses. In: SPIE Medical Imaging 2013: Physics of Medical Imaging, vol. 8668 (2013)

Density Assessment and Tissue Analysis

Mammographic Density Over Time in Women With and Without Breast Cancer

Abigail Humphrey[1], Elaine F. Harkness[2,3,4(✉)], Emmanouil Moschidis[2], Emma Hurley[3],
Philip Foden[5], Megan Bydder[3], Mary Wilson[3], Soujanya Gadde[3], Anthony Maxwell[2,3,4],
Yit Y. Lim[3], Ursula Beetles[3], Anthony Howell[3,6], D. Gareth Evans[3,7],
and Susan M. Astley[2,3,4]

[1] Manchester Medical School, University of Manchester,
Stopford Building, Oxford Road, Manchester M13 9PT, UK
[2] Centre for Imaging Sciences, Institute of Population Health, University of Manchester,
Stopford Building, Oxford Road, Manchester M13 9PT, UK
Elaine.F.Harkness@manchester.ac.uk
[3] Genesis Breast Cancer Prevention Centre and Nightingale Breast Screening Centre,
University Hospital of South Manchester NHS Trust, Wythenshawe, Manchester M23 9LT, UK
[4] Manchester Academic Health Science Centre, University Hospital of South Manchester,
The University of Manchester, Wythenshawe, Manchester M23 9LT, UK
[5] Centre for Biostatistics, Institute of Population Health, University of Manchester,
Oxford Road, Manchester M13 9PT, UK
[6] The Christie NHS Foundation, Withington, Manchester M20 4BX, UK
[7] Genomic Medicine, Manchester Academic Health Sciences Centre,
University of Manchester and Central Manchester Foundation Trust, Manchester M13 9WL, UK

Abstract. This study compared mammographic density over time between
women who developed breast cancer (cases) and women who did not (controls).
Cases had an initial negative mammographic screen and another three years later
when cancer was diagnosed. Cases were matched to three controls with two
successive negative screens by age, year of mammogram, BMI, parity, menopausal status and HRT use. Mammographic density was measured by Volpara^{TM}.
There was a significant reduction in percentage density in the affected breast for
cases (5.2 to 4.8 %, $p < 0.001$) and for the same matched breast in controls (4.9
to 4.5, $p < 0.001$). Similar results were found for the unaffected breast. After
adjusting for density measures at the initial screen, case-control status was only
significantly associated with fibroglandular volume in the unaffected breast
(adjusted mean 45.8 cm^3 in cases, 44.0 cm^3 in controls, $p = 0.008$). The results
suggest changes in mammographic density may be less important than initial
mammographic density.

Keywords: Breast cancer · Mammography · Digital · Breast density · Case-
control study

© Springer International Publishing Switzerland 2016
A. Tingberg et al. (Eds.): IWDM 2016, LNCS 9699, pp. 291–298, 2016.
DOI: 10.1007/978-3-319-41546-8_37

1   Introduction

Mammographic density has consistently been shown to be a strong independent risk factor for the development of breast cancer [1], and also has a significant attributable risk [2]. There is considerable variation in mammographic density amongst women and this can be attributed to many factors including heredity, age and menopausal status [3].

Pike et al. (1983) suggest it is not the chronological age of a women that puts her at increased risk of breast cancer, but the rate of exposure to "breast tissue ageing". It is believed that breast tissue ageing is associated with hormones affecting cell proliferation within the breast tissue, and that the cumulative exposure to breast tissue ageing increases susceptibility to breast cancer. The breast tissue ageing process starts during menarche, slows during pregnancy, slows further during the peri-menopausal period and is lowest post-menopausally [4, 5]. The fitted model by Pike et al. (1983) showed that women with an earlier age of menarche, nulliparity or later age of first full term pregnancy, and later age of menopause had an increased risk of breast cancer, suggesting hormones play a major role [4].

If changes in mammographic density were found to be associated with breast cancer this could potentially allow for identification of women at high risk of developing the disease, which in turn could lead to more intensive screening to aid earlier detection, or the introduction of preventative measures for reducing breast density, including chemo-preventive drugs such as tamoxifen or raloxifene, and lifestyle interventions. Furthermore mammographic density could be incorporated into risk stratification tools to improve their predictive accuracy.

There have been a number of studies examining the change in breast density longitudinally. However, the results have been mixed and the majority of studies have used qualitative (e.g. BIRADS) or semi-automated (e.g. Cumulus) density assessments based on film or digitized film mammograms [6]. In this study we aim to investigate changes in mammographic density measures using Volpara^{TM}, an automated method for assessing mammographic density in digital mammograms, in women with and without breast cancer.

2   Methods

Between October 2009 and April 2015 women attending the Greater Manchester National Health Screening Breast Screening Programme (NHSBSP) in the UK were invited to take part in the Predicting Risk Of Cancer At Screening (PROCAS) study [7]. Approximately 58,000 women consented to participate in PROCAS and provided additional information on risk factors for breast cancer by completing a 2-page questionnaire at the time of screening. Ethical approval for the study was given by the North Manchester Research Committee (09/H1008/81).

Cases in the current study had a negative screen at entry to PROCAS, and a subsequent screen when breast cancer was diagnosed (n = 175). Each case was matched to three controls based on age (within a year), year of mammogram, Body Mass Index (on kg/m^2), parity (nulliparous or parous), menopausal status (pre, peri, post-menopausal or unknown) and Hormone Replacement Therapy (HRT) use (current or never/previous).

Mammographic breast density measurements were made on all screening mammograms (Volpara^{TM} version 1.5.0) to assess the percentage of fibroglandular tissue and total fibroglandular volume (FGV). Results were produced for each mammographic view (left mediolateral oblique, right mediolateral oblique, left cranio-caudial and right cranio-caudial) and the average for each breast was obtained for each individual. The data for the density measures were found to be positively skewed and therefore the log of density measures were used. Results are presented for the affected and unaffected breast for cases, and the same matched breast for controls (also referred to as the affected and unaffected breast in the results).

We used paired t-tests to examine the difference in density measures between screen 1 and screen 2 for the affected and unaffected breast for cases and controls. To examine the relationship between density and case control status generalized estimating equations (GEEs) were used. GEEs were used due to the matched nature of the dataset where the subject variable was the identifier for each case-control set and the within-subject variable was the case-control identifier. An exchangeable correlation matrix, which assumes equal correlations between cases and controls, was used. The dependent variable was the log of the density measure from the diagnostic screen (screen 2) and this was adjusted for the log of the density measure from the prior negative screen (screen 1). Case-control status (cancer or control) was entered as an independent variable to determine whether there was a difference between cases and controls.

3   Results

Five cases were excluded (1 bilateral breast cancer, 4 with no details on BMI) leaving 170 cases and 510 matched controls eligible for the study. Cases and controls were well matched as shown in Table 1. The mean age was 60 years in both groups, and mean BMI was similar in both groups (28.7 in cases, 28.5 in controls). In both groups 77 % were postmenopausal and 12 % reported being current HRT users. The majority of women had children (87 % in both groups).

Table 2 shows the mean fibroglandular volume and percentage density for cases and controls for the affected and unaffected breast at screen 1 and screen 2. Paired t-tests showed statistically significant reductions in percentage density from screen 1 to screen 2 for cases in the affected and unaffected breast (5.2 to 4.8, p < 0.001 and 5.1 to 4.8, p < 0.001 respectively) and controls (4.9 to 4.5, p < 0.001 and 5.0 to 4.5, p < 0.001 respectively). There was little difference between screens in the gland volume for cases and controls for the affected and unaffected breast.

Table 1. Demographics for cases and controls

	Cases		Controls	
	Mean	SD	Mean	SD
Age	60.1	6.0	60.1	5.9
BMI	28.7	5.4	28.5	5.3
	n	%	n	%
Menopausal status				
Postmenopausal	131	77	393	77
Pre-menopausal	8	5	24	5
Peri-menopausal	27	16	81	16
Unknown	4	2	12	2
HRT use				
Current	21	12	63	12
Previous	60	35	177	35
Never	88	52	269	53
Unknown	1	0	1	0
Children				
Nulliparous	22	13	64	13
Parous	148	87	446	87

The paired t-tests show the general trend between cases and controls between screen 1 and screen 2, however this does not take into account the matched nature of the dataset and therefore we also used GEEs (as described above). Results from the GEEs demonstrated that, with the exception of fibroglandular volume in the unaffected breast, there were no statistically significant differences between cases and controls after adjusting for the relevant density measure at the inital screen (screen 1). Figure 1 shows the estimated marginal mean for fibroglandular volume was significantly higher for cases (45.8 cm^3) compared to controls (44.0 cm^3) in the unaffected breast ($p = 0.008$).

Table 2. Changes in Volpara™ fibroglandular volume (FGV in cm^3) and percentage density (PD - %) for cases and controls

	Screen 1		Screen 2		
	Mean	95 % CI	Mean	95 % CI	p-value
Affected breast					
FGV cases	48.0	45.1–51.1	48.1	45.1–51.5	0.785
FGV controls	43.3	41.8–44.9	42.7	41.2–44.3	0.084
PD cases	5.2	4.8–5.6	4.8	4.5–5.2	<0.001
PD controls	4.9	4.7–5.2	4.5	4.3–4.7	<0.001
Unaffected breast					
FGV cases	47.7	44.7–50.9	48.5	45.5–51.8	0.222
FGV controls	43.8	42.4–45.4	43.2	41.7–44.8	0.085
PD cases	5.1	4.7–5.5	4.8	4.4–5.2	<0.001
PD controls	5.0	4.8–5.2	4.5	4.4–4.7	<0.001

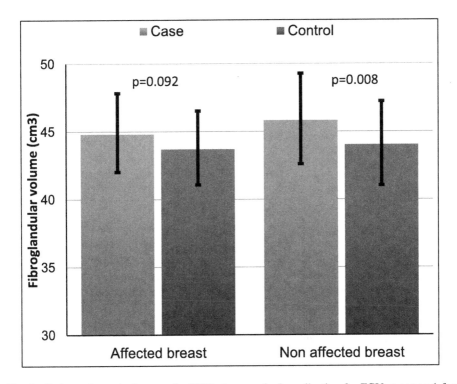

Fig. 1. Estimated marginal means for FGV at screen 2 after adjusting for FGV at screen 1 for cases and controls and for affected and non-affected breast (Color figure online)

We also added breast volume at screen 1 and screen 2 as a surrogate for weight change over time. Similar results were found, with the exception of percentage density where the difference in the adjusted means between cases and controls for the non-affected breast became statistically significant being higher in cases (4.7 %) than controls (4.6 %) (p = 0.008), the estimated marginal means were similar to those without adjusting for breast volume.

Mammograms were also reviewed retrospectively by consultant radiologists to determine whether there was evidence of any abnormalities on the prior negative screening mammogram (screen 1) for cancer cases. Signs of any of the following abnormalities were recorded: architectural distortion, asymmetry, lymph node presence, nipple retraction or evidence of the presence of a mass or calcification. On review a large proportion of cases (76/170, 45 %) were found to have evidence of an abnormality on screen 1. We therefore conducted a subgroup analysis in cases, and their matched controls, with no evidence of prior abnormality, to determine whether this had any effect on the results.

Results from the subgroup analysis were similar to those for the total group. Paired t-tests showed there were significant reductions in percentage density for both cases and controls from screen 1 to screen 2 for both the affected and unaffacted breasts [cases: 5.0 to 4.6, p < 0.001 and 5.0 to 4.7, p = 0.010 respectively; controls: 4.9 to 4.4, p < 0.001

and 4.9 to 4.5, p < 0.001 respectively]. There were no significant differences in gland volume between screen 1 and screen 2 for the affected or unaffected breast for either cases or controls.

Similarly results from the GEEs demonstrated that, with the exception of fibro-glandular volume in the unaffected breast, there were no statistically significant differences between cases and controls after adjusting for the relevant density measure at the inital screen (screen 1). The estimated marginal mean for fibroglandular volume was significantly higher for cases (45.3 cm^3) compared to controls (43.5 cm^3) in the unaffected breast (p = 0.023).

4 Discussion

Percentage density was significantly reduced from screen 1 to screen 2 for both cases and controls. There were no statistically significant differences in gland volume between screen 1 and screen 2. After accounting for the matching procedure and adjusting for fibroglandular volume at screen 1 there was a significant difference between cases and controls in fibroglandular volume for the unaffected breast with cases having significantly higher gland volume than controls at screen 2.

The strengths of this study include the matching of cases to three controls on a number of risk factors known to contribute to increased mammographic density. In a few instances it was not possible to obtain an exact match, for example there were some cases with particularly high BMIs for whom it was difficult to obtain an exact match. Nonetheless, matching appeared to be successful and we did not further consider the variables on which matching was performed as potential confounders in the analysis.

A further strength of this study was the retrospective review of first mammograms to confirm whether there were any abnormalities in cancer cases, thus we were able to carry out a subgroup analysis in those without any signs of abnormality in the previous screening round. Results from the subgroup analysis were similar to those in the main analysis. This is perhaps not surprising given the objective nature of the density assessment, however it may be more important where density is assessed visually and may explain the mixed results from earlier studies [6].

Limitations of the study include the relatively small number of cancers with previous digital mammograms available for the study. It would also be interesting to know whether other methods of density assessment, such as Quantra^{TM}, produce the same sort of results. Furthermore we did not have information in relation to change in weight over the two screens, however we adjusted for breast volume at screen 1 and screen 2, as a potential surrogate for weight change, and the results were broadly similar to those without adjustment.

The majority of women in this study were postmenopausal (77 %) and therefore no change in mammographic density over a relatively short period of time (three years approximately) may not be unsurprising. As hypothesized by Pike et al. (1983) the greatest reduction in mammographic density occurs when women are going through the menopause. Information on menopausal status was self-reported at the initial screen and although the majority of women who reported being pre- or peri-menopausal at screen

1 were likely to be post-menopausal at the time of screen 2 the number of women was relatively small and therefore we did not conduct a subgroup analysis for this group.

Case-control status was a significant predictor of fibroglandular volume in the unaffected breast at screen 2 after adjusting for fibroglandular volume at screen 1. However, although the difference in the estimated marginal means between cases and controls was statistically significant, the magnitude of the difference was relatively small, and it is questionable whether such a difference would be considered as clinically significant.

5   Conclusions

This is the first study to assess changes in mammographic density in digital mammograms in women with and without breast cancer. A subgroup analysis was also performed, after a retrospective review of mammograms to identify early signs of cancer, in women who had no abnormalities. There was a significant reduction in percentage density between screens in both cases and controls, however case-control status was not significantly associated with the majority of density measures at screen 2 after adjusting for baseline measures at screen 1. These results suggest that changes in mammographic density may not be as important as initial mammographic density.

Acknowledgements. We acknowledge the support of the National Institute for Health Research (NIHR) and the Genesis Prevention Appeal for their funding of the PROCAS study. We would like to thank the women who agreed to take part in the study and the study staff for recruitment and data collection. We also thank Matakina Technology Limited for providing Volpara™. This paper presents independent research funded by the National Institute for Health Research (NIHR) under its Programme Grants for Applied Research programme (reference number RP-PG-0707-10031: "Improvement in risk prediction, early detection and prevention of breast cancer"). The views expressed are those of the author(s) and not necessarily those of the NHS, the NIHR, or the Department of Health.

References

1. Vachon, C.M., van Gils, C.H., Sellers, T.A., Ghosh, K., Pruthi, S., Brandt, K.R., Pankratz, V.S.: Mammographic density, breast cancer risk and risk prediction. Breast Cancer Res. **9**(6), 217 (2007)
2. Boyd, N.F., Guo, H., Martin, L.J., Sun, L., Stone, J., Fishell, E., Jong, R.A., Hislop, G., Chiarelli, A., Minkin, S., Yaffe, M.J.: Mammographic density and the risk and detection of breast cancer. N. Engl. J. Med. **356**(3), 227–236 (2007)
3. Hutson, S.W., Cowen, P.N., Bird, C.C.: Morphometric studies of age related changes in normal human breast and their significance for evolution of mammary cancer. J. Clin. Pathol. **38**(3), 281–287 (1985)
4. Pike, M.C., Krailo, M.D., Henderson, B.F., Casagrande, J.T., Hoel, D.G.: Hormonal' risk factors, 'breast tissue age' and the age-incidence of breast cancer. Nature **303**, 767–770 (1983)
5. Boyd, N., Martin, L., Chavez, S., Gunasekara, A., Salleh, A., Melnichouk, O., Yaffe, M., Friedenreich, C., Minkin, S., Bronskill, M.: Breast-tissue composition and other risk factors for breast cancer in young women: a cross-sectional study. Lancet Oncol. **10**(6), 569–580 (2009)

6. Busana, M.C., DeStavola, B.L., Sovio, U., Jingmei, L., Moss, S., Humphreys, K., Dos-Santos-Silva, I.: Assessing within-women changes in mammographic density: a comparison of fully versus semi-automated area-based approaches. Cancer Causes Control **27**(4), 481–491 (2016)

7. Evans, D.G.R., Warwick, J., Astley, S.M., Stavrinos, P., Sahin, S., Ingham, S., McBurney, H., Eckersley, B., Harvie, M., Wilson, M., Beetles, U., Warren, R., Hufton, A., Sergeant, J.C., Newman, W.G., Buchan, I., Cuzick, J., Howell, A.: Assessing individual breast cancer risk within the U.K. national health service breast screening program: a new paradigm for cancer prevention. Cancer Prev Res. **5**(7), 943–951 (2012)

Learning Density Independent Texture Features

Michiel Kallenberg[1,2(✉)], Mads Nielsen[1,2], Katharina Holland[3],
Nico Karssemeijer[3], Christian Igel[1], and Martin Lillholm[1,2]

[1] University of Copenhagen, 2100 Copenhagen OE, Denmark
m.kallenberg@biomediq.com
[2] Biomediq A/S, 2100 Copenhagen OE, Denmark
[3] Radboud University Medical Centre, 6525 Nijmegen, Netherlands

Abstract. Breast cancer risk assessment is becoming increasingly important in clinical practice. It has been suggested that features that characterize mammographic texture are more predictive for breast cancer than breast density. Yet, strong correlation between both types of features is an issue in many studies. In this work we investigate a method to generate texture features and/or scores that are independent of breast density. The method is especially useful in settings where features are learned from the data itself. We evaluate our method on a case control set comprising 394 cancers, and 1182 healthy controls. We show that the learned density independent texture features are significantly associated with breast cancer risk. As such it may aid in exploring breast characteristics that are predictive of breast cancer irrespective of breast density. Furthermore it offers opportunities to enhance personalized breast cancer screening beyond breast density.

Keywords: Texture · Breast density · Deep learning · Breast cancer risk assessment

1 Introduction

In order to further optimize breast cancer screening personalized breast cancer screening has been proposed. In personalized breast cancer screening a subpopulation of women is offered alternative screening options that are known to be more sensitive to detect breast cancer. A key point in personalized breast cancer screening is risk assessment.

One of the strongest known risk factors for breast cancer after gender, age, gene mutations, and family history is the relative amount of radiodense tissue in the breast, expressed as mammographic density (MD). It has been suggested, however, that MD is a too coarse descriptor for breast cancer risk. Several authors have developed methods that aim to find breast tissue patterns (or textures, MT) that are potentially more predictive of breast cancer [2,6,7,9,14]. In general these methods operate by generating a (large) set of texture features that are subsequently combined with a classifier into a single texture score per

© Springer International Publishing Switzerland 2016
A. Tingberg et al. (Eds.): IWDM 2016, LNCS 9699, pp. 299–306, 2016.
DOI: 10.1007/978-3-319-41546-8_38

image. Intuitively, their goal is to characterize breast heterogeneity instead of breast density.

Although these works on texture scoring have shown that density and texture are independently associated with cancer risk, correlation between texture and density is still an issue: Häberle et al. [2], for example, noted that most of their texture features appeared to reflect mammographic density. Manduca et al. [7] reported that simultaneous inclusion of their texture features in a model with breast density did not significantly improve the ability to predict breast cancer.

Generally spoken two traditional approaches could be taken to generate texture features and/or scores that are independent of breast density: (i) *invariant scores:* ensure that the classifier that combines the texture features into a texture score does not select features that are highly correlated to density, or (ii) *invariant features:* ensure that the employed texture features are uncorrelated to density. An example of the first approach is to apply correlation based feature selection [3] and its variants as is done in e.g. [2]. A classic example of the second approach is to handcraft features that do not make use of first-order statistics, as is done in e.g. [9].

A problem with the employment of handcrafted features is that these features are not guaranteed to capture the salient information of the data. An increasing number of papers demonstrate that comparable or even better results are achieved by learning features directly from the data. Especially deep nonlinear models have been proven to generate descriptors that are extremely effective in object recognition and localization in natural images [1,12]. A problem with learning texture features directly from the data is, however, that they may very well be correlated to density, as could be observed in e.g. [5,6,10], as no restrictions are imposed.

In this work we present a means to generate density independent texture features and scores in a setting where features are learned from the data itself. The method follows the same principle as the one of a matched case control study. That is: in the feature learning phase we balance breast density over the two classes we want to discriminate between (i.e. cancer cases and controls). Since, as a result of the matching, no difference occurs in breast density between both classes the learned texture features and scores are determined to be independent of density.

2   Materials and Methods

We used a case control set consisting of 394 cancers, and 1182 healthy controls from a previous study on breast cancer risk assessment [6]. Initially controls were matched on age and acquisition date. The images were recorded between 2003 and 2012 on a Hologic Selenia FFDM system, using standard clinical settings. To exclude signs of cancerous tissue we took the contralateral mammograms. We used the raw image data. For each image the volumetric percentage of breast density (PMD), and the Volpara density grade (VDG) was computed using automated software (Volpara, Matakina Technology Limited, New Zealand).

As breast density is a risk factor for breast cancer, in the initial matching breast density was on average higher in the cases than in the controls ($8.89 \pm 5.62\%$ vs 7.60 ± 4.76, $p < 0.001$). In order to balance breast density over the cases and the controls we performed a rematching based on breast density. Rematching was done by the full matching algorithm described in [4]. We subsequently excluded controls that were 0.05 percent points less dense than their matched case. Cases for which no matching controls were available were excluded as well. Non-matching cases and controls were only excluded during training; in the testing phase all images were scored. After rematching the average breast density was $8.15 \pm 4.59\%$ and 7.84 ± 4.31 for cases and controls, respectively ($p = 0.44$). The discriminative power of breast density was AUC=0.509 (95% CI 0.472-0.546) in the rematched set, as opposed to 0.578 (0.546-0.611) in the original set.

In this work we train and test our texture based risk assessment machinery presented elsewhere [5,6,10] with the modification that here we train on density balanced data. The machinery comprises a multilayer convolutional architecture consisting of a stack of sparse autoencoders [8,11,13]. Features are initially learned in an unsupervised way, followed by fine-tuning with a supervised signal. Features are learned on multiple scales. Results are obtained by performing 5-fold cross-validation by image to estimate the generalization ability of our machinery. We compare the results of training on the original dataset (MT_{orig}) with training on the density balanced dataset (MT_{bal}).

3   Results

Figure 1 shows scatter plots between volumetric breast density (PMD) and texture scores for the two training regimes MT_{orig}, and MT_{bal}. Spearman's rank correlation between density and texture is $r = 0.81$ (0.79-0.83) for the original matching and $r = -0.0042$ (−0.057- 0.045) for training on the density balanced dataset.

Table 1 lists the odds ratios (OR) for each quartile of the texture scores for both MT_{orig} and MT_{bal}. Logistic regression is used to correct for age and breast density. As for MT_{bal} the scores are uncorrelated to breast density, correcting for breast density does not impact the ORs. The adjusted odds ratio for the highest texture category as compared to the lowest texture category is 1.39 (95% CI 0.92-2.09) for MT_{orig} and 1.48 (1.07-2.06) for MT_{bal}.

Figure 2 shows the ORs for MT_{bal} split out per density category (i.e. Volpara density grades (VDG)). In order to preserve a substantial number of cases in each category the texture scores are divided in tertiles. The tertiles were established on the whole dataset. We took VDG2-MT1 as a reference category in order to be on the conservative site. Obviously if e.g. VDG1-MT1 is taken ORs are higher. Note that texture is able to "unfold" the density axis. For example, woman who are classified as medium dense but have a high texture score (i.e. VDG2-MT3) have an approximately equal risk of getting breast cancer as women with high dense but a low texture score (i.e. VDG3/4-MT1) (OR = 1.16 (0.74-1.81)).

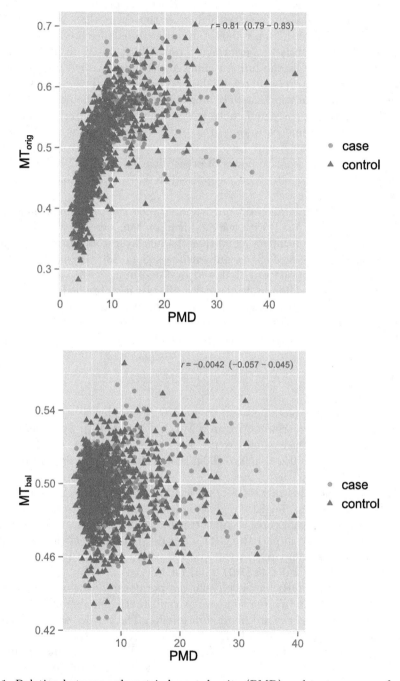

Fig. 1. Relation between volumetric breast density (PMD) and texture scores for two training regimes (MT_{orig}, and MT_{bal})

Table 1. Odds ratios for quartiles of MT_{orig} and MT_{bal}

MT_{orig}	OR	95% CI	OR*	95% CI
1	REF	-	REF	-
2	1.23	(0.86-1.76)	1.15	(0.81-1.65)
3	1.59	(1.13-2.24)	1.40	(0.98-2.00)
4	1.81	(1.30-2.53)	1.39	(0.92-2.09)

*adjusted for density and age

MT_{bal}	OR	95% CI	OR*	95% CI
1	REF	-	REF	-
2	1.15	(0.82-1.62)	1.21	(0.86-1.71)
3	1.33	(1.96-1.86)	1.46	(1.04-2.05)
4	1.45	(1.05-2.01)	1.48	(1.07-2.06)

*adjusted for density and age

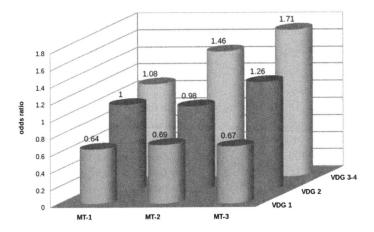

Fig. 2. Age adjusted odds ratios for tertiles of MT_{bal} for various density categories. It can be seen that texture is able to "unfold" the density axis. The association between texture and breast cancer risk is limited in VDG 1, but strong in VDG 3/4.

We also estimated the merits of the different texture scores in a combination model that included breast density. To that end we fitted a logit model on the texture scores, breast density and age. The parameters of the logit model were learned on the whole dataset, and not in a cross validation scheme. As such results may be slightly biased. For percent density alone the AUC is 0.578 (0.546-0.611). For the combination model including MT_{orig} the AUC is 0.589 (0.557-0.621) ($p = 0.40$). For the combination model including MT_{bal} the AUC is 0.587 (0.555-0.620) ($p = 0.45$).

In this work features are automatically generated with both unsupervised and supervised feature learning. Since we use deep nets, features are generated at multiple levels. In deep nets that are trained on natural images, one typically

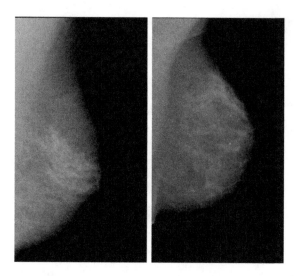

Fig. 3. Two example mammograms, both from VDG 3. The left mammogram has a low texture score (MT_{bal}=0.443), whereas the right mammogram has a high texture score (MT_{bal}=0.527).

finds edge detectors in the first layer. In our experiments we did not find such typical features, though, which could be explained by the fact that the mammographic appearance of the breast tissue does not contain that much of structure. Features in the second layer and beyond comprise descriptors that build upon the features of the previous layer(s). As such it is difficult to interpret the features of the layers beyond the first layer. In order to give an impression of what our texture scores reflect Fig. 3 shows two example mammograms with a similar volumetric breast density (PMD=8.18 %, and 8.00 % (i.e. VDG 3)), but different texture scores (MT_{bal}=0.443 (Q1), and 0.527 (Q4)).

4 Discussion

In many studies on breast cancer risk assessment texture features are highly correlated with density. It is therefore not clear what signal of breast cancer texture is actually picking up on. In this work we investigated a means to generate texture features and/or scores that are independent of breast density. The method is especially useful in settings where features are learned from the data itself. As such it may aid in identifying breast characteristics that are predictive of breast cancer irrespective of breast density. We showed that the generated density independent texture scores were significantly associated with breast cancer risk.

The association between texture and breast cancer risk was limited in VDG 1, but strong in VDG 3/4. We have seen such an interaction between texture and density in previous experiments as well. One hypothesis is that there are different patterns in which the fibroglandular tissue is distributed and organized, and that these patterns, which are reflected in our texture scores, are predictive of breast cancer risk. In fatty breasts the variation in the way fibroglandular tissue is organized may be limited, which may limit the role of texture in this category. In VDG 3/4 variation is potentially larger and as such the association between texture and breast cancer is more profound.

The texture based risk model offers opportunities to further enhance personalized breast cancer screening, beyond breast density. Future work will focus on the employment of combination models that have the capacity to model nonlinear interactions between density and texture.

References

1. Bengio, Y., Courville, A., Vincent, P.: Representation learning: a review and new perspectives. IEEE Trans. Pattern Anal. Mach. Intell. **35**(8), 1798–1828 (2013)
2. Häberle, L., Wagner, F., Fasching, P.A., Jud, S.M., Heusinger, K., Loehberg, C.R., Hein, A., Bayer, C.M., Hack, C.C., Lux, M.P., et al.: Characterizing mammographic images by using generic texture features. Breast Cancer Res. **14**(2), R59 (2012)
3. Hall, M.A.: Correlation-based feature selection for machine learning. Ph.D. thesis, The University of Waikato (1999)
4. Hansen, B.B., Klopfer, S.O.: Optimal full matching and related designs via network flows. J. Comput. Graph. Stat. **15**, 609–627 (2012)
5. Kallenberg, M., Lilholm, M., Diao, P., Petersen, K., Holland, K., Karssemeijer, N., Igel, C., Nielsen, M.: Assessing breast cancer masking risk with automated texture analysis in full field digital mammography. In: Annual Meeting of the Radiological Society of North America (2015)
6. Kallenberg, M., Petersen, K., Lilholm, M., Jørgensen, D., Diao, P., Holland, K., Karssemeijer, N., Igel, C., Nielsen, M.: Automated texture scoring for assessing breast cancer masking risk in full field digital mammography. In: ECR (2015)
7. Manduca, A., Carston, M., Heine, J., Scott, C., Pankratz, V., Brandt, K., Sellers, T., Vachon, C., Cerhan, J.: Texture features from mammographic images and risk of breast cancer. Cancer Epidemiol. Biomarkers Prev. **18**, 837–845 (2009). http://dx.doi.org/10.1158/1055-9965.EPI-08-0631
8. Masci, J., Meier, U., Cireşan, D., Schmidhuber, J.: Stacked convolutional auto-encoders for hierarchical feature extraction. In: Honkela, T. (ed.) ICANN 2011, Part I. LNCS, vol. 6791, pp. 52–59. Springer, Heidelberg (2011)
9. Nielsen, M., Vachon, C.M., Scott, C.G., Chernoff, K., Karemore, G., Karssemeijer, N., Lillholm, M., Karsdal, M.A.: Mammographic texture resemblance generalizes as an independent risk factor for breast cancer. Breast Cancer Res. **16**, R37 (2014). http://dx.doi.org/10.1186/bcr3641
10. Petersen, K., Chernoff, K., Nielsen, M., Ng, A.: Breast density scoring with multiscale denoising autoencoders. In: Proceedings Sparsity Techniques in Medical Imaging 2012, in conjunction with MICCAI 2012 (2012)
11. Ranzato, M., Poultney, C.S., Chopra, S., LeCun, Y.: Efficient learning of sparse representations with an energy-based model. In: Advances in Neural Information Processing Systems, pp. 1137–1144 (2007)
12. Schmidhuber, J.: Deep learning in neural networks: an overview. Neural Netw. **61**, 85–117 (2015)

13. Vincent, P., Larochelle, H., Bengio, Y., Manzagol, P.A.: Extracting and composing robust features with denoising autoencoders. In: International Conference on Machine Learning, pp. 1096–1103 (2008)
14. Zheng, Y., Keller, B.M., Ray, S., Wang, Y., Conant, E.F., Gee, J.C., Kontos, D.: Parenchymal texture analysis in digital mammography: a fully automated pipeline for breast cancer risk assessment. Med. Phys. **42**(7), 4149–4160 (2015)

Breast Asymmetry, Distortion and Density Are Key Factors for False Positive Decisions

Zoey Z.Y. Ang[1]([✉]), Rob Heard[2], Mohammad A. Rawashdeh[3],
Patrick C. Brennan[4], Warwick Lee[4], and Sarah J. Lewis[4]

[1] National Healthcare Group Diagnostics, Singapore, Singapore
zang6391@uni.sydney.edu.au
[2] Health Systems and Global Populations Research Group,
Faculty of Health Sciences, The University of Sydney, Sydney, Australia
[3] Faculty of Applied Medical Sciences,
Jordan University of Science and Technology, Irbid, Jordan
[4] Medical Imaging Optimisation and Perception Group (MIOPeG),
Discipline of Medical Radiation Sciences, Faculty of Health Sciences,
The University of Sydney, Sydney, Australia

Abstract. *Aim:* Understanding both normal mammographic appearance and how false positive (FP) errors occur is paramount to improving the efficiency and diagnostic accuracy of screening mammography services. While much of the focus of research is on increasing knowledge about the appearances and imaging of breast cancers, this study reports on findings where breast screen readers are asked to comment on past incorrect decisions by assigning a lexicon that best describes a known FP region. *Method:* Fifteen breast screen readers were given two tasks. The first was to assess nine normal screening cases which had attracted a high number of FP decisions in a test set of 60 cases in a previous study with 129 readers. In the second task, the 15 readers in this study, who were made aware that the nine cases were normal, were directed to view distinct regions of interest (ROI) that represented the FP markings from past readings in the blinded observer performance study. A list of descriptors derived from literature was used to assist readers to describe the mammographic appearance within those ROIs. *Results:* In the first task, readers identified breast density as the greatest difficulty in determining normality. In the second task, asymmetry of breast tissue and a suspicion of architectural distortion (AD) were the top two reasons our readers gave to explain the high number of past FP decisions. Additionally, our readers believed past FP decisions were less likely to reflect a suspicion of breast lesions or masses (second task). *Conclusion:* The classification of normal cases remains a challenging task, influenced by asymmetry and breast density. FP decisions may reflect a suspicion of AD and appear less related to suspicion of masses.

Keywords: Mammography · Normal mammograms · False positive · Breast density · Breast tissue asymmetry

© Springer International Publishing Switzerland 2016
A. Tingberg et al. (Eds.): IWDM 2016, LNCS 9699, pp. 307–315, 2016.
DOI: 10.1007/978-3-319-41546-8_39

1 Introduction

In Australia, breast cancer is the most common cancer affecting women [1], with one in eight diagnosed with the disease before the age of 85 [2]. The aim of BreastScreen Australia, the national breast cancer screening program, is to detect breast cancer in asymptomatic women at an early stage [1]. However, such programs have drawbacks through false positive (FP) results, in which women with normal mammograms are recalled for further assessment on the basis of suspicion of cancer [3]. Having a higher than expected FP rate lowers the specificity of breast cancer screening programs and may reduce confidence in the screening service. Understanding why FP decisions are made is paramount to increasing the effectiveness of screening since approximately 98 % of all presenting cases are normal [4].

In a study in 2013 by Rawashdeh et al. [5], 129 breast screen readers were asked to interpret a test set of 60 cases, identifying and marking the location of any suspected malignancies. A number of normal cases in the Rawashdeh study were noted as having a higher than expected FP rate, however, those cases were not individually analysed to establish the mammographic feature that may be responsible for the error. This study builds upon the 2013 research by investigating the reasons responsible for FP decisions, using a purpose designed lexicon and a review of the cases by 15 experienced breast screen readers.

2 Methods

2.1 Sample

Institutional ethics approval was granted by The University of Sydney Human Research ethics committee (Project no. 2015/327) and the need for patient consent to use the de-identified images was waived. This study included 15 breast screen readers (13 radiologists and two breast physicians) recruited at the Royal Australian and New Zealand College of Radiologists 10th General Breast Imaging Meeting on the Gold Coast, Queensland, Australia in July 2015. Demographics related to the number of years qualified, the number of years specialized in reading mammograms and the number of mammograms read per year were collected as shown in Table 1.

Table 1. Self-reported characteristics of readers.

	Years of qualification	Years of mammogram reading	Mammograms read per year
Median	28	20	7500
First quartile	15	10	2000
Third quartile	38	26	27500
Standard deviation	11.5	10.3	9402

2.2   Study Design

Cases. Nine normal cases were identified in the Rawashdeh 2013 study [5] as having considerably more FP markings than expected and those nine women would have been recalled by the readers in Rawashdeh study. Hence those cases were chosen for further analysis in this study as they represent error present in breast cancer screening. These cases were extracted to form the test set for our study. Each case consisted of a medio-lateral oblique (MLO) and a cranio-caudual (CC) view of each breast and were obtained from BreastScreen Australia in standardized Digital Imaging and Communications in Medicine (DICOM) format. These cases had been verified as normal by two independent radiologists and had a negative follow-up screening mammogram two years later.

Cases were displayed using high resolution images from a workstation (Sectra, Linköping, Sweden) connected to two 5-megapixels medical diagnostic monochrome liquid crystal display EIZO Radiforce G51 (EIZO, Japan) monitors. Both monitors were calibrated to the DICOM gray-scale standard display function. The study was carried out in a room measuring 15 m^2 with ambient lighting of approximately 20 lux measured using a calibrated photometer (model CL-200, Konic1a Minolta, Ramsey, USA) and walls were painted light grey with minimum specular reflection. The readers were allowed to use typical post processing tools such as zooming, panning and windowing with no time limit imposed.

Tasks. The readers in this study were informed that all nine cases were normal and then given two tasks. Firstly, they were asked to identify the key mammographic features of that case that allowed them to determine a "normal" or "no-recall" status. A list of descriptors was compiled from seven key publications on normal breast mammographic appearances [6–12] and readers were instructed to record their responses on paper (see Appendix A). At the same time, readers were asked to indicate if they believed each case would be suitable for a single reading strategy as opposed to the blinded double-reading strategy currently employed in BreastScreen Australia [4].

In the second task, the readers were again provided with the same nine normal cases but this time regions of interest (ROIs) that had attracted more than 10 FP markings from the Rawashdeh et al. [5] study were demarcated on the images (Fig. 1). The readers were asked to assess the ROIs and select the key mammographic features they believed would represent the incorrect FP decision (see Appendix A).

Data was analysed descriptively, feature by feature, to identify obvious trends. For each feature the total number of "Agree" and "Disagree" ratings by the 15 readers were summed across the nine cases, and expressed as percentages. To assess the association between the features of a case readers indicated it was normal, and the features they believed were responsible for its FP rating, Pearson correlations were calculated across cases (n = 9) between the number of "Agree" ratings for "normal" features and those for "FP responsible" features.

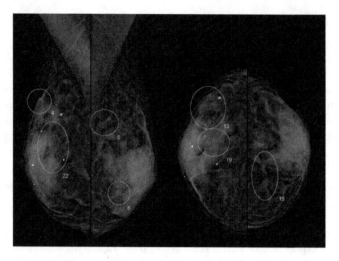

Fig. 1. Image marked with circle to highlight ROIs.

3   Results

The decisions of readers in the first task is summarised in Table 2. The top three features for agreeing a case was normal included symmetrical mammographic features, absence of micro-calcifications and regular ductal pattern. It was also highlighted that the majority of the responses indicated that the nine cases showed dense breasts.

Table 2. Percentage values indicate actual agree and disagree ratings for of the cases (Task 1).

Lexicon	Agree (%)	Disagree (%)
Regular ductal pattern	51.9	24.4
Uniform density	40.7	40.7
Non-dense breasts	26.7	65.9
Symmetrical mammographic features	55.6	33.3
Smooth, sharp, circumscribed margins	16.3	34.1
Spherical/round/radiolucent lesions	10.4	38.5
Absence of micro-calcifications	54.1	25.2
Overlapped density	37.0	40.0
"Benign" calcifications	17.8	37.0
Normal variant	18.5	34.1

Overall, the responses from the readers indicated that the nine cases were generally not suitable for a single reading strategy (Table 3). There was no difference in response to the single-double reading question when splitting the 15 readers into two groups using the number of mammograms they read a year.

Table 3. Suitability of cases for a single reading strategy.

All		Mammograms read per year			
		≤ 5000		>5000	
Yes (%)	No (%)	Yes (%)	No (%)	Yes (%)	No (%)
27.4	72.6	17.5	82.5	36.1	63.9

The percentage of "Agree" rating that a specific feature is responsible for attracting false positive decisions for the nine cases is summarised in Table 4. Overwhelmingly, asymmetrical density and perceived architecture distortion (AD) were the more prominent mammographic features attributed to another reader's FP decision. Conversely, features related to lesion suspicion, breast density, ductal pattern and calcifications were less likely to be chosen as the prime reason to account for the FP decisions previously made for the cases.

Table 4. Percentage values indicate actual agree and disagree ratings of the cases (Task 2).

Lexicon	Agree (%)	Disagree (%)
Irregular ductal pattern	14.1	20.0
Dense breasts	20.0	20.0
Asymmetrical density	74.8	7.4
Architecture distortion	40.0	21.5
Irregular or ill-defined margin	21.5	26.7
Ill-defined shape	18.5	50.0
Spiculated lesion	20.7	30.4
Radiopaque/hyperdense lesion	11.9	31.9
Cluster of micro-calcifications	8.9	34.8

There were few very strong associations between cases "Agree" ratings on features indicating they were normal (task 1), and features held responsible for their FP ratings (task 2). Not surprising, there was a strong association ($r = -0.75$, $p = 0.02$) between agreement ratings on cases representing breasts as "non-dense" in task 1 and "dense" in task 2. (The negative correlation here simply reflects the reversal in direction of wording between tasks 1 and 2 questionnaires. Please see the Appendix for the task instructions). The "Benign calcifications" agreement rating from task 1 was strongly associated with the ratings of "Cluster of micro-calcifications" from task 2 ($r = 0.71$, $p = 0.03$), indicating that the radiologists noted the calcifications in both tasks and the challenge they pose to readers. From task 1, agreement ratings that features of "Smooth, sharp and circumscribed margins" indicated the case was normal, showed a strong positive correlation with task 2 agreement ratings that "Speculated lesions" were responsible for the FP rating ($r = 0.75$, $p = 0.02$) (Table 5).

Table 5. Correlation between agreement scores of features indicating normal screening mammogram with features causing false positive (FP) decisions.

Normal mammographic features	Mammographic features that caused FP decisions								
	Irregular ductal pattern	Dense breasts	Asymmetrical density	Architecture distortion	Irregular or ill-defined margin	Ill-defined shape	Spiculated lesion	Radiopaque/hyperdense lesion	Cluster of micro-calcifications
Regular ductal pattern	0.36	−0.28	−0.03	0.18	−0.13	0.34	−0.06	0.10	−0.05
Uniform density	0.22	−0.48	−0.12	−0.29	−0.01	0.54	0.38	−0.07	0.02
Non-dense breasts	0.26	−0.75*	0.13	−0.16	−0.13	0.34	0.23	−0.11	−0.10
Symmetrical mammographic features	−0.08	−0.12	0.32	0.48	−0.52	−0.22	−0.60	−0.06	−0.32
Smooth, sharp, circumscribed margins	0.06	−0.39	−0.38	−0.41	0.47	0.20	0.75*	0.06	−0.15
Spherical/round/radio-lucent lesions	−0.12	−0.43	−0.22	−0.18	0.19	0.20	0.49	0.13	−0.05
Absence of micro-calcifications	0.10	−0.53	0.29	−0.43	−0.04	0.04	0.14	0.03	−0.65
Overlapped density	−0.43	0.48	0.21	−0.34	0.12	−0.47	−0.11	0.19	−0.46
"Benign" calcifications	0.13	0.48	−0.17	0.48	−0.01	0.10	−0.27	0.12	0.71*
Normal variant	0.26	0.28	−0.41	0.52	−0.06	0.07	−0.13	−0.37	0.28

* p < 0.05

4   Discussion and Conclusion

Asymmetrical density and AD were the top two reasons identified in a retrospective analysis of FP decisions by readers in this study. Our findings concur with other recent studies noting that symmetry of breast tissue is often taken as a bench mark for normal cases and, conversely, asymmetrical density usually calls for suspicion [8, 10, 12]. Moreover, previous work by our group has reported that symmetrical mammographic features was an important feature readers considered before coming to a conclusion that a case is normal [13].

The finding that AD could account for most of the FP decisions made concurred with other studies. In a study by Suleiman et al. [14], it was found that even with the availability of digital mammography, AD remains as a challenging feature to read and a feature of breast cancer that is most likely to be missed. Studies looking at AD have reported that breast screen readers often overlooked the mammographic features of AD and our study may be illustrating an awareness of this common error [14, 15].

It is interesting to note that the 15 readers initially had the impression that the nine cases were normal because of symmetrical mammographic features, an absence of micro-calcifications and regular ductal pattern. Additionally, cases with high breast density were considered difficult to mark as normal and not suitable for single reading strategy. However, in the second task when the ROIs were given to the readers, asymmetrical density was the leading reason for those cases to have such high number of FP decisions.

The lack of prior mammograms and inclusion of only nine normal cases could potentially skew the results with limited generalisability. The small number of cases might have also affected the statistical significance of the results and meant that only very strong correlations between features of cases that marked them as normal, and features responsible for their FP, would be significant. The two features most responsible for FP ratings also had correlations with "normal" features in this sample in the moderate-to-large range. If this study was reproduced in a larger sample, correlations of similar value may be significant, and may indicate areas for further exploration.

In conclusion, the findings from this study demonstrated that asymmetrical density and AD are two leading reasons to explain FP decisions from past readers. These findings may help educational and technological strategies aimed at reducing unnecessary recalls in screening mammography.

Acknowledgements. This study was supported by the National Breast Cancer Foundation (Australia), the Breastscreen Reader Assessment Strategy (BREAST), RANZCR, The University of Sydney and National Healthcare Group Diagnostic (Singapore).

A Appendix

Example of questionnaire for first task

Case Number 1: TSAB

1. My reason(s) for considering this case normal:

• Regular ductal patterns	Agree	Disagree	Not sure
• Uniform density	Agree	Disagree	Not sure
• Non-dense breasts	Agree	Disagree	Not sure
• Symmetrical mammographic features	Agree	Disagree	Not sure
• Smooth, sharp and/or circumscribed margins	Agree	Disagree	Not sure
• Spherical/round/radiolucent lesions	Agree	Disagree	Not sure
• Absence of micro-calcifications	Agree	Disagree	Not sure
• Overlapped density	Agree	Disagree	Not sure
• "Benign" calcifications	Agree	Disagree	Not sure
• Normal variant (accessory tissue/global asymmetry/scars)	Agree	Disagree	Not sure
• Others:			

2. In your opinion, would you consider this case to be suitable for reading by a single reader (as opposed to requiring a double reader strategy)?
   Yes   No

Example of questionnaire for second task
Please tell us the reason(s) why the circled areas on these NORMAL cases attracted false positives.

Case Number 1: TSAB

• Irregular ductal patterns	Agree	Disagree	Not sure
• Dense breasts	Agree	Disagree	Not sure
• Asymmetrical density	Agree	Disagree	Not sure
• Architecture distortion	Agree	Disagree	Not sure
• Irregular or ill-defined margin	Agree	Disagree	Not sure
• Ill-defined shape	Agree	Disagree	Not sure
• Spiculated lesion	Agree	Disagree	Not sure
• Radiopaque/hyperdense lesion	Agree	Disagree	Not sure
• Cluster of micro-calcifications	Agree	Disagree	Not sure
• Irregular ductal patterns	Agree	Disagree	Not sure
• Others:			

References

1. Australian Institute of Health and Welfare: BreastScreen Australia monitoring report 2011–2012 (2014). http://www.aihw.gov.au/WorkArea/DownloadAsset.aspx?id=60129548882. Accessed 15 May 2015
2. Australian Institute of Health and Welfare: Australian Cancer Incidence and Mortality (ACIM) books, Breast cancer (2015). http://www.aihw.gov.au/acim-books/. Accessed 10 Apr 2015
3. National Cancer Institute: Breast Cancer Screening (PDQ®) - Breast Cancer Screening Concepts (2015). http://www.cancer.gov/cancertopics/pdq/screening/breast/healthprofessional/Page4#_49. Accessed 11 Apr 2015
4. Lee, W.B., Peters, G.: Mammographic screening for breast cancer: a review. J. Med. Radiat. Sci. **60**(1), 35–39 (2013). doi:10.1002/jmrs.6
5. Rawashdeh, M.A., Bourne, R.M., Ryan, E.A., Lee, W.B., Pietrzyk, M.W., Reed, W.M., Borecky, N., Brennan, P.C.: Quantitative measures confirm the inverse relationship between lesion spiculation and detection of breast masses. Acad. Radiol. **20**(5), 576–580 (2013). doi:10.1016/j.acra.2012.12.010
6. American College of Radiology: ACR BI-RADS® Atlas Fifth Edition, Quick reference (2013). http://www.acr.org/∼/media/ACR/Documents/PDF/QualitySafety/Resources/BIRADS/Posters/BIRADS%20Reference%20Card_web_F.pdf. Accessed 2 Apr 2015
7. D'Orsi, C.J., Kopans, D.B.: Mammographic feature analysis. Semin. Roentgenol. **28**(3), 204–230 (1993). doi:10.1016/S0037-198X(05)80080-X
8. De Paredes, E.S.: Atlas of Mammography, 3rd edn. Wolters Kluwer Health/Lippincott Williams & Wilkins, Philadelphia (2007)
9. Guinebretière, J.M., Menet, E., Tardivon, A., Cherel, P., Vanel, D.: Normal and pathological breast, the histological basis. Eur. J. Radiol. **54**(1), 6–14 (2005). doi:10.1016/j.ejrad.2004.11.020
10. Kopans, D.B.: Breast Imaging, 3rd edn. Lippincott Williams & Wilkins, Baltimore (2006)
11. Shetty, M.: Breast Cancer Screening and Diagnosis, pp. 119–130. Springer, New York (2014)
12. Stines, J., Tristant, H.: The normal breast and its variations in mammography. Eur. J. Radiol. **54**(1), 26–36 (2005). doi:10.1016/j.ejrad.2004.11.017
13. Ang Z.Z.Y., Rawashdeh, M.A., Heard, R., Brennan, P.C., Lee, W.B., Lewis, S.J.: The classification of normal screening mammograms. In: SPIE Medical Imaging: Image Perception, Observer Performance, and Technology Assessment, vol. 9787, 97870I (2016). doi:10.1117/12.2216626
14. Suleiman, W.I., McEntee, M.F., Lewis, S.J., Rawashdeh, M.A., Georgian-Smith, D., Heard, R., Brennan, P.C.: In the digital era, architectural distortion remains a challenging radiological task. Clin. Radiol. **71**(1), e35 (2016)
15. Ayres, F.J., Rangayyan, R.M.: Characterization of architectural distortion in mammograms. IEEE Eng. Med. Biol. Mag. **24**(1), 59–67 (2005). doi:10.1109/MEMB.2005.1384102

Estimation of Perceived Background Tissue Complexity in Mammograms

Ali R.N. Avanaki[1(✉)], Kathryn S. Espig[1], Albert Xthona[1], and Tom R.L. Kimpe[2]

[1] Barco Healthcare, Beaverton, OR, USA
ali.avanaki@barco.com
[2] Barco N.V., Healthcare Division, Kortrijk, Belgium

Abstract. Two methods for estimation of location-dependent background tissue complexity (BTC) are proposed. The methods operate by calculating the lowest possible amplitude for which a small superimposed lesion remains visible at a given location in a mammogram: the higher BTC, the larger lesion insertion threshold amplitude. The visibility analysis is based on comparing a region of interest pre- and post-lesion using structural similarity metric (SSIM) in one method. The other proposed estimator is based on just noticeable difference (JND) notion Barten used in modeling contrast sensitivity function (we theorize that lesion detection is equivalent to detection of one cycle of a sinusoid). The proposed BTC estimators are evaluated by comparing them against the lesion insertion amplitude required for visibility set by a human observer. Our results indicate that both estimators correlate with each other (Spearman rank correlation coefficient r_s of 0.76) and outperform constant insertion amplitude in terms of correlation with perceived tissue complexity. The SSIM-based estimator has a higher correlation with the human observer over 24 locales that the estimators disagreed most or both predicted large BTC (r_s of 0.73, vs. 0.34 for JND-based estimator). The proposed estimators may be used to construct a BTC-aware model observer with applications such as optimization of contrast-enhanced medical imaging systems, and creation of an image dataset to match the characteristics of a given population.

1 Description of Purpose

Validation of a medical imaging system is challenging due to the large number of system parameters that must be considered. Conventional methods involving clinical trials are limited by cost and duration, and in the instance of systems using ionizing radiation, the requirement for the repeated irradiation of volunteers. We are proponents of an alternative, in the form of virtual clinical trials based on models of human anatomy, image acquisition, display and processing, and image analysis and interpretation. We have developed anthropomorphic model observers that better predict typical human observers than commonly used model observers which are designed after ideal observers with some concessions for computational tractability.

Previously, we reported [1, 2] that by embedding properties of human visual system (HVS) as pre-processing steps to a commonly used model observer (multi-slice channelized Hotelling observer [3]– msCHO), the model observer can better track the

© Springer International Publishing Switzerland 2016
A. Tingberg et al. (Eds.): IWDM 2016, LNCS 9699, pp. 316–323, 2016.
DOI: 10.1007/978-3-319-41546-8_40

performance of a human observer with changes in viewing distance, browsing speed, and display contrast when reading digital breast tomosynthesis (DBT) images.

In this paper, we explore the estimation of the background tissue complexity (a.k.a. anatomical clutter or noise; BTC hereafter) in mammograms, as it pertains to an anthropomorphic model observer. An automatic BTC estimator is necessary in tracking the performance of a human observer in reading images at various BTC levels. This is because the human observer's performance, unlike that of the existing model observers, varies considerably with BTC in a signal and location known exactly (SKE/LKE) paradigm [4]. The methods developed for BTC estimation may have applications in automatic estimation of breast density [8]. Moreover, a model observer's capability of tracking the human observer performance with BTC is especially important when using VCT for design and/or optimization of imaging modalities with significant variation in background complexity. A specific example is contrast enhanced (CE) breast imaging systems. In such systems, the uptake of the lesion relative to that of the normal fibroglandular tissue and the dose of injected contrast agent affect the perceived BTC and thus lesion visibility [5–7].

A visual example is provided in Fig. 1: the same round object (one cycle of a 2D radial cosine pattern) is added to 29×29 non-overlapping tiles of a mammogram. Care was taken to perform the addition in the luminance domain and to avoid clipping. It is clear that the visibility of the object is a function of its location in the background. We attribute lower visibility to higher perceived BTC, which we aim to estimate in this paper. If the insertion amplitudes were set using an ideal BTC estimator, the visibility of all lesions in Fig. 1 would be the same.

Fig. 1. Copies of the same "lesion" are added to non-overlapping tiles of a mammogram. Some are harder to see than others.

1.1 Prior Work

There has been prior research on this topic. Representative examples of recent work are briefly discussed below.

We introduced a supervised method of background complexity estimation for DBT stacks [9]. The differences between consecutive slices, measured in peak signal-to-noise ratio (PSNR), were used as the input to the estimator. A Hotelling observer trained with perceived BTC values (one per DBT stack) for a subset of input was used as the estimator. The problems with this approach are as follows. (i) Supervised training of the estimator may not be practical or desirable for most VCT scenarios. (ii) This method yields only one estimate of BTC per DBT stack. Hence, it is unusable for mammograms, as it cannot predict lesion visibility in different locations.

Mainprize *et al.* proposed a local signal to noise ratio, d_{local}, as a metric of the apparent density in mammograms [8], hence a metric for potential masking of a lesion. d_{local} is calculated for non-overlapping regions of interest (ROIs) of the input mammogram. Note that this method is unsupervised and provides local complexity information but the estimator from this method performed worse than our supervised estimator mentioned in the last paragraph.

2   Methods

2.1   Just Noticeable Difference (JND) Analysis

Barten modeled the visibility of a spatial sinusoidal luminance pattern as follows [10]:

$$\frac{\Delta L}{\bar{L}} > m_t \tag{1}$$

where ΔL is the sinusoid amplitude of variation required for visibility with a 50 % probability or more, $\bar{L}$ is the average luminance, and m_t is a threshold predicted by Barten's formulas and is mainly a function of spatial frequency of the pattern.

Now, consider an object that spans one cycle of a 2D radial cosine luminance pattern (Fig. 2). We theorize that visibility of this object may be also predicted by Barten's model, since it also involves distinguishing a luminance peak from a luminance valley. Thus, we have,

$$\frac{2(L_p - \bar{L})}{\bar{L}} > m_t \tag{2}$$

where ΔL in (1) is substituted by twice the difference of L_p, object's peak luminance, with the average luminance $\bar{L}$. Solving (2) for L_p yields

$$L_p > \left(1 + 0.5 m_t\right)\bar{L} \tag{3}$$

Without loss of generality, we can normalize the object to have a unit luminance. When such lesion is superimposed to the background with an insertion amplitude L_a, we have $L_p = L_a + L_0$, in which L_0 is the luminance of (before-lesion) background at the point that lesion peaks. We also have to consider that lesion insertion increases $\bar{L}$:

$$\Delta \bar{L} = \frac{A_o}{2A_{ROI}} L_a \tag{4}$$

in which A_o and A_{ROI} are the object and ROI (on which $\bar{L}$ was calculated) areas in pixels. By updating L_p and $\bar{L}$ in (3), we have:

$$L_a > \frac{\left(1 + 0.5m_t\right)\bar{L} - L_0}{1 - \left(1 + 0.5m_t\right)\dfrac{A_o}{2A_{ROI}}} \tag{5}$$

which gives the threshold insertion amplitude required for the lesion to be visible with a 50 % probability or better. $\bar{L}$ and L_0 may be readily calculated from the background at any given location. m_t may be calculated from Barten's model, or hand tuned to the desired degree of visibility.

2.2 Structural Similarity (SSIM) Analysis

Wang *et al.* introduced structural similarity index (SSIM) as metric for perceptual similarity of visual signals [11]:

$$SSIM(x, y) = \frac{(2\mu_x\mu_y + C_1)(2\sigma_{xy} + C_2)}{(\mu_x^2 + \mu_y^2 + C_1)(\sigma_x^2 + \sigma_y^2 + C_2)} \tag{6}$$

where x and y are input signals (e.g., image ROIs), μ and σ indicate average and standard deviation, σ_{xy} is the signals covariance, and C_1 and C_2 are small positive constants keeping the denominator non-zero.

To estimate BTC at a specific location, consider superimposing the given lesion at that location. Then, we adjust the insertion amplitude, L_a, for the lesion to become visible: That is when SSIM between (before-lesion) background and after-lesion ROIs reaches some set threshold.

2.3 BTC Measurement by a Human Observer

To estimate BTC at a specific location p, a human observer may adjust the insertion amplitude of the given lesion until it becomes visible. To measure the threshold insertion amplitude, we use QUEST [12], an adaptive threshold seeking procedure. As compared to adjusting the amplitude manually, QUEST is more convenient for the user and yields a more accurate threshold as well as its confidence interval. We use a Matlab

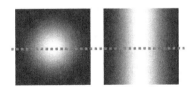

Fig. 2. One cycle of a radial cosine (left) vs. one cycle of a spatial sinusoidal luminance (right), with the same spatial frequency, used in derivation of contrast sensitivity function. The luminance profile along the dotted line is the same in both patterns.

implementation of QUEST available from http://psychtoolbox.org with the default value of parameters and 26 trials per threshold measurement. The number of trials per measurement is selected to strike a balance between experiment runtime and threshold measurement accuracy.

The experiments are conducted on a Barco Uniti display (MDMC-12133) to ensure low noise and consistent presentation, provided by RapidFrame™, and Color Per-Pixel-Uniformity™. In each trial, two panels are displayed; on one panel a square mammogram region centered at p is shown, and on the other panel the same region with lesion superimposed to the center at the insertion amplitude being tested is shown (Fig. 3). When p is too close to mammogram margin, the rest of the square region is filled with a mirror of mammogram along the nearest edge, using Matlab's padarray symmetric option, to preserve the observed texture continuity (Fig. 3). The two panels are separated by one fifth of a panel width. The panels together with margins extend to about fifteen visual degrees and are uniformly filled with average luminance of the region being displayed where there is no visual information for optimal eye adaptation. Lesion apparent size is about one fourth a degree which is the target object size for optimal visibility (spatial CSF remains flat and at its peak at about 0.1 to 1 degrees in typical viewing conditions [10]).

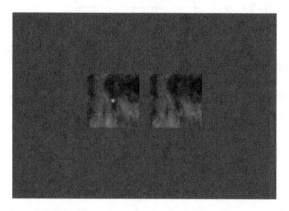

Fig. 3. An example screen for one trial of human measurement of BTC. Apparent size is about 15°. Observer's task is to pick the panel that has a lesion at the center (the right panel in this case).

In the first trial of each experiment the lesion is shown with maximum possible amplitude to familiarize observer with the shape, size and location (i.e., center of panel) of lesion. When adding lesion, care was taken to avoid clipping (all pixel values remain between 0 and 1), and that scaling (to modulate insertion amplitude) and addition are performed in luminance domain (not in pixel value). The task assigned to the human observer is to pick the panel with the lesion. Input choices are left, right or 'don't know.' The order of the panels (left or right) is chosen randomly by the experiment program, which compares observer's input to the actual location of lesion panel and based on this information (i.e., answered correct or incorrect) generates the next amplitude to be tested. A 'don't know' input is assumed to be an incorrect response.

2.4   Evaluation

We use the JND- and SSIM-based BTC estimation methods of Sects. 2.1 and 2.2 to derive two insertion amplitudes for each of the 29×29 non-overlapping tiles of the mammogram shown in Fig. 1. For benchmarking the performance of the proposed estimators, we use a human observer to measure BTC (Sect. 2.3). Since human measurement of BTC is time consuming, we select a few tiles as follows: the tiles whose JND- and SSIM-based BTC estimates (BTC_{JND} and BTC_{SSIM} hereafter) differ most (8 tiles with highest $BTC_{SSIM} - BTC_{JND}$, and 8 with highest $BTC_{JND} - BTC_{SSIM}$), as well as the tiles with large BTC_{SSIM} *and* BTC_{JND} (8 with highest $BTC_{JND} + BTC_{SSIM}$). To ensure BTC_{SSIM} and BTC_{JND} are comparable, we perform histogram equalization prior to $BTC_{SSIM} \pm BTC_{JND}$ calculations above. The selection of tiles to be measured by human is based on the premise that there is little disagreement between the estimation methods in low BTC areas (e.g., the three dark corners in Fig. 1). To evaluate the performance of the proposed BTC estimation methods, we calculate the rank correlation of human measured BTC values for the select tiles with the corresponding BTC values estimated by the proposed methods.

3   Results

We used JND- and SSIM-based methods of Sects. 2.1 and 2.2 to estimate BTC and modulate insertion amplitude accordingly so that we have a grid (lesions in the centers of 29×29 non-overlapping tiles) of evenly visible lesions in the same mammogram that was used in Fig. 1. The results are shown in Fig. 4. We also used the method of Sect. 2.4 to quantitatively evaluate the proposed estimators, and reached the following results. The rank correlation coefficients between human-measured BTC and BTC_{SSIM} and BTC_{JND} are 0.73 (p-value < 1e-4, for statistically significant difference from zero [13]) and 0.34 (p-value = 0.1) respectively calculated over 24 tiles selected per Sect. 2.4 procedure. The rank correlation coefficient between the BTC_{SSIM} and BTC_{JND} over 1012 tiles (i.e., the whole grid) is 0.76 (p-value < 1e-4).

4   Discussion

When comparing Fig. 4 to Fig. 1, it may be observed that both JND and SSIM analysis provide reasonably good BTC estimates. As expected, both methods assign lower insertion amplitude in the three darker corners (top-right, top-left and bottom-right). Based on the results shown in Fig. 4, neither of the methods has a clear advantage over the other: the arrows point to the prominent lesions with counterparts that are barely visible in the opposite panel. This observation is further confirmed by the considerable correlation between the estimators over the whole grid (0.76).

To break the tie, we compared the proposed estimators against a human observer over a set of contentious tiles selected according to Sect. 2.4 procedure. For such tiles, the human observer has significant correlation with the SSIM-based estimator (0.73, cf. 0.34 with JND-based method).

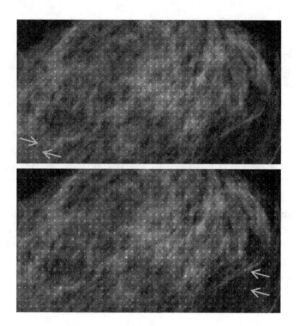

Fig. 4. Copies of the same lesion are added to non-overlapping tiles of a mammogram, with insertion amplitudes calculated using JND analysis (top; Sect. 2.1) or SSIM analysis (bottom; Sect. 2.2). Arrows point to locations where the underlying method performed better.

5   Conclusion

JND- and SSIM-based proposed BTC estimation methods correlate with each other and with the notion of perceptual background complexity introduced herein. The SSIM-based estimator has a higher correlation with the human observer where the proposed estimators disagreed or both predicted large BTC. Therefore, the proposed methods may be used to construct a BTC-aware model observer, with applications such as optimization of contrast-enhanced medical imaging systems, and creation of a diversified image dataset matching a desired population.

When measuring BTC by human both speed and precision are desirable, allowing for better understanding of human notion of background complexity and therefore designing better computational BTC estimators. However, we suspect simultaneous improvement in precision and speed of measurement may not be possible for the notion of BTC introduced herein, though each can be improved at the expense of the other (e.g., increasing the number of trials in a QUEST run increases precision *and* experiment runtime).

Acknowledgement.   Ali Avanaki would like to thank Eddie Knippel for his comments.

References

1. Avanaki, A.N., Espig, K.S., Maidment, A.D.A., Marchessoux, C., Bakic, P.R., Kimpe, T.R.L.: Development and evaluation of a 3D model observer with nonlinear spatiotemporal contrast sensitivity. In: Proceedings of SPIE Medical Imaging (2014)
2. Avanaki, A.N., Espig, K.S., Marchessoux, C., Krupinski, E.A., Bakic, P.R., Kimpe, T.R.L., Maidment, A.D.A.: Integration of spatio-temporal contrast sensitivity with a multi-slice channelized Hotelling observer. In: Proceedings of SPIE Medical Imaging (2013)
3. Platiša, L., Goossens, B., Vansteenkiste, E., Park, S., Gallas, B., Badano, A., Philips, W.: Channelized hotelling observers for the assessment of volumetric imaging data sets. J. Opt. Soc. Am. A: **28**, 1145–1163 (2011)
4. Avanaki, A.R.N., Espig, K.S., Xthona, A., Kimpe, T.R.L., Bakic, P.R., Maidment, A.D.A.: It is hard to see a needle in a haystack: modeling contrast masking effect in a numerical observer. In: Fujita, Hiroshi, Hara, Takeshi, Muramatsu, Chisako (eds.) IWDM 2014. LNCS, vol. 8539, pp. 723–730. Springer, Heidelberg (2014)
5. Chen, S.C., Carton, A.K., Albert, M., Conant, E.F., Schnall, M.D., Maidment, A.D.: Initial clinical experience with contrast-enhanced digital breast tomosynthesis. Acad. Radiol. **14**(2), 229–238 (2007)
6. Hill, M.L., Mainprize, J.G., Yaffe, M.J.: An observer model for lesion detectability in contrast-enhanced digital mammography. In: Martí, J., Oliver, A., Freixenet, J., Martí, R. (eds.) IWDM 2010. LNCS, vol. 6136, pp. 720–727. Springer, Heidelberg (2010)
7. Hill, M. L., Mainprize, J. G., Jong, R. A., Yaffe, M. J.: Design and validation of a mathematical breast phantom for contrast-enhanced digital mammography. In: SPIE Medical Imaging, pp. 79615E-79615E. International Society for Optics and Photonics (2011)
8. Mainprize, J.G., Wang, X., Ge, M., Yaffe, M.J.: Towards a quantitative measure of radiographic masking by dense tissue in mammography. In: Fujita, H., Hara, T., Muramatsu, C. (eds.) IWDM 2014. LNCS, vol. 8539, pp. 181–186. Springer, Heidelberg (2014)
9. Avanaki, A. R., Espig, K. S., Kimpe, T. R., Maidment, A. D.: On anthropomorphic decision making in a model observer. In: SPIE Medical Imaging, pp. 941610–941610. International Society for Optics and Photonics (2015)
10. Barten, P.G.: Contrast sensitivity of the human eye and its effects on image quality, vol. 72. SPIE press, Bellingham (1999)
11. Wang, Z., Bovik, A.C., Sheikh, H.R., Simoncelli, E.P.: Image quality assessment: from error visibility to structural similarity. IEEE Trans. Image Process. **13**(4), 600–612 (2004)
12. Watson, A.B., Pelli, D.G.: QUEST: a Bayesian adaptive psychometric method. Percept. Psychophys. **33**(2), 113–120 (1983)
13. http://vassarstats.net/rsig.html. Accessed Mar 2016

Dose and Classification

Patient Dose Survey of Mammography Systems in the UK in 2013–2015

Jennifer Oduko[1(✉)] and Kenneth Young[1,2]

[1] National Coordinating Centre for the Physics of Mammography,
Guildford, UK
{jenny.oduko,ken.young}@nhs.net
[2] Department of Physics, University of Surrey, Guildford, UK

Abstract. A nation-wide survey of patient dose data was carried out, using data recorded in 2013–2015. Data from 32,000 women were collected. The average dose for oblique views, for DR systems, was 1.65 mGy for all women, and 1.35 mGy for 50–60 mm breasts. There was a wide range of doses for different systems, with the highest more than twice the dose of the lowest (2.03 mGy and 0.91 mGy respectively for the Hologic Dimensions and Philips MicroDose L30 systems, averaged over all breasts). Image quality, as indicated by the threshold gold thickness for 0.25 mm details, was better (0.21 µm) for the Hologic systems; for all the others it was practically the same (0.28 µm), although their doses to the average breast varied over a wide range.

Keywords: Mammography · Patient dose · DR systems

1 Introduction

The National Health Service Breast Screening Programme in the United Kingdom invites all women aged 50 to 70 years to attend for screening every three years. Older women are screened on request and some younger and older women (ages 47–49 and 71–73) are also invited as part of an age extension trial. As part of the quality system, patient dose data is collected at least once every three years, for each X-ray set, for fifty or more women. The purpose is to ensure that doses are within the limits, and to facilitate comparison of different systems. The process of changing from film-screen to direct digital radiology (DR) systems in the UK was completed in 2015, and 91 % of the systems for which data is presented here are DR systems.

2 Method

All the physics services working with the breast screening programme sent patient dose data, from surveys carried out in 2013–15, to a central service. These were combined into a single database for analysis. In some cases the exposure parameters for individual patients were recorded by the radiographers who performed the mammography examinations. Alternatively, data was extracted from the DICOM headers of digital images using appropriate software. Data for women with implants, and from DR systems with less than ten dose surveys, were excluded from the analysis.

© Springer International Publishing Switzerland 2016
A. Tingberg et al. (Eds.): IWDM 2016, LNCS 9699, pp. 327–334, 2016.
DOI: 10.1007/978-3-319-41546-8_41

The physics services provided results of measurements from their own regular equipment surveys. These included the mean glandular dose (MGD) to the standard breast for each system, and the X-ray output and half-value layer at each kV, target, filter combination occurring in the patient dose data. The standard breast is a 45 mm thick block of polymethyl methacrylate (PMMA), and is exposed under automatic exposure control (AEC). All physics services used the same database to record the data; this also calculates the MGD for real breasts, using the Dance et al. method [1].

Physics services also provided values of threshold gold thickness for each model of X-ray set, in a separate national survey of the performance of digital mammography systems. Eight or sixteen images of the CDMAM 3.4 contrast detail test object were acquired, with 20 mm thick PMMA above and below the test object. The images were analysed using CDCOM [2] and CDMAM analysis [3] software to produce contrast-detail curves. Further details of all the measurement techniques are described in the UK guidance for testing DR systems [4].

3   Results

3.1   Numbers of Systems and MGD to the Standard Breast

Table 1 shows the numbers of DR and film-screen systems for which data was recorded and the average MGD to the standard breast for each system. Errors shown are 2 SEM (standard error of the mean).

Table 1. Numbers of systems and average MGD to the standard breast.

Manufacturer and model	Number of systems	Average MGD to standard breast (mGy)
GE Essential	92	1.27 ± 0.01
GE DS	23	1.19 ± 0.03
Siemens Inspiration	82	1.06 ± 0.01
Philips MicroDose L30	52	0.72 ± 0.01
Hologic Selenia W	73	1.41 ± 0.02
Hologic Dimensions	117	1.43 ± 0.01
Total/mean of all DR	439	1.22 ± 0.01
Film-screen (all)	43	1.51 ± 0.07

3.2   Average MGD for Oblique Views, for All Breasts

Figure 1 shows the distribution of average MGD for all DR and all film-screen systems.

Data were recorded for approximately 32,000 women. The MGD for oblique views, averaged over all breasts, ranged from 0.91 to 2.03 mGy for the DR systems, and the average thickness was 60 mm. Results are shown in Table 2, with the average for film-screen systems shown for comparison. Errors shown are 2 SEM (but where 2 SEM for average MGD is less than 0.01 it is not shown).

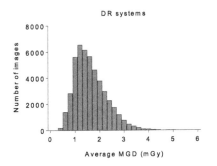
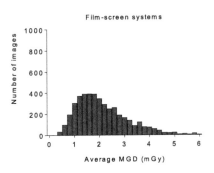

Fig. 1. Distribution of average MGD for all oblique views, for DR and film-screen systems.

Table 2. Average MGD and compressed breast thickness for oblique views of all breasts.

Manufacturer and model	Average MGD to all breasts, oblique views (mGy)	Number of images	Average compressed breast thickness (mm)
GE Essential	1.54	8180	63.8 ± 0.3
GE DS	1.46	1375	54.9 ± 0.5
Siemens Inspiration	1.37	6853	59.3 ± 0.4
Philips MicroDose L30	0.91	5081	63.0 ± 0.4
Hologic Selenia W	1.64	20891	56.6 ± 0.2
Hologic Dimensions	2.03	19179	62.3 ± 0.2
Mean for DR systems	1.65	61559	60.0 ± 0.1
Film-screen (all)	2.18 ± 0.03	4715	58.0 ± 0.4

3.3 Average MGD for Oblique Views, for 50–60 mm Thick Breasts

Calculating the average MGD for oblique views, for compressed breast thickness 50–60 mm, is generally used for comparison between different imaging systems. Average MGDs for this range of thickness are shown in Table 3. Errors shown are 2 SEM (but where 2 SEM for average MGD is less than 0.01 it is not shown).

Figure 2 shows, for all DR and film-screen systems, the average MGD for 50–60 mm breasts plotted against MGD to the standard breast. The national diagnostic reference level (NDRL) of 3.5 mGy for the average MGD for 50–60 mm breasts, and the remedial value of 2.5 mGy for dose to the standard breast are also shown.

Figure 3 shows similar data for two individual DR systems. The wide spread of points shown on the left-hand graph is typical of all the other DR systems except the MicroDose L30, shown on the right.

Table 3. Average MGD and compressed breast thickness for oblique views of 50–60 mm thick breasts. (The ratio shown is to the MGD to standard breast values from Table 1.)

Manufacturer and model	Number of images	Average MGD to 50–60 mm breasts, oblique views (mGy)	Ratio of avg. MGD (50–60 mm) to MGD to std. breast	Average compressed breast thickness (mm)
GE Essential	1935	1.25	0.98	55.4 ± 0.1
GE DS	422	1.37	1.15	55.2 ± 0.2
Siemens Inspiration	1749	1.22	1.15	55.3 ± 0.1
Philips M-Dose L30	1277	0.72	1.00	55.6 ± 0.2
Hologic Selenia W	6418	1.59	1.13	55.3 ± 0.1
Hologic Dimensions	4741	1.68	1.17	55.4 ± 0.1
Mean of DR systems	16542	1.46		55.4 ± 0.05
Film-screen (all)	1463	1.95		55.4 ± 0.2

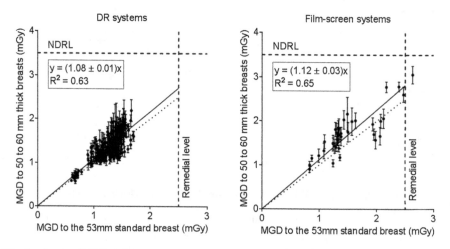

Fig. 2. Average MGD for oblique views of 50–60 mm thick breasts plotted against MGD to the standard breast for all DR and all film-screen systems. Dotted line shows equality. Error bars are 2 SEM.

3.4   Variation of MGD (for Oblique Views) with Thickness

Figure 4 shows, for all DR and all film-screen systems, the average MGD plotted against breast thickness. The dose limit as a function of thickness is also shown. Figure 5 shows similar data for all DR systems. Some error bars are too small to be seen.

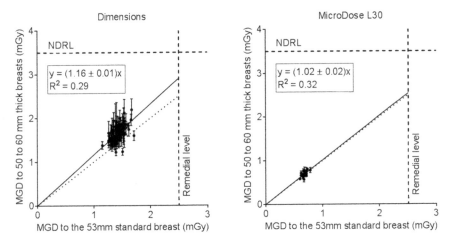

Fig. 3. Average MGD for oblique views of 50–60 mm thick breasts plotted against MGD to the standard breast for two DR systems. Error bars are 2 SEM.

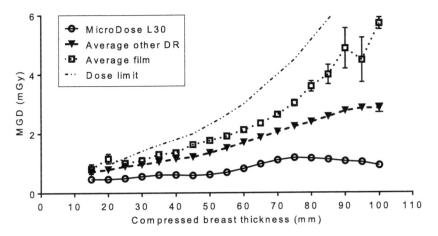

Fig. 4. Average MGD for oblique views plotted against thickness for all DR and all film-screen systems, and for the MicroDose L30. Error bars are 2 SEM.

3.5   Threshold Gold Thickness

Table 4 shows the average MGD for 50–60 mm breasts (from Table 2), with the average threshold gold thickness for 0.25 mm details as an indication of image quality.

4   Discussion

For DR systems, the average MGD for oblique views of all breasts was 1.65 ± 0.01 mGy. This is a 24 % dose saving over the average value for film-screen images 2.18 ± 0.02 mGy). For 50–60 mm thick breasts, the average MGD values

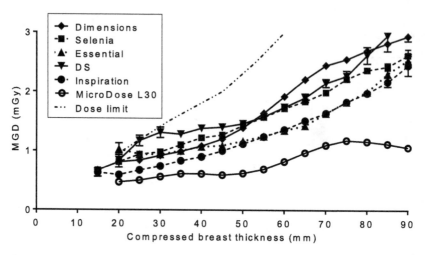

Fig. 5. Average MGD for oblique views plotted against thickness for six different DR systems. Error bars are 2 SEM.

Table 4. MGD to 50–60 mm breasts and average threshold gold thickness.

Manufacturer and model	Average MGD, oblique views, for 50–60 mm breasts (mGy)	Threshold gold thickness (μm) for 0.25 mm details
GE Essential	1.25	0.29 ± 0.01
GE DS	1.37	0.29 ± 0.01
Siemens Inspiration	1.22	0.27 ± 0.01
Philips MicroDose L30	0.72	0.28 ± 0.01
Hologic Selenia W	1.59	0.21 ± 0.01
Hologic Dimensions	1.95	0.20 ± 0.01

were up to 20 % lower (Tables 2 and 3). The average MGD for DR systems (oblique views of all breasts) in this survey was higher than values measured in the last two UK dose surveys, 1.46 ± 0.02 mGy in 2007–9 [5] and 1.58 ± 0.04 mGy in 2010–12 [6]. The film-screen images had a broader distribution than the DR images, with a longer tail extending to higher dose, as shown in Fig. 1. The current dose survey is based on a much larger sample of DR images, approximately 64,000, compared with 4,000 in 2007–9 and 25,000 in 2010–12.

The standard breast (45 mm thickness of PMMA) is intended to give a measure of the average MGD to oblique views of 50–60 mm thick breasts. For the average over many images acquired on many systems, the ratio of these quantities ranges from 0.98 to 1.17, as shown in Table 3. However, for individual systems there is a much wider variation, as shown by the scatter of points around the lines of equality in Figs. 2 and 3. The scatter of points in the Dimensions graph in Fig. 3 is typical of all the systems in this survey, except the MicroDose L30 for which there is little spread. Several possible factors may contribute to this variation. Breast density might contribute to the variation (if it differs for different samples of women), but it is not normally measured in the UK so this cannot be quantified. Radiographers may follow different local policies on what compression force to apply, as well as using a flexible paddle in many cases. Physics tests are normally performed with a fixed paddle, and often with a fixed compression force; the PMMA does not behave like a breast under compression. In addition, many manufacturers' systems now offer "smart AECs", which detect denser areas in the breast and set the exposure parameters accordingly. In view of these complications, it is unlikely that a uniform PMMA phantom, the standard breast, could accurately good model the average 50–60 mm breast for all systems. Patient dose surveys are still needed, and are carried out in the UK for newly installed systems, after major changes (e.g. to the AEC) and every three years if nothing has changed.

MGD increased with thickness, as shown in Figs. 4 and 5. All the DR systems, except one, are averaged in Fig. 4 for clarity. Most DR systems operate at about half of the dose limit, with the MGD higher for film-screen systems. The MGD for the Philips MicroDose L30 was much lower at all thicknesses, and showed an unusual trend of decreasing with thickness above about 75 mm breast thickness. A similar trend was observed in measurements with different thicknesses of PMMA in a technical report on this system [7]. There was little difference in the variation of MGD with thickness for the other DR systems, as shown in Fig. 5.

Perhaps surprisingly, there was little correlation of average MGD with image quality, as shown in Table 4. Threshold gold thickness for 0.25 mm details was lower (about 0.21 µm) for the two Hologic systems, but almost the same (about 0.28 µm) for all the others, despite a wide range of MGD. The lower value indicates better image quality. Measurements on single imaging systems have consistently shown that lowering the dose (with the same kV, target and filter) causes an increase in threshold gold thickness, but such a trend is not apparent over different systems.

Acknowledgments. The data collection was conducted under the auspices of the UK National Breast Screening Quality Assurance Coordinating Group for Physics. The authors are grateful to the NHSBSP radiographers who recorded data in the breast screening centres, and the physicists involved in the NHSBSP who provided technical data relating to the systems.

References

1. Dance, D.R., Skinner, C.L., Young, K.C., Beckett, J.R., Kotre, C.J.: Additional factors for the estimation of mean glandular breast dose using the UK mammography dosimetry protocol. Phys. Med. Biol. **45**, 3225–3240 (2000)
2. CDCOM version 1.6 software. EUREF. www.euref.org
3. CDMAM analysis UK version 1.4 software, NCCPM, Guildford, UK. www.nccpm.org
4. Kulama, E., Burch, A., Castellano, I., Lawinski, C.P., Marshall, N., Young, K.C.: Commissioning and Routine Testing of Full Field Digital Mammography Systems (NHSBSP Equipment report 0604). Sheffield: NHS Cancer Screening Programmes (2009)
5. Oduko, J.M., Young, K.C., Burch, A.: A survey of patient doses from digital mammography systems in the UK in 2007 to 2009. In: Martí, J., Oliver, A., Freixenet, J., Martí, R. (eds.) IWDM 2010. LNCS, vol. 6136, pp. 365–370. Springer, Heidelberg (2010)

6. Young, K.C., Oduko, J.M.: Radiation doses received in the United Kingdom breast screening programme in 2010 to 2012. Br. J. Radiol. **89**, 01508312 (2016)
7. Strudley, C.J., Young, K.C.: Technical Evaluation of Philips MicroDose SI digital mammography system (NHSBSP Equipment Report 1310). London: Public Health England, NHS Cancer Screening Programmes (2016)

A Pilot Study on Radiation Dose from Combined Mammography Screening in Australia

Jason Tse[1,2(✉)], Roger Fulton[1], Mary Rickard[1,3], Patrick Brennan[1], and Donald McLean[1,2]

[1] Faculty of Health Sciences, University of Sydney, Sydney, Australia
ttse4243@uni.sydney.edu.au
[2] Medical Physics and Radiation Engineering, Canberra Hospital, Canberra, Australia
[3] Sydney Breast Clinic, Sydney, Australia

Abstract. This article presents the results of a pilot dose survey including fifty patients who underwent combined screening: full field digital mammography (FFDM) plus digital breast tomosynthesis (DBT). The study also aimed to demonstrate the different dosimetric outcome from using different glandularity assumptions and dosimetry methods. The mean glandular dose to each patient was computed using Dance's method with UK glandularity assumption. The calculations were repeated using Wu/Boone's method with the "50–50" breast assumption and the results compared to those using Dance's method. For the typical breasts, the dose from combined examination was around 9.56 mGy: 4.26 mGy from two-view FFDM and 5.30 mGy from two-view DBT. Adopting UK glandularity assumption was believed to more realistically reflect the population dose. The comparison between Dance's and Wu/Boone's methods indicated that the latter tended to show lower dose values with mean differences of −3.6 % for FFDM and −5.5 % for DBT.

Keywords: Radiation dose · Digital mammography · Tomosynthesis

1 Introduction

Clinical studies [1–3] have shown that both the sensitivity and specificity of mammography screening would be generally improved when digital breast tomosynthesis (DBT) was used in combination to full field digital mammography (FFDM) (referred as combined mammography screening). It has been questioned whether the extra radiation dose associated with combined imaging would be adequately justified for population-based screening, particularly as the effect on breast cancer mortality is as yet unproven. Therefore, BreastScreen Australia has yet to recommend the inclusion of DBT in mammography screening awaiting further national clinical evidence and a better knowledge about the radiation dose from combined examinations to ensure patient safety.

The situation in Australia is additionally complicated as there is yet no national consensus regarding the standard method to determine radiation dose for DBT exposures

© Springer International Publishing Switzerland 2016
A. Tingberg et al. (Eds.): IWDM 2016, LNCS 9699, pp. 335–342, 2016.
DOI: 10.1007/978-3-319-41546-8_42

nor in fact for patient dose surveys in mammography. At present, there are two main schools of mammographic dosimetry formalism respectively advocated by Europe and North America: The former is based on the works by Dance [4, 5] (referred to as the Dance's method) which incorporates both FFDM and DBT methodologies and the latter is from the original works by Wu [6, 7], later extended by Boone [8] who worked on FFDM methodologies, and the work of Sechopoulos [9, 10] which developed into the American Association of Physicists in Medicine (AAPM) protocol for DBT dosimetry [11] (overall referred to as the Wu/Boone's method). All systems rely on Monte Carlo simulation techniques to estimate the mean glandular dose, a dose metric to characterize the risk of radiation-induced breast cancer, but with different simulation details leading to the expectation of different dosimetric outcomes.

Importantly the assumptions of breast density, used in dose estimation, need to be examined. For dosimetry, breast density is referred as "glandularity" which describes the proportional mass content of fibro-glandular tissues in the tissue core of the sim- ulated breast model, excluding a relatively thin layer of adipose tissue on the surface. In Dance's method, polynomial functions were derived from the screening data in the United Kingdom (UK) to estimate the average glandularity of the imaged breasts by their compressed thicknesses (referred as UK glandularity assumption) for two age groups of women and such estimations can be directly incorporated into dose calcu- lations [12]. Despite the potential errors, this approach is believed to be able to more realistically reflect the mean glandular dose to the screening population. In comparison, the Wu/Boone's method does not provide a specific guideline and assumes equal proportion of fibro-glandular and adipose tissues (referred as 50–50 breast assumption) in any dose calculation. This specific composition was conventionally believed to represent an average breast but recent works by Yaffe et al. [13] and Vedantham et al. [14] have added weight to previous work casting doubt on the validity of the 50–50 breast assumption by demonstrating that the fibro-glandular tissue composition is more typically in the range of around 20 %, depending on the definition of fibro-glandular tissue composition employed and the profile of women surveyed.

The study below presents the pilot dose data from combined mammography screening in Australia. It also aims to investigate the dosimetric outcome as a result of using different dosimetry methods and different assumptions on glandularity. The outcome of this study will be valuable when evaluating the introduction of DBT into the screening practice.

2   Methods and Materials

This pilot dose survey utilized patient data generated by a Hologic Selenia Dimensions (Hologic, Bedford, USA) mammographic unit with DBT functionality. Fifty asymp- tomatic female patients (average age of 54) who attended for screening for breast cancer in a private centre were randomly sampled from PACS records. Combined examinations, which composed of both FFDM and DBT acquisitions under the same compressed breast thickness, were performed at two views [cranio-caudal (CC) and mediolateral oblique (MLO)] on both breasts. Eight images were acquired for each patient, constituting a total of 400 images in this study. All examinations were performed using the automatic exposure control (AEC) setting: "Autofilter" that automatically selects suitable tube voltage (kV), anode/filter combinations and current-time product (mAs) depending on the compressed thickness of the breast and its attenuation to x-ray determined by the pre-pulse x-ray exposure.

From the patients' images, the acquisition parameters and characteristic of the breasts were extracted from the relevant DICOM tags. The volumetric breast density was also estimated for each patient using commercial software: Quantra^{TM} (Version 2.0). The radiation output and the beam qualities of the mammographic unit were measured using a dedicated mammography ionization chamber (Model $10 \times 6\text{-}6M$; Radcal, Monrovia, USA) and aluminum foils of high purity, respectively.

Combining the measurement results and the data collected for each patient, the associated mean glandular dose was computed using Dance's method for both FFDM and DBT acquisitions with the UK glandularity assumptions to study the typical dose from a combined examination. Subsequently, the calculations were repeated with the 50–50 breast assumption to study its impact on the dosimetric outcome and to allow direct comparison with the results calculated with Wu/Boone's methods.

3   Results and Discussion

3.1   Radiation Dose from Combined Examination

The demographics of the sampled patients were presented in Fig. 1, illustrating the distribution of compressed breast thickness. The average compressed thicknesses for CC and MLO view are 52.83 ± 15.18 mm and 52.89 ± 17.16 mm. Owing to the similar distributions of thickness, the respective radiation doses from these two views were not differentiated. The radiation dose from FFDM and DBT was presented in Table 1, as a function of compressed breast thickness and upon the UK glandularity assumption. On average, DBT delivers approximately 27 % more radiation dose to the imaged breast than FFDM which is comparable with the published results in the literature [15]. For the median compressed thickness between 50 and 60 mm, the mean glandular dose to the imaged breasts from a combined examination is approximately 9.56 mGy: 4.26 mGy from two-view FFDM and 5.30 mGy from two-view DBT.

The combined examinations have been shown to improve the effectiveness of mammography screening but at the expense of roughly doubling the radiation dose as demonstrated in the present survey. It is clear that the total dose to patients undergoing mammography screening will be determined by the clinical role of DBT in the future – whether it will be used solely or adjunct to FFDM and whether one-view DBT is adequate for accurate screening and diagnosis. In that regard, the clinical usefulness of synthetic 2D images reconstructed from DBT slice images would also require further investigation.

3.2   Impact of Glandularity Assumption

When compared to the results based upon the UK glandularity assumption (Table 1), using the 50–50 breast assumption would overestimate the dose for thinner breasts

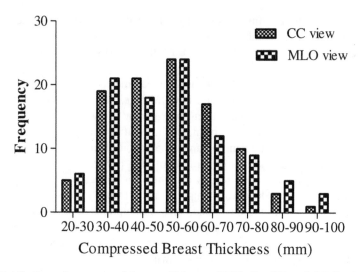

Fig. 1. Distribution of compressed breast thickness (CBT) for CC and MLO view in the sampled population

Table 1. Average radiation dose from FFDM and DBT (per acquisition) as a function of compressed breast thickness (CBT) calculated with Dance's method using the UK glandularity assumption.

CBT range (mm)	Sample size	FFDM (mGy)	DBT (mGy)	Ratio (DBT/FFDM)
20–30	11	1.29 ± 0.30	1.66 ± 0.24	1.34
30–40	40	1.41 ± 0.28	1.78 ± 0.27	1.27
40–0	39	1.59 ± 0.38	2.00 ± 0.21	1.30
50–60	48	2.13 ± 0.49	2.65 ± 0.24	1.29
60–70	31	3.12 ± 0.69	3.50 ± 0.41	1.14
70–80	19	4.58 ± 1.87	4.76 ± 0.70	1.13
80–90	8	5.47 ± 2.67	6.10 ± 1.01	1.25
90–100	4	4.27 ± 0.06	6.16 ± 0.35	1.44

(thickness: 20 to 40 mm) and underestimate the values for the thicker ones (thickness: 50 to 100 mm) (Table 2). These results were expected as breast glandularity was assumed to decline in a polynomial fashion with compressed breast thickness (left y-axis of Fig. 2): the thinner breasts would have glandularity greater than 50 % and vice versa for thicker ones as indicated by the dotted line in Fig. 3. Two polynomial curves are presented, representing the estimations for age groups: 40 to 49 (upper curve) and 50 to 64 (lower curve).

The present results are limited by the relatively small sample size in the survey and thus the glandularity distribution might not be representative owing to the variation in average glandularity within a sampled breast thickness and age group. Also, as discussed by Beckett and Kotre [16], the estimated glandularity from the UK assumption

Table 2. The same data as Table 1 recalculated with Dance's method using the 50–50 breast assumption.

CBT range (mm)	FFDM (mGy)	DBT (mGy)	Ratio (DBT/FFDM)
20–30	1.39 ± 0.33	1.80 ± 0.27	1.35
30–40	1.47 ± 0.28	1.85 ± 0.26	1.27
40–0	1.56 ± 0.37	1.97 ± 0.19	1.30
50–60	1.95 ± 0.47	2.42 ± 0.20	1.29
60–70	2.71 ± 0.63	3.04 ± 0.31	1.15
70–80	3.87 ± 1.60	4.03 ± 0.58	1.13
80–90	4.46 ± 2.21	5.02 ± 0.85	1.26
90–100	3.44 ± 0.04	5.04 ± 0.29	1.47

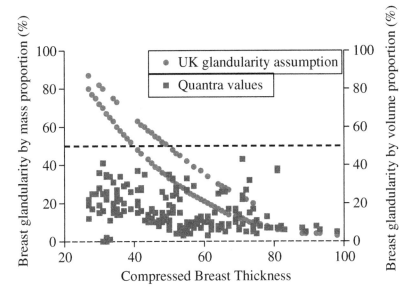

Fig. 2. The breast glandularity by mass proportion (left y-axis values) predicted by the UK glandularity assumption: two polynomial curves are presented, representing the estimations for age groups: 40 to 49 (upper curve) and 50 to 64 (lower curve). Also presented in the graph are the volumetric estimations by Quantra^TM (right y-axis values)

in theory would only be referring to the column of tissues above the AEC chamber and might not be directly comparable to the volumetric glandularity reported by automated software (e.g. Quantra^TM), in addition to the different definitions used which will be detailed next. This was evident in the right y-axis values of Fig. 2 which demonstrated that the individual volumetric glandularity, independently measured by Quantra^TM, in general deviated from the polynomial relationships with compressed thickness.

Incorporating individual glandularity information into dose calculation is not straight-forward in clinical settings as the information is not always available. Moreover, the values reported by radiologists or automated software are based on tissue area

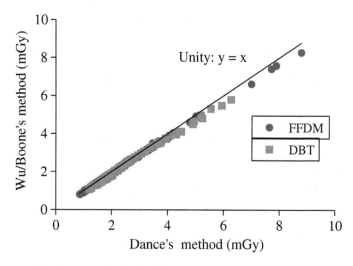

Fig. 3. A comparison between the dosimetric outcome using Dance's and Wu/Boone's methods for FFDM calculation and Dance's and AAPM methods for DBT exposures

or volumetric proportion as opposed to the mass proportion used in context of dosimetry. Additionally, the former estimates often include the subcutaneous adipose tissue, which is however excluded in dosimetry. Conversion between the two definitions is possible but access to the images would be necessary for further image processing. Commercial software is now available to perform "personalized" dose estimation taking into account the volumetric glandularity measured, and its impact on clinical practice would require further investigation [17].

3.3   Comparison of Dosimetry Methods

Linear relationships were observed between the dosimetry methods for both FFDM and DBT acquisitions (Fig. 3). Moreover, high correlations were also demonstrated with respective Pearson coefficients of 0.999 and 0.957. Further, compared to Dance's methodology, the Wu/Boone method tended to show lower dose values with the maximum difference of -10.8 % (mean = -3.6 %) for FFDM and -11.0 % (mean = -5.5 %) for DBT acquisitions. From the paired t-test, these differences were statistically significant ($p < 0.0001$).

This difference is mainly attributed to the different simulated breast models adopted in the two methods. In Dance's work, the breast was simulated as a symmetric semi-circular cylinder with an outer layer of adipose tissue (a surrogate of subcutaneous adipose tissue and skin) of thickness 4 mm enclosing a central region comprising a uniform mixture of breast tissues. Wu/Boone have utilized a similar breast model except with an outer adipose layer of 5 mm. This slight thickness variation of the outermost adipose would constitute a prominent dosimetric difference especially for the low x-ray energies utilized in mammography. This was evident that the largest deviations were from acquisitions with low kV settings. Other contributing factors include the different photon interaction cross-sectional areas (maximum alternations up to 10 %) as well as the difference in the irradiation geometry (maximum alternations up to 2.3 %). These small but significant differences must be recognized by users when interpreting dose values in reports and literature for risk assessment.

4 Conclusion

It was revealed in the pilot survey that the mean glandular dose to the imaged breasts from two-view combined examinations, as measured by mean glandular dose, would range from 5.90 to 23.14 mGy. For the median breasts in this survey, the total dose was approximately 9.56 mGy: 4.26 mGy from two-view FFDM and 5.30 mGy from two-view DBT. It was further demonstrated that these dose values would vary with the glandularity assumptions as well as the dosimetry methods and such dosimetric differences must be well recognized.

The results from this pilot study are inherently limited by its sample size and the fact that only one mammography unit is included. These limitations will be addressed in a follow-up study involving a larger sample size and multiple clinics using mammography units from different vendors.

References

1. Rose, S.L., et al.: Implementation of breast tomosynthesis in a routine screening practice: an observational study. AJR Am. J. Roentgenol. **200**, 1401–1408 (2013)
2. Ciatto, S., et al.: Integration of 3D digital mammography with tomosynthesis for population breast-cancer screening (STORM): a prospective comparison study. Lancet Oncol. **14**, 583–589 (2013)
3. Skaane, P., et al.: Comparison of digital mammography alone and digital mammography plus tomosynthesis in a population-based screening program. Radiology **267**, 47–56 (2013)
4. Dance, D.R., Young, K.C., van Engen, R.E.: Further factors for the estimation of mean glandular dose using the United Kingdom, European and IAEA breast dosimetry protocols. Phys. Med. Biol. **54**, 4361–4372 (2009)
5. Dance, D.R., Young, K.C., van Engen, R.E.: Estimation of mean glandular dose for breast tomosynthesis: factors for use with the UK, European and IAEA breast dosimetry protocols. Phys. Med. Biol. **56**, 453–471 (2011)
6. Wu, X., Barnes, G.T., Tucker, D.M.: Spectral dependence of glandular tissue dose in screen-film mammography. Radiology **179**, 143–148 (1991)
7. Wu, X., Gingold, E.L., Barnes, G.T., Tucker, D.M.: Normalized average glandular dose in molybdenum target-rhodium filter and rhodium target-rhodium filter mammography. Radiology **193**, 83–89 (1994)
8. Boone, J.M.: Normalized glandular dose (DgN) coefficients for arbitrary X-ray spectra in mammography: computer-fit values of Monte Carlo derived data. Med. Phys. **29**, 869–875 (2002)
9. Sechopoulos, I., Suryanarayanan, S., Vedantham, S., D'Orsi, C., Karellas, A.: Computation of the glandular radiation dose in digital tomosynthesis of the breast. Med. Phys. **34**, 221–232 (2007)

10. Sechopoulos, I., D'Orsi, C.: Glandular radiation dose in tomosynthesis of the breast using tungsten targets. J. Appl. Clin. Med. Phys. **9**, 161–171 (2008)
11. Sechopoulos, I., et al.: Radiation dosimetry in digital breast tomosynthesis: report of AAPM tomosynthesis subcommittee task group 223. Med. Phys. **41**, 091501 (2014)
12. Dance, D.R., Skinner, C.L., Young, K.C., Beckett, J.R., Kotre, C.J.: Additional factors for the estimation of mean glandular breast dose using the UK mammography dosimetry protocol. Phys. Med. Biol. **45**, 3225–3240 (2000)
13. Yaffe, M.J., et al.: The myth of the 50–50 breast. Med. Phys. **36**, 5437–5443 (2009)
14. Vedantham, S., Shi, L., Karellas, A., O'Connell, A.M.: Dedicated breast CT: fibroglandular volume measurements in a diagnostic population. Med. Phys. **39**, 7317–7328 (2012)
15. Dance, D.R., Strudley, C.J., Young, K.C., Oduko, J.M., Whelehan, P.J., Mungutroy, E.: Comparison of breast doses for digital tomosynthesis estimated from patient exposures and using PMMA breast phantoms. In: Maidment, A.D., Bakic, P.R., Gavenonis, S. (eds.) IWDM 2012. LNCS, vol. 7361, pp. 316–321. Springer, Heidelberg (2012)
16. Beckett, J.R., Kotre, C.J.: Dosimetric implications of age related glandular changes in screening mammography. Phys. Med. Biol. **45**, 801–813 (2000)
17. Tromans, C.E., Highnam, R., Morrish, O., Black, R., Tucker, L., Gilbert, F., Brady, S.M.: Patient specific dose calculation using volumetric breast density for mammography and tomosynthesis. In: Fujita, H., Hara, T., Muramatsu, C. (eds.) IWDM 2014. LNCS, vol. 8539, pp. 158–165. Springer, Heidelberg (2014)

Simulation of Dose Reduction in Digital Breast Tomosynthesis

Lucas R. Borges[1,2(✉)], Igor Guerrero[1], Predrag R. Bakic[2],
Andrew D.A. Maidment[2], Homero Schiabel[1],
and Marcelo A.C. Vieira[1]

[1] Department of Electrical Engineering, University of São Paulo,
São Carlos, Brazil
{lucas.rodrigues.borges,igor.guerrero}@usp.br,
{homero,mvieira}@sc.usp.br
[2] Department of Radiology, University of Pennsylvania, Philadelphia, USA
{Predrag.Bakic,Andrew.Maidment}@uphs.upenn.edu

Abstract. Clinical evaluation of dose reduction studies in x-ray breast imaging is problematic because it is difficult to justify imaging the same patient at a variety of radiation doses. One common alternative is to use simulation algorithms to manipulate a standard-dose exam to mimic reduced doses. Although there are several dose-reduction simulation methods for full-field digital mammography, the availability of similar methods for digital breast tomosynthesis (DBT) is limited. This work proposes a method for simulating dose reductions in DBT, based on the insertion of noise in a variance-stabilized domain. The proposed method has the advantage of performing signal-dependent noise injection without knowledge of the noiseless signal. We compared clinical low-dose DBT projections and reconstructed slices to simulated ones by means of power spectra, mean pixel values, and local standard deviations. The results of our simulations demonstrate low error (<5 %) between real and simulated images.

Keywords: Noise simulation · Dose reduction · Digital breast tomosynthesis · Anscombe transformation

1 Introduction

The ultimate study of radiation dose reduction in medical x-ray imaging requires images from the same patient at different radiation doses. In practice, such images cannot be obtained because of radiation risks. One way to overcome this limitation is to use anthropomorphic phantoms; phantom images can be acquired at various conditions without concern. However, physical phantoms do not simulate a sufficiently wide variety of breasts, which may negatively influence studies of radiologists' performance [1]. Another common approach is to manipulate standard dose images to exhibit the noise properties of an image acquired at lower radiation dose. In medical x-ray imaging, several methods have been proposed to simulate dose reduction [2–9]. However, the applicability of such methods to simulate dose reduction in digital breast tomosynthesis (DBT) is unknown.

© Springer International Publishing Switzerland 2016
A. Tingberg et al. (Eds.): IWDM 2016, LNCS 9699, pp. 343–350, 2016.
DOI: 10.1007/978-3-319-41546-8_43

Recently, we proposed a novel method of simulating dose reduction in full field digital mammography (FFDM) [9], based on noise insertion in a variance-stabilized domain, where no approximation of the noiseless signal is necessary. The method can be applied to flat fielded images. In this work, we evaluate our method to manipulate standard-dose DBT projections to mimic the noise characteristics of reduced-dose DBT projections.

2 Method

The proposed method for simulating dose reduction in DBT projections requires three sets of projection images as input: the standard-dose clinical exam and two uniform images at different doses. The two uniform images must be acquired using a uniform PMMA block, corresponding to the same kV and filtration as the clinical image. One uniform acquisition must be performed using the same exposure (mAs) as the standard-dose image; the other uniform image must be acquired using a reduced exposure time for the desired dose reduction. The three sets of images are used to generate simulated projections, which are then reconstructed to produce the reduced-dose DBT slices. Figure 1 presents the workflow used in this method.

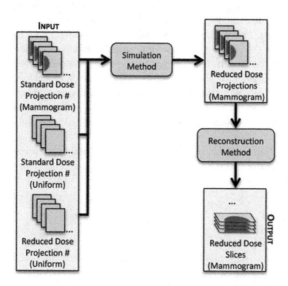

Fig. 1. Schematic of the simulation process adopted in this work.

The first stage of the simulation algorithm consists of linearizing all input images with respect to the entrance dose to the detector, and scaling the signal to the desired range. Since in this work we only consider reductions in exposure, scaling can be done simply by multiplying the original projections by the dose reduction factor (e.g., 0.7 for simulating 70 % of the dose).

The second stage of the simulation method is the noise injection. To calculate how much noise should be added to the scaled image to mimic the noise at the reduced dose, we estimate the local standard deviation on both uniform images. The difference between these estimates is then used to modulate a mask of Gaussian noise with zero mean and unity variance.

The final step is to incorporate this noise mask to the scaled image. Since the added noise must be signal-dependent, its standard deviation depends on the underlying noiseless signal. To avoid making approximations of the signal, we perform the noise insertion in a variance-stabilized domain, the Anscombe domain, where no previous knowledge of the underlying signal is necessary. Importantly, the standard deviation mask calculated previously accounts for trends in the noise statistics caused by corrections such as the flat fielding. A detailed methodology is given in [9].

3 Materials

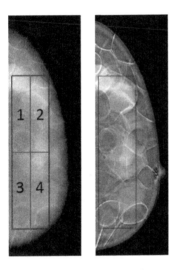

Fig. 2. Example of phantom images. Left: central raw projection. Right: central slice of the 3D reconstructed volume. The rectangles identify the ROI's used for the results. (Color figure online)

In this work we used a clinical Selenia Dimensions system (Hologic, Bedford, MA), at the Hospital of the University of Pennsylvania to assess the performance of the simulation method. Sets of DBT images were acquired using a physical anthropomorphic breast phantom, manufactured by CIRS, Inc. (Reston, VA) under license from the University of Pennsylvania [10]. The breast phantom consists of six slabs, each containing simulated anatomical structures manufactured using tissue mimicking materials, based upon a realization of the companion software phantom.

Images were acquired using a fixed tube voltage of 31 kVp, with a tungsten target, filtered with aluminum. The exposure was decreased from 60 to 30 mAs in four steps to simulate different doses. The average incident air kerma to the phantom provided by the DICOM header for each radiographic setting was: 5.62 mGy,   4.78 mGy,   3.94 mGy   and 2.81 mGy. Five acquisitions were performed for each configuration, resulting in 300 phantom projections (a set of 15 projections for each acquisition). Figure 2 shows examples of a central projection before reconstruction and a central slice of the reconstructed 3D volume.

Each exposure configuration was repeated to image a uniform 4 cm thick PMMA block, commonly used for flat-field correction. Two acquisitions were performed for each exposure configuration, resulting in 120 uniform projections.

Real and simulated projections were reconstructed using the Briona reconstruction software (Real Time Tomography, Villanova, PA). Each volume was generated using 1 mm spacing, resulting in 2040 DBT slices, 1020 of them real and 1020 simulated.

To assess the simulation method we analysed images both before and after reconstruction. For the projections prior to reconstruction, three metrics were used: power spectrum (PS), local mean, and local standard deviation. The PS was calculated as the average PS of non-overlapping 64×64 regions within a 14.3 cm $\times$ 3.5 cm (1024×256 pixels) ROI containing as much breast tissue as possible, as shown by the red rectangle in Fig. 2. The spatial dependence of the PS was explored by repeating the calculations in the four non-overlapping quadrants inside the ROI, as defined by the blue lines in Fig. 2. Spatial metrics, including the mean and standard deviation were calculated inside the large ROI using 256 non-overlapping 0.45 cm $\times$ 0.45 cm (32×32 pixels) windows. After reconstruction of the 3D volume, we analysed mean and standard deviation of each slice, using an ROI of the same size and position as above.

The average absolute error between each simulated image and the corresponding real image was calculated for each metric at each simulated dose. The results reported are the crossed comparison between all five real and five simulated images, resulting in 25 comparisons for each metric at each dose.

4 Results

After the simulation method was applied to the DBT projections, we reconstructed the 3D volume and performed tests on both raw projections and processed slices. Figure 3 shows examples of simulated and real images.

The first metric analysed was the global PS, calculated inside the entire ROI taken from the central projection. In Fig. 4(a) it is possible to evaluate the similarity between the PS of the real and the simulated images acquired using three different doses. Figure 4(b) shows the average error between simulated and real images.

The PS was also calculated locally in four quadrants of the global ROI. This metric allows the evaluation of the spectrum of the simulated noise in different regions of the breast. Figure 4(c) shows the

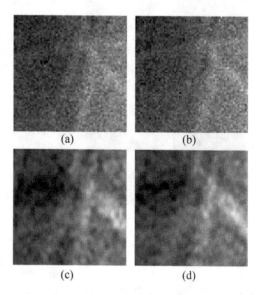

(a)   (b)

(c)   (d)

Fig. 3. Examples of real and simulated images (2.81 mGy, 50 % dose). (a) Real central projection, (b) Simulated central projection, (c) Real central slice, (d) Simulated central slice.

average absolute error at each quadrant. Note that the region used to calculate the PS on Fig. 4(c) is different in size to that used in Fig. 4(a), (b); therefore, the spectral resolution differs in the two experiments.

In the next experiment, we calculated the mean pixel value at each radiation dose and each projection before reconstruction. Figure 5(a) shows one example of the mean pixel value calculated at the central projection. Figure 5(b) is the average absolute error for each projection. Although we calculated the mean pixel value at 256 different ROIs as described in the methods section, we performed down sampling to allow better visualization of the data in Fig. 5(a); however, the errors calculated in Fig. 5(b) account for all 256 samples.

The last metric calculated on the DBT projections was the standard deviation. Similar to previous results, we give an example of the standard deviation calculated on the central slice in Fig. 6(a), and the average absolute error is reported in Fig. 6(b). Again, we performed down sampling to allow better visualization of Fig. 6(a), but the error reported in Fig. 6(b) accounts for all 256 samples.

Additional tests were performed on the reconstructed slices of the 3D volume. Figure 7(a) shows the average absolute error between the mean pixel value of the simulated and real reconstructed slices. Figure 7(b) shows the equivalent calculation for the standard deviation.

5 Discussion and Conclusions

In this work, we propose a new method for simulating dose reduction in DBT images. A number of existing dose-reduction simulation methods [2–6, 9] are based on a two-step approach: signal scaling, and noise insertion. Adding signal dependent noise to an already noisy image is a challenging task, since the noise statistics depend on the noiseless underlying signal, which is not available in most clinical cases. With the proposed method, noise insertion is performed in a variance-stabilized domain, where no knowledge of the noiseless signal is necessary. Furthermore, the method simulates noise locally; therefore, it can be applied to flat-fielded images and reproduce statistical trends, such as those generated by the heel effect.

A preliminary assessment was performed on the projection images and on the reconstructed slices. Power spectral analysis demonstrated that the noise was correctly simulated in terms of spatial frequency, with average absolute error below 3.5 % for every projection, as shown in Fig. 4(b). The average absolute error of the local power spectra reported on Fig. 4(c) shows the simulation could replicate the global and local dependencies of the clinical PS. As seen in Figs. 5 and 6, the local spatial statistics on raw projections also show small errors (<2.5 %) for every image.

The final experiment was performed on reconstructed slices. Figure 7 shows that the pixel values of the reconstruction images were very similar to the real reconstruction images, with errors below 0.5 %, and the standard deviation showed errors below 4.5 %. It is interesting to notice that in Fig. 7(a), although the errors are extremely low, it is possible to notice a trend in the results, with higher dose reductions resulting in higher errors. Furthermore, Fig. 7(b) shows that the noise was simulated

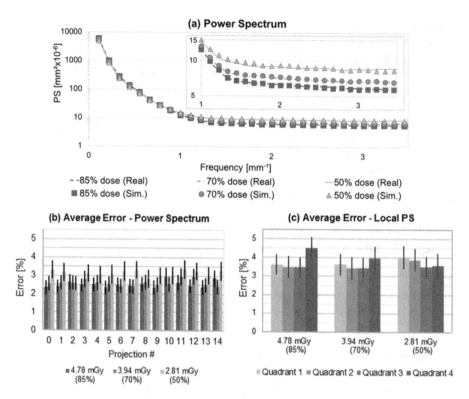

Fig. 4. Power spectra calculated from real and simulated central projections at different entrance doses to the phantom. (a) Entire spectra and high frequencies in detail, (b) average absolute error for each projection, (c) average absolute error for each quadrant. Error bars are the standard error. (Color figure online)

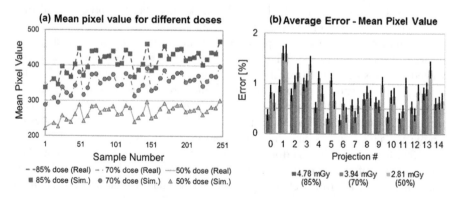

Fig. 5. Comparison between real and simulated mean pixel value at various doses to the phantom. (a) Example of the mean pixel value calculated in a central projection. (b) Average absolute error for each projection. Error bars represent the standard error. (Color figure online)

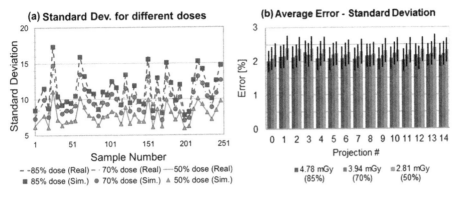

Fig. 6. Comparison between real and simulated standard deviation at various doses to the phantom. (a) Example of the standard deviation calculated in a central projection. (b) Average absolute error for each projection. Error bars represent the standard error. (Color figure online)

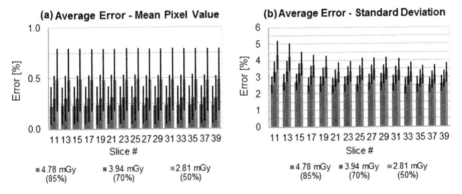

Fig. 7. Local metrics calculated from real and simulated slices at various doses to the phantom: (a) average absolute error of the mean pixel value, (b) average absolute error of the standard deviation. (Color figure online)

with higher precision in slices farther from the detector plate. Further tests are necessary to understand this behaviour.

Some limitations and future work are now addressed. In this work, we used a clinical unit with an amorphous-selenium (a-Se) detector with minimally correlated noise. Further analysis is necessary to simulate systems with highly correlated noise. In this work, we considered dose reductions achieved exclusively by reduction of the exposure. Further analysis is necessary for simulating changes on other radiographic factors, such as kV, target, and filtration. The PMMA blocks used for the uniform images were chosen to mimic the filtration of the breast. Future work should include analysis of the dependency between the thickness of the PMMA and the accuracy of the simulation method.

Acknowledgements. The authors would like to thank São Paulo Research Foundation (FAPESP grant# 2013/18915-5) and the Brazilian Foundation for the Coordination of Improvement of Higher Education Personnel (CAPES grant# 88881.030443/2013-01) for the financial support given to this project. The authors would also like to acknowledge the support of the National Institutes of Health/National Cancer Institute grant 1R01-CA154444. The content of this paper is solely the responsibility of the authors and does not necessarily represent the official views of the funding agencies. We thank Real Time Tomography (RTT) for providing assistance with image reconstruction. ADAM is a member of the scientific advisory board and shareholder of RTT.

References

1. Samei, E., Eyler, W., Baron, L.: Effects of anatomical structure on signal detection. In: Handbook of Medical Imaging, pp. 655–682 (2000)
2. Saunders, R.S., Samei, E.: A method for modifying the image quality parameters of digital radiographic images. Med. Phys. **30**, 3006–3017 (2003)
3. Båth, M., Håkansson, M., Tingberg, A., Månsson, L.G.: Method of simulating dose reduction for digital radiographic systems. Radiat. Prot. Dosimetry **114**, 253–259 (2005)
4. Kroft, L.J.M., Veldkamp, W.J.H., Mertens, B.J.A., Van Delft, J.P.A., Geleijns, J.: Detection of simulated nodules on clinical radiographs: dose reduction at digital posteroanterior chest radiography. Radiology **241**(2), 392–398 (2006)
5. Veldkamp, W.J.H., Kroft, L.J.M., Van Delft, J.P.A., Geleijns, J.: A technique for simulating the effect of dose reduction on image quality in digital chest radiography. J. Digit. Imaging **22**(2), 114–125 (2009)
6. Svalkvist, A., Båth, M.: Simulation of dose reduction in tomosynthesis. Med. Phys. **37**, 258–269 (2010)
7. Mackenzie, A., Dance, D.R., Workman, A., Yip, M., Wells, K., Young, K.C.: Conversion of mammographic images to appear with the noise and sharpness characteristics of a different detector and x-ray system. Med. Phys. **39**, 2721 (2012)
8. Mackenzie, A., Dance, D.R., Diaz, O., Young, K.C.: Image simulation and a model of noise power spectra across a range of mammographic beam qualities. Med. Phys. **41**, 121901-1–121901-14 (2014)
9. Borges, L.R., Oliveira, H.C.R., Nunes, P.F., Vieira, M.A.C.: Method for inserting noise in digital mammography to simulate reduction in radiation dose. In: Proceedings of the SPIE 9412, Medical Imaging, 94125J (2015)
10. Cockmartin, L., Bakic, P.R., Bosmans, H., Maidment, A.D., Gall, H., Zerhouni, M., Marshall, N.W.: Power spectrum analysis of an anthropomorphic breast phantom compared to patient data in 2D digital mammography and breast tomosynthesis. In: Fujita, H., Hara, T., Muramatsu, C. (eds.) IWDM 2014. LNCS, vol. 8539, pp. 423–429. Springer, Heidelberg (2014)

Non-expert Classification of Microcalcification Clusters Using Mereotopological Barcodes

Harry Strange[1]([✉]) and Reyer Zwiggelaar[2]

[1] Department of Computer Science, University College London,
Gower Street, London WE12 1HG, UK
h.strange@ucl.ac.uk
[2] Department of Computer Science, Aberystwyth University,
Aberystwyth SY23 3DB, UK
rrz@aber.ac.uk

Abstract. This paper investigates the use of mereotopological barcodes to help non-experts classify microcalcification clusters as either benign or malignant. When compared against classification using the microcalcification cluster segmentation maps, the use of barcodes is able to see a significant improvement in classification performance with the AUC significantly increasing ($p < 0.01$) from 0.62 for images to 0.82 for barcodes on the MIAS dataset. This shows that barcodes could prove useful to aid clinicians with interpreting and classifying mammographic microcalcifications.

Keywords: Mammography · Microcalcification classification · Mereotopological barcodes · Visualisation

1 Background

Microcalcification clusters are a primary indicator of breast cancer [1]. Clinically, benign and malignant microcalcification clusters can be identified via the morphology of individual microcalcifications and the distribution pattern of the cluster as a whole [2,3]. Benign microcalcifications will typically be larger than those associated with malignancy and exhibit a more spread out distribution. Malignant microcalcification clusters will tend to contain smaller microcalcifications and be more tightly clustered [3]. Due to the fact that microcalcifications and their associated clusters exhibit identifiable shape and distribution properties, numerous approaches have been developed to automatically classify a microcalcification cluster as either benign or malignant using aspects such as topology [4], shape features [5,6], or varied features with different classifiers [7].

One other recent approach used to automatically analyse and classify microcalcification clusters is based on the use of mereotopological barcodes to capture the distribution information of a cluster [1]. The approach works by capturing the change in mereotopological relationships among the microcalcifications in a cluster. Mereotopoly defines a language for describing the relationships between

© Springer International Publishing Switzerland 2016
A. Tingberg et al. (Eds.): IWDM 2016, LNCS 9699, pp. 351–358, 2016.
DOI: 10.1007/978-3-319-41546-8_44

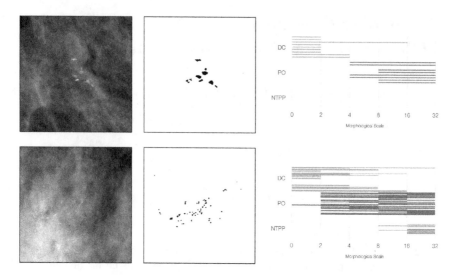

Fig. 1. Examples of benign (top row) and malignant (bottom row) microcalcification clusters. Shown are the raw ROI (left), the microcalcification segmentation map (centre) and the associated barcode (right).

two objects based on region connection calculus [8,9]. The relationships used for microcalcification cluster classification are disconnected (DC), edge connected (EC), partial overlap (PO), tangential proper part (TPP), non-tangential proper part (NTPP), and equal (EQ). As such, the mereotopological barcodes algorithm takes a segmentation mask as input (i.e. Fig. 1) where the foreground regions correspond to identified microcalcifications. These regions are then "grown" over a range of scales using mathematical morphology and the mereotopological relations among the regions are recorded at each scale in the form of intervals within a barcode (i.e. Fig. 1). Barcodes for benign and malignant cases exhibit different properties and so can be used as a feature for automatic classification [1]. However, they could also be used as a novel way of visualising the distribution of the microcalcifications within a cluster, a property that might lead to clinical benefit. Therefore, this paper describes an experiment where both microcalcification cluster segmentation maps and microcalcification barcodes (such as those in Fig. 1) were used by a group of non-experts to classify the underlying case as either benign or malignant. With minimal training, the non-experts were able to perform better using the barcodes than the segmented images and were also able to closely match the performance of the automatic barcode classification approach.

2   Methods

The aim of the experiment was to ascertain whether non-experts could use mereotopological barcodes to classify microcalcification clusters as either benign or malignant. If so, then this could indicate that using mereotopological barcodes to visualise the distribution of a microcalcification cluster could potentially help clinicians with the task of microcalcification classification. To compare the non-expert classification performance using mereotopological barcodes, a baseline classification performance was produced by asking the participants to classify the microcalcification cluster segmentation map images (Fig. 1). For both the barcodes and the images, a simple set of classification rules were given and a small training phase was used.

2.1   Experimental Setup

Data. The cases used for this experiment were taken from the MIAS dataset [10] consisting of 20 microcalcification clusters; 11 benign and 9 malignant. These patches were manually identified and annotated by expert radiologists. For each of the microcalcification clusters, a binary segmentation was produced using the method of Oliver et al. [11] and a mereotopological barcode over six scales was produced following the methodology of Strange et al. [1]. A binary segmentation was used as opposed to the mammographic ROI to try and reduce the need for the participants to both detect and classify microcalcification clusters. The presence of microcalcifications within a cluster when viewed as a mammographic patch can be subtle and difficult to identify; removing this task will help the results to be focused solely on classification by using the same starting point for both approaches (i.e. the microcalcification cluster segmentation maps). For the mereotopological barcodes, only the disconnected (DC), partial overlap (PO), and non-tangential proper part (NTPP) relations were included to save space and remove redundant relations. The dataset of 20 microcalcification clusters was then split into two subsets, A and B, using a stratified cross-validation approach such that each set contained roughly equal proportions of benign and malignant cases. These two subsets were used to produce the image and barcode sets given to the participants. Each participant was given a sheet of paper with ten microcalcification cluster images and ten microcalcification barcodes. To ensure that all images and barcodes were classified at least once, two sets of images/barcodes were produced. The first set contained the images from subset A and the barcodes from subset B; the second set contained the images from subset B and the barcodes from subset A. Each participant was randomly assigned to one of these two sets.

Participants. The participants were all part of a Science Café meeting which took place on the 9th December, 2015. Ethical clearance was gained for the experiment and all results were fully anonymised. None of the participants were clinicians and none had any previous expertise in classifying microcalcifications or mereotopological barcodes.

Participant Training. The participants were shown an example benign and malignant case (barcode and microcalcification segmentation) from the DDSM database [12] as initial training. As well as this, the participants were told the following classification rules:

Barcodes Benign: Fewer lines. Lines appear disconnected (DC) for longer.
Barcodes Malignant: More lines. More likely to move quickly from partial overlap (PO) to non-tangential proper part (NTPP).
Images Benign: Lager "blobs". More spread out.
Images Malignant: Tightly clustered in a smaller area

The descriptions given for the images were taken from the Pocket Radiologist definition of benign and malignant clusters [3]. The participants were also given the opportunity to ask any questions about the classification rules prior to the experiment beginning.

Classification. As well as a sheet of cases (segmentations and barcodes), the participants were also given a score sheet for classification. This sheet allowed the participants to enter a confidence score for whether they thought each image/barcode was benign or malignant. Each image/barcode was assigned a benign or malignant confidence score along the following scale:

Image 01	Benign									Malignant
	5	4	3	2	1	1	2	3	4	5

A score of "Benign 5" would indicate that the participant was sure that Image 01 was benign; a score "Malignant 5" would indicate that the participant was sure that Image 01 was malignant. Conversely, a score of 1 on either the benign or malignant scale would indicate that the participant was unsure about the classification. Notice that there is no middle ground, the participants had to assign each image/barcode to either the benign or malignant class even if they were not sure about the classification.

2.2 Analysis

The results were compared using classification accuracy and the area under the ROC curve (AUC), denoted A_z [13], along with the standard error [14]. The classification accuracy is defined as the percentage of true positives and true negatives with respect to the total number of samples in the dataset. The AUC is used to assess the predictive ability of a classifier and is equivalent to the Wilcoxon signed ranks test [15].

3 Results

A total of 32 participants took part in the experiment; however, 6 of those participants provided classification scores for only one of the groups (i.e. images

Table 1. Confusion matrices for the two non-expert classification approaches. The overall classification accuracies, A_z, and standard error for each approach are (a), CA = 72 %, A_z = 0.82, SE = 0.025, (b) CA = 59 %, A_z = 0.62, SE = 0.035.

<table>
<tr><td></td><td colspan="2" align="center">Truth</td><td></td><td colspan="2" align="center">Truth</td></tr>
<tr><td></td><td>Malignant</td><td>Benign</td><td></td><td>Malignant</td><td>Benign</td></tr>
<tr><td>Malignant</td><td>**102**</td><td>58</td><td>Malignant</td><td>**68**</td><td>58</td></tr>
<tr><td>Benign</td><td>16</td><td>**84**</td><td>Benign</td><td>48</td><td>**86**</td></tr>
<tr><td></td><td colspan="2" align="center">(a) Barcodes</td><td></td><td colspan="2" align="center">(b) Images</td></tr>
</table>

only or barcodes only) and so were removed from the results. This led to a final set of results from 26 participants. Therefore, each image/barcode was classified on average 13 times. Due to two unintelligible benign barcode results and two unintelligible malignant image results, the total number of samples for each class are 142 benign barcodes, 118 malignant barcodes, 144 benign images, and 116 malignant images.

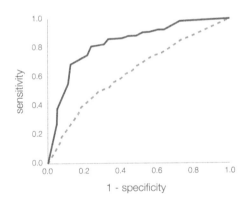

Fig. 2. ROC curves for non-expert classification of the MIAS database using segmentation map images (- - -) and barcodes (—). The A_z values for each curve are A_z = 0.62 (SE = 0.035) for images and A_z = 0.82 (SE = 0.025) for barcodes.

The confusion matrices for each approach are shown in Table 1. The barcodes show an improvement over images with the classification accuracy rising from 59 % to 72 % and the A_z value increasing from A_z = 0.62 for images to A_z = 0.82 for barcodes. Figure 2 shows the ROC curves for each of the approaches.

A comparison with automatic approaches to microcalcification classification on the MIAS dataset is given in Table 2. The two non-expert classification results are compared against existing topological, shape based, and feature based methods. Of particular interest is the comparison with Strange et al. [1] who use

Table 2. Comparison of classification accuracy and A_z between non-expert classification, using segmentation map images or barcodes, and various automatic approaches using the MIAS dataset. The approach of Strange et al. [1] is an automatic approach using mereotopological barcodes.

	Images	Barcodes	Strange [1]	Ma [5]	Ren [7]	Chen [4]
CA	59 %	72 %	95 %	80 %	85 %	95 %
A_z	0.62	0.82	0.80	0.76	0.91	0.96

mereotopological barcodes as the feature descriptor for automatic classification on the MIAS dataset.

4   Discussion

As can be seen from Table 1 and Fig. 2, the use of barcodes helps improve non-expert classification of microcalcification clusters when compared to using standard microcalcification cluster segmentation images. Classification accuracy increases from 60 % to 72 % and A_z increases from 0.62 to 0.82. This increase in A_z is a statistically significant improvement ($p < 0.01$).

Comparing with automatic approaches (Table 2), both non-expert approaches achieve far lower classification accuracy than the automatic methods. However, the A_z for the non-expert barcodes approach is an improvement over two of the automatic methods. Of particular interest is the fact that the A_z for the non-experts using barcodes is higher than the A_z value for the automatic barcode approach. This suggests that the current automatic barcode classification approach, using a greedy matching algorithm [1], does not sufficiently capture all of the discriminatory information contained in the mereotopological barcodes. The fact that non-experts are able to achieve improved A_z scores indicates that different automatic classification methods using barcodes may lead to improved results.

One of the questions posited in the original mereotopological barcodes paper was whether barcodes could be used in a clinical setting to help improve diagnostic accuracy. To help begin to answer that question, this experiment sought to investigate whether barcodes could be used as alternative visual descriptors of a microcalcification cluster. As the results show, for non-experts the improvements in classification performance when using barcodes as opposed to segmented images are significant. This suggests that barcodes are a viable alternative visual descriptor as they capture topological (distribution) properties of the clusters and display them in an easy to interpret manner. This work also fits into a new body of research that investigates alternative approaches to medical image analysis to help understand medical image perception and existing analysis systems (i.e. [16]).

By performing a larger experiment involving experienced radiologists it will be possible to see whether mereotopological barcodes can serve a diagnostic purpose within a clinical setting. Comparing the performance of experts on a set of real microcalcification cluster images and a set of equivalent mereotopological barcodes will enable a more rigorous conclusion to be drawn as to the efficacy of barcodes when used as an alternative visual descriptor of microcalcification clusters.

5   Conclusions

In summary, this paper has presented an experiment whereby non-experts classified a set of microcalcification clusters using both segmentation maps and mereotopological barcodes as the objects to be classified. Using a minimal amount of training, the non-experts were able to classify a set of microcalcification clusters taken from the MIAS dataset with a classification accuracy of 72% and an A_z value of 0.82. This is an improvement over classification using the segmentation images (CA of 59% and A_z of 0.62). This result suggests that mereotopological barcodes do indeed capture some of the distribution features of a microcalcification cluster that are important for classification purposes. It is expected that this result would transfer to other digital datasets since existing automatic detection and classification methods show little difference in performance across different digital datasets [4,11].

Future work will be focused on using mereotopological barcodes within a clinical setting. Although this work has shown that the use of barcodes can improve non-expert classification performance, it remains to be seen if the same outcome is true for expert readers. Therefore, future experimentation will look at how well radiologists (both junior and expert) perform when using mereotopological barcodes compared to mammographic images and segmentation maps.

Acknowledgments. The authors would like to thank the organisers of the Science Café for the opportunity to conduct this experiment. They would also like to extend their gratitude to all the participants for their willingness to be involved.

References

1. Strange, H., Chen, Z., Denton, E.R.E., Zwiggelaar, R.: Modelling mammographic microcalcification clusters using persistent mereotopology. Pattern Recogn. Lett. **47**, 157–163 (2014)
2. American College of Radiology: Illustrated Breast Imaging Reporting and Data System BIRADS. Third edn. American College of Radiology (1998)
3. Birdwell, R.L., Morris, E.A., Wang, S.C., Parkinson, B.T.: Pocket Radiologist: Breast Top 100 Diagnoses. Amirsys, Salt Lake City (2003)
4. Chen, Z., Strange, H., Oliver, A., Denton, E.R.E., Boggis, C., Zwiggelaar, R.: Topological modeling and classification of mammographic microcalcification clusters. IEEE Trans. Biomed. Eng. **62**(4), 1203–1214 (2015)
5. Ma, Y., Tay, P.C., Adams, R.D., Zhang, J.Z.: A novel shape feature to classify microcalcifications. In: Proceedings of the 17th IEEE International Conference on Image Processing (ICIP), pp. 2265–2268 (2010)

6. Shen, L., Rangayyan, R.M., Desautels, J.E.L.: Application of shape analysis to mammographic calcifications. IEEE Trans. Med. Imaging **13**, 263–274 (1994)
7. Ren, B., Smith, A., Jing, Z.: Measurement of breast density with digital breast tomosynthesis. In: Proceedings of Medical Imaging 2012: Physics of Medical Imaging (2012)
8. Galton, Antony: The mereotopology of discrete space. In: Freksa, Christian, Mark, David M. (eds.) COSIT 1999. LNCS, vol. 1661, p. 251. Springer, Heidelberg (1999)
9. Randell, D.A., Cui, Z., Cohn, A.G.: A spatial logic based on regions and connections. In: Proceedings of the 3rd International Conference on Knowledge Representation and Reasoning (1992)
10. Suckling, J., Parker, J., Dance, D., Astley, S., Hutt, I., Boggis, C., Ricketts, I., Stamatakis, E., Cerneaz, N., Kok, S., Taylor, P., Betal, D., Savage, J.:The mammographic images analysis society digital mammogram database. In: Digital Mammography, pp. 375–378 (1994)
11. Oliver, A., Torrent, A., Lladó, X., Tortajada, M., Tortajada, L., Sentís, M., Freixenet, J., Zwiggelaar, R.: Automatic microcalcification and cluster detection for digital and digitised mammograms. Knowl.-Based Syst. **28**, 68–75 (2012)
12. Heath, M., Bowyer, K., Kopans, D., Moore, R., Kegelmeye, W.P.: The digital database for screening mammography. In: Proceedings of the Fifth International Workshop on Digital Mammography, pp. 212–218 (2001)
13. Huang, J., Ling, C.: Using AUC and accuracy in evaluating learning algorithms. IEEE Trans. Knowl. Data Eng. **17**, 299–310 (2005)
14. Hanley, J.A., McNeil, B.J.: The meaning and use of the area under a Receiver Operating Characteristic (ROC) curve. Radiology **143**(1), 29–36 (1982)
15. Mason, S.J., Grahan, N.E.: Areas beneath the relative operating characteristics (ROC) and relative operating levels (ROL) curves: statistical significance and interpretation. Q. J. Royal Meteorol. Soc. **128**, 2145–2166 (2002)
16. Levenson, R.M., Krupinski, E.A., Navarro, V.M., Wasserman, E.A.: Pigeons (Columb livia) as trainable observers of pathology and radiology breast cancer images. PLoS ONE **10**(11), e0141357 (2015)

Mammographic Segmentation and Density Classification: A Fractal Inspired Approach

Wenda He[1($\boxtimes$)], Sam Harvey[2], Arne Juette[3], Erika R.E. Denton[3], and Reyer Zwiggelaar[1]

[1] Department of Computer Science, Aberystwyth University,
Aberystwyth SY23 3DB, UK
{weh,rrz}@aber.ac.uk
[2] School of Physics and Astronomy, University of Manchester,
Manchester M13 9PL, UK
sam.harvey-2@student.manchester.ac.uk
[3] Department of Radiology, Norfolk and Norwich University Hospital,
Norwich NR4 7UY, UK
{arne.juette,erika.denton}@nnuh.nhs.uk

Abstract. Breast cancer is the most frequently diagnosed cancer in women. To date, the exact cause(s) of breast cancer still remains unknown. The most effective way to tackle the disease is early detection through breast screening programmes. Breast density is a well established image based risk factor. An accurate dense breast tissue segmentation can play a vital role in precise identification of women at risk, and determining appropriate measures for disease prevention. Fractal techniques have been used in many biomedical image processing applications with varying degrees of success. This paper describes a fractal inspired approach to mammographic tissue segmentation. A multiresolution stack representation and 3D histogram features (extended from 2D) are proposed. Quantitative and qualitative evaluation was performed including mammographic tissue segmentation and density classification. Results showed that the developed methodology was able to differentiate between breast tissue variations. The achieved density classification accuracy for 360 digital mammograms is 78 % based on the BI-RADS scheme. The developed fractal inspired approach in conjunction with the stack representation and 3D histogram features has demonstrated an ability to produce quality mammographic tissue segmentation. This in turn can be found useful in early breast cancer detection, risk-stratified screening, and aiding radiologists in the process of decision making prior to surgery and/or treatment.

Keywords: Fractal · Mammographic tissue segmentation · Mammographic density classification · BI-RADS · Tabár

1 Introduction

Fractal dimension (FD) has been used to describe objects that possess self-similarity at all scales and levels of magnification. Such a (semi) self-similarity

© Springer International Publishing Switzerland 2016
A. Tingberg et al. (Eds.): IWDM 2016, LNCS 9699, pp. 359–366, 2016.
DOI: 10.1007/978-3-319-41546-8_45

to arbitrarily small scales can be found in many natural phenomena [1]. The Hausdorff dimension has been widely used for calculating highly irregular sets [2]. Existing fractal analysis techniques may try to characterise fractal behaviour by finding a set of appropriate scales which exhibit scaling behaviour; however, it has been observed that FD may have been misinterpreted and applied to some biomedical images where fractal behaviours are not present over a predetermined scale [3].

A popular way to calculate FD is the box-counting (BC) method [4]. Such a method uses the best fitting procedure and involves recursively partitioning the structural space with a fixed square grid in quadrants, each fractal structure under different scales is a quasi-copy of the whole. The number of non-empty boxes required to cover the fractal structure depends on the box size (scale). The implementation is flexible and can be robust. However, the process of non-empty boxes implies its use only for binary images, and is not applicable for analysing 2D grey-level images. Differential box counting (DBC) was proposed as an extension to BC for processing grey-scale images [5], where image intensity is considered as a 3D spatial surface during the fractal calculation. Such techniques have been applied to breast tumour classification [6] and micro-calcification detection [7]. Oliver *et al.* [8] investigated the use of FD for mammographic density segmentation (*e.g.* [9] and [10]), where an image is iteratively split into four equal size blocks if the local histogram covers a wide intensity range. The iteration stops when the decision function meets the criteria which indicates the current quadrant consists of uniform tissue. This resulted in rather large and coarse pixelated segmentation due to its quad tree structure based splitting and block tissue analysis. The approach may be less effective when tissue variations are small, and has a tendency to over or under estimate the number of boxes needed to cover a surface. Several DBC computational related issues were addressed in [11], including box scale selection, box number determination, and image intensity surface partition, whilst border effect and non-integer values of selected scales were investigated in [12]. Different improvements and their variations has led to a group of statistically self-similar fractal analysis approaches, the design of which may be suitable only for specific applications. As for a statistically self-affine fractal, fractional Brownian motion has been proven useful in characterising breast masses and tumours [13].

As a generalisation of the intuitive notion of topological dimension [14], FD can be used to measure the complexity of density variations and their association with breast tissue heterogeneity/homogeneity. Noise and artefacts may be introduced during mammographic image acquisition, despite that there is an intrinsic problem with mammograms in general; X-ray mammograms are 2D projections of 3D anatomical structures. Tissue superimposing as seen in such a modality may exhibit no local self-similarity in mammographic parenchyma, nor showing possession of basic fractal properties at any scale. However, certain structural similarities at different spatial scales are evident. This paper proposes a fractal inspired feature to characterise breast parenchyma roughness (complexity) for mammographic tissue segmentation. Based on the Hausdorff dimension,

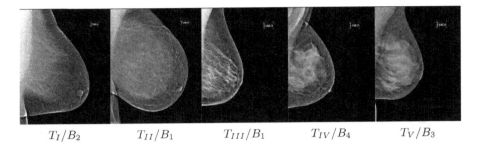

T_I/B_2 T_{II}/B_1 T_{III}/B_1 T_{IV}/B_4 T_V/B_3

Fig. 1. Example mammographic images; Tabár (T) and BI-RADS (B).

the approach is distinctively different to other existing fractal methods (*e.g.* BC and DBC) for surface roughness estimation. Such an approach analyses local fractal like properties and self-similarity is measured using the intensity distribution at different grey scale intervals. A multiresolution stack representation and 3D histogram features are incorporated to facilitate mammographic tissue segmentation and subsequent density/risk classification.

BI-RADS (Breast Imaging Reporting and Data System) 5th edition [15] indicates the importance of the association of estimated breast density with changes in the sensitivity of mammography. Breast composition is used to reflect the masking effect of dense fibroglandular tissue on mammographic depiction of noncalcified lesions; B_1 is almost entirely fat ($\lesssim 25\%$ glandular), B_2 has scattered fibroglandular densities $\approx(25\% - 50\%)$, B_3 consists of heterogeneously dense breast tissue $\approx(51\% - 75\%)$, and B_4 is extremely dense ($\gtrsim 75\%$ glandular). Alternatively, Tabár *et al.* [16] suggested that breast tissue composition based on mixtures of mammographic building blocks (i.e. [nodular%, linear%, homogeneous%, radiolucent%]) can be used to indicate mammographic risk; T_I [25\%, 15\%, 35\%, 25\%], T_{II} [2\%, 14\%, 2\%, 82\%], T_{III} is similar in composition to T_{II} except that the retroareolar prominent ducts are often associated with periductal fibrosis, T_{IV} [49\%, 19\%, 15\%, 17\%], and T_V [2\%, 2\%, 89\%, 7\%]. Figure 1 shows example mammographic images with Tabár risk classifications and their equivalent according to the BI-RADS density categories.

2   Data and Method

A total of 360 digital mammographic images (from 90 patients) were processed for optimal visual appearance to radiologists. The dataset containing 180 Mediolateral Oblique (MLO) and 180 Cranio-Caudal (CC) views. A consensus ground truth (i.e. density/risk labels) was obtained from three radiologists with mammographic reading experiences at the levels of junior, expert, and consultant.

The developed methodology has three steps; (1) generating a multiresolution stack representation, (2) feature extraction, and (3) clustering based segmentation. The workflow is illustrated in Fig. 2 and covered in subsequent subsections.

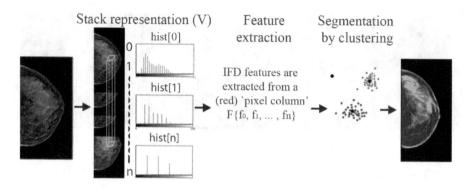

Fig. 2. Illustrated workflow for the developed methodology. (Color figure online)

2.1   Stack Representation

When an image is subjected to intensity binning, the number of grey values used to display local breast tissue is also reduced, correlated with the number of intensity bins used and shows regression. The proposed fractal inspired approach uses such a principle to calculate an intensity related "fractal dimension" (IFD) for local breast tissue. A multiresolution mammographic stack representation V is constructed to facilitate the calculation of IFD and 3D histogram features. Such a representation consists of a set of images with varying greylevel details, Fig. 2 shows an illustration for a V and the corresponding histograms. V can be constructed by first predefining a grey value interval T, which determines the number of sub-images Img_s and the number of available grey values nGV can be used by a sub-image. For example, the original image (Img_0) is used at the first level in V, which has intensity I ranging from I_{min} to I_{max} with one greylevel increment $inc = 1$ (*e.g.* $10, 11, 12, \ldots, 255$) and $nGV = I_{max} - I_{min}$. The image at the second level (Img_1) is constructed to the same I range but with $inc = T$ (*e.g.* $10, 10 + T, 10 + 2 \times T, \ldots, 10 + n \times T; 10 + n \times T \leq I_{max}$), resulting $nGV = (I_{max} - I_{min})/inc$. Empirical testing indicated that to construct a sufficient and statistically meaningful V, the nGV should be constrained to $10 \leq nGV \leq (I_{max} - I_{min})$. Therefore, $V(T) = \{Img_0, \ldots, Img_s\}$.

2.2   Features Extraction

Traditional FD can be calculated as

$$D = \lim_{s \to 0} \frac{log(N_s)}{log(1/S)}, \tag{1}$$

where N is the number of semi-similar structures in which an object can be subdivided and S is the scaling. By considering the number of grey values used to represent local breast tissue and the number of intensity bins used as "scaling", we can hypothesise that mammographic tissue roughness can be estimated from the log-log relationship commonly used to estimate FD. Note that this application specific approach is within the concept of the Hausdorff dimension as it obeys a power-law relation. The IFD for each pixel column in V (*e.g.* red column in Fig. 2) can be calculated as follows: (1) starting from the top level (sub image), count the number of pixels used to display the local breast tissue within a square window w, $W \in \{5, 7, 9\}$ was empirically defined to cover small to large anatomical structures; (2) plot the log of counted pixels against the log of the nGV index for each level; (3) repeat (1) and (2) for all the levels, yielding a set of points on a line; and (4) calculate the slope of the best-fitting straight line to the plot gives the IFD of the pattern, see Fig. 3 for example plots with corresponding local mammographic patches. The expectation of using such a stack representation for calculating IFD is to reduce anatomical noise (overlapping of fine structures) at low nGV levels which can affect clustering based segmentation, but at the same time V still conveys meaningful changes in surface roughness as (pixel) resolution reduces.

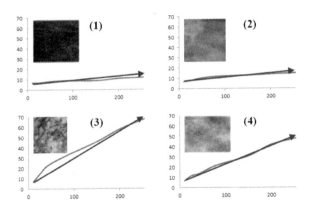

Fig. 3. Illustrative plots showing the slopes for (1) fatty, (2) high density, (3) fibroglandular and (4) heterogeneous tissue. X-axis and Y-axis are the number of pixels used to display the breast tissue and intensity scaling (nGV index), respectively.

The IFD feature is specifically designed to measure breast tissue surface roughness. In addition, six pseudo 3D texture features were calculated for each pixel column. Extended from classic 2D first-order statistics, these features tend to correlate to mammographic density [17], including

$$mean(\mu_w) = \frac{\sum\limits_{i=0,j=0}^{W_w} \sum\limits_{k=0}^{S} V(i,j,k)}{W_w^2 \times S} \tag{2}$$

$$standard\ deviation(\sigma_w) = \frac{\sum\limits_{i=0,j=0}^{W_w} \sum\limits_{k=0}^{S} (V(i,j,k) - \mu_w)}{W_w^2 \times S} \tag{3}$$

$$energy(\epsilon_w) = \frac{\sum\limits_{i=0,j=0}^{W_w} \sum\limits_{k=0}^{S} V^2(i,j,k)}{W_w^2 \times S} \tag{4}$$

$$entropy(\varepsilon_w) = \frac{\sum\limits_{i=0,j=0}^{W_w} \sum\limits_{k=0}^{S} V(i,j,k)(-ln\,V(i,j,k))}{W_w^2 \times S} \tag{5}$$

$$skewness(\lambda_w) = \frac{\sum\limits_{i=0,j=0}^{W_w} \sum\limits_{k=0}^{S} (V(i,j,k)-\mu_w)^3}{W_w^2 \times S \times \mu^3} \tag{6}$$

$$kurtosis(\tau_w) = \frac{\sum\limits_{i=0,j=0}^{W_w} \sum\limits_{k=0}^{S} (V(i,j,k)-\mu_w)^4}{W_w^2 \times S \times \mu^4} - 3 \tag{7}$$

where w and S denote the current window size and the sub images, respectively. Therefore, for each pixel column $V(i,j,k)$, a linear feature $F = \{\mu_w, \sigma_w, \epsilon_w, \varepsilon_w, \lambda_w, \tau_w\}$ concatenated with $IFD = \{ifd_w\}$ was constructed. The additional 3D histogram features are designed to enhance the overall statistical variations in the feature space.

2.3 Mammographic Segmentation and Density/Risk Classification

Clustering (K-means) based segmentation was used where the number of density classes $k = 4$, corresponding to fatty, semi-fatty (*e.g.* fibroglandular), semi-dense (*e.g.* heterogeneous densities), and dense tissue. For each segmented image, the breast tissue composition was calculated. Subsequent mammographic density and risk classifications were performed based on BI-RADS and Tabár scheme, respectively, using a leave one (woman) out methodology.

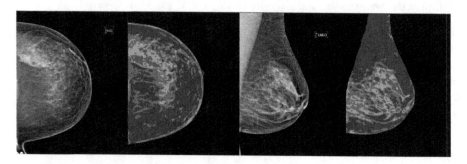

Fig. 4. Mammographic segmentation examples. Colour coding; fatty (navy), semi-fatty (grey), semi-dense (yellow), and high dense (red) tissue. (Color figure online)

3   Results and Discussion

Segmentation results show realistic tissue separations over anatomical structures, see Fig. 4 for examples. The developed IFD can be used to describe local breast tissue composition complexity, which reflects intensity surface roughness and texture heterogeneity/homogeneity at different level of grey scales. For local breast tissue where the intensity is heterogeneously distributed in the spatial structure, the IFD becomes smaller as the number of grey values decreases, indicating that homogeneity of the spatial structure is increasing. Note that heterogeneity at small scales can be quite homogeneous when examined at larger scales or vice versa. The additional 3D histogram features worked well with IFD in describing breast parenchyma. The experiment did not include analysis on cases of benign or malignant lesions. However, the proposed IFD is expected to be able to differentiate lesions with different surface roughness associated with different malignancies and intensity variations. The 3D measurement may be suitable for analysing tomosynthesis (DBT) data. It is because tomographic separation of the breast tissue as seen in such a modality, allows volumetric parenchymal properties such as self-similarity being reflected in IFD and applicable for the true 3D texture measurement. Caution is needed when extending the approach to DBT, as the pseudo 3D texture features are extracted column-wise through the entire stack. In a true 3D analysis this may include multiple tissue types to be analysed which is not ideal. The density classification accuracy was 78 % (CC 77 % and MLO 79 %) for the BI-RADS scheme and the risk classification was 74 % (CC 72 % and MLO 75 %) for the Tabár scheme. Table 1 shows the confusion matrices. In both cases, mammographic images in high density/risk classes seem to have more misclassification (percentage wise). Current grey value scaling was set up to use an even interval, an objective approach to this IFD based segmentation would be to assess the clinical relevance of different scale ranges, and determine the appropriate scales at which the IFD is more relevant for the application.

Table 1. Classification confusion matrices for BI-RADS and Tabár scheme.

BI-RADS	B_1	B_2	B_3	B_4
B_1	95	29	13	0
B_2	14	143	1	0
B_3	8	3	41	2
B_4	1	1	4	5

Tabár	T_I	$T_{II/III}$	T_{IV}	T_V
T_I	154	12	0	4
$T_{II/III}$	34	74	10	5
T_{IV}	0	12	26	5
T_V	1	2	8	11

4   Conclusions

The developed mammographic segmentation methodology is inspired by traditional fractal methods. The results show anatomically accurate segmentation over the breast parenchyma, leading to satisfactory density/risk classification accuracies. The discussed methodology shortcomings warrant further investigations, especially in the areas of quantification of change of relative proportion of breast tissue, for aiding radiologists' estimation in mammographic density/risk assessment, and providing risk-stratified screening to patients.

References

1. Lopes, R., Betrouni, N.: Fractal and multifractal analysis: a review. Med. Image Anal. **13**(4), 634–649 (2009)
2. Theiler, J.: Estimating fractal dimension. J. Opt. Soc. Am. A **7**(6), 1055–1073 (1990)
3. Ciccotti, M., Mulargia, F.: Pernicious effect of physical cutoffs in fractal analysis. Phys. Rev. E **65**, 037201 (2002)
4. Napolitana, A., Ungania, S., Cannata, V. (eds.): Fractal dimension estimation methods for biomedical images. In: INTECH 2012 (2012)
5. Sarker, N., Chaudhuri, B.B.: An efficient differential box-counting approach to compute fractal dimension of image. IEEE Trans. Syst. Man Cybern. **24**, 115–120 (1994)
6. Dobrescu, R., Ichim, L., Crian, D.: Diagnosis of breast cancer from mammograms by using fractal measures. Int. J. Med. Imaging **1**(2), 32–38 (2013)
7. Zhang, P., Agyepong, K.: Wavelet-based fractal feature extraction for microcalcification detection in mammograms. In: IEEE SoutheastCon, pp. 147–150 (2010)
8. Oliver, A., Freixenet, J., Martí, R., Zwiggelaar, R.: A comparison of breast tissue classification techniques. In: Larsen, R., Nielsen, M., Sporring, J. (eds.) MICCAI 2006. LNCS, vol. 4191, pp. 872–879. Springer, Heidelberg (2006)
9. Oliver, A., Freixenet, J., Marti, R., Pont, J., Pérez, E., Denton, E.R.E., Zwiggelaar, R.: A novel breast tissue density classification methodology. IEEE Trans. Inf. Technol. Biomed. **12**(1), 55–65 (2008)
10. He, W., Juette, A., Denton, E.R.E., Oliver, A., Marti, R., Zwiggelaar, R.: A review on automatic mammographic density and parenchymal segmentation. Int. J. Breast Cancer, Article ID 276217 (2015)
11. Li, J., Du, Q., Sun, C.: An improved box-counting method for image fractaldimension estimation. Pattern Recogn. **42**(11), 2460–2469 (2009)
12. Buczkowski, S., Kyriacos, S., Nekka, F., Cartilier, L.: The modified box-counting method: analysis of some characteristics parameters. Pattern Recogn. **3**, 411–418 (1998)
13. Voss, R.F.: Random fractal forgeries. Fundam. Algorithms Comput. Graph. **17**, 805–835 (1991)
14. Fernández-Martínez, M., Sánchez-Granero, M.A.: Fractal dimension for fractal structures. Topology Appl. **163**, 93–111 (2014)
15. American College of Radiology: Breast Imaging Reporting, Data System BI-RADS, 5th edn. American College of Radiology, Reston (2013)
16. Tabár, L., Tot, T., Dean, P.B., Cancer, B.: The Art And Science Of Early Detection With Mamography: Perception, Interpretation, Histopatholigic Correlation, 1st edn. Georg Thieme, Stuttgart (2004)
17. He, W., Juette, A., Denton, E.R.E., Zwiggelaara, R.: Novel multiresolution mammographic density segmentation using pseudo 3D features, adaptive cluster merging. In: SPIE Proceedings: Medical Imaging, vol. 9413, pp. 94133I-1–94133I-6 (2015)

Whole Mastectomy Volume Reconstruction from 2D Radiographs and Its Mapping to Histology

Thomy Mertzanidou[1]([⊠]), John H. Hipwell[1], Sara Reis[1],
Babak Ehteshami Bejnordi[2], Meyke Hermsen[4], Mehmet Dalmis[2],
Suzan Vreemann[2], Bram Platel[2], Jeroen van der Laak[2], Nico Karssemeijer[2],
Ritse Mann[3], Peter Bult[4], and David J. Hawkes[1]

[1] Centre for Medical Image Computing, University College London,
Gower Street, London WC1E 6BT, UK
t.mertzanidou@cs.ucl.ac.uk
[2] Diagnostic Image Analysis Group, Radboud University Medical Centre,
P.O. Box 9101, 6500 HB Nijmegen, The Netherlands
[3] Department of Radiology, Radboud University Medical Centre,
P.O. Box 9101, 6500 HB Nijmegen, The Netherlands
[4] Department of Pathology, Radboud University Medical Centre,
P.O. Box 9101, 6500 HB Nijmegen, The Netherlands

Abstract. Women that are diagnosed with breast cancer often undergo surgery to remove either the tumour and some of the surrounding tissue (lumpectomy) or the whole breast (mastectomy). After surgery, the excised tissue is sliced at the pathology department, where specimen radiographs of the slices are typically acquired. Representative parts of the tissue are then sampled for further processing, staining and examination under the microscope. The results of histopathological imaging are used for tumour characterisation. As the 3D structure of the specimen is inevitably lost during specimen handling, reconstructing a volume from individual specimen slices could facilitate the correlation of histology to radiological imaging. This work proposes a novel method for a whole specimen volume reconstruction and is validated on six mastectomy cases. We also demonstrate how these volumes can be used as a means to map multiple histology slides to a whole mastectomy image (MRI or CT).

Keywords: 3D volume reconstruction · Breast histology-radiology registration

1 Introduction

Spatial correspondence between radiological and histopathological breast imaging would be a valuable research tool, as it could lead to better interpretation of the in-vivo radiological images (such as MRIs and X-ray mammograms), routinely acquired for breast cancer detection, diagnosis and therapy monitoring.

© Springer International Publishing Switzerland 2016
A. Tingberg et al. (Eds.): IWDM 2016, LNCS 9699, pp. 367–374, 2016.
DOI: 10.1007/978-3-319-41546-8_46

Correlation of features extracted from the same locations in radiological and histological images has the potential to enable better in-vivo tumour characterisation, which could provide prognostic information and have a significant impact on patient stratification. Linking the radiological images to pathology could also be beneficial for pathologists, for example to assist them in selecting representative parts of the tissue for sampling and staining, that can then be used for tumour characterisation.

The tissue undergoes a number of severe deformations from the in-vivo state, when imaged in radiology, to the ex-vivo histological slide. In particular when the specimen is sliced after surgery, the coherence of the 3D structures within the breast tissue is lost. There has been increased interest within the medical image community in reconstructing a whole specimen volume, as this is key in relating the information from the microscopic to the macroscopic scale. Previous works were primarily focused on animal studies or organs that are less deformable than the breast; for example the brain and the prostate.

In pre-clinical studies, a number of previously proposed volume reconstruction techniques have used either a global or a local rigid transformation model to deform each slice in the volume [1–3]. This was often performed in combination with pairwise registrations, where each slice in the stack was aligned to its adjacent slice. The use of more than one slice in the local neighbourhood during alignment has been proposed [4–8] to favour smoothness of the reconstructed volume and coherence of the structures across slices.

In breast cancer studies, a 3D volume of a mouse's mammary gland was reconstructed from 2D histology images using rigid and elastic transformations [9]. In clinical studies, a volume was reconstructed from histology images either using manual interaction and pairwise affine transformations [10], or a pairwise rigid block-matching registration [11]. We have presented previously preliminary results that illustrated the benefit of using neighbourhood slice information in combination with a rigid transformation in order to reconstruct a whole breast specimen volume [12].

In this work, we propose the use of Free-Form Deformations (FFD) in combination with neighbourhood information from two adjacent slices for the 3D volume reconstruction of whole mastectomy samples from specimen slice radiographs. The main contribution of this work is algorithmic, as the proposed methodology combines the benefits of two previously proposed 3D volume reconstruction techniques applied on brain data [1,4] and further extends them, by incorporating a flexible non-linear transformation model [13], instead of the rigid transformation originally used. The combination of using two target adjacent slices with a non-linear transformation during alignment, results in more coherent reconstructed volumes, as demonstrated in the experiments and validated using whole specimen images (MRI and CT).

2   Methodology

The data used for the mastectomy volume reconstruction consist of 2D digital radiographs of the fresh specimen slices (before formalin fixation) that are acquired routinely in pathology at the hospital's mammography station (GE Medical Systems 147 Senograph 2000D). The slices are typically 4–5 mm thick. The individual slices are initially stacked and aligned using 2D pairwise registrations, as previously proposed for the animal brain volume reconstruction [1]. The mid-slice is chosen as a reference and remains unchanged. Each slice is aligned to its adjacent neighbouring slice towards the centre of the stack, using a 2D registration. For this task, an intensity-based approach in combination with a rigid block-matching transformation is used, providing the advantage of using the local similarity within blocks in the two images for the alignment, rather than the overall similarity across the whole images.

After the pairwise registrations, we apply an additional registration step, where the alignment of each slice I_i is driven by its similarity to both adjacent slices in the stack, one towards the centre and one towards the end of the stack (I_{i-1} and I_{i+1}). This approach has been proposed previously for the reconstruction of a rat's brain [4]. However, its flexibility was limited due to the use of a rigid transformation model. We propose deforming each slice using a non-linear transformation, based on B-splines (FFD) [13]. The combination of a non-linear transformation with the alignment of each slice to both its adjacent neighbours simultaneously favours the reconstruction of coherent breast tissue structures across the direction of the specimen slicing. As in the pairwise registrations, the mid-slice in the volume I_r is used as reference and it is not being deformed. For N slices in the volume, we seek the optimal parameters $\Phi = \{\Phi_1, ..., \Phi_{r-1}, \Phi_{r+1}, ..., \Phi_N\}$, where Φ_i are the transformation parameters corresponding to each 2D slice. For a 2D FFD these are the displacements in x and y of the control points in the mesh. Thus Φ_i denotes the $n_x^i \times n_y^i$ mesh of control points $\phi_{j,k}^i$ defined on image I_i. The FFD is then defined as:

$$T_{\Phi_i}(p) = \sum_{m=0}^{3}\sum_{n=0}^{3} B_m(u)B_n(v)\phi_{j+m,k+n}^i, \tag{1}$$

where $p = (x, y)$, $j = \lfloor x/n_x \rfloor - 1$, $k = \lfloor y/n_y \rfloor - 1$, $u = x/n_x - \lfloor x/n_x \rfloor$, $v = y/n_y - \lfloor y/n_y \rfloor$ and B_m is the m-th basis function of the B-splines.

If S is the similarity across all 2D slices in the volume, we can define the optimisation problem of the global energy function $E(\Phi)$ as: $\hat{\Phi} = \underset{\Phi}{\mathrm{argmax}}(E(\Phi))$, where

$$E(\Phi) = \sum_{i=1}^{N-1} E_i(\Phi_i) = \sum_{i=1}^{N-1}\sum_{j\in R_i}\sum_{p\in\Omega} S(I_i(T_{\Phi_i}(p)), I_j(T_{\Phi_j}(p))). \tag{2}$$

R_i denotes the neighbouring slices of image I_i (in our case its two adjacent slices) and $I_i(T_{\Phi_i}(p))$ is the image I_i at the transformed position $T_{\Phi_i}(p)$ using the parameters Φ_i. We optimise the local energy E_i sequentially for each 2D slice in the stack. In all registrations, we use Normalised Cross Correlation as a cost function and a gradient descent optimisation scheme.

3 Experiments

For validation we firstly assess the smoothness of the reconstruction using six mastectomy samples. For this task we use the distance of each 2D slice contour from the contour of its two adjacent neighbouring images. For each slice i in the stack this distance is $d_i = \frac{d_{i,i-1}+d_{i,i+1}}{2}$, where $d_{i,j}$ is the mean Euclidean distance between the points in the contour corresponding to slice i and the closest points in the contour of slice j. For each reconstructed volume, the mean distance for all N 2D slices is $d = \frac{1}{N}\sum_{i=1}^{N} d_i$. This value represents the mean distance of each slice contour from its two adjacent slices and it provides a metric of surface smoothness in the volume reconstruction. The results are shown in Fig. 1a. Each mastectomy sample has been reconstructed using three separate techniques: (1) The initialisation before registration, where the slices are translated across the X-axis using their centre of mass (X-TR volume), (2) A pairwise rigid block-matching algorithm (P-BM volume) and (3) Our proposed volume reconstruction with FFD and simultaneous alignment of each slice to its two adjacent neighbours (FFD-N2 volume). The mean contour distance has been computed for each of these three volume reconstruction approaches. For all patients, the mean, standard deviation, minimum and maximum distance values were lower for our approach. Examples of the reconstructed volumes are shown in Figs. 2 and 3.

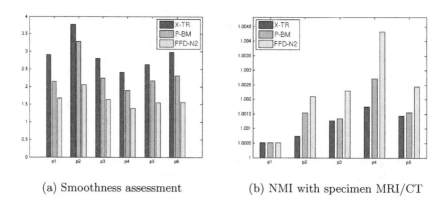

(a) Smoothness assessment   (b) NMI with specimen MRI/CT

Fig. 1. Validation of the proposed algorithm using (a) the outer contours of the slices and (b) the internal intensities. (a) Mean contour distances for each of the three reconstruction methods: X-TR, P-BM and FFD-N2. (b) NMI value between the whole specimen image and each of the three reconstructed volumes. (Color figure online)

After a quantitative assessment based on the outer boundaries of the 2D slices, we assess how well the internal breast tissue structures are reconstructed. For this task a whole specimen image was acquired for five cases before slicing and was used as ground truth for validation (this was an MRI for p1 and a CT for p2-p5). The MRI and the CT images were acquired at clinical scanners, a 3T

Siemens TrioTim and a Toshiba Aquilion ONE respectively. The whole specimen image was registered independently, to each of the three reconstructed mastectomy samples (X-TR, P-BM and FFD-N2) using a 3D rigid registration followed by FFD. The final value of the similarity measure – Normalised Mutual Information (NMI) – computed by the registration, provides a quantitative measure of the similarity in the appearance of the internal tissue structures between the reconstruction and the specimen volume before slicing. The results for all five cases are illustrated in Fig. 1b. For four patients FFD-N2 provides an improvement in the similarity measure compared to X-TR and P-BM, while for p1 all three reconstruction techniques produce similar results. Figure 2f illustrates the whole specimen image of p2 aligned with the 3D volume reconstruction in Fig. 2d. Similarly, Figs. 3e and f display the results for patients p1 and p3 respectively.

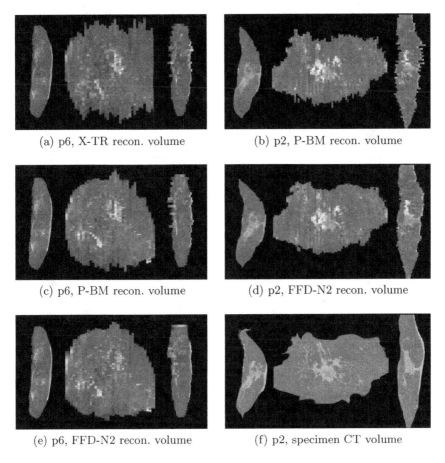

(a) p6, X-TR recon. volume   (b) p2, P-BM recon. volume

(c) p6, P-BM recon. volume   (d) p2, FFD-N2 recon. volume

(e) p6, FFD-N2 recon. volume   (f) p2, specimen CT volume

Fig. 2. Reconstructed mastectomy samples for p6 (a, c and e) and p2 (b and d) using different methods. (f) shows the specimen CT of p2. In all images, from left to right: axial, coronal and sagittal planes.

372 T. Mertzanidou et al.

Finally, we illustrate how a mastectomy volume, reconstructed from the 2D slice radiographs, can be used as a means to align multiple histology slides to a whole specimen image. For this task, multiple digitised H&E images of cases p1 and p3 were initially registered to the 2D specimen radiographs. The 3D volumes were then reconstructed using FFD-N2 and the whole specimen volumes were aligned to them (Fig. 3). We can see in the example images that the H&E sections do not cover the complete specimen, as the volumes are typically only sparsely sampled.

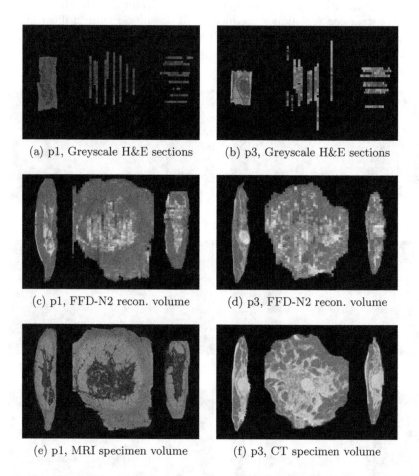

(a) p1, Greyscale H&E sections   (b) p3, Greyscale H&E sections

(c) p1, FFD-N2 recon. volume   (d) p3, FFD-N2 recon. volume

(e) p1, MRI specimen volume   (f) p3, CT specimen volume

Fig. 3. Mapping digitised histological sections to a whole specimen image (MRI and CT) via the reconstructed volume: for p1 (a, c and e) and p3 (b, d and f). In all images, from left to right: axial, coronal and sagittal planes.

4 Discussion

We have presented a novel method for the 3D volume reconstruction of a whole specimen from individual 2D slice radiographs. The proposed algorithm combines a flexible transformation model with neighbourhood information from the adjacent slices when transforming each slice in the volume, thus favouring coherency of the 3D structures across the slices. The smoothness of the reconstruction was validated on six mastectomy cases. For five of these cases, a whole specimen image (MRI or CT) was acquired. This was used as a ground truth image of the 3D breast anatomy before slicing and enabled the validation of the reconstruction with respect to the internal breast structures. We also demonstrated how the reconstructed volume can be used as a means to map H&E slides to a radiological image of the whole specimen. This is an important step towards mapping microscopic features in histology to macroscopic features in in-vivo radiological imaging. Future work will be focused on aligning the whole specimen image to an in-vivo breast MRI, completing the registration pipeline from histology to in-vivo imaging.

Acknowledgements. This study was funded by the European 7th Framework Program grant VPH-PRISM (FP7-ICT-2011-9, 601040) and the Engineering and Physical Sciences Research Council grant MIMIC (EP/K020439/1).

References

1. Ourselin, S., Roche, A., Subsol, G., Pennec, X., Ayache, N.: Reconstructing a 3D structure from serial histological sections. Image Vis. Comput. **19**(1), 25–31 (2001)
2. Pitiot, A., Guimond, A.: Geometrical regularization of displacement fields for histological image registration. Med. Image Anal. **12**(1), 16–25 (2008)
3. Alic, L., Haeck, J.C., Bol, K., Klein, S., van Tiel, S.T., Wielepolski, P.A., de Jong, M., Niessen, W.J., Bernsen, M., Veenland, J.F.: Facilitating tumor functional assessment by spatially relating 3D tumor histology and in vivo MRI: image registration approach. PloS ONE **6**(8), e22835 (2011)
4. Nikou, C., Heitz, F., Nehlig, A., Namer, I., Armspach, J.: A robust statistics-based global energy function for the alignment of serially acquired autoradiographic sections. J. Neurosci. Methods **124**(1), 93–102 (2003)
5. Yushkevich, P.A., Avants, B.B., Ng, L., Hawrylycz, M., Burstein, P.D., Zhang, H., Gee, J.C.: 3D mouse brain reconstruction from histology using a coarse-to-fine approach. In: Pluim, J.P.W., Likar, B., Gerritsen, F.A. (eds.) WBIR 2006. LNCS, vol. 4057, pp. 230–237. Springer, Heidelberg (2006)
6. Bagci, U., Bai, L.: Automatic best reference slice selection for smooth volume reconstruction of a mouse brain from histological images. Med. Imaging, IEEE Trans. **29**(9), 1688–1696 (2010)
7. Feuerstein, M., Heibel, H., Gardiazabal, J., Navab, N., Groher, M.: Reconstruction of 3-D histology images by simultaneous deformable registration. In: Fichtinger, G., Martel, A., Peters, T. (eds.) MICCAI 2011, Part II. LNCS, vol. 6892, pp. 582–589. Springer, Heidelberg (2011)

8. Cifor, A., Bai, L., Pitiot, A.: Smoothness-guided 3-D reconstruction of 2-D histological images. Neuroimage **56**(1), 197–211 (2011)
9. Arganda-Carreras, I., Fernández-González, R., Muñoz-Barrutia, A., Ortiz-De-Solorzano, C.: 3D reconstruction of histological sections: application to mammary gland tissue. Microsc. Res. Tech. **73**(11), 1019–1029 (2010)
10. Clarke, G., Murray, M., Holloway, C., Liu, K., Zubovits, J., Yaffe, M.: 3D pathology volumetric technique: a method for calculating breast tumour volume from whole-mount serial section images. Int. J. Breast Cancer **2012**, 691205 (2012)
11. Reis, S., Eiben, B., Mertzanidou, T., Hipwell, J., Hermsen, M., van der Laak, J., Pinder, S., Bult, P., Hawkes, D.: Minimum slice spacing required to reconstruct 3D shape for serial sections of breast tissue for comparison with medical imaging. In: SPIE Medical Imaging, p. 94200K. International Society for Optics and Photonics (2015)
12. Mertzanidou, T., Hipwell, J., Dalmis, M., Platel, B., van der Laak, J., Mann, R., Karssemeijer, N., Bult, P., Hawkes, D.: Towards spatial correspondence between specimen and in-vivo breast imaging. In: Fujita, H., Hara, T., Muramatsu, C. (eds.) IWDM 2014. LNCS, vol. 8539, pp. 674–680. Springer, Heidelberg (2014)
13. Rueckert, D., Sonoda, L., Hayes, C., Hill, D., Leach, M., Hawkes, D.: Nonrigid registration using free-form deformations: application to breast mr images. Med. Imaging, IEEE Trans. **18**(8), 712–721 (1999)

Image Processing, CAD, Breast Density
and New Technology

Accurate Quantification of Glandularity and Its Applications with Regard to Breast Radiation Doses and Missed Lesion Rates During Individualized Screening Mammography

Mika Yamamuro[1(✉)], Kanako Yamada[1], Yoshiyuki Asai[1], Koji Yamada[1], Yoshiaki Ozaki[2], Masao Matsumoto[3], and Takamichi Murakami[4]

[1] Department of Central Radiology, Kindai University Hospital, Osaka-sayama, Japan
yamamuro@radt.med.kindai.ac.jp
[2] Research Institute of Scientific Investigation,
Kyoto Prefectural Police Headquarters, Osaka-sayama, Japan
[3] Division of Health Sciences, Graduate School of Medicine, Osaka University,
Osaka-sayama, Japan
[4] Department of Radiology, Kindai University Faculty of Medicine, Osaka-sayama, Japan

Abstract. Mammography, the most effective early breast cancer detection technique, is associated with the risk of missed lesions in dense breasts, and excessive X-ray exposure. Accurate estimations of glandularity and radiation dose are important during screening. We propose a novel, inexpensive method for accurate glandularity quantification using pixel values in clinical digital mammograms and X-ray exposure spectra. Glandularities were calculated for 314 mammograms in Japanese women, and the Dance formula c-factor was applied to estimate breast doses. To investigate the relationship between breast thickness and missed lesions, images were classified into four categories based on the rate of missed lesions, and correlated with breast thickness. Glandularity decreased with increasing compressed breast thickness, indicating that commonly used breast doses (assumed 50% glandularity) significantly overestimate thin breasts and underestimate thick breasts. The missed lesion rate was higher for thinner compressed breast thicknesses. Accurate glandularity estimation could thus promote individualized screening mammography.

Keywords: Individualized screening mammography · Glandularity · Breast dose · X-ray spectrum · Missed lesion rate

1 Introduction

Breast cancer is among the most common causes of death in women [1, 2], and early detection is required to reduce the incidence of fatality. Currently, mammography is the most effective modality for the early detection of breast cancer and has been accepted by many countries worldwide [3, 4]; this modality is associated with issues such as the risk of missed lesions in dense breasts and X-ray exposure. Therefore, those examined should receive accurate information about breast dose values and recommendations of

© Springer International Publishing Switzerland 2016
A. Tingberg et al. (Eds.): IWDM 2016, LNCS 9699, pp. 377–384, 2016.
DOI: 10.1007/978-3-319-41546-8_47

other modalities based on individual glandularity; in other words, individualized screening mammography.

In this study, we proposed a novel method to quantify glandularity in the breasts of individual Japanese women using pixel values in digital mammogram and X-ray exposure spectra, measured under actual mammographic exposure conditions [5, 6]. Subsequently, quantified glandularity was substituted into the Dance formula c-factor [7] to accurately estimate the breast dose. Furthermore, we clarified the relationship between glandularity and the degree of missed lesions within a comprehensive approach to clinical application. This study aimed to support individualized screening mammography from the viewpoints of quantitative glandularity analysis, accurate breast dose estimation, and elucidation of the relationship between compressed breast thickness and missed lesions during mammography.

2   Materials and Methods

The outline of this study is shown in Fig. 1. A total of 314 mediolateral oblique-view mammograms from Japanese women aged 25–85 years with apparently normal breasts were used in this study. We selected the contralateral breasts to involved side. All images were radiographed by the Toshiba Pe-ru-ru mammographic system, equipped with a target/filter of molybdenum/molybdenum (for less than 20 mm breast thickness) or molybdenum/rhodium (for over 20 mm breast thickness). The evaluation was conducted in the following three stages.

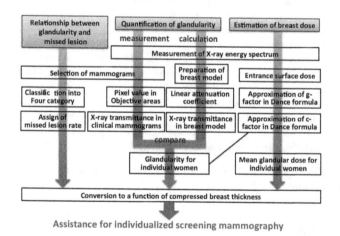

Fig. 1. Outline of this study

2.1   Quantification of Glandularity

We assumed that the breast consists of only two components: glandular and adipose tissue. Pixel values were measured at two locations on clinical mammograms (one with only adipose tissue, and the other with both adipose and glandular tissue), using a histogram function incorporated in Image J software (Fig. 2). Two expert radiological technologists, who have over 7 years experience in mammography, performed these measurements. A set of pixel values was converted to an X-ray intensity attenuation ratio using a characteristic curve. In addition, the theoretical attenuation ratio values for every combination of adipose and glandular tissue thicknesses were calculated using measured X-ray spectra and linear attenuation coefficients [5, 6, 8]. To quantify glandularity, we compared both the attenuation ratios to identify a combination with an attenuation ratio closest to that of a clinical mammogram. In this study, a breast model surrounded by a 2.5-mm adipose layer was assumed for a compressed breast thickness ranging from 2 cm to 5 cm, and glandularity was defined as the fraction of glandular tissue by weight within the central region, excluding the 2.5-mm adipose layer.

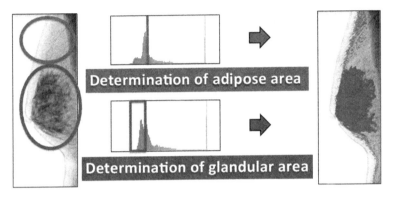

Fig. 2. The central figure shows the distribution of the pixels values, that is, the histogram corresponding to the circled area in the left image. The adipose and glandular tissues are colored red and blue, respectively, in the right side image (Color figure online)

2.2 Estimation of the Breast Dose

Rather than an assumed constant glandularity of 50%, the quantitative glandularity, determined as described in Sect. 2.1, was applied to the c-factor in the Dance formula [7] to estimate an accurate mean glandular dose (MGD). The compressed breast thickness range was the same as that described in Sect. 2.1. The entrance surface dose in air kerma (ESD) under clinical mammographic exposure conditions was also obtained from the X-ray spectra using the mAs (exposure current × exposure second) value.

2.3 Relationship Between Glandularity and Missed Lesion Rate

In mammography, the missed lesion is one of the most important problems related to a patient's liability, and false negatives are especially significant for dense breasts [9, 10]. To investigate the relationship between glandularity and missed lesion rate during clinical mammography, all images used in Sect. 2.1 were also classified by a radiologist into the following four categories based on the recommendations of the Japan Central Organization on Quality Assurance of Breast Cancer Screening: (1) dense breast, (2) homogeneous high density, (3) scattered glandular, and (4) fatty breast. The average glandularity was determined in each category. Although this classification correlates with the basic level of ease with which lesions are missed during clinical mammograms, it does not correspond to the quantitative missed lesion rate. We utilized mammographic sensitivity values to resolve this issue, as the value of 1−mammographic sensitivity is equal to the false-negative rate (i.e., missed lesion rate) of clinical mammograms. In this study, previously described mammographic sensitivities of 51.1%, 68.3%, 79.2%, and 90.7% were used for the above-described categories (1) to (4) [10]. The weighted average method, according to the occupancy rate of each category, was used to identify the relationship between the compressed breast thickness and the missed lesion rate in clinical mammograms.

3   Results and Discussion

We have restricted glandularity measurements to the area indicated by the blue circle in Fig. 2. This is based on subjective classifications for breast composition by the Japan Central Organization on Quality Assurance of Breast Cancer Screening. We believe this method is more suitable to obtain accurate estimations of glandularity, since it is clinically important to know how much adipose tissue is included in the densely packed glandular tissue.

Figure 3 shows that glandularity decreases with increasing patient's age. This tendency indicates that glandular tissue is replaced by the adipose tissue during the aging process. In Japanese women, the typical glandularity of a breast of 4 cm thickness was 51.0%. As shown in Fig. 4, glandularity increased as the compressed breast thickness decreased, in accordance with the assumed breast model and glandularity calculation described in Sect. 2.1. Thus, a breast thickness of 2 cm corresponded to a significantly higher glandularity. Consequently, thinner breasts were more strongly affected by the adipose layer. To resolve this issue, further research regarding the adipose layer thickness, corresponding to each compressed breast thickness, will be required.

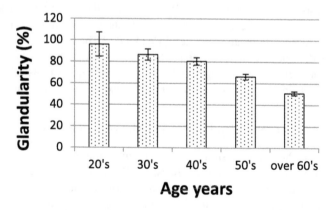

Fig. 3. Dependence of glandularity on participant age

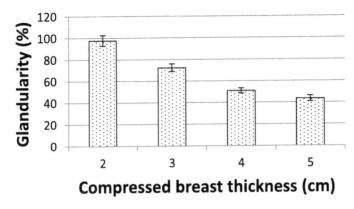

Fig. 4. Dependence of glandularity on compressed breast thickness

Figure 5 shows the MGD (per 1 mGy of ESD) as a function of compressed breast thickness. The dotted and solid lines indicate the results obtained with a simple 50% constant glandularity, and with quantitatively determined glandularity, respectively. The decreasing slope in both lines was due to the effect of the Dance formula g-factor (breast thickness conversion factor). Because the g-factor was identical for both conditions, the difference between MGD values was attributable to the effect of the Dance formula c-factor. Therefore, as shown in Fig. 5, the use of a simple 50% constant glandularity leads to a 13% overestimation at a breast thickness of 2 cm, and a 4% underestimation at 5 cm, underscoring that the appropriate use of the c-factor is an important step in accurate breast dose estimation.

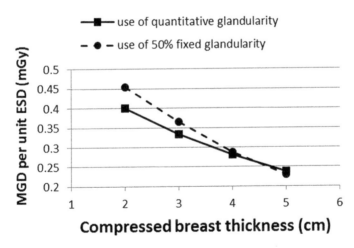

Fig. 5. Difference in mean glandular dose (MGD; per 1 mGy of entrance surface dose [ESD]) by compressed breast thickness, calculated using the Dance formula with either fixed or quantitative glandularity values. Differences are attributable to the effect of the c-factor in the Dance formula. Currently, a fixed value of 50% is used worldwide.

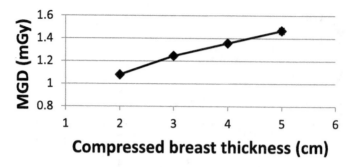

Fig. 6. Effect of compressed breast thickness on actual mean glandular dose (MGD) in clinical mammography

In actual clinical mammography, the ESD is adjusted using the automatic exposure control to maintain a constant X-ray energy per unit area for the detector. Figure 6 shows the actual MGD incurred by mammography. The actual MGD increased as compressed breast thickness increased; the increase in ESD that corresponded to compressed breast thickness was greater than the decrease in g-factor.

It should be noted that we do not intend here to suggest exposure doses for individual women. The exposure doses in this study are statistically averaged under the assumed condition that the adipose and glandular tissues are uniformly mixed. The elemental composition and distributions of glandular tissues within the breast are simply not known for any individual woman. Any changes in glandular tissue distribution will lead to changes in individual MGD value [11, 12].

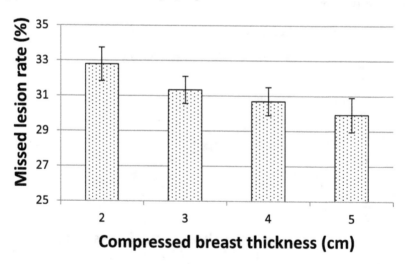

Fig. 7. Dependence of the missed lesion rate during clinical mammogram on compressed breast thickness

Both the breast radiation dose and missed lesion rate represent liabilities in screening mammography. Figure 7 presents the missed lesion rate during screening mammography as a function of compressed breast thickness; specifically, this rate decreased as the compressed breast thickness increased, because high glandularity within thinner breasts increased the difficulty of discriminating lesions that overlapped normal glandular tissues. The missed lesion rate for a 2-cm breast was approximately 10% higher than that of a 5-cm breast, because of this higher glandularity. Given the popularization of individualized screening mammography, it is important to have a clear understanding of these factors, and desirable for radiologists to provide this information to examinees promptly and accurately.

4   Conclusion

We proposed a novel method to quantitatively determine glandularity using pixel values and X-ray exposure spectra that does not require expensive software. By applying quantitative glandularity to the Dance formula, we could accurately determine the breast dose incurred during screening mammography. We therefore established that the use of a constant 50% glandularity in the Dance formula leads to significant overestimation of the radiation doses incurred in thin breasts. Furthermore, we quantitatively determined the relationship between the missed lesion rate during clinical mammography and compressed breast thickness.

In the near future, the establishment of a prediction formula for an accurate determination of glandularity, based on the results described in this study, will enable the prevention of liabilities associated with screening mammography, such as over- or underestimation of X-ray radiation doses, and the risk of missed lesions.

References

1. Paul, S., Solanki, P.P., Shahi, U.P., Srikrishna, S.: Epidemiological study on breast cancer associated risk factors and screening: practices among women in the holy city of Varanasi, Uttar Pradesh, India. Asian Pac. J. Cancer Prev. **16**, 8163–8171 (2015)
2. Braithwaite, D., Demb, J., Henderson, L.M.: Optimal breast cancer screening strategies for older women: current perspectives. Clin. Interv. Aging. **11**, 111–125 (2016)
3. Haddad, F.G., Kourie, H.R., Adib, S.M.: Trends in mammography utilization for breast cancer screening in a Middle-Eastern country: Lebanon 2005–2013. Cancer Epidemiol. **39**, 819–824 (2015)
4. Jayadevan, R., Armada, M.J., Shaheen, R., Mulcahy, C., Slanetz, P.J.: Optimizing digital mammographic image quality for full-field digital detectors: artifacts encountered during the QC process. Radiographics **35**, 2080–2089 (2015)
5. Maeda, K., Matsumoto, M., Taniguchi, A.: Compton-scattering measurement of diagnostic X-ray spectrum using high-resolution Schottky CdTe detector. Med. Phys. **32**, 1542–1547 (2005)
6. Tomal, A., Cunha, D.M., Antoniassi, M., Poletti, M.E.: Response functions of Si(Li), SDD and CdTe detectors for mammographic X-ray spectroscopy. Appl. Radiat. Isot. **70**, 1355–1359 (2012)
7. Dance, D.R., Skinner, C.L., Young, K.C., Beckett, J.R., Kotre, J.C.: Additional factors for the estimation of mean glandular breast dose using the UK mammography dosimetry protocol. Phys. Med. Biol. **45**, 3225–3240 (2000)

8. Hubbell, J.H., Seltzer, S.M.: Tables of X-ray mass attenuation coefficients and mass energy-absorption coefficients 1 keV to 20 MeV for elements Z1 to 92 and 48 additional substances of dosimetric interest. Technology Administration. USGPO Washington, D.C. (1995)

9. Peters, G., Jones, C.M., Daniels, K.: Why is microcalcification missed on mammography? J. Med. Imaging Radiat. Oncol. **57**, 32–37 (2013)

10. Suzuki, A., Kuriyama, S., Kawai, M., Amari, M., Takeda, M., et al.: Age-specific interval breast cancers in Japan: estimation of the proper sensitivity of screening using a population-based cancer registry. Cancer Sci. **99**, 2264–2267 (2008)

11. Dance, D.R., Hunt, R.A., Bakic, P.R., Maidment, A.D.A., Sandborg, M., Ullman, G., Carlsson, G.A.: Breast dosimetry using high-resolution voxel phantoms. Radiat. Prot. Dosim. **114**, 359–363 (2005)

12. Dance, D.R., Skinner, C.L., Carlsson, G.A.: Breast dosimetry. Appl. Radiat. Isot. **50**, 185–203 (1999)

A Preliminary Study on Breast Cancer Risk Analysis Using Deep Neural Network

Wenqing Sun[1], Tzu-Liang (Bill) Tseng[1], Bin Zheng[2,3], and Wei Qian[1,3(✉)]

[1] College of Engineering, University of Texas at El Paso, El Paso, TX, USA
weiqian188188@gmail.com
[2] College of Engineering, University of Oklahoma, Norman, OK, USA
[3] College of Biological Sciences, University of Texas at El Paso, El Paso, TX, USA

Abstract. Deep learning is a powerful tool in computer vision areas, but it is most effective when applied to large training sets. However, large dataset are not always available for medical images. In this study we proposed a new method to use deep neural network for near-term breast cancer risk analysis. In our data base, we have 420 cases with two sequential mammogram screenings, and half of the cases were diagnosed as positive in the second screening and the other half remained negative. Instead of using human designed features, we designed a deep neural network (DNN) with four pairs of convolution neural network and one fully connected layer. Every breast image were divided into 100 ROIs with 52 by 52 pixels, and each ROI were trained with the DNN individually, and the final predictions of each case were based on the overall risk scores of all the 100 ROIs. And the ROI based area under the curve (AUC) is 0.6982, and the case based AUC is 0.7173 using our proposed scheme. The results showed our proposed scheme is promising to apply deep learning algorithms in predicting near-term breast cancer risk with limited data size.

Keywords: Breast cancer · Risk analysis · Deep learning · Deep neural network · Convolutional neural network

1 Introduction

Breast cancer is one of leading death causes all over the world and predicting breast cancer risk has been studied more than 30 years [1]. Breast density has been treated as one of the most important and effective image based breast cancer risk measurements, and higher breast density usually means higher breast cancer risk [2]. However, the measurements of breast density are based on visual assessment of mammographic density by radiologists, and the density is rated and grouped into four American College of Radiology Breast Imaging Reporting and Data System (BI-RADS) density categories [3]. But these subjective ratings are inaccurate or inconsistent due to the large intra- and inter-observer variability [4]. From our previous research we also noticed that except density information, other image based features, like texture features, are also important to analyze breast cancer risk [5]. So how to efficiently design the reliable features is a great challenge for all the breast cancer risk researchers [6–8].

© Springer International Publishing Switzerland 2016
A. Tingberg et al. (Eds.): IWDM 2016, LNCS 9699, pp. 385–391, 2016.
DOI: 10.1007/978-3-319-41546-8_48

Recent three years, deep neural network (DNN) [9, 10] has been showing dramatic power in improving the performance of the state of the art computer vision tasks, including from segmentation to classification. Instead of designing and extracting the computational features from images manually, DNN can use the image itself as input and learn the features from the training images itself. We observed this opportunity in improving the performance of near-term breast cancer risk prediction, but like most deep learning algorithms, DNN requires a large number of training data for tuning parameters [11]. To collect data for breast cancer risk analysis research, we need the participants have at least two screening mammograms: the "prior" screening with negative diagnosis result, and "current" screening or medical report after 6 to 24 months after "prior" screening. In clinic, the majority women remain negative in the second screening, and to build a balanced dataset, we generally use same amount of negative and positive data. For these reasons, it is extremely hard to generate a large enough dataset for DNN. In this study, we developed a new scheme to use DNN on a limited data set for risk analysis, the details and results are listed below.

2   Materials and Methods

2.1   Dataset

Our dataset includes 420 pair of full-field digital mammography (FFDM) images from 420 women. All these data are randomly selected from pre-established data base, and all the participants have at least two screening mammography with the intervals between 6 months to 24 months. All "prior" mammograms were interpreted as normal by the radiologists at the time of screening, and half of the "current" mammograms are diagnosed as positive and the other half are diagnosed as benign or normal. For the positive cases, we used the "prior" mammograms from the same side of breast with later cancer diagnosis; for the negative cases, we randomly choose either right or left side mammograms. So for each case, we get two mammograms from one side, one mediolateral oblique (MLO) view and one craniocaudual (CC) view mammogram. In this study, we treat each mammogram as an independent and individual image, but we always put the mammograms from the same woman together for the training or testing (i.e. we will never use one mammogram for training and the other mammogram from the same case for testing).

2.2   Method

2.2.1   Mammogram Preprocessing

From these 420 cases, we get 840 mammograms altogether. The first step is to remove the mammogram labels and background, then we used computer to find the largest containing rectangular in each breast image. The size of these rectangular varies according to the size and shape of the original breast image. From each of the rectangular, we selected 100 52 pixel by 52 pixel region of interests (ROIs). To make these ROIs as much evenly distributed as possible, we meshed each rectangular with a 10 by 10 grid, and the center of each grid is the center of a ROI. If the rectangular is big, there would be some gap among the ROIs; if the rectangular is small, there would be some overlaps. After this step, 84000 ROIs were extracted and used as input for next step. Figure 1 showed an example of the ROIs extracted from one mammogram.

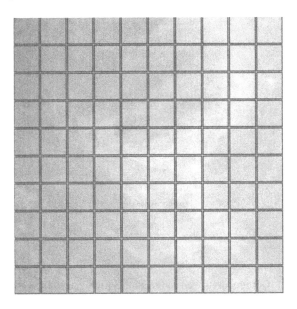

Fig. 1. An example of dividing 100 ROIs from one rectangular on mammogram

2.2.2 Convolutional Neural Network

Our deep neural network has eight convolutional neural network layers and one fully connected layer. The input image starts with the convolutional layer: a bank of 5 by 5 kernels is convolved with the original ROI in a moving window fashion. These kernels are randomly generated from uniform distribution with zero mean of unit norm. The second layer is the max-pooling layer, the bank of convolved images output the maximum activations in every non-overlapped square regions. In convolution layers of our proposed scheme, every odd number layers are convolutional layers, and every even number layers are max-pooling layers. The first two convolutional layers used 5 by 5 kernels, and the last two layers used 3 by 3 kernels. Also, the first and last convolutional layers have six output maps, and the two middle layers have twelve output maps. The fully connected layer transforms the output of the previous layer into a feature vector, and they are fully connected with the two classes (low risk and high risk classes) with a softmax function. The convolutional architecture is shown in Fig. 2.

2.2.3 Experimental Design and Evaluation

To develop and analyze the best way to use DNN in predicting the near-term breast cancer, we conducted two experiments for comparison. In the first experiment, we used the largest rectangular extracted from the breast area as the input to DNN, and all the rectangular are downsampled to the size of 52 by 52. So the 840 samples will be the

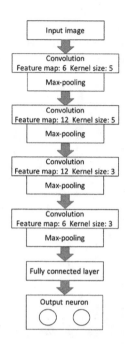

Fig. 2. Our proposed deep convolutional neural network structure

used for the training and testing. In the second experiment, we used all ROIs extracted from every rectangular to train and test the DNN. The total sample size is 84000. Since we divided one rectangular into many ROIs, we also tested and compared the DNN performance on different number of ROIs extracted from each rectangular at three different levels: 16, 64, 100. The 10-fold cross validation method is used for all experiments.

3   Results

For the first experiment, the DNN didn't converge; for the second experiment, the averaged accuracy is 0.6707 for all the 84000 ROIs (ROI based accuracy) using 10-fold cross validation. Since every breast image has 100 ROIs, and not every ROI has the same predicted risk label, so we set a percentage threshold t. If more than t ROIs from one image were predicted as high risk, we regarded this case as high risk case; otherwise, it was treated as low risk case. Based on different threshold t, we plotted the ROC curve in Fig. 3, and the threshold maximize the area of the containing rectangular under the curve is 0.5200. Using this threshold (t = 0.5200), the case based accuracy is 0.6972 and the ROI based accuracy is 0.6707, while the area under the curve (AUC) is 0.7173 and 0.6982 respectively. We also compared the different number of ROIs at three different levels: 16, 64, and 100 ROIs for each breast image. We compared the case based accuracy and ROI based accuracy, and the results are shown in the Table 1.

Table 1. Prediction accuracies using different amount of ROIs

	ROI amount in each breast image		
	16 (4 by 4)	64 (8 by 8)	100 (10 by 10)
ROI based accuracy	0.6590	0.6664	0.6707
Case based accuracy	0.6134	0.6523	0.6972

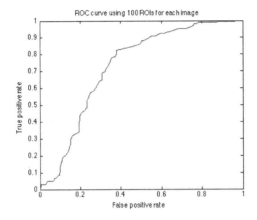

Fig. 3. ROC curve using 100 ROIs for each breast image

Figure 4 shows the some of the examples of feature maps from our DNN structure. These feature maps were generated by computer itself, and it is more representative than human-designed features. Intuitively, they are the combination of density, texture and orientations.

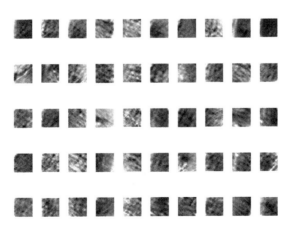

Fig. 4. Some examples of feature maps generated from our DNN algorithm

4   Discussions

From the results discussed above, it is very promising to use our proposed method to predict near-term breast cancer risk, and the case based accuracy is as high as 0.6972. To the best of our knowledge, this is the first study using deep learning algorithms in breast cancer risk prediction. Usually, deep learning methods require a large dataset to train numerous parameters inside the structure, and it is not easy to collect tens of thousands of medical image labeled data since it is a great burden for radiologists to mark the ground truth. And in most situations, one medical image need three or four radiologists to make sure the group truth is as objective as possible. For breast cancer risk analysis, the data is even harder to collect because each case need two successive screening results ranging from 6 months to 24 months, and the majority of the data remained normal or benign in the second screening that makes most of these cases have to be removed from the dataset to keep its balance. In this situation, we designed a DNN based deep learning structure and divide each image into 100 ROIs, the final results are based on the overall predictions on all these 100 ROIs in one image. We also compared the scheme using the raw data only without dividing them into multiple ROIs, the classifier cannot converge on this limited dataset.

In our proposed method, we predict each case's cancer risk score based on the percentage of the ROIs with its score surpassed the threshold. Based on different thresholds, we plotted the ROC curve and find the best threshold that maximizes the area of containing rectangular under the curve. Under this threshold the cased based accuracy is 0.6972 and ROI based accuracy is 0.6707. We also compared the number of ROIs being divided for each image at three different levels, the we found the using 100 ROIs is better than 64 and 16 ROIs, and we observed a sharp decrease of case based accuracy when using 16 ROIs for each image.

In our opinion, our proposed method has the potential to be used in other medical imaging data when the overall information is dominated over the local information. In future, we aimed at testing this proposed method on other deep learning algorithms and also other dataset.

References

1. Smith, R.A., Duffy, S., Tabar, L.: Breast cancer screening: the evolving evidence. Oncology **26**(5), 471–486 (2012)
2. Amir, E., Freedman, O.C., Seruga, B., Evans, D.G.: Assessing women at high risk of breast cancer: a review of risk assessment models. J. Natl. Cancer Inst. **102**(10), 680–691 (2010)
3. Nelson, H.D., Tyne, K., Naik, A., Bougatsos, C., Chan, B.K., Humphrey, L.: Screening for breast cancer: an update for the U.S. preventive services task force. Ann. Intern. Med. **151**(10), 727–737 (2009)
4. Kopans, D.B.: Basic physics and doubts about relationship between mammographically determined tissue density and breast cancer risk. Radiology **246**(2), 348–353 (2008)
5. Sun, W., Tseng, T.-L.B., Qian, W., Zhang, J., Saltzstein, E.C., Zheng, B., Lure, F., Yu, H., Zhou, S.: Using multiscale texture and density features for near-term breast cancer risk analysis. Med. Phys. **42**(6), 2853–2862 (2015)

6. Qian, W., Sun, W., Zheng, B.: Improving the efficacy of mammography screening: the potential and challenge of developing new computer-aided detection approaches. Expert Rev. Med. Devices **12**(5), 497–499 (2015)
7. Sun, W., Zheng, B., Lure, F., Wu, T., Zhang, J., Wang, B.Y., Saltzstein, E.C., Qian, W.: Prediction of near-term risk of developing breast cancer using computerized features from bilateral mammograms. Comput. Med. Imaging Graph. **38**(5), 348–357 (2014)
8. Sun, W., Tseng, T.-L.B., Zheng, B., Zhang, J., Qian, W.: A new breast cancer risk analysis approach using features extracted from multiple sub-regions on bilateral mammograms. In: SPIE Medical Imaging, vol. 9414, p. 941422. International Society for Optics and Photonics (2015)
9. LeCun, Y., Kavukcuoglu, K., Farabet, C.: Convolutional networks and applications in vision. In: ISCAS 2010 - 2010 IEEE International Symposium on Circuits and Systems: Nano-Bio Circuit Fabrics and Systems, pp. 253–256 (2010)
10. Simard, P.Y., Steinkraus, D., Platt, J.C.: Best practices for convolutional neural networks applied to visual document analysis. In: Proceedings of the Seventh International Conference on Document Analysis and Recognition, pp. 1–6 (2003)
11. Bengio, Y.: Learning deep architectures for AI. Found. Trends® Mach. Learn. **2**(1), 1–127 (2009)

A Novel Breast Cancer Risk Assessment Scheme Design Using Dual View Mammograms

Wenqing Sun[1], Tzu-Liang (Bill) Tseng[1], Bin Zheng[2,3],
Jiangying Zhang[4], and Wei Qian[1,3(✉)]

[1] College of Engineering, University of Texas at El Paso, El Paso, TX, USA
wqian@utep.edu
[2] College of Engineering, University of Oklahoma, Norman, OK, USA
[3] Sino-Dutch Biomedical and Information Engineering School,
Northeastern University, Shenyang, China
[4] College of Biological Sciences, University of Texas at El Paso,
El Paso, TX, USA

Abstract. Computer aided diagnosis (CADx) schemes based on dual view mammograms are able to provide extra information compared to single view schemes. To explore an efficient and effective way for combining the information from different views, a new breast cancer risk analysis scheme was developed and tested in this study. 120 pairs of dual view mammograms from 120 women were used in this study. Three different groups of texture features and density features were extracted from both MLO view and CC view mammograms. The asymmetry score that measures the asymmetry levels of these two view mammograms was considered in our proposed scheme. 91 computational features on each view and 3 asymmetry measurements were computed and used for the proposed scheme. Three classifiers were used in our proposed scheme, one for each of the dual view mammograms, and the third one combined dual view scores with asymmetry measurements. The highest area under the curve (AUC) we obtained was 0.753 ± 0.039.

Keywords: Breast cancer · Dual-view mammogram · Risk analysis · Asymmetry measurements

1 Introduction

Evaluating the risk of getting breast cancer has been a hot topic in recent years. It has been reported that colorectal cancer and lung cancer incidence rates have been slow to decline, while breast cancer rate has remained relatively flat since 2003 [1]. To find a reliable predictor of near-term breast cancer, many studies have reported the relation between breast tissue density patterns and cancer risks. After the pioneering work Wolfe Pattern [2], many models and systems like Gail model [3], Claus model [4], BRCAPRO model [5], Jonker model [6], Breast Imaging Report and Data System (BI-RADS) [7] were proposed.

© Springer International Publishing Switzerland 2016
A. Tingberg et al. (Eds.): IWDM 2016, LNCS 9699, pp. 392–399, 2016.
DOI: 10.1007/978-3-319-41546-8_49

However, the large inter-observer variability makes these subjectively rated methodologies unreliable [8]. To achieve more reliable and accurate results, several studies including our previous researches have already investigated and tested the possibility of developing computerized schemes to automatically quantify mammographic density and to predict breast cancer risks using computed mammographic image features [9, 10]. To the best of our knowledge, all these researches only used single view mammograms, i.e. either Cranial-Caudal (CC) or Mediolateral Oblique (MLO) view mammograms, an example of CC and MLO view mammogram was shown in Fig. 1. Physically, women's breasts are three-dimensional (3D) objects, after projecting them into two-dimensional (2D) mammograms, the actual percentage of dense tissues are less accurate to measure. Moreover, some structural information of the breast tissue is missing due to the overlapping on the projections. For example, a shell shaped dense tissue may have significant different appearance if observed from side to side (CC view) and from top to bottom (MLO view) [11]. In clinic, the evaluation of cancer risk is based on radiologists' subjective assessment on both CC and MLO view mammograms.

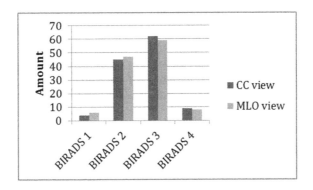

Fig. 1. The BIRADS rate distribution of our dataset.

In this study, we developed a computerized scheme to predict breast cancer risk using features extracted from both MLO and CC view mammograms, and we compared the performance of using only one view and both views mammograms. Several feature groups and feature extraction methods were explored and discussed to find an efficient and effective way to utilize the features from dual views. The details are listed in the following sections.

2   Materials and Methods

2.1   Dataset

Our dataset consists of 120 women derives from an established in-house full-field digital mammography (FFDM) image database, and all these cases were selected only if screen-negative mammograms from at least two routine screening examinations preceding diagnosis were available. For each case, it contains two CC view and two MLO view mammograms from both right and left breast. Among the 120 cases, we either chose right or left breast mammogram from each case, and 60 pairs of mammograms from each side were used in this study. The BIRADS rate of every mammogram was evaluated by the radiologists individually and the density distributions of CC and MLO mammograms were shown in Fig. 1. From the sequential screening results, half of the 120 participants were diagnosed as cancer in the next sequential screening and the rest remained cancer-free and not recalled by radiologists.

2.2   Scheme Design

To analyze these data, we first implemented some computational features to quantitatively measure each image. At the first stage, features were extracted from single view mammograms respectively and the feature selection method was used to reduce the dimension of the features. Then the selected features from each of dual view mammogram were sent to two classifiers for classification, and two scores will be generated from CC and MLO view mammograms. The asymmetry of CC view and MLO view mammograms were measured by three asymmetry features, and all the three features will be sent to the third classifier alone with two single view scores calculated from previous step. The first two classifiers are support vector machine (SVM) and the third classifier is artificial neural network (ANN). All the single view features and asymmetry features will be described in Sect. 2.3. The flowchart of our proposed scheme is shown in Fig. 2.

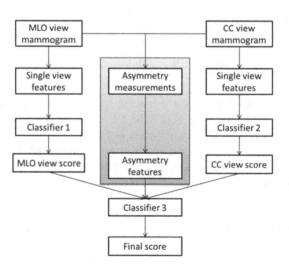

Fig. 2. The flowchart of our proposed scheme

2.3   Computational Features

In this study, we implemented and tested run-length features, sum and different histograms (SDHs) [12], and gray value features. Many texture features were used here to detect the subtle texture changes in mammograms, as an abnormality or distortion found on a mammogram can also be a possible indicator for cancer risk [13].

Run length statistics describe the coarseness of a texture in a specific direction, and run-length matrix count the occurrence of runs for each gray levels and length in certain direction. In this study, eleven run-length features were calculated at two directions (horizontal and vertical): short run emphasis, long run emphasis, high gray-level run emphasis, low gray-level run emphasis, short run low gray-level emphasis, short run high gray-level emphasis, long run low gray-level emphasis, long run high gray-level emphasis, gray-level non-uniformity, run length non-uniformity, run percentage [14].

SHDs features are another group of statistic features and highly correlated with mammographic density. From SDHs, three different relative displacements (d = 1, 3, 5 pixels) and four different angels ($\theta = 0, 45, 90, 135$) were considered for computational feature extraction. For each pair of parameters, the mean, variance, entropy, correlation, and homogeneity were calculated.

Gray value features are the most commonly used features in breast cancer risk analysis. The distribution of pixel intensity can mimic the density BIRADS rated by radiologists, which is currently being treated as cancer risk indicator. For gray value features, we calculated the energy, entropy, inertial, mean value, standard deviation, skewness, kurtosis, smoothness, mean gradient.

Asymmetry features are important in our proposed scheme because it is the link of CC view and MLO view mammograms. In this study, we used three asymmetry features: the first one measures the histogram differences of CC and MLO view mammograms, the second feature compares the area differences of dense region of two mammograms, the third feature calculated the reciprocal of correlation of the single view feature vectors extracted from each view. The details of the asymmetry features were listed in Table 1.

Table 1. The descriptions of the asymmetry used in our proposed dual view scheme

Asymmetry feature	Descriptions
Histogram difference	The summation of absolute differences of the value on each corresponding histogram bins
Dense area difference	The absolute value of dense area differences
Feature vector asymmetry	The reciprocal of the correlation of the feature vectors from each view

2.4   Classification and Evaluation

For each of the single view mammogram, 91 features were extracted from all three feature groups. To reduce the dimension of the feature, sequential floating forward selection (SFFS) was used as our feature selection method. The selected features were sent to the first two classifiers. Three classifiers were used in our scheme, two SVMs were trained for CC and MLO view mammograms and each gives a predicted score from the information on each of the CC and MLO view mammograms individually. And another ANN was used to combine the two predicted scores and three asymmetry features, the final risk core will be generated by this ANN classifier.

Since we have a limited dataset for this experiment, we used leave one out fashion for evaluation. The area under the curve (AUC) and true positive were calculated for comparison. All the t tests are two sided and the p value less than 0.05 were considered as statistically significant.

3   Results

After feature selection 9 features were remained from the original 91 features, these 9 features were sent to the first two classifiers. The original number of features in each feature group and number of selected features for each classifier are shown in Table 2.

Table 2. Feature amount before and after feature selection for each classifier and feature group

Feature type	Count				
	Classifier 1		Classifier 2		Classifier 3
	Original	After SFFS	Original	After SFFS	
Run-length	22	2	22	2	0
SDHs	60	4	60	4	0
Gray value	9	3	9	3	0
Asymmetry	0	0	0	0	3
Classifier score	0	0	0	0	2
Total	91	9	91	9	5

To evaluate the discriminative power of the implemented features, we calculated the AUC using each feature group from single view mammograms. These features were extracted from both MLO and CC views, the results comparison is shown in Table 3. Overall the CC view mammograms outperform MLO view mammograms, and run-length features on CC view mammograms yield highest AUC.

Table 3. Performance comparison using different feature groups from CC and MLO mammograms

Feature group	AUC_{MLO}	AUC_{CC}
Run-length	0.649±0.047	0.714±0.032
SDHs	0.672±0.071	0.705±0.043
Gray value	0.661±0.039	0.703±0.022

We also tested the necessity of asymmetry features, by removing the three designed asymmetry features from our scheme we get the AUC of 0.711 ± 0.077, compared the

AUC of 0.753 ± 0.039 using the asymmetry features. The MLO single view scheme gives the lowest AUC value among the four candidates. And the proposed dual view scheme gives the highest truth positive (TP) too. By analyzing and comparing the p values, we noticed the performance of dual view scheme in terms of predicted risk scores are significantly different from MLO single view scheme (p value 0.04).

4 Discussions

The results discussed above demonstrated that our proposed dual view scheme can predict the risk of near-term breast cancer based on "prior" normal screening mammograms. This study is based on our previous work using single view mammograms to predict cancer risk [9], and the experimental results showed it is very promising to combine dual view mammograms for cancer risk prediction. To the best of our knowledge, this is the first breast cancer risk analysis scheme based both CC and MLO view mammograms, and it outperforms single view mammogram schemes. The higher AUC values and true positive rate are important to lead this project to our ultimate goal: develop a personalized screening recommendation system based on previous patient screening history and to stratify the patients into high risk group and low risk group, so that the higher risk group can be screened more often for early detection purpose while the lower risk group can be screened less often to avoid the side effect.

The design and implementation of asymmetry features are important to combine and utilize the information from dual view mammograms. Since women's breast are naturally soft object and CC view and MLO view are the projections from different angles. So comparing and integrating the features from the different sources are challenging. The features extracted from CC view and MLO view mammograms have a high correlation, simply merge the feature sets together generated no better results compared to single view. In this study, we used two classifiers to train CC and MLO view mammogram features respectively, and a third classifier was used to combine the classification scores and asymmetry features together. In this study, we also tested the importance of the asymmetry features, by removing them from our proposed scheme, and we found the performance was even slightly worse than CC view scheme, but still better than MLO single view scheme (Table 4). Another important find is our proposed scheme has higher TP values than single view schemes. For a clinical acceptable

Table 4. AUC comparison for each feature group on MLO view and CC view mammograms

	AUC	P value (compare with MLO view)	P value (compare with CC view)	TP
MLO view	0.682 ± 0.050	N/A	0.27	0.70
CC view	0.729 ± 0.023	0.27	N/A	0.74
Dual view scheme	0.753 ± 0.039	0.04	0.14	0.77
Dual view scheme (without asymmetry features)	0.711 ± 0.077	0.24	0.58	0.72

system, high true positive values are important because the false positive predictions may increase the unnecessary financial and mental burden for the women [15].

Despite of the encouraging results, this study still has some limitations. First, the dataset is very limited, and only 120 cases were investigated in this study. Second, we only tested three groups of computational features extracted from each mammogram, and the best combination of bigger feature set for dual view mammogram schemes still need to be investigated. Third, we only investigated three asymmetry features in this study, and more potential asymmetry measurements should be computed and analyzed. In future, we will focus on how to better incorporate the dual view mammogram information on a larger dataset.

References

1. Siegel, R., Ma, J., Zou, Z., Jemal, A.: Cancer statistics, 2014. CA Cancer J. Clin. **64**(1), 9–29 (2014)
2. Wolfe, J.N.: Breast patterns as an index of risk for developing breast cancer. Am. J. Roentgenol. **126**(6), 1130–1137 (1976)
3. Gail, M.H., Brinton, L.A., Byar, D.P., et al.: Projecting individualized probabilities of developing breast cancer for white females who are being examined annually. J. Natl. Cancer Inst. **81**(24), 1879–1886 (1989)
4. Claus, E.B., Risch, N., Thompson, W.D.: Genetic analysis of breast cancer in the cancer and steroid hormone study. Am. J. Hum. Genet. **48**(2), 232–242 (1991)
5. Parmigiani, G., Berry, D.A., Aquilar, O.: Determining carrier probabilities for breast cancer susceptibility genes BRCA1 and BRCA2. Am. J. Hum. Genet. **62**(1), 145–148 (1998)
6. Jonker, M.A., Jacobi, C.E., Hoogendoorn, W.E., Nagelkerke, N.J., de Bock, G.H., van Houwelingen, J.C.: Modeling familial clustered breast cancer using published data. Cancer Epidemiol. Biomark. Prev. **12**(12), 1479–1485 (2003)
7. American College of Radiology (ACR). Breast Imaging Reporting and Data System Atlas (BI-RADS® Atlas). American College of Radiology, Reston, VA (2003)
8. Berg, W.A., Campassi, C., Langenberg, P., et al.: Breast imaging reporting and data system: inter- and intraobserver variability in feature analysis and final assessment. AJR Am. J. Roentgenol. **174**(6), 1769–1777 (2000)
9. Sun, W., Zheng, B., Lure, F., Wu, T., Zhang, J., Wang, B.Y., Qian, W.: Prediction of near-term risk of developing breast cancer using computerized features from bilateral mammograms. Comput. Med. Imaging Graph. **38**(5), 348–357 (2014)
10. Sun, W., Tseng, T.L.B., Qian, W., Zhang, J., Saltzstein, E.C., Zheng, B., Zhou, S.: Using multiscale texture and density features for near-term breast cancer risk analysis. Med. Phy. **42**(6), 2853–2862 (2015)
11. Kopans, D.B.: Basic physics and doubts about relationship between mammographically determined tissue density and breast cancer risk 1. Radiology **246**(2), 348–353 (2008)
12. Unser, M.: Sum and difference histograms for texture classification. IEEE Trans. Pattern Anal. Mach. Intell. **1**, 118–125 (1986)
13. Tice, J.A., O'Meara, E.S., Weaver, D.L., Vachon, C., Ballard-Barbash, R., Kerlikowske, K.: Benign breast disease, mammographic breast density, and the risk of breast cancer. J. Natl. Cancer Inst. **105**(14), 1043–1049 (2013)

14. Xu, D.H., Kurani, A.S., Furst, J.D., Raicu, D.S.: Run-length encoding for volumetric texture. Heart **27**, 25 (2004)
15. Qian, W., Sun, W., Zheng, B.: Improving the efficacy of mammography screening: the potential and challenge of developing new computer-aided detection approaches. Expert Rev. Med. Devices **12**(5), 497–499 (2015)

Automated Multimodal Computer Aided Detection Based on a 3D-2D Image Registration

T. Hopp[✉], B. Neupane, and N.V. Ruiter

Institute for Data Processing and Electronics, Karlsruhe Institute of Technology,
Kaiserstr. 12, 76131 Karlsruhe, Germany
torsten.hopp@kit.edu
http://www.ipe.kit.edu

Abstract. Computer aided detection (CADe) of breast cancer is mainly focused on monomodal applications. We propose an automated multimodal CADe approach, which uses patient-specific image registration of MRI and X-ray mammography to estimate the spatial correspondence of tissue structures. Then, based on the spatial correspondence, features are extracted from both MRI and X-ray mammography. As proof of principle, distinct regions of interest (ROI) were classified into *normal* and *suspect* tissue. We investigated the performance of different classifiers, compare our combined approach against a classification with MRI features only and evaluate the influence of the registration error. Using the multimodal information, the sensitivity for detecting *suspect* ROIs improved by 7 % compared to MRI-only detection. The registration error influences the results: using only datasets with a registration error below 10 mm, the sensitivity for the multimodal detection increases by 10 % to a maximum of 88 %, while the specificity remains constant. We conclude that automatically combining MRI and X-ray can enhance the result of a CADe system.

Keywords: Computer aided detection · Multimodal image registration · X-ray mammography · MRI

1 Introduction

Computer aided detection (CADe) and diagnosis (CADx) systems for breast imaging have been widely studied in the last years. Most attention was drawn to X-ray mammography-based CADe systems [1]. Furthermore CADe has often been applied for breast magnetic resonance imaging (MRI) [2] and breast sonography [3]. Though it was shown in several studies, e.g. [4], that the combination of modalities can lead to better detection rates, there are only few approaches combining the diagnostic information of two imaging modalities for CADe, e.g. [5]. One reason is the challenging spatial correlation of tissue structures in different modalities due to the different patient positioning and compression state of the breast. For multimodal CADe systems this leads to complex manual annotation of corresponding tissue structures visible in both modalities [5] which limits their applicability.

© Springer International Publishing Switzerland 2016
A. Tingberg et al. (Eds.): IWDM 2016, LNCS 9699, pp. 400–407, 2016.
DOI: 10.1007/978-3-319-41546-8_50

In our previous work we developed and evaluated an automated method for MRI to X-ray mammography image registration based on a biomechanical model [6]. It allows calculating the position of a tissue structure in the X-ray mammogram given the location of this structure in the MRI by the estimated deformation field. Based on this registration we now propose an automated multimodal CADe approach using the combination of X-ray mammograms and MRI. In this paper we present a first feasibility study, compare multimodal against monomodal CADe and investigate the influence of the registration error on the detection performance.

2 Methods

2.1 Image Registration

To estimate the spatial correspondence between MRI and X-ray mammography, the image registration uses a biomechanical model of the breast to simulate the mammographic compression. The patient-specific biomechanical model is generated from the segmented MRI volume, for which a fuzzy C-means clustering similar to [7] and edge detection is used. The model geometry is assembled by a tetrahedral mesh differentiating fatty and glandular tissue. A hyperelastic neo-hookean material with individual material parameters for fatty and glandular tissue is applied. Mammographic compression is simulated using compression plates and formulating a contact problem which is solved by the Finite Element method. Based on the estimated deformation field, each three-dimensional point in the MRI volume can be mapped to a two-dimensional point in the X-ray mammogram. For more details refer to our earlier publications [6,8].

2.2 Computer Aided Detection System

To test the feasibility of a CADe system using multimodal information, the breast in the MRI volume is quantized into distinct, cubic regions of interest (ROIs). The aim of our CADe system is to classify each ROI into one of the categories *normal* or *suspect*. To extract multimodal information, the eight vertices of the MRI ROI are mapped to the X-ray mammogram. The mammography ROI is then formed by the convex hull of these eight automatically mapped points (Fig. 1).

For the 3D MRI ROI, 64 features are extracted. Intensity based features include e.g. mean intensity and variance for three time points pre-contrast, 1 min and 6–7 min post-contrast. Texture features are based on 3D gray-level co-occurence matrices [9]. Temporal features analyze the contrast enhancement by measuring the slope from pre-contrast to 1 min post-contrast and from 1 min post-contrast to the last time point similar to the three time points method [10].

For the mapped mammography ROIs, 43 features are extracted. Similar to the MRI intensity features e.g. the mean intensity, median and variance in the ROI are computed. Texture features are based on gray-level co-occurence matrices [11] and gray-level runlength matrices [12]. Furthermore a multilevel Otsu

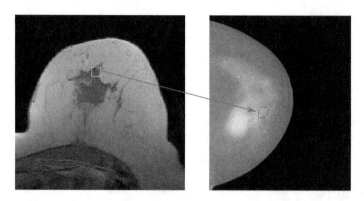

Fig. 1. Mapping from the MRI (left) to the mammogram (right) based on the estimated deformation field. The vertices of the MRI ROI (yellow rectangle) are mapped to the X-ray mammogram (yellow dots). The X-ray mammography ROI is formed by the convex hull of these points (green). (Color figure online)

thresholding [13] is applied and features based on morphological enhancement [14] are added. All features from MRI and mammography are gathered in a combined feature vector.

The classification problem is addressed by the WEKA pattern recognition toolbox [15]. A best-first feature selection is performed. Afterwards the classifier is trained and tested by a randomized 10-fold cross-validation. Experiments were performed with a selection of commonly used probabilistic, decision tree and instance-based classifiers [16]. As representative algorithms of these families, Naive Bayes, Random Forest and Nearest Neighbor were used. Additionally two and all three classifiers were combined using a meta classifier approach, which averages the predicted output class probabilities.

2.3 Clinical Datasets and Evaluation Methods

Evaluation of the method was performed with 65 patient datasets from a previous image registration study [6]. The average patient age was 58 years (min: 24 years, max: 82 years). Each dataset included a time series of T1-weighted dynamic contrast enhanced MRI volumes and the corresponding cranio-caudal mammogram of the same patient. MR images were acquired on 1.5 T scanners (Siemens Magnetom Symphony, Sonata, Avanto) with the patient in prone position using dedicated breast coils and a standardized protocol according to international guidelines. Full field digital mammograms were acquired on GE Senograph 2000D units.

As ground truth for the classifier training and evaluation, the 3D ROIs were labeled based on expert annotations. Each annotation circumscribes a visible lesion with a freehand tool. The annotated lesions included a mixture of malign and benign lesions verified by histology or follow-up diagnosis. The mammographic breast density was estimated using LIBRA [17] and datasets were grouped into density categories according to the American College of Radiology (ACR) [18]: the datasets included 34 ACR I, 22 ACR II, 8 ACR III and 1 ACR IV cases.

A ROI of our CADe approach was labeled as *suspicious* if at least 50 % of its volume was covered by the expert's lesion annotation. As a proof of principal, a ROI size in the MRI of $10 \times 10 \times 10\,mm^3$ was chosen as tradeoff between detectable lesion size and the currently time consuming mapping from MRI to the mammogram of each ROI. This resulted in a total of 45,723 ROIs of which 744 were labeled as *suspicious*. The registration of these datasets was performed in a previous study and resulted in an average target registration error (TRE) of approx. 14.0 mm (range: 1.5 mm - 42.7 mm)[6]. The cross-validation was repeated 32 times with different random seeds. The evaluation was carried out with the features from MRI only and with the combination of MRI and mammography features.

To analyze classifier performance, the error rate of incorrectly classified ROIs as well as ROI related sensitivity and specificity were calculated from the true/false positive/negative rates, where *suspicious* ROIs are positive. Furthermore the positive and negative predictive values (PPV, NPV) were computed.

3   Results

Figure 2 shows a bar plot of the evaluation for different classifiers and the MRI-only (gray) compared to the multimodal combination case (black). For MRI-only features, the sensitivity varies between 0.68 and 0.77 depending on the classifier. The specificity varies between 0.991 and 0.998. The best sensitivity, yet the worst specificity, is achieved with a Naive Bayes classifier. In contrast the Random Forest classifier achieves the best specificity. A tradeoff between sensitivity and specificity is achieved by the combination of Naive Bayes and Random Forest (NB + RF) with a sensitivity of 0.75 and a specificity of 0.996.

Throughout all classifiers, all metrics improve by the combination of MRI and mammography features. The best sensitivity of approximately 0.82 is achieved with the combined NB + RF classifier. For the same classifier the specificity is 0.996. Compared to the classification with only MRI features, the sensitivity increases for the NB + RF example by 0.07, while the specificity stays constant. The overall error rate decreases from 0.8 % to 0.6 %, while the PPV increases from 0.74 to 0.78 and the NPV remains approximately constant.

The results are consistent for different random seeds: the standard deviation of the sensitivity for repeated random cross validations was 0.003.

In order to analyze the influence of the TRE on the classification performance, datasets were grouped into two categories at a TRE threshold of 10 mm, which equals the size of a ROI in our evaluated scenario. This resulted in 27 datasets with a TRE below 10 mm and 38 datasets with a TRE above 10 mm.

Figure 3 shows the performance of the proposed CADe system for datasets with a TRE below 10 mm. The sensitivity for the MRI-only case as well as for the multimodal case is slightly higher than for all datasets, which might be

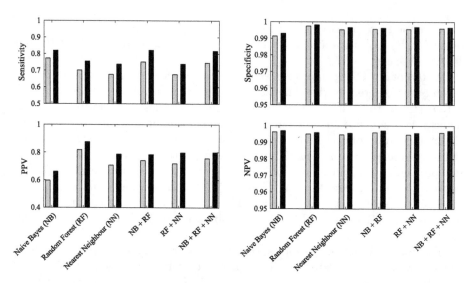

Fig. 2. Sensitivity, specificity, positive (PPV) and negative predictive value (NPV) for classification with different classifiers and comparing MRI-only (gray) to multimodal combination (black).

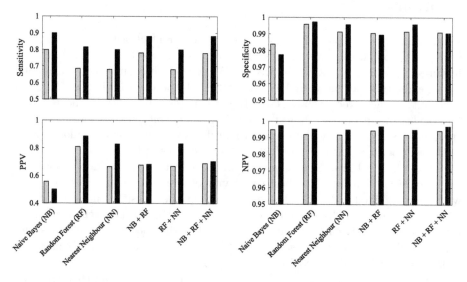

Fig. 3. Results for classification of datasets with a registration error below 10 mm: Sensitivity, specificity, PPV and NPV for different classifiers and comparing MRI-only (gray) to multimodal combination (black).

due to the smaller number of datasets. Yet, the sensitivity differences between MRI-only (gray) and multimodal combination (black) are considerably more pronounced: for the NB + RF combination, the sensitivity increases from 0.78 to 0.88 (difference 0.10 compared to a difference of 0.07 for all datasets).

In contrast, we observed mixed results for datasets with a TRE above $10\,mm$: the sensitivity and specificity stays approximately constant or even decreases from the multimodal to the MRI-only evaluation: e.g. for the combined NB + RF classifier, the sensitivity decreases from 0.70 to 0.68.

Figure 4 illustrates a detection result for one patient showing the quantization of the MRI into distinct ROIs and their classification. The true positive and false negative ROIs are displayed in the mammogram which allows observing the spatial correspondence between areas detected as *suspicious* in both imaging modalities.

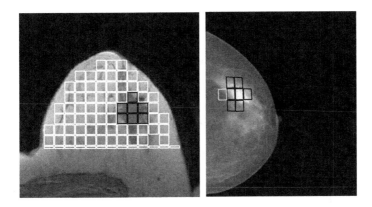

Fig. 4. Left: quantization of an MRI into distinct ROIs (green rectangles) and their classification given as color. True positive (TP) ROIs are displayed in red, false negative (FN) ROIs are displayed in yellow. Right: mapping of the TP and FN ROIs to the mammogram. (Color figure online)

4   Discussion and Conclusion

We presented a method for an automated multimodal CADe system based on a registration of MRI and X-ray mammography. To the best of our knowledge an automated combination of multimodal features for breast cancer detection has not been carried out before.

To check the feasibility of our approach, we applied a straightforward pattern recognition using distinct ROIs with a size of $10 \times 10 \times 10\,mm^3$ in our prototype implementation. In combination with our ROI labeling, which requires at least a 50 % volume overlap with the annotated ground truth to label the ROI as *suspicious*, the average lesion size which can be detected by our approach is approximately in the same range as the ROI size. Acceleration of the mapping between MRI and mammography by parallel processing will allow extending the method to smaller ROI sizes or a sliding window approach in future.

The feasibility study was carried out with datasets selected retrospectively from clinical routine. All MRI examinations were carried out with the same protocol and mammograms were all acquired with the same mammography system. Only cases in which a lesion could be delineated in both the MRI and X-ray mammogram by an expert were included to evaluate the TRE. Cranio-caudal mammograms were used as proof of principle. As the image registration was applied for oblique mammograms in a previous study as well, extending our approach to the combination of multiview mammograms and MRI in future might enhance the results further. For our first evaluation, a basic set of commonly used features was extracted for both MRI and X-ray mammography, which might not yet tap the full potential of a CADe system. We implemented a plugin-like software architecture to easily include more advanced features in future.

The results are promising: 88 % of the *suspect* labeled ROIs could be identified by our proposed multimodal method, which was not achieved without the combination of MRI and mammography features. Though adding MRI to mammography did not significantly increase the sensitivity in some previous clinical studies, e.g. for high risk populations [19], the additional information seems beneficial in our CADe scenario: as an improvement was observed across several classifier families, this indicates that the multimodal combination adds non-redundant information.

The TRE influences the results. Due to non-linear deformations, complex tissue structures and manual interactions during the patient positioning, the accurate registration of X-ray mammograms and MRI is challenging and a lively field of research. Yet a TRE in the range of current MRI to mammography registration approaches [6,20,21] already leads to improvements of the CADe performance. This leads us to the conclusion that automatically combining MRI and mammography can enhance the result of a CADe system.

References

1. Cheng, H., Shi, X., Min, R., Hu, L., Cai, X., Du, H.: Approaches for automated detection and classification of masses in mammograms. Pattern Recogn. **39**(4), 646–668 (2006)
2. Dorrius, M., der Weide, M.V., van Ooijen, P., Pijnappel, R., Oudkerk, M.: Computer-aided detection in breast MRI: a systematic review and meta-analysis. Eur. Radiol. **21**(8), 1600–1608 (2011)
3. Cheng, H., Shan, J., Ju, W., Guo, Y., Zhang, L.: Automated breast cancer detection and classification using ultrasound images: a survey. Pattern Recogn. **43**(1), 299–317 (2010)
4. Lord, S., Lei, W., Craft, P., Cawson, J., Morris, I., Walleser, S., Griffiths, A., Parker, S., Houssami, N.: A systematic review of the effectiveness of magnetic resonance imaging (MRI) as an addition to mammography and ultrasound in screening young women at high risk of breast cancer. Eur. J. Cancer **43**(13), 1905–1917 (2007)

5. Yuan, Y., Giger, M.L., Li, H., Bhooshan, N., Sennett, C.A.: Multimodality computer-aided breast cancer diagnosis with FFDM and DCE-MRI. Acad. Radiol. **17**(9), 1158–1167 (2010)
6. Hopp, T., Dietzel, M., Baltzer, P., Kreisel, P., Kaiser, W., Gemmeke, H., Ruiter, N.: Automatic multimodal 2D/3D breast image registration using biomechanical FEM models and intensity-based optimization. Med. Image Anal. **17**(2), 209–218 (2013)
7. Wu, S., Weinstein, S., Keller, B.M., Conant, E.F., Kontos, D.: Fully-automated fibroglandular tissue segmentation in breast MRI. In: Maidment, A.D.A., Bakic, P.R., Gavenonis, S. (eds.) IWDM 2012. LNCS, vol. 7361, pp. 244–251. Springer, Heidelberg (2012)
8. Hopp, T., de Barros Rupp. Simioni, W., Perez, J.E., Ruiter, N.: Comparison of biomechanical models for MRI to X-ray mammography registration. In: Proceedings 3rd MICCAI Workshop on Breast Image Analysis, pp. 81–88 (2015)
9. Chen, W., Giger, M.L., Li, H., Bick, U., Newstead, G.M.: Volumetric texture analysis of breast lesions on contrast-enhanced magnetic resonance images. Magn. Reson. Med. **58**(3), 562–571 (2007)
10. Degani, H., Gusis, V., Weinstein, D., Fields, S., Strano, S.: Mapping pathophysiological features of breast tumors by MRI at high spatial resolution. Nat. Med. **3**(7), 780–782 (1997)
11. Haralick, R.M., Shanmugam, K., Dinstein, I.: Textural features for image classification. IEEE Trans. Syst. Man Cybern. **3**(6), 610–621 (1973)
12. Galloway, M.M.: Texture analysis using gray level run lengths. Comput. Graphics Image Process. **4**(2), 172–179 (1975)
13. Otsu, N.: A threshold selection method from gray-level histograms. IEEE Trans. Syst. Man Cybern. **9**(1), 62–66 (1979)
14. Li, H., Wang, Y.J., Liu, K.J.R., Lo, S.C.B., Freedman, M.T.: Computerized radiographic mass detection - part i: lesion site selection by morphological enhancement and contextual segmentation. IEEE Trans. Med. Imaging **20**, 289–301 (2001)
15. Hall, M., Frank, E., Holmes, G., Pfahringer, B., Reutemann, P., Witten, I.H.: The WEKA data mining software: an update. SIGKDD Expl. **11**(1), 10–18 (2009)
16. Witten, I., Frank, E., Hall, M.A.: Data Mining, 3rd edn. Elsevier, Amsterdam (2011)
17. Keller, B.M., Nathan, D.L., Wang, Y., Zheng, Y., Gee, J.C., Conant, E.F., Kontos, D.: Estimation of breast percent density in raw and processed full field digital mammography images via adaptive fuzzy c-means clustering and support vector machine segmentation. Med. Phys. **39**(8), 4903–4917 (2012)
18. D'Orsi, C., Sickles, E., Mendelson, E., Morris, E.: ACR BI-RADS Atlas. Breast Imaging Reporting Data Syst. American College of Radiology (2013)
19. Kuhl, C.K., Schrading, S., Leutner, C.C., Morakkabati-Spitz, N., Wardelmann, E., Fimmers, R., Kuhn, W., Schild, H.H.: Mammography, breast ultrasound, and magnetic resonance imaging for surveillance of women at high familial risk for breast cancer. J. Clin. Oncol. **23**(33), 8469–8476 (2005)
20. Mertzanidou, T., Hipwell, J., Johnsen, S., Han, L., Eiben, B., Taylor, Z., Ourselin, S., Huisman, H., Mann, R., Bick, U., Karssemeijer, N., Hawkes, D.: MRI to x-ray mammography intensity-based registration with simultaneous optimisation of pose and biomechanical transformation parameters. Med. Image Anal. **18**(4), 674–683 (2014)
21. Lee, A., Rajagopal, V., Gamage, T.P.B., Doyle, A.J., Nielsen, P., Nash, M.: Breast lesion co-localisation between X-ray and MR images using finite element modelling. Med. Image Anal. **17**(8), 1256–1264 (2013)

Exposure Conditions According to Breast Thickness and Glandularity in Japanese Women

Hiroko Nishide[1,2(✉)], Kouji Ohta[3], Kaori Murata[3], and Yoshie Kodera[1]

[1] Radiological and Medical Laboratory Sciences, Nagoya University Graduate School of Medicine, Nagoya, Japan
kodera@met.nagoya-u.ac.jp
[2] Radiological Technology, Gifu University of Medical Science, Seki, Japan
hnishide@u-gifu-ms.ac.jp
[3] Fukui Prefectural Hospital, Fukui, Japan
kouji0470326@yahoo.co.jp,
k-murata-ef@pref.fukui.lg.jp

Abstract. We retrospectively collected data on patient age, exposure factors, and compressed breast thickness (CBT) from 7,566 mammograms, which were obtained in the medio-lateral oblique projection over a 1-year period. The mean CBT was 31.7 mm, and was <30 mm in 44.8 % of cases. In 93.1 % of the mammograms with CBT 20-29 mm, tube voltage was 24 kV. In 196 mammograms exposed at 24 kV, the CBT was 29 mm and a maximum mAs value was over than 270 mAs. In order to evaluate the dose reduction, the tube loading was measured, using the semi-automatic AEC mode, for the mammography phantoms with a thickness of 10 to 30 mm while varying the tube voltage from 24 to 27 kV. The tube loading at 27 kV was approximately 50 % lower than that at 24 kV, the average glandular dose calculated could be reduced by about 20 %.

Keywords: Exposure condition · Digital mammography · Breast glandularity · Thin breast

1 Introduction

In mammography, the exposure conditions are usually set by using an automatic exposure control (AEC) system. The settings depend on each AEC system. However, the target/filter combination and tube voltage are often determined by the compressed breast thickness (CBT). Japanese women have been reported to have breasts with low thickness and higher breast density. Usually, thin breasts are exposed at lower voltage. However, because the radiation dose is determined by attenuation in the regions with highest density by AEC, it may cause a high radiation dose. This study aims to estimate the average glandular dose and to consider the possibility of dose reduction in thin breasts in digital mammography.

© Springer International Publishing Switzerland 2016
A. Tingberg et al. (Eds.): IWDM 2016, LNCS 9699, pp. 408–414, 2016.
DOI: 10.1007/978-3-319-41546-8_51

2   Methods and Materials

2.1   Clinical Data

We retrospectively collected data from women who underwent screening and diagnostic mammography at Fukui Prefectural Hospital from April 2012 to March 2013.
They were 7,566 medio-lateral oblique views of 3,922 patients. The patient age, CBT,
target/filter combination, tube voltage, and tube loading (mAs) were collected. The
Lorad Selenia mammography system with a flat panel detector based on amorphous
selenium was used. The target/filter combination and tube voltage were almost determined by CBT. The mAs values were determined by using the AEC system to have
constant values of exposure index in regions that were automatically decided to have
the densest glandular tissue (Fig. 1).

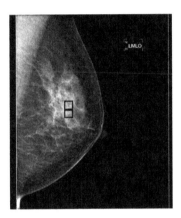

Fig. 1. Two areas (1 cm^2) were chosen automatically to determine the radiation dose

2.2   Methods and Materials

Clinical Data. The distribution and average thickness of 7,566 breasts were obtained.
At each tube voltage, the mean and standard deviation of the mAs values were calculated. For CBT of 20–29 mm, the relationship between the CBT and the mAs values
was determined for each tube voltage.

Phantom Study. Mammography phantom materials (total thickness 10, 15, 20, 25,
and 30 mm) of varying compositions (30 %, 50 %, and 70 % glandularity) were
exposed at 24–27 kV using a molybdenum target and filter (Mo/Mo). The mAs value
was set using the semiautomatic AEC mode. All phantoms were rectangular with
dimensions of 12.5 cm × 10 cm. The phantoms were positioned at the midline of the
breast support table and 1 cm outside from the chest wall edge with the paddle in
contact. The AEC detector was set at the centre of the phantom. The mammography
system used was the same as that used in the clinical study.

Dosimetry. To estimate the incident air kerma for the average glandular dose estimation, the entrance doses were measured at mAs values of 24–27 kV using Unfors Xi in the mammography mode. The chamber was positioned at the midline of the breast support table and at 60 mm from the chest wall edge with the paddle in contact [1].

Average Glandular Dose for Clinical Exposures. The average glandular dose was calculated in compliance with the European Guidelines for Quality Assurance in Breast Cancer Screening and Diagnosis [2]. The clinical data of breasts exposed at 24 kV for CBT of 29 mm were used. The data was calculated divided into age groups of the 40–49 and 50–64 years. The average glandular dose for each clinical exposure was calculated using the following formula [3–5].

$$D = Kgcs \tag{1}$$

where

    K - the incident air kerma calculated at the upper surface of the PMMA
    g - an index corresponding to 50 % glandularity
    c - an index referring to the tissue composition of the breast
    s - an index referring to the X-ray spectrum

3 Results

Figure 2 shows the number of each CBT of the 7,566 mammograms in increments of 1 mm. The Patients' average age was 57 years, and the tube voltage was 32-22 kV. The average CBT in clinical cases was 31.7 mm, and 44.8 % of CBTs were less than 30 mm (Fig. 2).

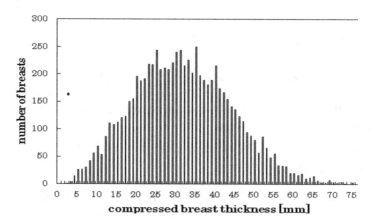

Fig. 2. The CBT was 2–77 mm, and the average CBT was 31.7 mm

Figure 3 shows the tube voltage for each CBT. In most mammograms, the tube voltage values were determined by the CBT. For CBT of 20–29 mm, the tube voltage was 24 kV; for CBT more than 30 mm, it was changed every 5 mm.

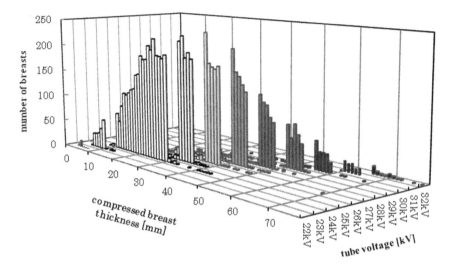

Fig. 3. Number of breasts with each CBT for each tube voltage

Figure 4 shows the relationship between the tube voltage and the average mAs values. A Comparison of the average mAs value for each tube voltage showed that the average mAs value was the highest at 25 kV, but the standard deviation was the highest at 24 kV.

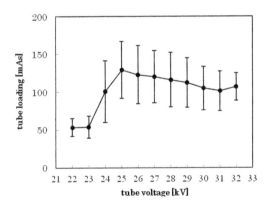

Fig. 4. Relationship between tube voltage and tube loading (average and standard deviation)

The mAs values were determined by the CBT in each image. In 93.1 % of mammograms with CBT of 20–29 mm, the tube voltage was 24 kV, and the target/filter combination was Mo/Mo. The mean mAs value increased as the CBT increased and the range of mAs values widened. For CBT of 29 mm, the maximum mAs value exceeded 270 mAs, and the average mAs value was 143.6 mAs higher than that at 25 kV (Fig. 5(a)). The mAs values of mammograms exposed at 25–27 kV were lower than those at 24 kV (Fig. 5 (b)).

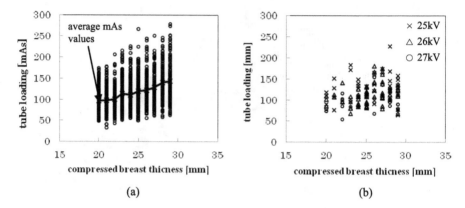

Fig. 5. Relationship between the CBT and the tube loading for CBT of 20–29 mm (exposed at (a) 24 kV and (b) 25–27 kV)

Figure 6 shows the mAs values at each tube voltage using the semiautomatic AEC mode in the mammographic phantom (BR12) of various compositions with phantom thickness of 30 mm. In the phantom exposure data, the mAs values decreased with an increase in the tube voltage. It was ∼50 % lower at 27 kV than at 24 kV.

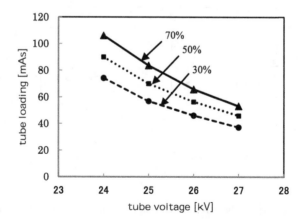

Fig. 6. Relationship between tube voltage and tube loading in phantoms with varying composition and 30-mm thickness; the mAs values decreased with an increase in the tube voltage

Table 1 shows the calculated average glandular doses for clinical exposure with CBT of 29 mm. In each group, the average glandular dose decreased with an increase in the tube voltage. The mean values of the average glandular doses at 27 kV were ∼20 % lower than those at 24 kV.

Table 1. Mean values of average glandular doses for clinical exposure with CBT of 29 mm

Age group	24 kV	25 kV	26 kV	27 kV
40–49 (n = 54)	2.48	2.33	2.15	2.02
50–64 (n = 97)	2.21	2.08	1.92	1.80

[mGy]

4 Discussion and Conclusion

In this study, we retrospectively collected data from 7,566 mammograms and evaluated the relationship between the CBT and the exposure conditions. In mammography, the exposure conditions were usually determined using the AEC system. In around half of the breasts examined in this study, the CBT was less than 30 mm. Most were exposed at 24 kV with high radiation dose.

We examined the reduction of dose by increasing the tube voltage. Increasing the tube voltage increases the penetrating beam quality and decreases attenuation by the breast. The mean values of average glandular doses at 27 kV were lower ∼20 % than those at 24 kV using the AEC.

Although the average glandular dose decreased with an increase in the tube voltage, it should be considered the changes in image quality. Subject contrast is important in mammography and increasing the penetrating quality of the beam decreases attenuation differences. In future work, we plan to reconsider the changes of image quality using the calculating of the threshold contrast visibility.

Because the mAs value differed significantly even with the same CBT, the tube voltage should be adjusted depending on the breast glandularity. However, there are no models for the glandularity in thin breasts. Therefore, a method to estimate the glandularity in thin breasts is needed.

References

1. Perry, N., Broeders, M., de Wolf, C.: European Guidelines for Quality Assurance in Breast Cancer Screening and Diagnosis 4th edn. Supplements. S1 Digital Mammography Update. EC, Luxembourg (2013)
2. Perry, N., Broeders, M., de Wolf, C.: European Guidelines for Quality Assurance in Breast Cancer Screening and Diagnosis, 4th edn. EC, Luxembourg (2006)
3. Dance, D.R.: Monte Carlo calculation of conversion factors for the estimation of mean glandular breast dose. Phys. Med. Biol. **35**, 1211–1219 (1990)

4. Dance, D.R., Skinner, C.L., Young, K.C., Beckett, J.R., Kotre, C.J.: Additional factors for the estimation of mean glandular breast dose using the UK mammography dosimetry protocol. Phys. Med. Biol. **45**, 3225–3240 (2000)
5. Biegała, M., Jakubowska, T., Markowska, K.: Effect of anode/filter combination on average glandular dose in mammography. J. Med. Phys. **40**, 45–51 (2015)

Deep Cascade Classifiers to Detect Clusters of Microcalcifications

Alessandro Bria[1(✉)], Claudio Marrocco[1], Nico Karssemeijer[2], Mario Molinara[1], and Francesco Tortorella[1]

[1] DIEI, University of Cassino and Southern Latium, Cassino, FR, Italy
{a.bria,c.marrocco,m.molinara,tortorella}@unicas.it
[2] DIAG, Radboud University Nijmegen Medical Centre, Nijmegen, The Netherlands
nico.karssemeijer@radboudumc.nl

Abstract. Recent advances in Computer-Aided Detection (CADe) for the automatic detection of clustered microcalcifications on mammograms show that cascade classifiers can compete with high-end commercial systems. In this paper, we introduce a deep cascade detector where the learning algorithm of each binary pixel classifier has been redesigned in the early stopping mechanism conventionally used to avoid overfitting to the training data. In this way, we strongly increase the number of features considered in each stage of the cascade (hence the term "deep"), yet we still benefit from the cascade framework by obtaining a very fast processing of mammograms (less than one second per image). We evaluated the proposed approach on a database of full-field digital mammograms; the experiments revealed a statistically significant improvement of deep cascade with respect to the traditional cascade framework. We also obtained statistically significantly higher performance than one of the most widespread commercial CADe systems, the Hologic R2CAD ImageChecker. Specifically, at the same number of false positives per image of R2CAD (0.21), the deep cascade detected 96 % of true lesions against the 90 % of R2CAD, whereas at the same lesion sensitivity of R2CAD (90 %), we obtained 0.05 false positives per image for the deep cascade against the 0.21 of R2CAD.

Keywords: Computer aided detection · Mammography · Clusters of microcalcifications · Cascade of classifiers

1 Introduction

The presence of clusters of microcalcifications (μCs) in mammograms is one of the earliest signs of breast cancer [1]. The small size of μCs and the low contrast of the image make particularly difficult the interpretation of screening mammograms even for an expert radiologist. To this end, the use of Computer-Aided Detection (CADe) systems is recently widespread among radiologists to improve their detection performance [2]. CADe systems are usually based on supervised learning techniques that classify each pixel of a mammographic image

© Springer International Publishing Switzerland 2016
A. Tingberg et al. (Eds.): IWDM 2016, LNCS 9699, pp. 415–422, 2016.
DOI: 10.1007/978-3-319-41546-8_52

as belonging to a μC or not [3–7]. These kinds of approaches, however, suffer from the high computational burden generated by the number of pixels to be processed and the high complexity of the classifiers to be employed.

An efficient solution to these drawbacks has been proposed in [8] where a multistage system for the automatic detection of clustered μCs in Full-Field Digital Mammograms (FFDM) was introduced. The rationale of their method is to build an ensemble of ranking-based boosting classifiers with increasing complexity and specificity connected in series as in the cascade face detector proposed by Viola and Jones [9].

In this paper we present an improvement of such system. The main novelty is the μC detector where the learning algorithm of each node classifier of the cascade is redesigned in the early stopping mechanism conventionally used to avoid overfitting to the training data when the learning goals of the node classifier cannot be met. In this way, we obtain a large increase of the number of pixel classifiers, and, at the same time, we keep unchanged the computational benefit of the cascade by maintaining a very low processing time per image. We named the new system *DeepCasCADe*, where the term "deep" indicates the high number of classifiers employed in each stage of the cascade. Even though this is a slight modification of the original system, we obtain a significant experimental improvement of the detection performance. In particular, experiments accomplished on a FFDM database show that not only the DeepCasCADe detector performs statistically significantly better than [8], but also that DeepCasCADe has statistically significantly higher performance than one of the most widespread high-end CADe commercial systems, the Hologic R2CAD ImageChecker.

2   Method

2.1   The CasCADe System

The CasCADe system recently proposed in [8] consists of three main phases: a preprocessing stage, a detection stage and a classification stage that reduces the number of false positive detected clusters.

The preprocessing phase is intended to rescale pixel intensities to a scale with uniform noise level. In the detection phase a cascade of two-class classifiers classifies each pixel of the mammogram as positive (i.e., belonging to a μC) or negative (i.e., not belonging to any μC). The cascade of dichotomizers is built as a sequence of node classifiers with increasing complexity. A given sample passes to the next node only if the current one classifies it as positive, otherwise it is rejected. The majority of samples belonging to easily detectable background tissue are discarded by the early nodes, while the most likely-μC samples go through the entire cascade. As a result, the detection rate D and the false positive rate F of a cascade composed by n nodes are given respectively by $D = \prod_{i=1}^{n} d_i$ and $F = \prod_{i=1}^{n} f_i$, being d_i and f_i the detection rate and the false positive rate of the ith node respectively. In this way, the cascade provides a high constant sensitivity and a growing specificity through the nodes obtained by connecting more simpler classifiers with high sensitivity and sufficient specificity. Specifically, the first stages of the cascade are built to reject the most distinguishable background samples, while the last stages are specialized to discriminate between the most likely-μCs and the most confusing background samples so as to reduce the number of false positives produced by the detector.

A particular strategy is adopted for the last node of the cascade that does not reject negative samples, but it merely associates to each pixel arriving to it a confidence degree about the presence of a μC. In this way, it is possible to implement a clustering algorithm to detect clustered μCs and a post-processing classification step (see [8] for more details) that exploits the topological features of the detected μC clusters to reduce the number of false positive findings.

2.2   Early Stopping Mechanism and DeepCasCADe

The cascade is built incrementally by adding node classifiers in subsequent stages $i = 1, 2, \ldots$ until the desired false positive rate is reached or the set of negative samples available for the classifiers (hereafter referred to as *pool*) is empty. To construct the ith node classifier, a training set and a validation set are used to set the decision threshold for which the node learning goals d and f are reached. Therefore, in principle, the training rounds for the ith node go on until the node learning goals d and f are met. In fact, the decision threshold of the ith node classifier is always chosen at each round for reaching the required d; hence, the number of rounds t is governed only by whether the condition $f_{i,t} \leq f$ is satisfied, being $f_{i,t}$ the actual false positive rate of the ith node achieved at round t.

When the classification task is getting more and more complex throughout the cascade, this condition might be too difficult to meet, and an early stopping mechanism is needed to avoid overfitting to the training data. To this end, when designing the CasCADe detector, a new training round is considered only if a significant reduction of $f_{i,t}$ can be achieved. Specifically, let $\psi_i(\Delta) = \{f_{i,\tau}\}_{\tau=t-\Delta, t-\Delta+1, \ldots, t}$ be the latest Δ achieved false positive rates of the ith node. We can evaluate the variance $\sigma^2_\psi = Var(\psi_i(\Delta))$ and define an early stopping mechanism if such variance is lower than a small quantity ϵ, i.e., $\sigma^2_\psi \leq \epsilon$. New features are therefore added to the node classifier of the CasCADe detector until the condition $f_{i,t} > f \wedge \sigma^2_\psi > \epsilon$ holds [10].

In the training phase of DeepCasCADe detector, instead, we redesigned the early stopping mechanism as follows. Firstly, we remove the condition on σ^2_ψ so that the training rounds go on until the learning goals are met. This usually happens in the first nodes of the cascade that easily discriminate the most distinguishable background regions, but this is hard to achieve in the last stages of the cascade where the detection problem becomes more challenging. In this case, the number of training rounds (and thus of employed features) considerably increases with respect to the CasCADe detector. However, when using a huge number of features, the detector can still suffer from overfitting. Therefore, we have to find a trade-off between the performance improvement and the overfitting risk; to this end, we establish a maximum number of iterations T to be executed. In summary, we can say that new features are added to the node classifier of the DeepCasCADe detector until the condition $f_{i,t} > f \wedge t \leq T$ holds. If the condition $t = T$ is reached, i.e., the learning goals are not met after T iterations, we revert to the training round t for which $f_{i,t}$ is minimum.

3   Results

3.1   Dataset

The performance of the proposed DeepCasCADe system was assessed on a private database containing more than 40,000 cases obtained in routine screening. All the images were acquired with a Hologic Selenia FFDM system with a resolution of $70\,\mu$m per pixel and 14-bit grayscale pixel depth. Malignant findings on the mammograms have been proven to be cancer through a biopsy.

Two datasets have been extracted from the database. The first dataset (named $\mathcal{A}$) consists of 252 raw mammograms from 129 abnormal cases (70 benign and 59 malignant) extracted by selecting all the available images with individual μCs manually labeled by an experienced reader (7,758 in total). The second dataset (named $\mathcal{B}$) consists of 374 cases not present in the first dataset consisting of 318 normal cases (1,152 raw mammograms) and 56 malignant cases containing 100 lesions.

3.2   Evaluation of the DeepCasCADe Detector

The first experiment is intended to evaluate the effectiveness of the DeepCas-CADe detector with respect to the original CasCADe detector. To this end, the detectors were evaluated on the 252 mammograms of dataset $\mathcal{A}$ at 7,758 pixel locations centered on labeled μCs (positive samples) and at 25,190,476 pixel locations on background tissue (negative samples), using a subwindow of size 12×12 pixels $(0.84\,\text{mm} \times 0.84\,\text{mm})$.

Ten-fold cross validation was performed considering 9 folds for training set, validation set and pool and the remaining fold as test set. In each cross validation step we used 6,982 positive samples equally parted between training and validation sets and 22,751,429 negative samples subdivided in 20,000, 60,000 and 22,671,429 respectively for training set, validation set and pool. After the 10-fold cross validation, the confidence degrees obtained for each sample in the test sets were pooled together.

The configuration of CasCADe detector was the same as in [8], with node detection rate equal to 0.99, node false positive rate equal to 0.3 and $\epsilon = 10^{-4}$ for the early stopping mechanism. For the DeepCasCADe detector, we employed the same learning goals, and we experimentally fixed the maximum number of iterations $T = 2000$ that represents a good trade-off between performance improvement and overfitting risk. Both the detectors were composed by 5 node classifiers for all the 10 cascades built in the 10-fold cross validation procedure. The average number of employed features were 88.6 and 1,120.0 respectively for the CasCADe and the DeepCasCADe detectors.

The detectors were evaluated in terms of Receiver Operating Characteristics (ROC) curve by plotting True Positive Rate (TPR) against False Positive Rate (FPR) for a series of thresholds on the confidence degree associated to each sample. In this case not all the ROC curve is of interest since only low values of FPR are acceptable. For this reason, our analysis was focused on the initial portion of the curve and, subsequently, we considered as performance measure the *Partial Area Under the ROC Curve* (PAUC) defined as $\mathrm{PAUC}(x) = \int_0^x \mathrm{TPR} \; d\mathrm{FPR}$ where $[0, x]$ is the range of interest for FPR [11].

To determine if the DeepCasCADe detector provided statistically significantly better performance than CasCADe detector, we applied the bootstrap procedure [12]. The test set was sampled with replacement 2,000 times so that each new set of sampled data contained the same number of examples as the original set. For each considered FPR range, the difference ΔPAUC in PAUC between the DeepCasCADe detector and the CasCADe detector was computed. Resampling 2,000 times resulted in 2,000 values for ΔPAUC, and the p-values were defined as the fraction of ΔPAUC values that were negative or zero (i.e., the cases in which DeepCasCADe detector did not provide any improvement). The statistical significance level was chosen as 0.05 and performance differences were statistically significant if $p < 0.05$.

Average ROC curves for the two detectors are reported in Fig. 1. We can see that the ROC curve of the DeepCasCADe detector always dominates the curve of CasCADe detector. Moreover, DeepCasCADe detector yielded a statistically

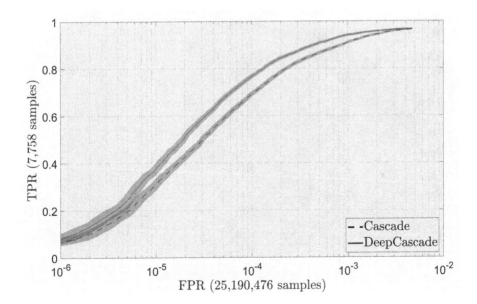

Fig. 1. Average ROC curves for CasCADe and DeepCasCADe detectors obtained from 2,000 bootstrap samples. Confidence bands indicate 95 % confidence intervals along the TPR axis.

significant increase in PAUC equal to 5.7 % ($p < 0.05$) and 14.7 % ($p < 0.05$) respectively for FPR equal to 10^{-3} and 10^{-4}.

3.3   Comparison with R2CAD

We compared the proposed DeepCasCADe system with one of the most wide-spread commercial CADe systems, the Hologic R2CAD ImageChecker on the detection of biopsy-proven malignant clusters of μCs. To this end, DeepCas-CADe detector trained on dataset $\mathcal{A}$ was applied on the 374 cases of dataset $\mathcal{B}$. Then, after clustering the detected μCs, a 10-fold cross validation was performed as in [8] to train and test a cluster classifier to discriminate abnormal versus non-abnormal clusters. For all the cases of dataset $\mathcal{B}$, we also used reports of R2CAD obtained with the following parameters: (i) algorithm version "R2 mammo calc 8.1"; (ii) configuration "[A] - high sensitivity", which was the highest sensitivity setting allowed by the system; (iii) "maximum inter-mc distance" equal to 10 mm, that is the same value we used for the DeepCasCADe.

A bootstrapping methodology suited for the comparison between CAD systems [13] was used. To this end, cases were sampled with replacement 2,000 times so that each new set of sampled cases contained the same number of cases as the original set. For each resampling, lesion-based Free-Response ROC (FROC) curves that plots TPR versus the False Positive per image (FPpi) were

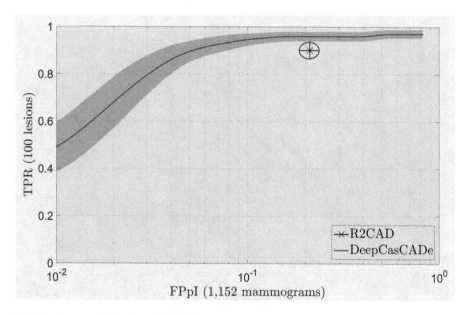

Fig. 2. Average lesion-based FROC curves of DeepCasCADe and R2CAD obtained fro 2,000 bootstrap samples. For DeepCasCADe, confidence bands indicate the standard deviation along the sensitivity axis. For R2CAD, the marks denote the average operating points and the ellipses indicate the standard deviation along both the axes.

constructed for both DeepCasCADe and R2CAD by counting true and false positives with a method partially inspired by [7] and described in [8]. For Deep-CasCADe, abnormality scores from the 10-fold cross validation were used to construct the FROC curves, whereas for R2CAD only one FROC point could be obtained, since no abnormality scores were present in the R2CAD reports. Resampling 2,000 times resulted in 2,000 values for each performance difference, and the p-values were defined as the fraction of the corresponding performance difference that were negative or zero. The statistical significance level was chosen equal to 0.05 and performance differences were considered as statistically significant if $p < 0.05$.

Average FROC curves of DeepCasCADe together with the average operating points of R2CAD are shown in Fig. 2. The results show that DeepCasCADe compared statistically significantly better than R2CAD both in sensitivity and in specificity. In particular, at the same lesion sensitivity of R2CAD (90 %) on biopsy proven malignant cases, FPpi decreased from 0.21 to 0.05 ($p < 0.05$), whereas at the same FPpi of R2CAD (0.21), the lesion sensitivity increased from 90 % to 96 % ($p < 0.05$).

4   Discussion

In this paper we have proposed an improvement of a well-known CADe system for the detection of clustered μCs based on a cascade architecture [8]. The novelty was to redesign the early stopping mechanism employed during the training of the node classifiers of the cascade and commonly used to reduce the overfitting on the training data. We obtained a deep cascade detector where the term "deep" indicates the high number of training rounds required to train each node classifier. More precisely, in the first stages of the cascade, where the classification task (i.e., the reject of the most distinguishable background regions) is quite simple, the learning goals of the node classifier can be met, and thus, the traditional cascade and the deep cascade produce very similar node classifiers. In the last stages, instead, where the node classifiers have to specialize in discriminating between actual μCs and the most confusing background configurations, the DeepCasCADe detector employs a very high number of features with respect to the traditional cascade detector.

An experimental analysis accomplished on a FFDM database revealed that DeepCasCADe detector trained on millions of image examples showed a significant increase of sensitivity and specificity (the 15 % of TPR for FPR $= 10^{-4}$) and, in general, statistically significantly higher PAUC than the traditional cascade. At the same time, the DeepCasCADe system still maintained the benefits of employing a traditional cascade framework which allowed very fast processing of the mammograms (less than one second per image).

The DeepCasCADe system also performed statistically significantly better than the Hologic R2CAD ImageChecker, one of the most widespread commercial CADe systems. DeepCasCADe achieved an increase of 6 % in the malignant lesion sensitivity and a decrease from 0.21 to 0.05 in the number of false positive lesions per image. In this way, we also improved the results obtained in [8] where the performance differences between CasCADe and R2CAD were not statistically significant. To our knowledge there are no other CADe systems presented in the literature that are able to overcome high-end commercial systems.

References

1. Kopans, D.B.: Breast Imaging. Lippincott Williams & Wilkins, Hagerstown (2007)
2. Eadie, L.H., Taylor, P., Gibson, A.P.: A systematic review of computer-assisted diagnosis in diagnostic cancer imaging. Eur. J. Radiol. **81**(1), e70–e76 (2012)
3. El Naqa, I., Yang, Y., Wernick, M.N., Galatsanos, N.P., Nishikawa, R.M.: A support vector machine approach for detection of microcalcifications. IEEE Trans. Med. Imaging **21**(12), 1552–1563 (2002)
4. Wei, L., Yang, Y., Nishikawa, R.M., Wernick, M.N., Edwards, A.: Relevance vector machine for automatic detection of clustered microcalcifications. IEEE Trans. Med. Imaging **24**(10), 1278–1285 (2005)
5. Marrocco, C., Molinara, M., D'Elia, C., Tortorella, F.: A computer-aided detection system for clustered microcalcifications. Artif. Intell. Med. **50**(1), 23–32 (2010)
6. Oliver, A., Torrent, A., Tortajada, M., Lladó, X., Peracaula, M., Tortajada, L., Sentís, M., Freixenet, J.: A boosting based approach for automatic microcalcification detection. In: Martí, J., Oliver, A., Freixenet, J., Martí, R. (eds.) IWDM 2010. LNCS, vol. 6136, pp. 251–258. Springer, Heidelberg (2010)
7. Jing, H., Yang, Y., Nishikawa, R.M.: Detection of clustered microcalcifications using spatial point process modeling. Phys. Med. Biol. **56**(1), 1–17 (2011)
8. Bria, A., Karssemeijer, N., Tortorella, F.: Learning from unbalanced data: a cascade-based approach for detecting clustered microcalcifications. Med. Image Anal. **18**(2), 241–252 (2014)
9. Viola, P., Jones, M.: Robust real-time object detection. Int. J. Comput. Vis. **57**(2), 137–154 (2001)
10. Bria, A., Marrocco, C., Molinara, M., Tortorella, F.: An effective learning strategy for cascaded object detection. Inf. Sci. **340–341**, 17–26 (2016)
11. Yousef, W.A.: Assessing classifiers in terms of the partial area under the ROC curve. Comput. Stat. Data Anal. **64**, 51–70 (2013)
12. Samuelson, F.W., Petrick, N.: Comparing image detection algorithms using resampling. In: IEEE International Symposium on Biomedical Imaging, pp. 1312–1315 (2006)
13. Samuelson, F.W., Petrick, N., Paquerault, S.: Advantages and examples of resampling for CAD evaluation. In: IEEE International Symposium on Biomedical Imaging, pp. 492–495 (2007)

Mammographic Ellipse Modelling Towards Birads Density Classification

Minu George[1]([✉]), Andrik Rampun[1], Erika Denton[2], and Reyer Zwiggelaar[1]

[1] Department of Computer Science, Aberystwyth University,
Aberystwyth SY23 3DB, UK
{mig24,yar,rrz}@aber.ac.uk
[2] Department of Radiology, Norfolk and Norwich University Hospital,
Norwich NR4 7UY, UK
erika.denton@nnuh.nhs.uk

Abstract. It has been shown that breast density and parenchymal patterns are important indicators in mammographic risk assessment. In addition, the accuracy of detecting abnormalities depends strongly on the structure and density of breast tissue. As such, mammographic parenchymal modelling and the related density estimation or classification are playing an important role in computer aided diagnosis. In this paper, we present a novel approach to the modelling of parenchymal tissue, which is directly linked to Tabar's normal breast tissue representation and based on the multi-scale distribution of dark ellipses, and the complementary distribution of bright ellipses which represent dense tissue. Our initial evaluation is based on the full MIAS database. We provide analysis of the separation between the Birads density classes, which indicates significant differences and a way towards automatic Birads based density classification.

Keywords: Breast density modelling · Blob and ellipse detection

1 Introduction

One of the major risk factors associated with breast cancer is breast tissue density and the appearance of the parenchymal tissue. It has a direct relation with the probability of developing breast cancer [1–3]. Examples of mammographic images illustrating various types of tissue densities as per Breast Imaging Reporting and Data System (BIRADS) density classification are illustrated in Fig. 1. The manual assessment of breast density and/or parenchymal patterns is covered in various classification schemes [1,2,4,5], which are all correlated [6]. The automatic segmentation of mammographic tissue and the related (BIRADS) density classification of the mammograms has been an active research area. In general this has concentrated on the modelling and detection of dense tissue [7,8,11]. The review by He et al. [10] demonstrated all recent approaches to finding the correlation between the breast density and its classification methods

© Springer International Publishing Switzerland 2016
A. Tingberg et al. (Eds.): IWDM 2016, LNCS 9699, pp. 423–430, 2016.
DOI: 10.1007/978-3-319-41546-8_53

in risk assessment. In [10] they showed that the main approaches in the literature use techniques like thresholding, clustering, and statistical model building.

In this study we look at incorporating the modelling of the complement of dense tissue: i.e. the modelling of the distribution of fatty tissue and how this can be exploited to provide BIRADS density classification. This work is closely related to that of Chen et al. [9], which developed a mammographic segmentation approach using topographic maps with an emphasis on the modelling and distribution of bright blobs in mammographic images.

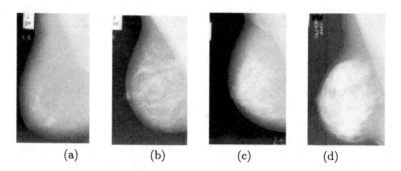

| (a) | (b) | (c) | (d) |

Fig. 1. Some example mammograms showing various BIRADS density classification based on Birads 4th edition. (a) BIRADS 1 (entirely fatty breast tissue), (b) BIRADS 2 (scattered fibro-glandular density), (c) BIRADS 3 (heterogeneously dense breast obscuring small masses), and (d) BIRADS 4 (extremely dense breast lowering the sensitivity of mammography).

2   Detecting Blobs in Images

In computer vision, blob detections refers to the identification of regions or points, which are either darker or brighter than the local area. The higher the contrast between the region and the surrounding tissue and the more blob-like the region is the higher the "blob probability" should be. Traditional approaches have concentrated on the detection of circular objects for which approach such as the Hough transform [12] and Laplacian of Gaussian (LoG) filtering [13] have been used. However, a lot of regions in natural images are not truly circular and as such ellipse detection might be a more appropriate approach. To facilitate detection of orientated ellipse-like structures in images, Kong et al. [14] introduced a generalized Laplacian of Gaussian (gLoG) based approach, which allows for the detection of asymmetric regions and includes directional estimation for such regions. The gLoG approach uses a set of orientation and scale dependent kernels. As with the LoG approach, the image, $f(x, y)$ is processed with a Gaussian and differential aspects as defined by

$$\nabla^2[G(x, y) * f(x, y)] = \nabla^2[G(x, y)] * f(x, y) \tag{1}$$

where

$$\nabla^2 G(x,y) = \frac{\partial^2 G}{\partial x^2} + \frac{\partial^2 G}{\partial y^2} \tag{2}$$

and

$$G(x,y) = A.e^{-\left(ax^2 + 2bxy + cy^2\right)} \tag{3}$$

In Eq. 3, the parameters are determined by

$$a = \frac{\cos^2 \theta}{2\sigma_x^2} + \frac{\sin^2 \theta}{2\sigma_y^2} \tag{4}$$

$$b = -\frac{\sin 2\theta}{4\sigma_x^2} + \frac{\sin 2\theta}{4\sigma_y^2} \tag{5}$$

$$c = \frac{\sin^2 \theta}{2\sigma_x^2} + \frac{\cos^2 \theta}{2\sigma_y^2} \tag{6}$$

where σ_x, σ_y and θ are respectively the standard deviation in the horizontal direction, the standard deviation in the vertical direction, and the orientation of the Gaussian kernel. The two σ_x, σ_y values determine the scale/width of the Gaussian kernel, and as there are two values this can now be asymmetrical. Some typical kernels can be found in Fig. 2.

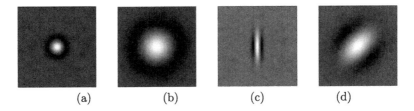

(a)   (b)   (c)   (d)

Fig. 2. A set of gLoG example kernels, where (a) $\{\sigma_x = 4, \sigma_y = 4\}$, (b) $\{\sigma_x = 10, \sigma_y = 10\}$, (c) $\{\sigma_x = 8, \sigma_y = 2, \theta = \pi/2\}$, and (d) $\{\sigma_x = 12, \sigma_y = 8, \theta = \pi/4\}$.

3   Data and Experimental Results

For this initial study we have used the MIAS dataset [15], which contains 322 digitised MLO mammograms. The database consists of left and right MLO mammograms of 161 women. The spatial resolution of images is $50\,\mu\text{m} \times 50\,\mu\text{m}$ quantised to 8 bits. All the mammograms were classified according to the BIRADS density classification scheme [4] by expert breast radiologists [16].

All the images are pre-processed and the breast area is separated from the background region and from the pectoral muscle. Blob-like structures detected outside the breast area are removed.

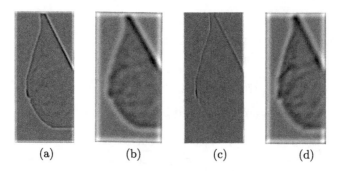

(a)   (b)   (c)   (d)

Fig. 3. Example gLoG processing based on the mammogram shown in Fig. 1(b) and the gLoG kernels shown in Fig. 2.

Subsequently, all the mammograms were processed with Eq. 1, using a variety of $\{\sigma_x, \sigma_y, \theta\}$ kernels. A few typical examples can be found in Fig. 3. This shows that different size and orientation structures are localized and enhanced by the different kernels.

Based on the gLoG results we identify local maxima, which indicate the central location of blob-like structures and thresholding could be used to select only those regions with a higher probability. Some blob detection results can be found in Fig. 4.

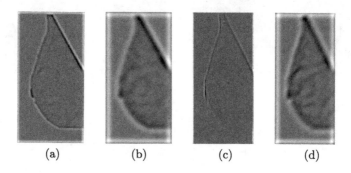

(a)   (b)   (c)   (d)

Fig. 4. Detected blobs super-imposed on the original mammogram based on the images shown in Fig. 3.

To demonstrate the working of blob detection on various density type mammograms from BIRADS I to BIRADS IV are taken into account and is shown by Fig. 1. The extrema of local regions in the image at different scales are estimated. Such detected blobs represent the approximate size of blob like fatty and dense tissue regions. To calculate the overall amount of blob like fatty/dense tissue structures from the image, the blobs are identified at multiple scales. All these blobs are merged together to represent the total amount of dense/fatty tissue in the image. On merging, blob overlapping occurs in areas where tissues are closely related. Blobs detected for fatty tissue from all the scales are represented in Fig. 5 and the problem of overlapping ellipses should be evident from Fig. 5. This is because the same blob like tissue structures are detected as blobs at different scales with their origin at a similar location. This problem of overlapping is solved by merging based on the qualitative relations between the blobs. The qualitative relations between two blobs (blob A and blob B) under consideration are the distance (d) between the centre points of blobs and the radius of each blob (rA and rB, where rA > rB). The three common relations found while merging are external where the distance between the blobs is greater than the sum of its radius(d > rA + rB), internal (d < rA − rB) and intersection (rA − rB < d < rA + rB).

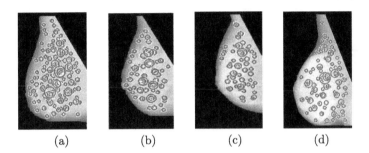

(a)   (b)   (c)   (d)

Fig. 5. Blobs detected fatty tissue at multi-scale for mammograms sorted from BIRADS I to BIRADS IV as per Fig. 1

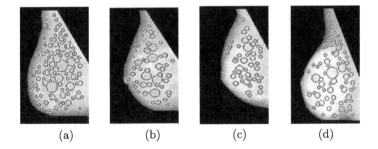

(a)   (b)   (c)   (d)

Fig. 6. Blobs detecting fatty tissue at multi-scale after merging based on qualitative relations for mammograms sorted from BIRADS I to BIRADS IV

The overlapped and intersected blobs are removed using the above qualitative relations. The merging procedure starts from the largest scale to the smallest scale. The external blobs are retained. If the distance between the blobs is less than the radius of the largest blob, the inner blob is eliminated. If they are

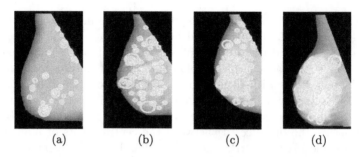

Fig. 7. Blobs detected dense tissue at multi-scale for mammograms sorted from BIRADS I to BIRADS IV

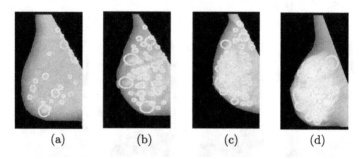

Fig. 8. Blobs detecting dense tissue at multi-scale after merging based on qualitative relations for mammograms sorted from BIRADS I to BIRADS IV

intersecting and if the distance between them is less than the radius of largest blob, it leads to its deletion. The final merged multi-scale blobs after the removal of additional blobs are illustrated in Fig. 6. The corresponding tissue area is normalized using the total breast area for the final estimation of tissue area.

As discussed before the same procedure can be used for estimating the blob like dense tissue structures in mammogram image. The sample images are shown in Figs. 7 and 8. Figure 7 illustrates the blobs detected at all scales and Fig. 8 illustrates the dense blob like structures where overlapped and intersected blobs have been removed through the qualitative measurements.

It is clear from the Figs. 6 and 8 that the number of blobs detecting fatty tissue area decreasing for BIRADS I to BIRADS IV while the amount of dense tissue inreases for BIRADS I to BIRADS IV.

While comparing the relationship between dense and fatty tissue in estimating Birads class, it is found from Fig. 9 that when relative dense tissue increases with Birads class, the fatty tissue area decreases with Birads class in correlation with the dense tissue. In addition it shows that there is a close relationship between fatty tissue area for Birads II and Birads III indicating that the fatty tissue pattern for Birads II and Birads III is nearly similar compared to the drastic change in structure between Birads I and Birads IV.

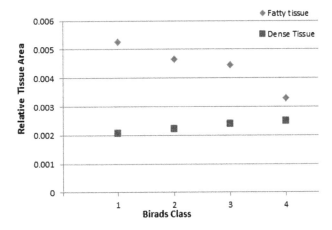

Fig. 9. Average relative tissue area for all the MIAS mammograms.

Although the Fig. 9 shows a average linear increase of dense tissue and decrease of fatty tissue respectively with Birads class, there is significant variation in the the dense/fatty tissue. This could be due to the over/under segmentation of tissue areas.Further investigation is needed to control the over/under segmentation while detecting the fatty/dense tissue area through multi-scale blobs.

4   Discussion and Conclusions

The main purpose of the paper has been in determining the fatty/dense tissue present in mammograms using multi-scale blob detection method and to find the relation between the Birads class and the fatty/dense tissue in mammograms.

We have shown that a generalized Laplacian of Gaussian based approach can be used to estimate the relative amount of fatty/dense tissue within the breast. As a compliment of the dense tissue within the breast, the fatty tissue can also be linked to the Birads density classification scheme. The investigation on the relationship between the area of fatty/dense tissue detected by the blob analysis with the BIRADS class version IV shows the results to be promising.

The future work will focus on implementing the multi-scale ellipse detection approach, which will be evaluated on larger digitised and digital datasets to estimate the relationship between dense/fatty tissue and Birads density classes. In addition, we will investigate the topology of detected blobs and how this might be related to density classification of mammographic images.

To summarize, it is found that the modelling the distribution of fatty/dense tissue could be exploited in providing the Birads density classification.

References

1. Wolfe, J.N.: Risk for breast cancer development determined by mammographic parenchymal pattern. Cancer **37**, 2486–2492 (1976)
2. Boyd, N.F., Byng, J.W., Jong, R.A., Fishell, E.K., Little, L.E., Miller, A.B., Lockwood, G.A., Tritchler, D.L., Yaffe, M.J.: Quantitative classification of mammographic densities and breast cancer risk: results from the Canadian National Breast Screening Study. J. Natl. Cancer Inst. **87**, 670–675 (1995)
3. Vachon, C.M., Van Gils, C.H., Sellers, T.A., Ghosh, K., Pruthi, S., Brandt, K.R., Pankratz, V.S.: Mammographic density, breast cancer risk and risk prediction. Breast Cancer Res. **9**, 217 (2007)
4. BI-RADS Committee and American College of Radiology: Breast imaging reporting and data system. American College of Radiology (1998)
5. Tabar, L., Tot, T., Dean, P.: Breast Cancer: The Art and Science of Early Detection with Mammography. Thieme, Stuttgart (2005)
6. Muhimmah, I., Oliver, A., Denton, E.R.E., Pont, J., Pérez, E., Zwiggelaar, R.: Comparison between Wolfe, Boyd, BI-RADS and Tabár based mammographic risk assessment. In: Astley, S.M., Brady, M., Rose, C., Zwiggelaar, R. (eds.) IWDM 2006. LNCS, vol. 4046, pp. 407–415. Springer, Heidelberg (2006)
7. He, W., Denton, E.R.E., Zwiggelaar, R.: Mammographic segmentation and risk classification using a novel binary model based bayes classifier. In: Maidment, A.D.A., Bakic, P.R., Gavenonis, S. (eds.) IWDM 2012. LNCS, vol. 7361, pp. 40–47. Springer, Heidelberg (2012)
8. Chen, Z., Zwiggelaar, R.: A modified fuzzy c-means algorithm for breast tissue density segmentation in mammograms. In: 10th IEEE International Conference on Information Technology and Applications in Biomedicine (ITAB), pp. 1–4. IEEE, Corfu (2010)
9. Chen, Z., Oliver, A., Denton, E., Zwiggelaar, R.: Automated mammographic risk classification based on breast density estimation. In: Sanches, J.M., Micó, L., Cardoso, J.S. (eds.) IbPRIA 2013. LNCS, vol. 7887, pp. 237–244. Springer, Heidelberg (2013)
10. He, W., Juette, A., Denton, E.R.E., Oliver, A., Mart, R., Zwiggelaar, R.: A review on automatic mammographic density and parenchymal segmentation. Int. J. Breast Cancer **2015**, 1–31 (2015)
11. Chen, Z., Wang, L., Denton, E., Zwiggelaar, R.: A multiscale blob representation of mammographic parenchymal patterns and mammographic risk assessment. In: Wilson, R., Hancock, E., Bors, A., Smith, W. (eds.) CAIP 2013, Part II. LNCS, vol. 8048, pp. 346–353. Springer, Heidelberg (2013)
12. Illingworth, J., Kittler, J.: A survey of the Hough transform. Comput. Vis. Graph. Image Process. **44**, 87–116 (1988). Elsevier
13. Gonzales, R., Woods, R., Eddins, S.: Digital Image Processing Using MATLAB. Pearson Education India, Delhi (2004)
14. Kong, H., Akakin, H.C., Sarma, S.E.: A generalized Laplacian of Gaussian filter for blob detection and its applications. IEEE Trans. Cybern. **43**, 1719–1733 (2013)
15. Suckling, J., Parker, J., Dance, D.R., Astley, S.M., Hutt, I., Boggis, C.R.M., Ricketts, I., Stamatakis, E., Cerneaz, N., Kok, S.L., Taylor, P., Betal, D., Savage, J.: The mammographic image analysis society digital mammogram database. In: Proceedings of International Workshop on Digital Mammography, pp. 211–221 (1994)
16. Oliver, A., Freixenet, J., Mart, R., Pont, J., Perez, E., Denton, E., Zwiggelaar, R.: A novel breast tissue density classification methodology. IEEE Trans. Inform. Technol. Biomed. **12**, 55–65 (2008)

Automatic Image Quality Assessment for Digital Pathology

Ali R.N. Avanaki[1(✉)], Kathryn S. Espig[1], Albert Xthona[1], Christian Lanciault[3], and Tom R.L. Kimpe[2]

[1] Barco Healthcare, Beaverton, OR, USA
Ali.Avanaki@Barco.com
[2] Healthcare Division, Barco N.V., Kortrijk, Belgium
[3] Department of Pathology, Oregon Health & Science University, Portland, OR, USA

Abstract. Slide quality is an important factor in pathology workflow and diagnosis. We examine the extent of quality variations in digitized hematoxylin-eosin (H&E) slides due to variations and errors in staining and/or scanning (e.g., out-of-focus blur & stitching). We propose two automatic quality estimators by adapting image quality assessment (IQA) methods that are originally developed for natural images. For the first estimator, we assume a gold-standard reference digital pathology slide is available. Quality of a given slide is estimated by comparing the slide to such a reference using a full-reference perceptual IQA method such as VIF (visual information fidelity) or SSIM (structural similarity metric). Our second estimator is based on IL-NIQE (integrated local natural image quality evaluator), a no-reference IQA, which we train using a set of artifact-free H&E high-power images (20× or 40×) from breast tissue. The first estimator (referenced) predicts marked quality reduction of images with simulated blurring as compared to the artifact-free originals used as references. The histograms of scores by the second estimator (no-reference) for images with artifact (blur, stitching, folded tissue, or air bubble artifacts) and for artifact-free images are highly separable. Moreover, the scores by the second estimator are correlated with the ratings given by a pathologist. We conclude that our approach is promising and further research is outlined for developing robust automatic quality estimators.

Keywords: Whole slide imaging (WSI)

1 Description of Purpose

The benefits of adopting a digital pathology whole slide imaging (WSI) workflow are numerous [1], and include the following.

- "Allowing multiple annotations as well as allowing multiple users to view the same image from different physical locations simultaneously," hence facilitating low-cost diagnosis quality assurance programs [5] which involve seeking the opinion of a second pathologist about a fraction of cases.
- "Continuous addition of material, ease of disease classification modification and faster distribution to a larger geographic area."

© Springer International Publishing Switzerland 2016
A. Tingberg et al. (Eds.): IWDM 2016, LNCS 9699, pp. 431–438, 2016.
DOI: 10.1007/978-3-319-41546-8_54

- Avoiding "the potential for discrepancy among slides due to loss of tissue in deeper sections and difficulty annotating glass slides."
- "Reducing the quantity of tissue and slides required," in teaching venues.

In this paper, we discuss image quality issues in WSI and propose automatic image quality estimators.

Staining procedures can go wrong in several ways, for example, bad mounting causing folded tissue, incomplete wax removal, weak differentiation, elevated eosin pH, hematoxylin break down, wrong stain timing, or insufficient dehydration [3]. In addition, H&E stain procedures vary from laboratory to laboratory and personal preference plays a large part in the final results [2].

The scanning process also introduces variations in digital slides [4]. Such variations stem from permissible differences among the manufactures, for example illumination, resolution, and image composition algorithm. In addition, failures can occur in focusing, which yields a blurred output, or stitching, which causes a visible border between scanned patches, especially in high-power views (Fig. 1).

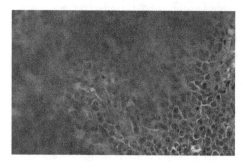 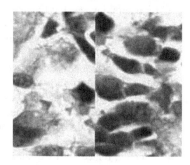

Fig. 1. Blur (left) and stitching error (right) artifacts. These small regions are cropped from breast slides publicly available at Leeds digital pathology library [21].

Given these facts, the importance of automatic quality assessment for digital pathology slides becomes clear. Measuring and/or detection of one type of WSI artifact (or one aspect of quality) have been studied. Ameisen *et al.* proposed a WSI quality estimator by automatic blur measurement based on calculating a map of edge sharpness, and aggregation of the sharpness map to a binary blur or crisp decision (e.g., considered crisp if less than 30 % of 10× level blurry) [6, 7]. Yagi and Hashimoto proposed a quality estimator based on edge thickness, independence from surround, blockiness, and difference within block [23]. To the best of our knowledge, no prior research addressed the problem of anthropomorphic WSI quality assessment. That is, to simulate a pathologist who is able to score the overall quality of a slide (and not with respect to the presence or extent of each artifact type) in terms of the utility of the slide in diagnosis.

The problem of image quality assessment (IQA) as a whole for natural (i.e., non-medical) images has been the subject of active research in recent years. IQA metrics may be categorized in two groups: referenced, and no-reference (a.k.a. blind). Referenced IQA metrics, in addition to the image under test (IUT), require the *corresponding original* (i.e., the reference) image as well. The metric consists of a comparison between the reference and IUT, and summarizing all perceptible differences due to degradations or artifacts (e.g., compression, noise, communication errors, etc.) as a measure of perceived quality. Examples of referenced IQA metrics are SSIM [8], VIF [9], HDR-VDP [10], JNDmetrix [11, 12]. To compensate for the lack of a reference image, the metrics in the no-reference category [13–20] include a training phase, which is implicit (i.e., the metric comes pre-trained to a set of images unavailable to the end user) in some cases. Blind IQA methods operate by calculating the statistical properties of IUT and comparing them against the distribution of such properties in the training images.

2   Methods

For automatic quality assessment of digital pathology images, we propose to adapt the metrics that are originally developed for quality assessment of natural images. We consider two assessment scenarios described below.

(i) **A reference digital pathology slide is available.** Such a reference slide may be generated by scanning a reference glass slide with a reference scanner. The quality of the reference scanner is assured by a different means (e.g., by several pathologists inspecting several outputs). In this scenario, one can assess the performance of any other scanner by comparing its output with the reference digital slide using a referenced IQA method (e.g., SSIM [8] or VIF [9]). Scanning artifacts such as blur (due to focus failure) or stitching errors will reduce the quality metric which may be used to quantify the scanning performance.

(ii) **No-reference slide assessment.** A no-reference IQA metric is used to detect artifacts in a digital slide. We have adapted IL-NIQE [17] since the training is not implicit and we can customize IL-NIQE by training it to pathology images with certain stain and tissue (e.g., H&E breast). IL-NIQE only needs "pristine" (i.e., artifact-free) images for training. Despite this, it is shown that IL-NIQE outperforms other methods that require images with various artifacts for training as well as other competing quality assessment methods (including full-reference methods).

A pathologist reviewed regions of interest (ROIs) from H&E digital slides of breast tissue and scored them in terms of slide quality and ease of diagnosis in a scale of 1 to 10. We used ROIs, instead of whole slides, so that we know what area of the slide is used for scoring.

3   Results

3.1   Pathology Reader Study

We selected six ROIs (about 1 mm × 2 mm each) from H&E digital slides of breast tissue from the University of Leeds virtual pathology slide library [21]. The selection process aimed to represent the diversity in morphology. Aperio's ImageScope "Extract region" tool was used to save ROIs, which were presented to a pathologist and a quality score was recorded for each (Table 1, right column).

Table 1. Quality scores for six ROIs from blind computational assessment and by pathologist. Higher pathologist scores and lower IL-NIQE scores indicate better quality.

ROI ID #	1082	31120	33542	33556	33561	37889
IL-NIQE scores	38	26	25	47	31	24
Pathologist scores (1–10)	8.5	10	7	9	9	10

3.2 No-Reference Computational Quality Assessment Using IL-NIQE

We extracted 112 artifact-free ROIs (about 900×1800 pixels each; at 20× or 40× powers) from Leeds H&E breast digital slides and used them as the pristine images for training IL-NIQE. The selected ROIs represented the variety of morphology and staining in among the available slides and number of ROIs was picked to be close to the size of the training set that comes with IL-NIQE release (i.e., 90).

Then, we used this breast-H&E-trained IL-NIQE* to estimate the quality of 112 ROIs in its training set as well as that of 15 ROIs, also from Leeds library, suffering from blur, stitching, folded tissue, or air bubble artifacts. The histograms of quality estimates for both sets are shown in Fig. 2. The same method is used to estimate the quality for the six ROIs that were presented to the pathologist (Table 1, middle column).

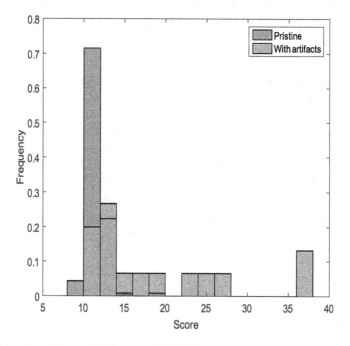

Fig. 2. Histograms of breast-H&E-trained IL-NIQE scores for pristine (i.e., artifact-free) and images with artifacts. Lower score means better quality. (Color figure online)

3.3 Referenced Computational Quality Assessment

The blur artifact was simulated (Fig. 3) for the abovementioned 112 artifact-free ROIs using a 7 × 7 box filter [24][1]. Matlab's implementation of SSIM and pixel domain VIF [22] were used to calculate the perceived similarity (to be used as a quality indicator) between the blurred ROIs (used as IUT) and the corresponding original artifact-free ROI (used as reference). The histograms of quality estimates for both metrics are shown in Fig. 4. With both metrics, the perfect similarity between IUT and reference (i.e., when IUT is identical to the reference) yields output of 1, while other levels of similarity yield a positive number under 1.

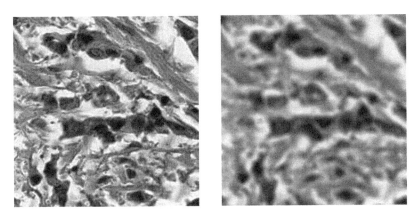

Fig. 3. Portion of a ROI before (left) and after applying blur (right).

4   Discussion

The histograms of IL-NIQE scores for with artifact images and for pristine images (Fig. 2) are highly separable. This indicates that IL-NIQE is rather successful in recognizing the artifact cases in our simple setup. The performance of this quality estimator may be improved using a more sophisticated scoring algorithm. For example, by application of IL-NIQE to a sliding window over the image, a "quality map" for a large image may be generated. Assigning a single score to the large image may be based on such map (e.g., for a conservative scoring, the image quality score may be set as the global minimum of the map). Moreover, one can examine the artifact cases received low IL-NIQE scores (i.e., recognized as pristine) and the pristine cases received high scores (i.e., recognized as artifact) and amend the assessment and scoring algorithms accordingly.

Spearman rank correlation between pathologist and IL-NIQE scores is −0.26, at a p-value of 0.3. The correlation coefficient is negative as expected (because pathologist

---

[1] The actual blur may be caused by a different kernel and is a function of scanner modulation transfer function, (auto-)focus quality and method, and vary with location, due to specimen height variations.

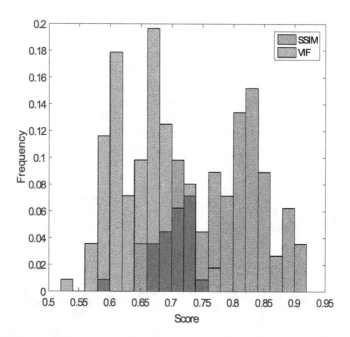

Fig. 4. Histograms of SSIM and VIF scores (i.e., estimated perceived similarity with the reference) for blurred ROIs. Lower score means worse quality. (Color figure online)

and IL-NIQE scoring are in opposite directions). We would expect a statistically stronger conclusion would be reached if more ROIs are scored. The weakness of correlation may be attributed to the fact that the six ROIs scored by pathologists are much larger than those used for training IL-NIQE. The pathologist might have scored the quality based on availability of diagnostically relevant information *somewhere* on the ROI. A blind IQA method such as IL-NIQE, however, summarizes the *overall* ROI quality. To enhance the correlation between the computational quality estimates and pathologist scores, in addition to improved scoring described in the last paragraph, we plan to ask a pathologist to score several smaller ROIs independently, or to localize the artifacts in the image. Given such information, the automatic quality estimator may be evaluated by comparing its estimated quality map, defined in the last paragraph, against the pathologist produced artifact map.

The inputs to both SSIM and VIF must be gray-scale images. Thus, only the luminance component of ROIs was used as inputs. When assessing slide quality that is possibly affected by color artifacts, SSIM and VIF should be amended to include color or replaced by a color-aware method (e.g., JNDmetrix). From Fig. 4, it maybe observed that despite the fact that all 112 images suffered from the same blurring, SSIM and VIF estimate of the resulted degradation was widely varied (VIF score range was slightly smaller than that of SSIM). This may not be an undesirable outcome though: a more detailed (i.e., structure-rich) image may suffer more by adding blur than a flat-field image. In continuation of this research, a pathologist opinion may be sought to quantify the impact of additional blur and correlation of such impact with the estimate of referenced computational quality metrics. Moreover, we would like to simulate stitching error and other WSI artifacts in a realistic way and investigate the utility of referenced and blind computational metrics in estimating their resulting degradations in slide quality.

In the draft guidance document issued by US Food and Drug Adminstration [4], the following system-level assessments for WSI are listed: color reproducibility, spatial resolution, focusing test, whole slide tissue coverage, and stitching error. The results presented herein pertain to spatial resolution and focusing. We plan to study whether all aspects of assessment are addressed by the proposed methods in continuation of our research.

5 Conclusion

The proposed computational quality assessment metrics for digital pathology slides hold promise. However, further research is needed to make such metrics practical.

Acknowledgement.   Ali Avanaki would like to thank Eddie Knippel for his comments.

References

1. Barr, T., Nicol, K., Billiter, D., Wohlever, K., Baker, P., Prasad, V.: Utility of VIPER (virtual imaging for pathology, education and research) in continuing medical education and slide surveys. Lab. Invest. **89**, 298A–298A (2009). 75 Varick St, 9th Flr, New York, NY 10013-1917 USA: Nature Publishing Group
2. Henwood, A.: Microscopic quality control of haematoxylin and eosin – know your histology. Connection **14**, 115–120 (2010). 6392 Via Real Carpinteria, CA 93013 USA: DAKO
3. Brown, S.: The Science and Application of Hematoxylin and Eosin Staining. http://mhpl.facilities.northwestern.edu/files/2013/10/The-Science-and-Application-of-Hematoxylin-and-Eosin-Staining-6-5-2012.pdf. Accessed 21 Oct 2015
4. Anderson, N., Badano, A.: Technical Performance Assessment of Digital Pathology Whole Slide Imaging Devices, Draft Guidance for Industry and FDA Staff. http://www.fda.gov/ucm/groups/fdagov-public/@fdagov-meddev-gen/documents/document/ucm435355.pdf. Accessed 21 Oct 2015
5. Ghaznavi, F., Evans, A., Madabhushi, A., Feldman, M.: Digital imaging in pathology: whole-slide imaging and beyond. Annu. Rev. Pathol. Mech. Dis. **8**, 331–359 (2013)
6. Ameisen, D., Deroulers, C., Perrier, V., Bouhidel, F., Battistella, M., Legrès, L., Janin, A., Bertheau, P., Yunès, J.B.: Towards better digital pathology workflows: programming libraries for high-speed sharpness assessment of Whole Slide Images. Diagn. Pathol. **9**(Suppl 1), S3 (2014)
7. Bertheau, P., Ameisen, D.: U.S. Patent Application 13/993,988 (2011)
8. Wang, Z., Bovik, A.C., Sheikh, H.R., Simoncelli, E.P.: Image quality assessment: from error visibility to structural similarity. IEEE Trans. Image Process. **13**(4), 600–612 (2004)
9. Sheikh, H.R., Bovik, A.C.: Image information and visual quality. IEEE Trans. Image Process. **15**(2), 430–444 (2006)

10. Mantiuk, R., Kim, K.J., Rempel, A.G., Heidrich, W.: HDR-VDP-2: a calibrated visual metric for visibility and quality predictions in all luminance conditions. ACM Trans. Graph. (TOG) **30**(4), 40 (2011). ACM

11. Lubin, J.: The use of psychophysical data and models in the analysis of display system performance. In: Digital Images and Human Vision, pp. 163–178. MIT Press, Cambridge, October 1993

12. Lubin, J.: A visual discrimination model for imaging system design and evaluation. Vis. Models Target Detect. Recogn. **2**, 245–357 (1995)

13. Gu, K., Zhai, G., Yang, X., Zhang, W.: Using free energy principle for blind image quality assessment. IEEE Trans. Multimedia **17**(1), 50–63 (2015)

14. Gu, K., Zhai, G., Lin, W., Yang, X., Zhang, W.: No-reference image sharpness assessment in autoregressive parameter space. IEEE Trans. Image Process. **24**(10), 3218–3231 (2015)

15. Liu, Y., Wang, J., Cho, S., Finkelstein, A., Rusinkiewicz, S.: A no-reference metric for evaluating the quality of motion deblurring. ACM Trans. Graph. **32**(6), 175 (2013)

16. Xue, W., Mou, X., Zhang, L., Bovik, A.C., Feng, X.: Blind image quality assessment using joint statistics of gradient magnitude and Laplacian features. IEEE Trans. Image Process. **23**(11), 4850–4862 (2014)

17. Zhang, L., Zhang, L., Bovik, A.C.: A feature-enriched completely blind image quality evaluator. IEEE Trans. Image Process. **24**(8), 2579–2591 (2015)

18. Mittal, A., Soundararajan, R., Bovik, A.C.: Making a "completely blind" image quality analyzer. IEEE Signal Process. Lett. **20**(3), 209–212 (2013)

19. Mittal, A., Moorthy, A.K., Bovik, A.C.: No-reference image quality assessment in the spatial domain. IEEE Trans. Image Process. **21**(12), 4695–4708 (2012)

20. Ye, P., Doermann, D.: No-reference image quality assessment based on visual codebook. In: 2011 18th IEEE International Conference on Image Processing (ICIP), pp. 3089–3092. IEEE, September 2011

21. http://www.virtualpathology.leeds.ac.uk/slidelibrary/. Accessed Oct 2015

22. http://live.ece.utexas.edu/research/quality/vifp_release.zip. Accessed Oct 2015

23. Yagi, Y., Hashimoto, N.: Real Time Image Quality Assessment for WSI. Presentation at Pathology Visions, Boston, MA, October 2015

24. https://en.wikipedia.org/wiki/Box_blur/. Accessed Nov 2015

Automated Analysis of Breast Tumour in the Breast DCE-MR Images Using Level Set Method and Selective Enhancement of Invasive Regions

Atsushi Teramoto[1(✉)], Satomi Miyajo[2], Hiroshi Fujita[3],
Osamu Yamamuro[2], Kumiko Omi[2], and Masami Nishio[4]

[1] School of Health Sciences, Fujita Health University, Aichi, Japan
teramoto@fujita-hu.ac.jp
[2] East Nagoya Imaging Diagnosis Center, Aichi, Japan
[3] Graduate School of Medicine, Gifu University, Gifu, Japan
[4] Nagoya Radiological Diagnosis Center, Aichi, Japan

Abstract. Analysis of invasive regions using breast magnetic resonance (MR) images plays an important role in diagnosis and decision-making regarding the treatment method. However, many images are obtained by MR imaging (MRI); development of an automated analysis method for breast tumours is desired. The main purpose of this study was to develop a novel method for automated analysis of the tumour region in breast MR images. First, early and late-subtraction images were obtained by subtracting early- and late-contrast-enhanced MR images, respectively, from the pre-contrast ones. Then, tumours in the images were enhanced based on the signal values of the normal mammary regions. Subsequently, using the level set method, a type of dynamic contour extraction, the outline of the tumour in the tumour-enhanced images was obtained. In order to evaluate the usefulness of the analysis method, we compared the tumour size listed in the interpretation report by a physician and analyzed the results obtained from the proposed method using clinical images from 10 cases. The mean absolute error of the size of tumours in all cases was less than 3.0 mm. These results indicate that the proposed method may be useful for the automated analysis of invasive breast tumours using breast MR images.

Keywords: Breast tumour · Analysis · Magnetic resonance imaging · Level set

1 Introduction

Breast cancer is the most common cancer among women worldwide, with approximately 1.7 million new cases diagnosed in 2012 [1]. This is about 12 % of all new cancer cases and 25 % of all cancers in women. There are two main types of surgery for treating breast cancer – mastectomy and breast-conserving surgery. In the latter, only the part of the breast containing the cancer is removed. It has been adapted widely from the point of view of quality of life of patients with breast cancer.

© Springer International Publishing Switzerland 2016
A. Tingberg et al. (Eds.): IWDM 2016, LNCS 9699, pp. 439–445, 2016.
DOI: 10.1007/978-3-319-41546-8_55

Currently, various modalities are used as diagnosis methods for breast cancer. These include mammography, breast ultrasound, and breast magnetic resonance imaging (MRI). Mammography and breast ultrasound are mainly used for screening, localization of tumour, and evaluation of malignancy. Breast MRI is often used to decide the appropriate form of surgery, and accurate analysis of the invasive region of tumours using breast MR images has become important in the diagnosis [2–4]. In this study, we focus on tumour analysis using breast MRI.

In breast MRI examinations, dynamic scans using contrast material are commonly used. Physicians identify the range of tumour by focusing on the time intensity curve obtained from multi-phase T1 weighted images. However, the burden of analysis with large amount of images should be released. Regarding the analysis of breast tumour, many automated analysis methods using time intensity curves have been developed for breast MR images [5–7].

Here, the increased pattern of signal value in the malignant region is not consistent. Furthermore, an increase in signal is also observed in normal tissue. Therefore, accurate identification of the range of tumour is often difficult; a method using the signal value of normal tissue is desirable.

In this study, we describe a novel automated analysis of the tumour region using the level-set method and selective enhancement of invasive regions in the dynamic contrast-enhanced breast MR images.

2 Materials and Methods

2.1 Materials

We collected breast MR images of 10 cases. They include T1-weighted MR images of precontrast, early-contrast (45 s after injection), and post-contrast (315 s after injection) enhanced breast MR images. These images were acquired using a 3-T unit (Signa HDXT 3.0T; GE Healthcare) at the East Nagoya Imaging Diagnosis Center (Nagoya, Japan). Fields of view ranged from 320–360 × 320–360 × 190 mm^3, and voxel size ranged from 0.625 × 0.625 × 1.8–0.703 × 0.703 × 1.8 mm^3. In all cases, the bounding boxes of invasive regions were determined by a physician. This study was approved by our institutional review board and patient agreement was based on the assumption that all data were anonymized.

2.2 Automated Analysis of Breast Tumours

The outline of the automated analysis is shown in Fig. 1. Proposed method consists of image alignment, subtraction, tumour enhancement, and tumour segmentation. Through these processing, the bounding box, which has x, y, and z coordinates, are obtained.

(1) Position alignment
   During the dynamic scan in the breast MRI examination, position miss-alignment often occurs. Since this causes an error of automated analysis of invasive regions,

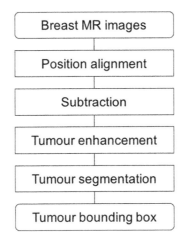

Breast MR images

Position alignment

Subtraction

Tumour enhancement

Tumour segmentation

Tumour bounding box

Fig. 1. Flow-chart of the analysis method

image alignment was conducted as pre-processing. We first defined the two kinds of images as $S(x, y, z)$ and $T(x, y, z)$, respectively. We then simply moved the $T(x, y, z)$ over each (x, y, z) point in the $S(x, y, z)$, and calculated the mean absolute error between $S(x, y, z)$ and the moved $T(x, y, z)$. Among all possible positions of $T(x, y, z)$, the position with the lowest error was determined as the best position.

(2) Subtraction

Thereafter, early- and late-subtraction images were obtained by subtracting early- and late-contrast–enhanced images, respectively, from the pre-contrast ones. Figure 2 shows the example of subtraction images.

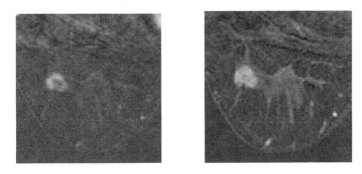

(a) Early phase subtraction image   (b) Delay phase subtraction image

Fig. 2. Subtraction images

(3) Tumour enhancement

In the late-phase T1-weighted image, the signal value of the normal mammary gland was increased as well as that of the tumours. Therefore, regions in the late-subtraction images with a pixel value below a predetermined threshold were excluded in order to eliminate the influence of the normal mammary glands. Higher pixel values were then output by comparing the pixel values of the early- and late-subtraction images. In this way, the exact region of tumour invasion was obtained.

(4) Tumour segmentation

Outline of the tumour in the tumour-enhanced image was obtained using the level set method, which is a type of dynamic contour extraction technique [8]. In this study, we introduced ITK SNAP for the processing of the level set method [9]. Finally, the bounding box of the tumour was calculated using the contour-extracted images; this was considered as the result of the automated analysis of tumour invasion.

3   Results

In order to evaluate the usefulness of the analysis method, we applied it to breast MR images from 10 cases. We compared the tumour size listed in the interpretation report by a physician and analyzed the results obtained from the proposed method.

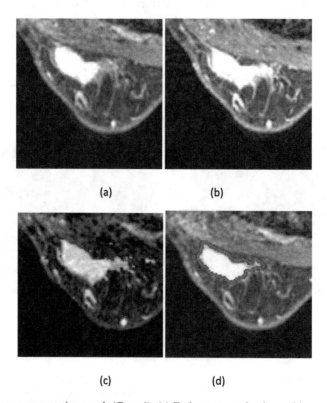

(a)   (b)

(c)   (d)

Fig. 3. Tumour segmentation result (Case 4). (a) Early contrasted enhanced image, (b) Delayed contrast enhanced image, (c) Tumour enhanced image, (d) Tumour segmented image (Red) (Color figure online)

Figures 3 and 4 show examples of tumour segmentation result where the tumour contour was traced correctly. The calculated tumour sizes for all cases are shown in Table 1. In eight out of 10 cases, measurement errors were less than 5 mm; the mean absolute error in the size of tumours was less than 3.0 mm.

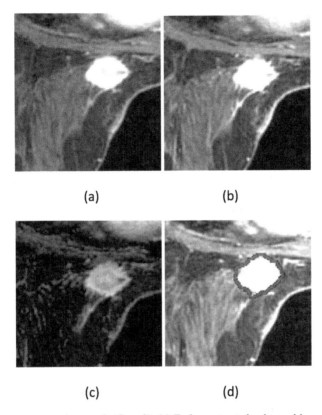

(a)   (b)

(c)   (d)

Fig. 4. Tumour segmentation result (Case 3). (a) Early contrasted enhanced image, (b) Delayed contrast enhanced image, (c) Tumour enhanced image, (d) Tumour segmented image (Red) (Color figure online)

4   Discussion

The mean absolute error of the measured size of invasive regions was less than 3.0 mm. However, there were two cases of overestimation (cases 2 and 9). In these cases, most of the normal mammary gland was recognized as a invasive region. Our method calculated the threshold based on the signal value on the normal mammary gland. However, the signal value on the normal mammary gland often fluctuates due to the influence of an abnormal lesion. Therefore, the threshold value was deviated from the appropriate value, resulting in the overestimation. We should improve the calculation method for the threshold from the normal mammary glands.

Table 1. Tumour measurement results

	X [mm]			Y [mm]			Z [mm]		
	Physician	Measured	Error	Physician	Measured	Error	Physician	Measured	Error
Case 1	11	10	−1	10	10	0	8	8	0
Case 2	10	16	+6	9	14	+5	7	10	+3
Case 3	20	18	−2	20	16	−4	15	15	0
Case 4	21	24	+3	17	16	−1	13	14	+1
Case 5	16	14	−2	13	14	+1	10	13	+3
Case 6	7	10	+3	6	7	+1	4	6	+2
Case 7	10	13	+3	10	10	0	9	9	0
Case 8	26	26	0	22	24	+2	21	21	0
Case 9	31	37	+6	21	29	+8	20	27	+7
Case 10	27	25	−2	18	22	+4	10	14	+4
MAE [mm]			2.8			2.6			2.0

MAE: mean absolute error

5 Conclusions

In this study, we proposed a novel method of automated analysis to quantify the tumour region using dynamic contrast-enhanced breast MR images. High accuracy was obtained in the evaluation using the clinical images. These results indicate that the proposed method may be useful for the automated analysis of invasive breast tumour using breast MR images.

Acknowledgment. The authors are grateful to Toshiki Kobayashi, Tsuneo Tamaki, and Masami Nishio of the Nagoya Radiological Diagnosis Foundation. This research was supported in part by a Grant-in-Aid for Scientific Research on Innovative Areas (#26108005), MEXT, Japan.

References

1. Breast Cancer Statistics, World Cancer Research Fund International. http://www.wcrf.org/int/cancer-facts-figures/data-specific-cancers/breast-cancer-statistics
2. Kuhl, C.: The current status of breast MR imaging. Part I. Choice of technique, image interpretation, diagnostic accuracy, and transfer to clinical practice. Radiology **244**(2), 356–378 (2007)
3. Mann, R.M., Kuhl, C.K., Kinkel, K., et al.: Breast MRI: guidelines from the European society of breast imaging. Eur. Radiol. **18**, 1307–1318 (2008)
4. ACR practice guideline for the performance of contrast-enhanced magnetic resonance imaging (MRI) of the breast. American college of radiology. http://www.acr.org/~/media/ACR/Documents/PGTS/guidelines/MRI_Breast.pdf. Accessed 12 Sept 2015
5. Chen, W., Giger, M.L., Bick, U., Newstead, G.M.: Automatic identification and classification of characteristic kinetic curves of breast lesions on DCE-MRI. Med. Phys. **33**(8), 2878–2887 (2006)
6. Bhooshan, N., Giger, M.L., Jansen, S.A., Li, H., Lan, L., Newstead, G.M.: Cancerous breast lesions on dynamic contrast-enhanced MR images: computerized characterization for image-based prognostic markers. Radiology **254**(3), 680–690 (2010)

7. Dorrius, M.D., Weide, M.C., Ooijen, P.M., Pijnappel, R.M., Oudkerk, M.: Computer-aided detection in breast MRI: a systematic review and meta-analysis. Eur. Radiol. **21**(8), 1600–1608 (2011)
8. Malladi, R., Sethian, J.A., Vemuri, B.C.: Shape modeling with front propagation: a level set approach. IEEE Trans. Pattern Anal. Mach. Intell. **17**(2), 158–175 (1995)
9. ITK SNAP. http://www.itksnap.org/pmwiki/pmwiki.php. Accessed 12 Sept 2015

Feasibility of Depth Sensors to Study Breast Deformation During Mammography Procedures

Oliver Díaz[1](✉), Arnau Oliver[1], Sergi Ganau[2], Eloy García[1], Joan Martí[1], Melcior Sentís[2], and Robert Martí[1]

[1] ViCOROB Research Institute, University of Girona, Girona, Spain
{oliver.diaz,arnau.oliver,eloy.garcia,joan.marti,
robert.marti}@udg.edu
[2] UDIAT – Centre Diagnòstic, Institute Universitari Parc Taulí - UAB, Sabadell, Spain
{sganau,msentis}@tauli.cat

Abstract. Virtual clinical trials (VCT) currently represent key tools for breast imaging optimisation, especially in two-dimensional planar mammography and digital breast tomosynthesis. Voxelised breast models are a crucial part of VCT as they allow the generation of synthetic image projections of breast tissue distribution. Therefore, realistic breast models containing an accurate representation of women breasts are needed. Current voxelised breast models show, in their compressed version, a very round contour which might not be representative of the entire population. This work pretends to develop an imaging framework, based on depth cameras, to investigate breast deformation during mammographic compression. Preliminary results show the feasibility of depth sensors for such task, however post-processing steps are needed to smooth the models. The proposed framework can be used in the future to produce more accurate compressed breast models, which will eventually generate more realistic images in VCT.

Keywords: Breast imaging · Breast compression · Mammography · DBT · Microsoft Kinect · Virtual clinical trials · Breast phantom

1 Introduction

Traditionally, large clinical trials are used to evaluate the performance of new x-ray mammography systems or even to optimise image acquisition parameters (e.g. beam quality, projection angle, detector characterisation, etc.). However, clinical trials involve irradiation of asymptomatic women and, at the same time, the entire process becomes expensive and very time consuming. Furthermore, they require a large amount of specialised personnel, e.g. radiographers, radiologists, etc.

Recently, digital breast tomosynthesis (DBT) has been suggested as a replacement of planar x-ray mammography [1]. Furthermore, current DBT clinical trials (STORM [2], OSLO [3] and MBTST [4]) are investigating several approaches to replace conventional mammography in screening or to use DBT as an additional imaging modality. However, certain optimisations in DBT image acquisition parameters require faster,

© Springer International Publishing Switzerland 2016
A. Tingberg et al. (Eds.): IWDM 2016, LNCS 9699, pp. 446–453, 2016.
DOI: 10.1007/978-3-319-41546-8_56

cheaper and radiation-free approaches, e.g. optimal number of projections, projection angle, energy spectra, etc. For these reasons, virtual clinical trials (VCTs) represent a pivotal tool which allow large evaluation using synthetic images, i.e. without radiation.

VCTs highly rely on producing realistic images of the breast. Therefore, a large number of anthropomorphic breast models is needed to provide a population-based approximation of breast images. Frequently, these breast models are originally generated in an uncompressed form. Then, these are deformed to produce a compressed breast shape based on several parameters, including breast density or the mechanical properties of the different tissues among others [5].

Several compressed anthropomorphic breast models are available [6–8]. Two of these models are shown in Fig. 1 in their compressed form (sagittal plane), where a very round contour is observed. However, we suspect this contour shape might not be representative to the entire women population. Furthermore, compressed breast shape might be related to tissue properties, i.e. breast glandularity, or even breast size. For these reasons, we investigated tools which would allow future analysis of breast deformation during mammography compression in clinical scenarios.

   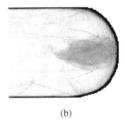

(a)   (b)

Fig. 1. Sample of compressed anthropomorphic breast models (sagittal plane) developed by (a) Bliznakova et al. [6] and (b) Bakic et al. [7]. Note the rounded contour of the breast models in both cases.

Agasthya and Sechopoulos [9] performed a similar study to characterise breast surface during compression using a pair of projector-camera setup. However, we investigate more affordable image sensors (150–200 euros) which provide depth information, as these might represent a low cost approach for this task.

The Microsoft Kinect sensor has been previously used for assessment of the breast for surgery planning and breast volume estimation [10–12]. Therefore, it is a good starting point for this investigation. This work presents an imaging framework to study breast deformation during mammography compression. Since the compression procedure is exactly the same, this could be applied to both conventional mammography and DBT. Results of this research can be useful to produce more accurate compressed breast models in the future, and therefore, generate more realistic images in VCTs. In addition, accurate knowledge of breast models can also improve scattered radiation estimation since breast curvature plays an important role [13] or even to develop more precise knowledge for mean glandular dose calculations.

The rest of the paper is structured as follows. Section 2 describes the measurements performed to estimate the accuracy of Kinect sensors as well as the clinical setup used to acquired breast contours during mammography image acquisition. The results section shows the precision's analysis of the Kinect sensor and several sample images of uncompressed and compressed breasts from participants. Observations and issues encounter during the Kinect image acquisition are described in the discussion section. Finally, the main outcomes of this work are reported in the conclusion section.

2 Methodology

In a first stage, a total of 4 women, of age 45 ± 4.5 years old, have volunteered to capture their breast shape during their routinely DBT acquisition at the clinic site. The Kinect for Xbox 360 sensor, Kinect v1, has been employed to image each breast before and after cranio-caudal (CC) compression. The Kinect device not only has an optical sensor to acquire colour images (RGB), but also an infrared emitter and sensor which allow generating images with depth information of the scene, so called RGB-D (RGB-Depth).

The first task undertaken was to quantify the correlation between the Kinect sensor and experimental measurements, and evaluate the Kinect performance for the task of this paper. In order to compare experimentally depth measures with Kinect measures, the following experiment was designed in the laboratory: a piece of cardboard (150×85 mm^2) was placed at a fixed distance from the Kinect sensor. The distance from the Kinect sensor to the cardboard was varied from 800 to 1200 mm, in steps of 10 mm. The distance produced by the Kinect sensor was calculated as the average distance value of a 10×10 pixel region of interest (ROI) within the cardboard depth image.

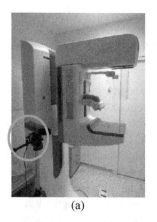
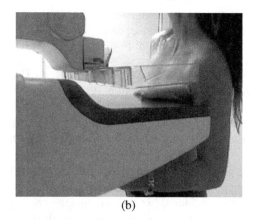

(a)   (b)

Fig. 2. (a) Clinical set up including the Kinect sensor (red circle). (b) shows a sample RGB image of a volunteer (compressed breast) acquired by the Kinect sensor. (Color figure online)

Secondly, the Kinect sensor was mounted in a tripod at the clinical site (UDIAT – Centre Diagnòstic - Institute Universitari Parc Taulí - UAB, Sabadell) as shown in Fig. 2a. The Kinect sensor was located at between 800 and 900 mm from the DBT/ mammography unit, i.e. Hologic Selenia Dimensions. Before entering the image acquisition room, the purpose of this experiment was explained to each of the partici-pants. A sample RGB image of a volunteer obtained from the Kinect point of view is shown in Fig. 2b. For the purpose of this work, breasts were imaged before and after compression prior image acquisition. As used in clinical practise at UDIAT, a flexible breast compression paddle was employed. Due to the fixed position of the Kinect sensor, only CC compression was investigated in this work. Three-dimensional (3D) triangular meshes, 3D point clouds and RGBD images of each breast were generated with the aid of the software tools Skanect (v1.8.3), KScan3D (v1.2.0.2) and Matlab (R2015b).

3 Results

The experiment to estimate the Kinect accuracy illustrates high correlation between experimentally and Kinect depth measures (slope = 1.0118, R^2 = 0.9999), as illustrated in Fig. 3. Regarding its precision, an average distance error of 3.6 ± 1.7 mm was observed. Within the ROI used to measure the Kinect distance, an average variance of 2.7 mm was found. Therefore, the Kinect sensor produces acceptable results for studying the curvature of the breast.

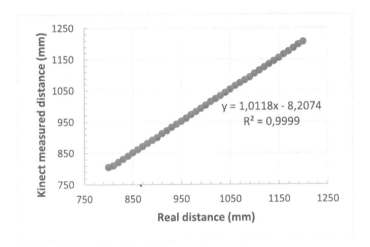

Fig. 3. Distance measured experimentally and using Kinect sensor.

Sample results using the clinical setting are illustrated in Fig. 4 for two participants. Three-dimensional triangle meshes of the breast are shown in Fig. 4a, b for an uncom-pressed and compressed breast, respectively. Note the tilt of the top surface of the compressed breast due to the flexible compression paddle used during compression. Depth images of the entire scenario and breast are illustrated in Fig. 4c, d, respectively.

Three-dimensional rendering surfaces of the clinical scenario are shown in Fig. 5, where both uncompressed and compressed breasts are highlighted in yellow. It can be observed that part of the mammography system, e.g. breast support, is also present.

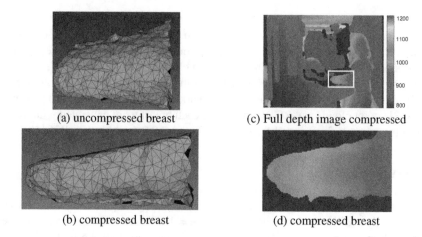

(a) uncompressed breast

(c) Full depth image compressed

(b) compressed breast

(d) compressed breast

Fig. 4. (a) and (b) correspond to the 3D meshes of an uncompressed and compressed breast, respectively. A full depth image is shown in (c) during compression for a different volunteer. Its corresponding compressed breast (white square) is depicted in (d).

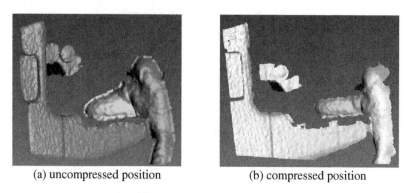

(a) uncompressed position

(b) compressed position

Fig. 5. Three-dimensional surface rendering of the clinical scenario for (a) uncompressed and (b) compressed breast. Breasts are highlighted in yellow. Note that part of the mammography system is also displayed. (Color figure online)

4   Discussion

Results presented in the previous section illustrate breast surface models with enough spatial information to analyse the deformation of the breast. Initial qualitative analysis demonstrates that the breast shape when compressing with a flexible paddle (Fig. 4b, d) is not considered in current anthropomorphic breast models, as observed in Fig. 1. However due to the small population used in this study, no general conclusions could be made regarding breast shape.

The Kinect sensor used has some limited resolution in the depth map (320×240 pixels) to capture small details. Therefore, further processing is needed for smoothing the breast models as well as user interaction to correct of imperfections. This has motivated a small experiment with the latest version of the Microsoft Kinect for Windows, i.e. Kinect v2. Figure 6 illustrates the breast surface captured by the Kinect v2 of an uncompressed and compressed breast.

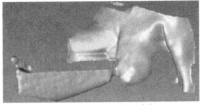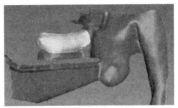

(a) uncompressed position   (b) compressed position

Fig. 6. Three-dimensional surface rendering capture by the Kinect sensor v2. (a) uncompressed and (b) compressed breasts are highlighted in yellow. Note that part of the mammography system is also shown. (Color figure online)

Compared with data from Kinect v1 (Fig. 5), the Kinect v2 sensor shows higher details of the breasts due to the improved depth image resolution (512×424 pixels). In addition to this, Kinect v2 sensor has wider horizontal and vertical field of view, which enable to capture more information in a single shot. However, the reflexion of the breast in the breast support adds inaccuracies to the reconstructed breast surface model. Also the transparency of the compression paddle might produce distortions in the top surface of the breast, creating a large hole.

One of the main limitations of this study was the analysis of only craniocaudal compression. The fixed position of the Kinect sensor in a tripod made difficult the capture of the breast for additional views, since the entire system rotates 45° for mediolateral oblique (MLO) and 90° for mediolateral (ML) view. A camera device mounted in the system as used by Tyson et al. [14] for breast thickness estimation might be a solution to capture breast surface images in more than one view.

Another limitation was the use of a single camera sensor. This setup might be sufficient to capture the breast contour, but two calibrated cameras must be employed to capture the entire breast organ as described by Agasthya and Sechopoulos [9].

5   Conclusions

This paper investigated an imaging framework which employs a Microsoft Kinect sensor to study breast shape during mammography compression. This has potential to be used for further analysis on breast deformation and eventually produce more accurately compression algorithms. This might lead to more realistic synthetic images in VCTs.

Although several limitations were previously described, the Kinect sensors provide depth images with enough resolution to investigate breast surface. Another potential application of such framework includes quality assessment of patient position to avoid repeated tests during mammography acquisition.

Further work will include the design of a more robust imaging framework which will allow to capture breast surface from a larger number of women, and analyse the possible correlation of breast compression with breast density and size. This will improve previously developed breast compression models developed within our research group [15]. Also, further modifications are needed to account for additional view compressions, i.e. MLO and ML views.

Acknowledgments. This work is part of the SCARtool project (H2020-MSCA-IF-2014, reference 657875), a research funded by the European Union within the Marie Sklodowska-Curie Innovative Training Networks. Also, some of the authors have been partially supported from the Ministry of Economy and Competitiveness of Spain, under project references TIN2012-37171-C02-01 and DPI2015-68442-R, and the FPI grant BES-2013-065314. The authors would also like to thank radiographers at UDIAT for their help during image acquisition.

References

1. Lång, K., Andersson, I., Rosso, A., Tinberg, A., Timberg, P., Zackrisson, S.: Performance of one-view breast tomosynthesis as a stand-alone breast cancer screening modality: results from the Malmö Breast Tomosynthesis Screening Trial, a population-based study. Eur. Radiol. **26**(1), 184–190 (2015)
2. Ciatto, S., Houssami, N., Bernardi, D., et al.: Integration of 3D digital mammography with tomosynthesis for population breast-cancer screening (STORM): a prospective comparison study. Lancet Oncol. **14**(7), 583–589 (2013)
3. Skaane, P., Bandos, A.I., Gullien, R., et al.: Comparison of digital mammography alone and digital mammography plus tomosynthesis in a population-based screening program. Radiology **267**(1), 47–56 (2013)
4. Tingberg, A., Fornvik, D., Mattsson, S., Svahn, T., Timberg, P., Zackrisson, S.: Breast cancer screening with tomosynthesis – initial experiences. Radiat. Prot. Dosim. **147**(1–2), 180–183 (2011)
5. Hsu, C.M.L., Palmeri, M.L., Segars, W.P., Veress, A.I., Dobbins, J.T.: An analysis of the mechanical parameters used for finite element compression of a high-resolution 3D breast phantom. Med. Phys. **38**(10), 5756–5770 (2011)
6. Bliznakova, K., Suryanarayanan, S., Karellas, A., Pallikarakis, N.: Evaluation of an improved algorithm for producing realistic 3D breast software phantoms: applications for mammography. Med. Phys. **37**(11), 5604–5617 (2010)
7. Bakic, P.R., Zhang, C., Maidment, A.D.A.: Development and characterization of an anthropomorphic breast software phantom based upon region-growing algorithm. Med. Phys. **38**(6), 3165–3176 (2011)
8. Li, C.M., Segars, W.P., Tourassi, G.D., Boone, J.M., Dobbins, J.T.: Methodology for generating a 3D computerized breast phantom from empirical data. Med. Phys. **36**(7), 3122–3131 (2009)
9. Agasthya, G., Sechopoulos, I.: TU-CD-207-09: analysis of the 3-D shape of patients' breast for breast imaging and surgery planning. Med. Phys. **42**, 3612 (2015). http://dx.doi.org/10.1118/1.4925628
10. Pöhlmann, S.T., Hewes, J., Williamson, A.I., Sergeant, J.C., Hufton, A., Gandhi, A., Taylor, C.J., Astley, S.M.: Breast volume measurement using a games console input device. In: Fujita, H., Hara, T., Muramatsu, C. (eds.) IWDM 2014. LNCS, vol. 8539, pp. 666–673. Springer, Heidelberg (2014)

11. Wheat, J.S., Choppin, S., Goyal, A.: Development and assessment of a Microsoft Kinect based system for imaging the breast in three dimensions. Med. Eng. Phys. **36**, 732–738 (2014)
12. Henseler, H., Kuznetsova, A., Vogy, P., Rosenhahn, B.: Validation of the Kinect device as a new portable imaging system for three-dimension breast assessment. J. Plast. Reconstr. Aesthet. Surg. **67**, 483–488 (2014)
13. Díaz, O., Dance, D.R., Young, K.C., Elangovan, P., Bakic, P.R., Wells, K.: Estimation of scattered radiation in digital breast tomosynthesis. Phys. Med. Biol. **59**(15), 4375–4390 (2014)
14. Tyson, A.H., Mawdsley, G.E., Yaffe, M.J.: Measurement of compressed breast thickness by optical stereoscopic photogrammetry. Med. Phys. **36**(2), 569–576 (2009)
15. García, E., Oliver, A., Díez, Y., Díaz, O., Georgii, J., Martí, R., Martí, J.: Comparing regional breast density using full-field mammograms and magnetic resonance imaging: a preleminary study. In: MICCAI-BIA 2015, Proceeding of the 3rd MICCAI Workshop on Breast Image Analysis, pp. 33–40 (2015)

Proposal of Semi-automatic Classification of Breast Lesions for Strain Sonoelastography Using a Dedicated CAD System

Karem D. Marcomini[1(✉)], Eduardo F.C. Fleury[2], Homero Schiabel[1], and Robert M. Nishikawa[3]

[1] Department of Electrical Engineering, University of São Paulo, São Carlos, Brazil
karem.dm@usp.br
[2] Brazilian Institute for Cancer Control, São Paulo, Brazil
[3] Department of Radiology, University of Pittsburgh, Pittsburgh, USA

Abstract. The aim of this study was to develop a tool to classify breast lesions using ultrasound elastography. Our dataset included a total of 78 patients enrolled for percutaneous biopsy of 85 breast lesions. These lesions were classified into three sonoelastographic scores, where scores of 1 and 2 were considered negative – soft and intermediate respectively; the score 3 was considered positive – hard. The visual classification of elastography performed by two radiologists was compared with our semi-automatic method. This classification aims to segment the red pixels found in the color elastography, quantify them and characterize the lesion by comparing the areas in red with the manually segmented lesion by the two radiologists. Our semi-automated technique had comparable performance to that of the two radiologists: sensitivity of 54.5 % and specificity of 90.5 %. The agreement kappa was greater than 0.8 for all observers. Thus, we concluded that the proposed method achieved a high rate of agreement between observers. In addition, the method presented high diagnostic specificity in classifying breast elastography images. By including more image features in the future, we expect our classifier can be use to standardize the classification of breast elastography.

Keywords: Breast cancer · Elastography · Classification · Color map

1 Introduction

The detection of abnormalities in medical images is an error-prone procedure, even for qualified and experienced radiologists. Breast biopsy is the current method used to distinguish between benign and malignant breast lesions seen at imaging. However, up to 75 % of these patients are benign by means of pathology [1, 2].

Elastography is an emerging imaging technique that may aid in differentiating benign from malignant solid breast masses. This technique quantifies the "stiffness" of a breast lesion in relation to the surrounding tissue. Stiffer areas deform less easily than do their surroundings and are depicted as specific colors on strain images, whereas softer areas deform more easily than do their surroundings [3]. Usually, malignant lesions tend to be harder than the benign lesions due to its high cellularity and surrounding desmoplasia.

© Springer International Publishing Switzerland 2016
A. Tingberg et al. (Eds.): IWDM 2016, LNCS 9699, pp. 454–460, 2016.
DOI: 10.1007/978-3-319-41546-8_57

Recently, manufacturers have equipped ultrasound devices with several image acquisition systems, which provide information regarding the strain. They include systems with strain elastography (SE), which requires manual compression vibration, and systems equipped with shear wave elastography (SWE) technology that supply vibration energy by means of ultrasound. These methods share the concept of providing qualitative and quantitative data to the diagnostic, i.e., imaging and numerical expression of the stiffness of a target, into the field of ultrasonography, which is primarily concerned with morphological diagnosis. However, these systems differ in terms of their theory, the direction of their development, and their accuracy [4].

However, the main limitation of this method is the inter-observer agreement in the results. Variability in the results may be a consequence of an operator's degree of compression and experience and because there is no current standard procedure for performing the exam.

The elastographic classification proposed by [5] included a three-point scale according to the color variation during compression and decompression of the region of interest (ROI). A score of 1 was assigned to lesions that, after decompression, presented variation to lighter strains of more than 50 % of the mass area when compared with the image acquired during compression. A score of 2 was assigned to lesions with color variation in less than 50 % of the lesion area (between 10 % and 50 %) after decompression. Finally, a score of 3 was assigned to lesions that did not present significant color variation during compression and after decompression of the parenchyma.

The goal of our study was to develop a method to classify breast lesions in elastography images using a semi-automatic method.

2   Data and Method

2.1   Patients

Investigators conducted this prospective and observational study from July to December 2015. The local ethics committee approved the study, and investigators obtained written informed consent from all included patients. Investigators included 83 patients who were referred to the IBCC (Brazilian Institute for Cancer Control, São Paulo, SP, Brazil) for percutaneous biopsy of breast nodules with 92 lesions. However, 5 patients, with 7 lesions, were excluded for presenting non-nodular lesions to the ultrasound. Of these cases, 33 findings were malignant and 52 benign.

2.2   Equipment

Ultrasound examinations and freehand strain elastography were performed using the Toshiba Aplio 400 (Toshiba, Japan) with a 5–10-MHz transducer. A previous work describes the technique used to acquire the images [5]. The images were stored and transferred to the computer for post-processing. All images obtained contained mass lesions and we chose the frame that showed the lesion in the major axis.

Figure 1 shows strain elastography and B-mode ultrasound on split-screen mode of lesions with different stiffness.

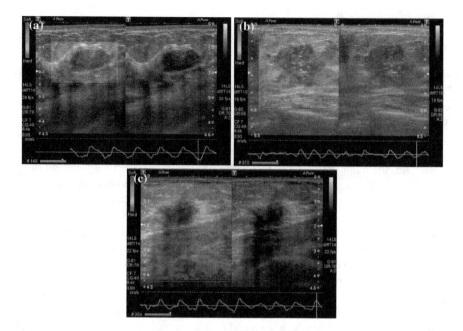

Fig. 1. Patients with invasive ductal carcinoma with different strain. (a) soft; (b) intermediate; and (c) hard.

2.3   Classification

For each lesion selected, two radiologists, one with 16 years of experience in breast imaging and the other one with 2 year experience, drew manually and arbitrarily the contour of the lesions, easily delimited, in ultrasound images using ImageJ software. Then, we positioned this same contour on the elastography image, keeping the aspect ratio and positioning. Black replaced the part represented by adjacent tissue and the inside of the lesion receive the colors contained in the original elastogram.

In order to distinguish the red color from the other colors in the elastogram, we used the method presented by [5]. CIE L*a*b* (CIELAB) is the most complete color space specified by the International Commission on Illumination because the Lab color is designed to approximate human vision. The three coordinates of CIELAB represent the lightness of the color (L* = 0 yields black and L* = 100 indicates diffuse white; specular white may be higher), its position between red/magenta and green (a*, negative values indicate green while positive values indicate magenta, from −127 to +127) and its position between yellow and blue (b*, negative values indicate blue and positive values indicate yellow, from −127 to +127). The CIELAB color space is based on the concept that colors can be considered as combinations of red and yellow, red and blue, green and yellow, and green and blue [6, 7]. In Fig. 2(d–f) we have an example of an ROI with the Lab channels shown separately.

To distinguish the red from the other colors, the user needs to manually delimit a single region that represents the red color in the elastography, creating a mask – Fig. 2(b, c). It is

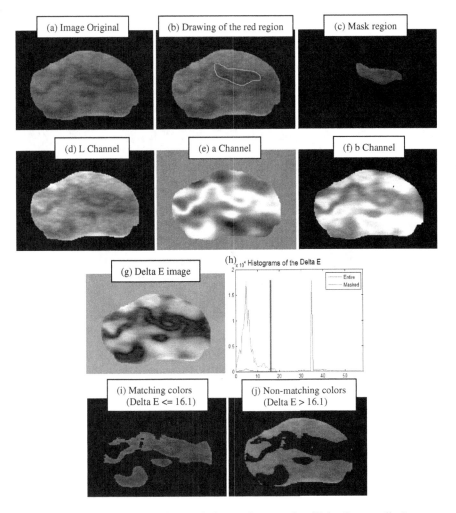

Fig. 2. Classification of lesions in breast elastography. (Color figure online)

important to note that it is not necessary to outline the whole area in red, just a region that contains the maximum and minimum red intensity.

After selecting the mask, we calculated the value of the Delta E according to Eq. 1. The results of the application on the ROI is illustrated in Fig. 2(g).

$$DeltaE = \sqrt{(LChannel - Lmean)^2 - (aChannel - a\_mean)^2 - (bChannel - b\_mean)^2} \tag{1}$$

where, *LChannel, aChannel* and *bChannel* are the images from Lab channels and *Lmean, a_mean* and *b_mean* are the mean values of the pixels in the mask.

Then, we calculated the tolerance value (Eq. 2). This value corresponds to the mean of the Delta E in the mask plus three times the standard deviations.

$$tolerance = meanMaskedDeltaE + 3 * stDevMaskedDeltaE \tag{2}$$

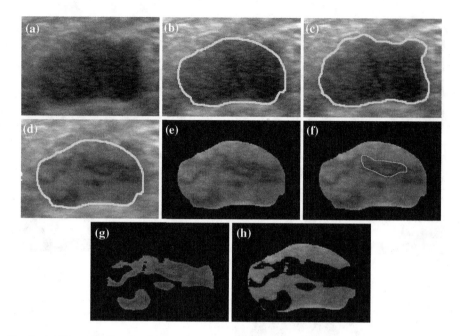

Fig. 3. (a) Ultrasound image; (b) contour outlined manually by the Radiologist 1 (R1); (c) contour outlined manually by the Radiologist 2 (R2); (d) contour R1 superimposed on the elastogram; (e) elastogram without background; (f) initial contour (CI) defined by the user; (g) regions classified as red; and (h) with other colors. (Color figure online)

Thus, the pixel will be set to red (matching color) if its value in the Delta E image is less or equal to the tolerance value. If its value is greater than the tolerance, it is set to non-matching color – Fig. 2(i, j). We can see from the histogram the use of this threshold – Fig. 2(h).

Based on the model proposed by [5] and according with the classification proposed by BI-RADS lexicon, we classify the lesion in three categories, which are: (1) soft for a lesion with red area lower than 50 % of the lesion area outlined by the radiologist; (2) intermediate for a lesion with red area between 50–75 %; and (3) hard for a lesion with red area higher than 75 % of the total lesion area. The lesions classified as soft and intermediate were considered negative and hard as positive.

We compared the results to the results of the percutaneous biopsies. Then, we evaluated the sensitivity, specificity and diagnostic accuracy of the method and the agreement with radiologists.

3   Results

We compared the manual delineation performed by Radiologist 1 (R1) with that performed by Radiologist 2 (R2), and obtained the following mean values: 74.72 %, 9.37 %, 18.14 % and 85.11 % for area overlap measure (AOM), undersegmentation measure (AUM) and oversegmentation measure (AVM) and Dice coefficient [8, 9].

After obtaining the contour of the lesion, we used the proposed approach to distinguish the red color of the remaining. Figure 3 shows the steps of an ROI when it is submitted to computational classification.

We show the results of the visual classification of Radiologist 1 (the higher performing) and using the proposed method in Tables 1 and 2.

Table 1. Data obtained with the breast lesions classification.

Observer	Sensitivity	Specificity	AUC
Radiologist (lesions seen on ultrasound)	97.0 %	59.6 %	0.861
Radiologist (lesions seen on ultrasound and elastography)	100.0 %	63.5 %	0.904
Radiologist (lesions seen just on elastography)	60.6 %	88.4 %	–
Classifier (outlined by the Radiologist 1)	54.5 %	90.5 %	0.837
Classifier (outlined by the Radiologist 2)	54.5 %	90.4 %	0.810

Table 2. Interobserver agreement.

Observer	Kappa
Radiologist 1 (visual analysis) and Classifier (outlined by the Radiologist 1)	0.898
Radiologist 1 (visual analysis) and Classifier (outlined by the Radiologist 2)	0.813
Classifiers (outlined by the Radiologist 1 and Radiologist 2)	0.867

4   Discussion and Conclusion

When we used our proposal to classify the elastogram based on color, we obtained AUC, sensitivity and specificity comparable with the visual classification of the radiologists. Therefore, we conclude that our method is comparable to a radiologist.

We must take into consideration that the low experience of the second specialist did not have significant influence on the results of the classification, achieving values close to those of the experienced radiologist. This shows that our method is not dependent on the contour and, hence, the exact morphology of the lesion. Note that in this study, we did not evaluate aspects related to the morphology of the lesions, such as whether oval or round lesions had the same accuracy as spiculated lesions. We assessed if the interobserver variability could influence the classification of the data.

In additional, it is possible to increase diagnostic specificity using the elastogram. However, elastography alone has low sensitivity. Therefore, elastography should complement the ultrasound exam for obtaining additional information and increasing the accuracy of the diagnosis.

One of the major clinical applications of elastography would be to reduce the number of breast biopsies in probably benign lesions, BI-RADS 3, increasing the specificity of the method.

Although it is a semi-automatic classification model, it is fast and relatively simple. Thus, the proposed method can be used in CAD systems to classify lesions in breast elastography images.

As future work, we intend to add to this study an automatic segmentation method and compare this result with our current results.

Acknowledgements. To FAPESP (2015/17302-5) for the financial support.

References

1. Kumm, T.R., Szabunio, M.M.: Elastography for the characterization of breast lesions: initial clinical experience. Control Cancer **17**, 156–161 (2010)
2. Au, F.W., Ghail, S., Moshonov, H., Kahn, H., Brennan, C., Dua, H., Crystal, P.: Diagnostic performance of quantitative shear wave elastography in the evaluation of solid breast masses: determination of the most discriminatory parameter. AJR Am. J. Roentgenol. **203**, W328–W336 (2014)
3. Awad, F.M.: Role of supersonic shear wave imaging quantitative elastography (SSI) in differentiating benign and malignant solid breast masses. Egypt. J. Radiol. Nucl. Med. **44**, 681–685 (2013)
4. Barr, R.G.: Breast Elastography. Thieme, New York (2015)
5. Fleury, E.F.C., Fleury, J.C.V., Piato, S., Roveda Jr., D.: New elastographic classification of breast lesions during and after compression. Diagn. Interv. Radiol. **15**, 96–103 (2009)
6. Ganesan, P., Rajini, V.: Segmentation and edge detection of color images using CIELAB color space and edge detectors. Emerg. Trends Robot. Commun. Technol. (INTERACT), 393–397 (2010)
7. Baldevbhai, P.J., Anand, R.S.: Color image segmentation for medical images using L*a*b* color space. Electron. Commun. Eng. **1**(2), 24–45 (2012)
8. Pei, C., Wang, C., Xu, S.: Segmentation of the breast region in mammograms using marker-controlled watershed transform. In: 2nd International Conference on Information Science and Engineering, pp. 2371–2374 (2010)
9. Egghe, L., Rousseau, R.: Classical retrieval and overlap measures satisfy the requirements for rankings based on a Lorenz curve. Inf. Process. Manag. **42**, 106–120 (2006)

Markovian Approach to Automatic Annotation of Breast Mass Spicules Using an *A Contrario* Model

Sègbédji R.T.J. Goubalan[1,2](✉), Yves Goussard[1], and Hichem Maaref[2]

[1] École Polytechnique de Montréal, Université de Montréal, Montréal, Canada
{segbedji-rethice-theophile-j.goubalan,yves.goussard}@polymtl.ca
[2] Laboratoire IBISC, Université d'Evry Val d'Essonne, Evry, France
{Junior.Goubalan,Hichem.Maaref}@ibisc.univ-evry.fr

Abstract. In this paper, we propose a new method for automatic extraction of breast mass spicules in 2-D mammography. Spicules are abnormal curvilinear structures which characterize most of malignant breast masses. They are important features for discrimination between benign and malignant masses. In our method, the curvilinear structures are first approximated by line segments derived from localized Radon transforms; then, the Markov random field is used to take into account the local interactions via the contextual information between these segments. Finally, detection of the curvilinear structures that most likely correspond to spicules is performed using an a contrario framework. Validation of the approach was performed on a large dataset of spiculated masses which were selected from a public digital database; the results showed a high agreement with manually annotated mammograms.

Keywords: Breast · Spicules · Localized radon transform · Markov random field · A contrario detection

1 Introduction

Breast cancer is among the leading causes of cancer deaths for women. In 2012, 522 000 deaths have been recorded worldwide, representing a 14% increase compared to 2008 [1]. Early diagnosis and treatment can improve survival rates among patients suffering from breast cancer. Despite the emergence of digital breast tomosynthesis (DBT), mammography is still the only recognized screening exam used in the clinic, because it allows for cancer detection at early stages, therefore reducing the mortality rate.

In 2-D mammography, image interpretation by radiologists is difficult, time-consuming, and sometimes increases the ratio of false positives (fps) due to tissue superimposition. This is even more apparent in the context of screening exams, because decisions that pose a threat to the patient's life should be avoided. Some studies shown that radiologists miss 10 % to 30 % of cancers during mammograms' interpretation [2]. Hence, to help radiologists improve detection and

© Springer International Publishing Switzerland 2016
A. Tingberg et al. (Eds.): IWDM 2016, LNCS 9699, pp. 461–468, 2016.
DOI: 10.1007/978-3-319-41546-8_58

diagnosis accuracy, all while limiting the rate of unnecessary biopsies, the design of computer aided detection (CADe) systems known a great leap forward in recent years due to their ability to provide an objective and reproducible second opinion.

This paper focuses on the detection of spicules, which are curvilinear structures in 2-D mammography. Among breast abnormalities, masses whose margins are spiculated have a stellate pattern and are highly suspicious. According to Liberman *et al.* [3], 81 % of malignant masses are spiculated. Thus, spicules are a leading discriminant factor in the classification of various masses. Their extraction is a complex task, because of their low contrast, variable widths and the overlapping of blood vessels, fibers and ducts. The case of spiculated masses is related to breast imaging reporting and data system (BI-RADS) V and defined by a palpable opacity with radiating lines towards the center of the mass.

Usually, detection methods for stellar lesions proceed in two stages: first, extraction of local features from the image, and second, classification of observations, such as assigning to each pixel a probability of belonging to a lesion. Many approaches are available for extraction of these features (see, *e.g.*, Kegelmeyer *et al.* [4], Karssemeijer and te Brake [5], Liu *et al.* [6]), but most of them only aim at separating suspicious anatomical structures from normal ones in mammographies (see, *e.g.*, Zwiggelaar *et al.* [7]). However, a limited number of research contributions (see, *e.g.*, Kobatake and Yoshinaga [8], Muralidhar *et al.* [9]) propose to extract the spicules from the mass image. Our approach pursues the same goal by attempting to capture the salient characteristics of spicules: after discretization of curvilinear structures into segments, the local interactions between segments that characterize curvilinear structures are accounted for through Markov modeling. Then, the geometric relationship between the spicules and the mass they originate from is taken into account by the *a contrario* detection method. This allows us to avoid computation and extraction of local image features, and to rely on general-purpose classification procedures whose performance and computational efficiency can greatly vary depending on design and image characteristics.

2   Method

The proposed method is based on several assumptions on the structure of spicules as they appear in mammograms which have been reported in the literature. The four more important ones are the following: (*a*) In 2-D mammography, the spicules, which are almost straight lines at a small scale in 3-D, have a curvilinear aspect due to tissue superimposition and partial occlusions caused by projection of a 3D object onto a 2-D plane; (*b*) in a whole mammogram, the spicules are not the most elongated structures due to the presence of blood vessels, mammary and lymphatic ducts, fibers and other structures; (*c*) all segments present in the image do not necessarily belong to the same structure, the discriminating factors being constraints on the orientations of neighboring segments and distance between their end-points; (*d*) spicules are structures which intersect the mass boundary and converge toward the mass center.

In order to make use of the above assumptions, the proposed method proceeds along the following steps: first, the mammogram is separated into patches onto which the curvilinear structures are discretized into segments. Then, Markov modeling and contextual information are used to refine the segment positions and associate segments into curvilinear structures. Finally, spicules are detected based on geometric assumptions (b) and (d).

The first part of our algorithm is similar to some research contributions in remote sensing such as those proposed by Lacoste et al. [10] and Gao et al. [12]. In order to perform detection of the spicules among all modeled curvilinear structures, the a contrario modeling proposed by Desolneux et al. [13] and used in the specific case of mammography by Palma et al. [14] for convergence areas, was adapted to the spicules detection. We now briefly describe the different steps of the proposed method.

2.1 Extraction of Elongated Structures

The general idea is to discretize the mammogram into slightly overlapping patches which contain exactly one segment. After an initialization stage, the position of the segment in each patch is estimated according to the observed mammogram and to the prior Markov model that accounts for the geometric properties of curvilinear structures. The segments are then clustered into curvilinear structures, which are processed for detection of those corresponding to spicules.

Discretization. As indicated above, the image is separated into patches which are allowed to overlap in order to facilitate the recovery of segments that belong to the same structure. The initial position of the segment in each patch is determined through local Radon transform. The latter maps a straight line in the original image to a point in the transformed space. As opposed to previous contributions [9] where the global Radon transform was employed, we use a local version on each patch, which allows us to take into account the curvature of anatomical structures. This method is similar to that proposed in [15], with the only difference that our scale is the size of our patch. Each initial segment corresponds to the point with maximal intensity in the Radon space. This initial configuration is then enhanced using contextual information as indicated in the next paragraph.

Combination of Curvilinear Line Segments. The probabilistic Markov model used to refine the segment positions is designed as follows: each patch s_n ; $1 \leq n \leq N$ is considered as a node of a cartesian lattice S whose probability is given by:

$$p(S) = 1/K \ \exp\left\{-\beta \sum_n \mathcal{U}(s_n)\right\} \tag{1}$$

$$\mathcal{U}(s_n) = \mathcal{V}(s_n, s_n^-) + \mathcal{V}(s_n, s_n^+) \tag{2}$$

where K, β and $\mathcal{U}(\cdot)$ respectively denote a normalizing factor, a weighting term and the energy term of each configuration. s_n^- and s_n^+ are the two neighboring nodes on a 8-neighborhood that best satisfy a continuity criterion between segments, and $\mathcal{V}(\cdot)$ is a continuity measure based on both curvature and distance between end-points, as proposed in Lacoste *et al.* [10,11] and Gao *et al.* [12] for remote sensing applications. Using the classical maximum *a posteriori* approach which is consistent with Markov modeling, estimation of the segment positions is performed through minimization of the following criterion:

$$\mathcal{J} = \underbrace{\sum_n \mathcal{D}(s_n)}_{unary\ data\ term} + \underbrace{\beta}_{weight\ term} \underbrace{\sum_n \mathcal{U}(s_n)}_{regularization\ term} \tag{3}$$

with the $\mathcal{D}(\cdot)$ term measuring the quality of segment s_n with respect to data. Due to the strong nonlinearities present in the expression of $\mathcal{J}$, optimization is performed through a simulated annealing (SA) algorithm whose convergence is favored by the relatively small number of patches.

After convergence of the procedure, clustering of the segments into curvilinear structures is performed via the assignment of specific display colors to the segments for which the fact of belonging to a curvilinear structure leads to the configuration of minimal energy, *i.e.*, the segments arrangement which minimizes $\mathcal{U}(\cdot)$.

2.2   Detection of Convergent Segments

In order to select the structures which are the spicules, we first segment the breast mass by using an almost unsupervised segmentation algorithm based on Pickard random fields (PRFs) and using the telegraph model developed by Goussard *et al.* [16] and extended by Idier *et al.* [17]. We redefined this method by introducing an inverse logarithmic transformation and a sparse dictionary learning approach [18] in order to enhance contrast and remove the noise. The employed data pre-processing considerably improved the performance of the PRFs. The segmentation is an important step which allows us to extract the breast mass margin with a good precision and also to determine an accurate mass center to which the spicules must converge.

Next, we used a method which is similar to that proposed by Palma *et al.* [14], who modeled converging areas by annuli composed of two concentric circles with radius r and αr ; $\alpha \in]0,1[$, in which a sufficient number of pixels are directed towards the inner disk. Here, we proceed differently by only taking into account the end-points' positions of the structures detected in the previous stage, compounded with a simple directional measurement of the orientation of the final segment of the curvilinear structure. This allows us to simplify the processing of the segments and thus to reduce the computation time. Due to the fact that the spicules are not present in the *naive* model, one needs to find a threshold for adverse values of the variables involved in the model proposed by Palma *et al.* The *a contrario* model is suitable for this purpose, and enables the computation of such thresholds, based on the number of false alarms we accept to generate [13]. In addition, in the proposed model, we take into account the intersection of the last segment of the curvilinear structure with the mass margin, in the aim to ensure the existence of a link between them.

It is important to notice that the mass segmentation and spicules extraction are performed separately in order to avoid the significant influence of the noise reduction and contrast enhancement on the *a contrario* detection scheme.

3   Database Description and Implementation

Protocol. We tested the proposed spicules detection method on the digital database for screening mammography (DDSM) [19] DDSM is the largest public database, with 2620 cases including two views of each breast: mediolateral oblique (MLO) and craniocaudal (CC), for a total of 10,480 images, with all types of findings from normal images to images with benign and malign lesions. In our case, we select 100 images with 5 containing malignant masses. For each image we extract a region of interest (ROI), which corresponds to the image region where the breast mass is located.

Numerical Details. Our method was implemented in Matlab ® and running times are given for a machine with a 2.2 GHz quad-core Intel Core i7 processor and 16 GiB RAM. Specifically, Matlab' Parallel Computing Toolbox was used to process the patches in parallel. The size of each ROI was of 300×300 pixels; next, patches of size s×s were extracted with $s = 20$ and $\delta = \frac{1}{4}$ was selected as the maximum intersection area between two patches. To produce the output of each image, we used the following parameters: $\beta_o = 3.0$ and $\beta_d = 0.2$ respectively for orientation and distance weights obtained empirically; and a number of 50 iterations for SA. Finally, for the Radon transform, we used $[0, 180[$ as the angle range and we allowed a minimum number of $k = 4$ segments to form a curvilinear structure.

4   Results and Discussion

In order to characterize the proposed approach, it was tested on a large mammogram dataset. Let TP the true positives (*i.e.*, number of curvilinear structures which are considered by the radiologists as a spicule), FN the false negatives (*i.e.*, number of obvious spicules that were missed by our method) and FP the false positives (*i.e.*, the number of curvilinear structures that were found by our method but did not correspond to spicules). We evaluate our approach by means of three figures of merit which are the *precision* ($\mathcal{P} = \frac{TP}{TP+FP}$), the *recall* ($\mathcal{R} = \frac{TP}{TP+FN}$) and rate of false positive per image (FPI) ($\frac{FP}{TP}$). The values obtained with our dataset and those reported by other authors are shown in Table 1.

Despite differences in the composition of the datasets and figures of merit, the results presented in Table 1 indicate that our method performs well compared to

Table 1. Descriptive statistics of the efficiency of our method

Methods	$\mathcal{P}$	$\mathcal{R}$	FPI
Ours	0.83	0.9	0.2
Muralidhar *et al.*	0.76	0.84	N/A
Zwiggelaar *et al.*	N/A	N/A	0.22
Karssemeijer *et al.*	N/A	N/A	1

approaches proposed in the literature, even though our results can only be considered as preliminary. So, with our dataset, we obtained a precision value of 0.83 and 0.9 for recall against respectively 0.76 and 0.84 for Muralidhar *et al.* [9], who tested their method on a dataset of 20 ROIs.

Our result is also favorably compared to those obtained by Zwiggelaar *et al.* [20] and Karssemeijer *et al.* [5] on different datasets who reported respectively a FPI of 0.22 for a region size of 12 mm and 1 FPI; whereas we reported a FPI of 0.20. It should be underlined that contrarily to [5], our method deals with all shapes of anatomical structures *i.e.*, both straight lines and curvilinear structures. Nevertheless, it is important to notice that contrarily to [5], we don't want to detect the suspicious area (malignant masses with a stelatte pattern) in a full mammogram, but only to detect the spicules related to the malignant mass previously extracted; that specificity can explain our result.

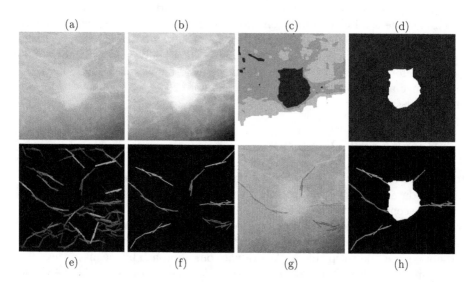

Fig. 1. Annotation of spicules : (a) mass ROI, (b) ROI after noise reduction and contrast enhancement, (c) mass segmentation via PRF algorithm, (d) binary version of (c), (e) curvilinear structure discretization, (f) annotated spicules, (g) superimposition of images (a, f) and (h) result of fps reduction.

A typical result is presented in Fig. 1. From a visual standpoint, the appropriate structures that seem to satisfy the proposed constraints were extracted. Thus, we provide a fast and powerful tool for spicule annotation without introducing additional artifacts by filtering the image.

5   Conclusion

In this paper, we designed and evaluated an automatic and accurate method for the extraction of spicules in 2D-mammography. We extended the idea of local Radon transform while introducing the local interaction between line segments via a MRF. We showed that the MRF-based regularization presented in this paper can improve the detection of curvilinear structures in general. It is a supervised approach with promising potential which takes into account the *a priori* information about the orientation and distance between the segments in order to select the most likely configuration of the curvilinear structures of the mammogram. Moreover, the usage of constraints on the orientation and distance of the recovered structures helped us identify the curvilinear structures which can be labeled as breast masses or architectural distorsion spicules (*i.e.*, converging towards the mass center and having an intersection with its margin). Finally, the consistency and accuracy of our method is confirmed by experimental results using the figures of merit, such as the *precision*, the *recall* and the FPI.

Acknowledgments. This work was supported by Mitacs and Campus France (Research Grant IT5501). The authors wish to thank Dr. Jérome Idier and Dr. Andrea Ridolfi for the practical implementation of the PRF-based segmentation algorithm and Dr. Stéphane Bedwani for its contribution of the realization of this work.

References

1. IARC, Globocan: observation of strains: Estimated cancer incidence, mortality and prevalence worldwide in 2012 (2011). http://globocan.iarc.fr/Default.aspx
2. Elter, M., Horsch, A.: CADx of mammographic masses and clustered microcalcifications: a review. Med. Phys. **36**(6), 2052–2068 (2009)
3. Liberman, L., Abramson, A.F., Squires, F.B., Glassman, J.R., Morris, E.A., Dershaw, D.D.: The breast imaging reporting and data system: positive predictive value of mammographic features and final assessment categories AJR. Am. J. Roentgenol. **171**(1), 35–40 (1998)
4. Kegelmeyer, W.P., Pruneda, J.M., Bourland, P.D., Hillis, A., Riggs, M.W., Nipper, M.L.: Computer-aided mammographic screening for spiculated lesions. Radiology **191**(2), 331–337 (1994)
5. Karssemeijer, N., te Brake, G.M.: Detection of stellate distortions in mammograms. IEEE Trans. Med. Imaging **15**(5), 611–619 (1996)
6. Liu, S., Babbs, C.F., Delp, E.J.: Multiresolution detection of spiculated lesions in digital mammograms. IEEE Trans. Image Process. **10**(6), 874–884 (2001)
7. Zwiggelaar, R., Astley, S.M., Boggis, C.R.M., Taylor, C.J.: Linear structures in mammographic images: detection and classification. IEEE Trans. Med. Imaging **23**(9), 1077–1086 (2004)

8. Kobatake, H., Yoshinaga, Y.: Detection of spicules on mammogram based on skeleton analysis. IEEE Trans. Med. Imaging **15**(3), 235–245 (1996)
9. Muralidhar, G.S., Bovik, A.C., Giese, J.D., Sampat, M.P., Whitman, G.J., Haygood, T.M., Stephens, T.W., Markey, M.K.: Snakules: a model-based active contour algorithm for the annotation of spicules on mammography. IEEE Trans. Med. Imaging **29**(10), 1768–1780 (2010)
10. Lacoste, C., Descombes, X., Zerubia, J.: Point processes for unsupervised line network extraction in remote sensing. IEEE Trans. Pattern Anal. Mach. Intell. **27**(10), 1568–1579 (2005)
11. Krylov, V.A., Nelson, J.D.B.: Stochastic extraction of elongated curvilinear structures with applications. IEEE Trans. Image Process. **23**(12), 5360–5373 (2014)
12. Gao, R., Bischof, W.F.: Detection of linear structures in remote-sensed images. In: Kamel, M., Campilho, A. (eds.) ICIAR 2009. LNCS, vol. 5627, pp. 896–905. Springer, Heidelberg (2009)
13. Desolneux, A., Moisan, L., Morel, J.-M.: Meaningful alignments. Int. J. Comput. Vis. **40**(1), 7–23 (2000)
14. Palma, G., Muller, S., Bloch, I., Iordache, R.: Convergence areas detection in digital breast tomosynthesis volumes using a contrario modeling. In: SPIE Symposium on Medical Imaging: Computer-Aided Diagnosis, Lake Buena Vista, FL, USA (2009)
15. Copeland, A.C., Ravichandran, G., Trivedi, M.M.: Localized radon transform-based detection of ship wakes in SAR images. IEEE Trans. Geosci. Remote Sens. **33**(1), 33–45 (1995)
16. Goussard, Y., Idier, J., De Cesare, A.: Unsupervised image segmentation using a telegraph parameterization of Pickard random fields, vol. 4, pp. 2777–2780. IEEE, Munich (1997)
17. Idier, J., Goussard, Y., Ridolfi, A.: Unsupervised image segmentation using a telegraph parameterization of Pickard random fields. In: Moore, M., Guyon, X. (eds.) CRM series in Statistics, pp. 115–140. Springer, New York (2000)
18. Goubalan, S.R.T.J., et al.: Optimization of the dictionary size selection: an efficient combination of K-SVD and PCA to denoise and enhance digital mammography contrast. In: Martin-Gonzalez, A., et al. (eds.) ISICS 2016. CCIS, vol. 597, pp. 1–15. Springer, Heidelberg (2016). doi:10.1007/978-3-319-30447-2_1
19. Heath, M., Bowyer, K., Kopans, D., Kegelmeyer Jr., P., Moore, R., Chang, K., Munishkumaran, S.: Current status of the digital database for screening mammography. In: Karssemeijer, N., Thijssen, M., Hendriks, J., van Erning, L. (eds.) Digital Mammography, pp. 457–460. Springer, Heidelberg (1998)
20. Zwiggelaar, R., Parr, T.C., Schumm, J.E., Hutt, I.W., Taylor, C.J., Astley, S.M., Boggis, C.R.M.: Model-based detection of spiculated lesions in mammograms. Med. Image Anal. **3**(1), 39–62 (1999)

Improving Mammographic Density Estimation in the Breast Periphery

Xin Chen[1(⊠)], Emmanouil Moschidis[2], Chris Taylor[2],
and Susan Astley[2]

[1] Division of Imaging Sciences and Biomedical Engineering,
King's College London, St Thomas' Hospital, Westminster SE1 7EH, UK
xin.chen@kcl.ac.uk
[2] Centre for Imaging Sciences, Institute of Population Health,
University of Manchester, Oxford Road, Manchester M13 9PT, UK

Abstract. Mammographic density is a strong risk factor for breast cancer. Volumetric breast density can be estimated from a digital mammogram by modelling the imaging process; this provides a more accurate assessment than subjective and 2D area-based methods. However, reliable density estimation in the uncompressed peripheral breast region and determination of compression paddle tilt are still open and challenging problems that affect the accuracy of measurement. Here we present a complete system that is able to perform thickness correction for both the compressed and uncompressed breast regions. The system was evaluated on a dataset of 208 mammograms, and compared with results from commercial software Volpara™ (version 1.5). The proposed method yielded Pearson correlation coefficients (PCC) of volumetric breast density (VBD) between left and right breasts of 0.88 (CC view) and 0.91 (MLO view). The PCC between Volpara™ VBD and our method is 0.93.

Keywords: Digital mammogram · Volumetric breast density · Thickness correction · Compression paddle tilt

1 Introduction

A major focus of breast cancer imaging research in recent years has been the estimation of mammographic breast density. Mammograms are x-ray images of the compressed breast, and differences in attenuation coefficients of the tissues in the breast permit quantitative analysis of composition. It has been shown that women with high mammographic density (MD), measured as the proportion of the breast area occupied by dense fibro-glandular tissue, have a two to six fold increased breast cancer risk compared to women with low MD [1, 2]. However, 2D area-based measures of density are dependent on the way in which the breast is imaged, since volumes of dense tissue are projected onto a plane and may overlap. Increasing interest in direct and objective measurement of volumes of fat and dense tissue from digital mammograms has led to the development of automated volumetric methods such as Cumulus V [3], Quantra™ [4] and Volpara™ [5]. However, accurate estimation of volumetric breast density (VBD) still remains an open and challenging problem as there is a lack of agreement

© Springer International Publishing Switzerland 2016
A. Tingberg et al. (Eds.): IWDM 2016, LNCS 9699, pp. 469–477, 2016.
DOI: 10.1007/978-3-319-41546-8_59

between automated methods and mammography systems are evolving to improve patient comfort, for example by allowing the paddle which compresses the breast during imaging to tilt. Accurate knowledge of the thickness of tissue at each pixel in the mammogram is necessary for volumetric density estimation. This is particularly difficult to estimate at the periphery of the breast where it loses contact with the compression paddle and support platform; we refer to this as the uncompressed region. For longitudinal studies assessing change in breast density over time, it is especially important to eliminate variation due to patient positioning or compression. In this paper, we propose a system that estimates VBD from digital mammograms, accounting for thickness in both the compressed and uncompressed regions.

For estimating thickness in the compressed region, the primary challenge is to estimate the angle of tilt of the compression paddle reliably. Kallenberg and Karssemeijer [6] proposed two methods based on segmentation of fatty tissue and minimising the entropy of image histogram respectively, which were found to have similar performance. Our method identifies fatty tissue using the method described in [7]. In the uncompressed region, the thickness varies across and around the periphery of the breast. Snoeren and Karssemeijer [8] used multiple semi-spheres to approximate the peripheral region and more recently they employed an anisotropic diffusion method [9]. Both methods are claimed to be generally robust, but the authors note that they may create artifacts in some cases. Stefanoyiannis *et al.* [10] described a line fitting method for peripheral region enhancement, but their method assumed constant thickness at any iso-distance from the breast edge; this assumption fails when paddle tilt occurs. Our method takes a novel approach to estimating thickness in the uncompressed region, making fewer assumptions about the shape whilst still obtaining robust results. The key ideas are to identify the compressed and uncompressed regions, and then propagate thickness from the compressed to the uncompressed region using image evidence, whilst imposing smoothness constraints. This allows us to compute a thickness-corrected image from which volumetric density can be calculated [9].

2   Overview and Preliminaries

A typical geometry of the digital mammographic acquisition process is illustrated in Fig. 1 (a). During mammogram acquisition, the breast is compressed by a tilting paddle with one degree of freedom (1-DoF), rotation angle α. Consequently, only part of the breast is fully compressed. The thickness h in Fig. 1(a) can be read out from the DICOM image header. In the following sections, we describe strategies to solve the following problems: estimation of the line that separates the compressed and uncompressed breast regions in the mammogram; estimation of paddle tilt angle and thickness correction of the compressed region; thickness correction of the uncompressed region; and VBD estimation.

As an initial step we represent each pixel location in the breast using a custom coordinate system (θ, d) (Fig. 1(b)), where d is the Euclidean distance between the current location and closest point on the breast edge (obtained by a segmentation method described below). The coordinate system origin is located at the row with maximum d, and the 1st column of the image. $\theta \in [0°, 180°]$ is the angle around the origin from the bottom half of the vertical axis in an anti-clockwise direction.

Chen *et al.* [7] proposed a machine learning method that is able to simultaneously segment the breast region, pectoral muscle, fatty tissue, glandular tissue and nipple. The method learns feature descriptors using the dual-tree complex wavelet transform and a random forest classifier. Here we extend it to classify the fibrous tissue as well. The segmentation method produces a label map and associated confidence map for each anatomical class. Figure 2 shows a digital mammogram, together with the resulting class labels, and the fatty tissue confidence map (brighter pixels represent higher confidence).

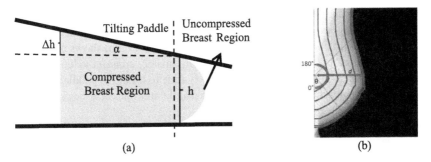

Fig. 1. (a) A typical geometry representing the mammographic acquisition process. (b) Digital mammogram represented in (θ, d) coordinate system.

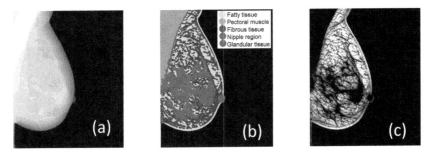

Fig. 2. (a) An example digital mammogram (b) Automatic segmentation – see colour version (c) Confidence map for fatty tissue: bright pixels represent high confidence. (Color figure online)

3   Methodology

Our approach follows that of previous work [9] in using fatty tissue to estimate breast thickness and correct estimates of dense tissue volume. Of the various tissues present in the mature female breast (lobules, ducts, fatty and fibrous connective tissue), fatty tissue is the most ubiquitous and homogenous. Since image intensity in digital mammograms is proportional to integrated tissue density, it can be used to estimate breast thickness in regions containing purely fatty tissue. To exploit this, we use the fatty tissue regions segmented using the method of [7], together with the corresponding confidence map to give greater weight to those points where the classification confidence is high.

3.1   Identifying the Compressed Region

Since we use different thickness estimation strategies for the compressed and uncompressed breast regions, the first task is to find the line d_p that separates the two regions. We define a quantity $R(d)$, the difference in weighted mean intensity between adjacent iso-distance lines:

$$R(d) = \sum_{\theta=0°}^{180°} I_{\theta,d+1} w_{\theta,d+1} - \sum_{\theta=0°}^{180°} I_{\theta,d} w_{\theta,d} \approx constant, \quad \text{for all } d > d_p \quad (1)$$

where $I_{\theta,d}$ is the image intensity at angle θ and distance d from the breast edge, and $w_{\theta,d}$ is its corresponding weighting parameter computed from the fatty tissue confidence map (Fig. 1(c)), normalized for each iso-distance line. Figure 3(a) shows a plot of $R(d)$ for a typical mammogram, exhibiting small, approximately constant values of R in the compressed region, where thickness varies slowly (due to tilt of the paddle), and a clear 'knee' where the breast loses contact with the paddle and thickness begins to change more rapidly.

To find d_p we fit a horizontal line (red dotted line in Fig. 3(a)) to the observed data points (blue line). The optimum position is defined as that which maximizes the number of data points within 0.002 (empirically determined which is not sensitive to image resolution) of the fitted line. Then d_p is the smallest distance value among the 'inlier' points. Figure 3 (b) shows an example segmented digital mammogram (excluding the pectoral muscle) with white and grey areas indicating the compressed and uncompressed regions respectively.

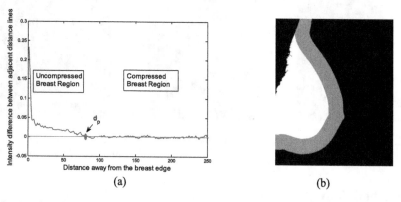

(a)   (b)

Fig. 3. (a) Plot of $R(d)$ for a typical mammogram, (b) Segmented mammogram, with white and grey areas indicating the compressed and uncompressed regions. (Color figure online)

3.2   Thickness Correction for the Compressed Breast Region

Since the compression paddle only tilts around the vertical axis of the image, we can limit our attention to variation in thickness across the image. To do so, we calculate the mean intensity in each image column within the compressed region, weighted by the fatty tissue confidence, normalized per column. An example plot is shown in Fig. 4(a).

The tilt angle is estimated by fitting a least squares straight line, as shown by the solid red line in the figure. Although there are relatively few fatty tissue pixels in some columns, the strong 1-DoF constraint delivers a robust estimate of tilt. This allows the intensity due to fatty tissue to be estimated for each column, and subtracted from the measured intensity at each pixel to give the intensity due to the thickness of dense tissue (so-called thickness correction). Ideally after correction the intensity values of fatty pixels within the compressed region should be zero, non-fatty pixel values should be positive, and the intensity of pixels in the uncompressed region should be negative. In practice, the presence of the pectoral muscle and skin folds result in variations in peripheral thickness. To compensate for this we re-define the uncorrected peripheral region by applying a threshold with a small tolerance (-0.05 in our experiments) to the corrected image (Fig. 4 (b)). It results in a new boundary d_{out} determined by the maximum distance of the uncorrected pixels.

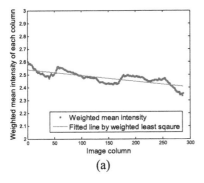

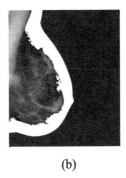

(a)   (b)

Fig. 4. (a) Weighted least square line fitting for paddle tilt angle estimation. (b) Image intensity corrected for the compressed region. The uncorrected region highlighted by white pixels. Red line indicates the maximum distance d_{out} of the uncorrected pixels. (Color figure online)

3.3   Thickness Correction for the Uncompressed Breast Region

Estimating thickness in the uncompressed region is more challenging, because it is unrealistic to assume a simple functional form for the variation of thickness with position. The situation is exacerbated by the fact that segmentation results tend to be least reliable in the uncompressed region, precisely because the thickness varies, so it is difficult to identify pixels that are unequivocally fatty tissue. To address this problem, we propose to propagate breast thickness from the compressed region to the uncompressed region using intensity change.

If we assume the tissue type composition at (θ, d) and $(\theta, d + 1)$ is very similar (identical), the image intensity difference between these two locations are only due to breast thickness change. Since the intensity due to fatty tissue (proportional to breast thickness) is known in the compressed region (Sect. 3.2), The intensity due to fatty tissue for the uncompressed region at (θ, d) can be estimated by:

$$T_{\theta,d} = I_{\theta,d} - (I_{\theta,d+1} - T_{\theta,d+1}) \tag{2}$$

where $I_{\theta,d}$ is the original image intensity at (θ, d). $T_{\theta,d+1}$ is the estimated intensity due to fatty tissue at $(\theta, d+1)$, and $I_{\theta,d+1}$ is the corresponding original image intensity. Hence we can estimate $T_{\theta,d}$ progressively for each radial line (at $1°$ intervals in our experiments), starting from the edge of the compressed region (d_{out} depicted as a red line in Fig. 4(b)) to the edge of the breast.

Since we expect thickness to vary smoothly, we can improve robustness by fitting smooth functions to the estimated $T_{\theta,d}$. We first performed a weighted 5-DoF polynomial fit to the estimated $T_{\theta,d}$ values along each iso-distance line, with weights based on normalized fatty tissue confidence values (Fig. 5(a)). We then sampled the resulting continuous functions at discrete points along each radial line, and fitted a 5-DoF polynomial $T_{\theta}(d)$ to those values (Fig. 5(b)), again using weights based on normalized fatty tissue confidence. In order to ensure the interpolation was smooth at the boundary between the compressed and uncompressed regions, we started fitting from the distance line at $d_{out} + 20$, with the 20 extra data points assigned to the maximum weight of 1. Value T at any non-integer position (θ, d) can be estimated by interpolating between $T_{\theta-}(d)$ and $T_{\theta+}(d)$, where $(\theta-,\theta+)$ are discrete values bracketing θ.

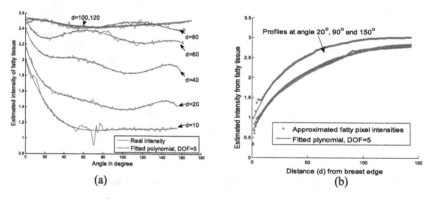

Fig. 5. (a) 5-DoF polynomial curves fitted to fatty pixel intensities along selected iso-distance lines. (b) 5-DoF polynomial curves fitted to approximated fatty pixel intensities from (a), along selected radial lines. (Color figure online)

Figure 6(a) shows the estimated thickness map (intensities only due to fatty tissues) obtained by combining the results for the compressed and uncompressed regions, for the digital mammogram shown in Fig. 2(a). Subtracting the thickness map from the original digital mammogram gives the corrected dense tissue thickness map shown in Fig. 6(b). Note that thickness T is represented by the intensity of fatty tissue, which can be proportionally transferred to physical thickness using h in Fig. 1(a). Based on the thickness map, a 3D breast geometry model (Fig. 6(c)) can be recovered by assuming symmetry of the upper and lower part of the uncompressed breast region.

3.4 Volumetric Breast Density Estimation

The 3D breast volume (BV) is obtained by summing all the thickness values in the thickness map (Fig. 6(a)) excluding the pectoral muscle region. In the corrected mammogram, any pixel intensity I_c can be represented by $I_c = \mu_{gf} h_g$, where μ_{gf} is the difference between the attenuation coefficients of fibro-glandular and fatty tissue, and h_g is the thickness of the fibro-glandular tissue. In our experiments we used values of μ_{gf} listed in [9]; these depend on the known anode target material, filter material, breast thickness, and kVP. The volume of dense tissue (VDT) is obtained by summing h_g across the mammogram. The volumetric breast density VBD is given by VDT/BV $\times$ 100 %.

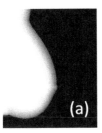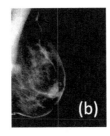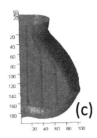

Fig. 6. (a) Estimated thickness map. (b) Digital mammogram after thickness correction. (c) Reconstructed 3D mesh model from thickness map.

4 Evaluation

In the absence of ground truth for volumetric breast density, we compared our method with validated commercial software Volpara™ (version 1.5) using 208 anonymised full field digital mammograms randomly selected from the National Health Service Breast Screening Programme of the Nightingale Centre of University Hospital of South Manchester. These originated from GE Senographe Essential systems with a pixel size of 94.1 μm. We also compared estimates for left and right breasts of the same subjects, which are expected to have similar volumes and densities. The Pearson correlation coefficients (PCC) of BV, VDT and VBD between left and right breasts for CC and MLO views for Volpara™ and the proposed method respectively are listed in Table 1. The PCC between Volpara™ and the proposed method for mean BV, VDT and VBD were 0.97, 0.85 and 0.93 respectively. A scatter plot of mean VBD for the proposed method and Volpara™ is shown in Fig. 7.

Table 1. The Pearson correlation coefficients of BV, VDT and VBD between left and right breasts for CC and MLO views repectively.

	BV		VDT		VBD	
	CC	MLO	CC	MLO	CC	MLO
Volpara™	0.9626	0.9707	0.8785	0.8602	0.9232	0.9311
Proposed	0.9624	0.9637	0.8878	0.8523	0.8829	0.9089

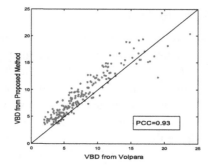

Fig. 7. Scatter plot of mean VBD for each woman (the proposed method against Volpara™).

5   Conclusions and Discussion

We have developed a methodology for digital mammogram thickness correction and volumetric breast density estimation. Our approach combines a machine-learning based segmentation and a new progressive thickness correction method in a custom coordinate system, and is appropriate for both MLO and CC views. Physical ground truth is not readily available for volumetric breast density and breast volume; surrogates such as MRI images may be used, but also require segmentation. In the absence of reliable ground truth the proposed system was evaluated against commercial breast density software (Volpara™) which has undergone clinical testing in relation to risk of developing breast cancer. Our method achieved comparable results (PCC of 0.93 for VBD); however it consistently produced slightly higher VBD values than Volpara™. This may be due to including the breast density additionally estimated from the peripheral region, and will be investigated in the future.

References

1. Boyd, N., Martin, L., Bronskill, M., Yaffe, M., Duric, N., Minkin, S.: Breast tissue composition and susceptibility to breast cancer. J. Nat. Cancer Inst. **102**(16), 1224–1237 (2010)
2. McCormack, V., Silva, I.: Breast density and parenchymal patterns as markers of breast cancer risk: a meta-analysis. Cancer Epidemiol. Biomark. Prev. **15**(6), 1159–1169 (2006)
3. Alonzo-Proulx, O., Packard, N., Boone, J., Al-Mayah, A., Brock, K., Shen, S., Yaffe, M.: Validation of a method for measuring the volumetric breast density from digital mammograms. Phys. Med. Biol. **55**(11), 3027–3044 (2010)
4. Hartman, K., Highnam, R., Warren, R., Jackson, V.: Volumetric assessment of breast tissue composition from FFDM images. In: IWDM 2010, pp. 408–413 (2008)
5. Jeffreys, M., Harvey, J., Highnam, R.: Comparing a new volumetric breast density method (VolparaTM) to cumulus. In: IWDM 2010, pp. 408–413 (2010)
6. Kallenberg, M., Karssemeijer, N.: Compression paddle tilt correction in full-field digital mammograms. Phys. Med. Biol. **57**(3), 703–715 (2012)

7. Chen, X., Moschidis, E., Taylor, C., Astley, S.: A novel framework for fat, glandular tissue, pectoral muscle and nipple segmentation in full field digital mammograms. In: Fujita, H., Hara, T., Muramatsu, C. (eds.) IWDM 2014. LNCS, vol. 8539, pp. 201–208. Springer, Heidelberg (2014)

8. Snoeren, P., Karssemeijer, N.: Thickness correction of mammographic images by means of a global parameter model of the compressed breast. IEEE Trans. Med. Imaging **23**, 799–806 (2004)

9. van Engeland, S., Snoeren, P., Huisman, H., Boetes, C., Karssemeijer, N.: Volumetric breast density estimation from full-field digital mammograms. IEEE Trans. Med. Imaging **25**(3), 273–282 (2006)

10. Stefanoyiannis, A., Costaridou, L., Skiadopoulos, S., Panayiotakis, G.: A digital equalisation technique improving visualisation of dense mammary gland and breast periphery in mammography. Eur. J. Radiol. **45**(2), 139–149 (2003)

Simulation of Breast Anatomy: Bridging the Radiology-Pathology Scale Gap

Predrag R. Bakic[1(✉)], David D. Pokrajac[2], Rebecca Batiste[3], Michael D. Feldman[3], and Andrew D.A. Maidment[1]

[1] Department of Radiology, University of Pennsylvania, Philadelphia, PA, USA
Predrag.Bakic@uphs.upenn.edu
[2] Computer and Information Sciences Department, Delaware State University, Dover, DE, USA
[3] Department of Pathology and Laboratory Medicine, University of Pennsylvania, Philadelphia, PA, USA

Abstract. We have developed an efficient simulation of breast anatomy over a range of spatial scales, covering tissue details seen in both radiology and pathology images. The simulation is based on recursive partitioning using octrees, and is performed in two stages. First, the macro- and meso-scale anatomical features are simulated: breast outline, skin, and the matrix of tissue compartments and subcompartments, outlined by Cooper's ligaments. These compartments are labeled as adipose or fibroglandular, according to the desired overall glandularity and the realistic distribution of dense tissue. Second, pathology images are generated to match selected region within the breast, by filling the region with simulated cells (adipocytes, ductal epithelium and myoepithelium, lymphocytes, and fibroblasts) and collagen fibers. Matched synthetic images can support discovery and virtual trials of image-based biomarkers for specific pathology findings. Our proof-of-concept is presented and further optimizations of the simulation discussed.

Keywords: Breast tissue simulation · Virtual clinical trials · Small scale tissue structures · Recursive partitioning · Octrees · Image-based biomarkers

1 Introduction

Computer simulations of breast anatomy have been used for pre-clinical testing of new breast imaging systems and image analysis methods. Breast images synthesized with simulated anatomy are used in virtual clinical trials (VCTs), which have gained significant attention among breast imaging researchers. With the development of digital pathology, and the close relationship between radiology and pathology, there is a growing need for the analysis and simulation of breast anatomy as visualized in radiology and pathology images (Fig. 1).

We have previously developed a method for real-time simulation of breast anatomy at the spatial macro- and meso-scale level [1–3]. Our software breast phantoms and imaging simulation methods have been used by numerous researchers in academia, industry, and government for preclinical trials of digital breast tomosynthesis acquisition

© Springer International Publishing Switzerland 2016
A. Tingberg et al. (Eds.): IWDM 2016, LNCS 9699, pp. 478–485, 2016.
DOI: 10.1007/978-3-319-41546-8_60

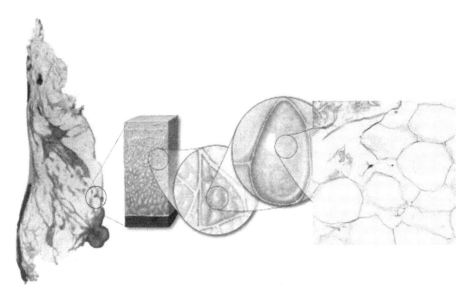

Fig. 1. Example of breast tissue sections at various spatial scales, from sub-gross, whole-breast section (left) to digitized histopathological section (right). (*Modified from* [4, 5].)

and reconstruction, image denoising methods, breast density and parenchymal complexity biomarkers, and for the development of anthropomorphic physical breast phantoms.

In this paper we describe the extension of our simulation to the cellular level, and its use to model breast anatomy over a range of spatial scales, from radiology to pathology. Section 2 briefly reviews the histopathology of the breast, identifying the anatomical structures to be simulated. Section 3 describes the simulation method and presents our proof-of-concept results. Advantages and limitations of the proposed method, and further optimization are discussed in Sect. 4.

2   Histopathology of the Breast

Figure 1 illustrates the organization of breast tissue at various spatial scales. Starting from a sub-gross, whole breast section (Fig. 1, left [4]), drawings of magnified tissue sections (Fig. 1, center) show fat compartments (or pearls) and subcompartments (or lobuli) [5], revealing individual cells in a pathology image (a digitized histopathological section, Fig. 1, right). Pathology images show a wide variation in the arrangement of different cell types, as seen in Fig. 2.

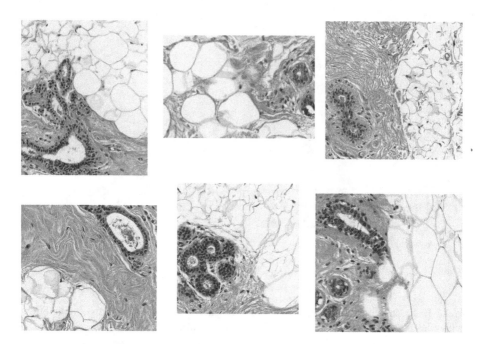

Fig. 2. Details of pathology images (H&E stained), showing regions of predominantly fibroglandular and predominantly adipose tissues.

In this paper, we have focused on the simulation of normal anatomy based upon its description in the literature, and the analysis of pathology images available from the Department of Pathology at the University of Pennsylvania. Simulation of breast abnormalities at the cellular level is our future research task.

Specifically, we simulate the following structures at the cellular scale:

- *Predominantly adipose regions* which consist of *adipocytes* (of size 70–120 μm), hierarchically organized into adipose compartments and subcompartments of decreasing size (*see* Fig. 1, *modified from* [5]), septated by *collagen fiber* ligaments and sparse *fibroblasts cells* (10–15 μm).
- *Predominantly fibroglandular regions* which consist of mammary ducts of irregular shape, lined with two layers of cells: *epithelial* (20–60 μm) and *myoepithelial*; terminal ductal lobular units (TDLUs) with terminal ducts and lobuli/acini (also lined with epithelial and myoepithelial cells), surrounded by basement membrane of *dense and loose fibrous tissue*, with sparse *fibroblast cells* and small *lymphocytes* (7–20 μm).

3   Simulation of the Breast Anatomy at the Cellular Scale

Our breast tissue simulation method is performed in two stages. First, macro- and meso-scale anatomical features are simulated to generate a software breast phantom at *the radiological scale (RS)*. This phantom includes the breast outline, a layer of skin, and the matrix of tissue compartments and subcompartments defined by a hierarchy of Cooper's ligaments [1, 6]. The compartments are labeled as predominantly adipose or fibroglandular, according to the overall breast glandularity, and the realistic distribution of dense tissue [7].

During the second stage, a region within the 3D volume of the RS phantom is selected, and used to simulate the matching pathology image. Figure 3 illustrates the process of selecting the region of the RS phantom to be simulated at the cellular scale.

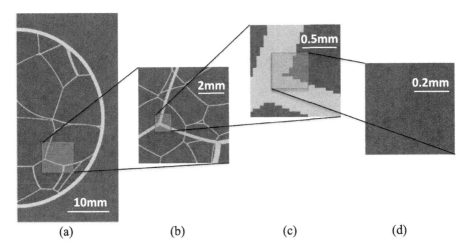

(a)   (b)   (c)   (d)

Fig. 3. A desired subvolume (a) within a RS breast phantom is identified and magnified (b and c) to select a small region (d) which will be used as a mask for simulating anatomical structures at the cellular scale.

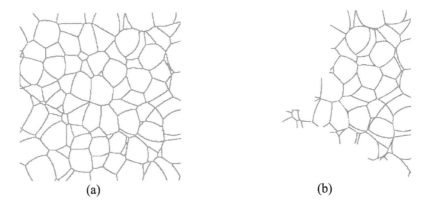

(a)   (b)

Fig. 4. A random collection of simulated adipocytes (a) is used to fill the adipose region of the matching pathology image (b), based upon the mask extracted from the radiology scale simulation, and resamples to match the pathology scale (Fig. 3(d)).

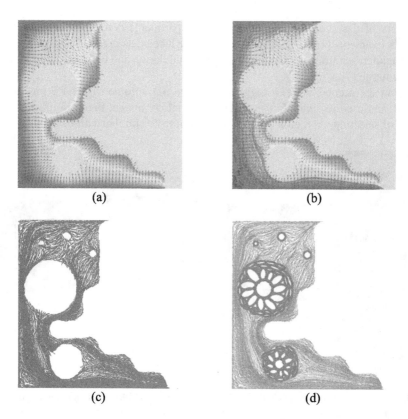

Fig. 5. (a) The region extracted from the RS phantom (Fig. 3(d)), is used for calculating the potential and its gradient to automatically place (b) ellipsoidal fiber bundles and fibroblasts (as illustrated in red) along the equipotential lines. (c) Simulated collagen fiber bundles and fibroblasts. (d) Completely simulated predominantly fibroglandular portion of the pathology image. (Color figure online)

The selected region is resampled to the spatial resolution of the pathology image, and filled with tissue structures simulated at the cellular scale. Appropriate cell types are selected among those listed in Sect. 1. Adipocytes, ductal epithelium and myoepithelium, lymphocytes, fibroblasts and collagen fiber bundles are simulated using recursive partitioning with octrees, [1] selecting appropriate parameters to control the compartment size and shape. Additional anatomical structures may be optionally simulated, e.g., collocated arteries, veins, and lymph vessels, with lumens lined by endothelium, and surrounded by smooth muscles.

For the purpose of this paper, we generated a proof-of-concept example of a pathology image, simulated at 1 µm spatial resolution, starting from an RS phantom simulated at 50 µm voxel size. The region in Fig. 3(d) contains a predominantly adipose portion (part of an adipose subcompartment from the RS phantom), and a predominantly fibroglandular portion (part of a ligament and a glandular tissue from the RS phantom).

The predominantly adipose portion in our example consist of a random collection of adipocytes, simulated using the recursive partitioning in the same fashion as for the adipose compartments of the RS phantom). Figure 4 illustrates the simulation of adipocytes within the predominantly adipose portion of the pathology image.

The predominantly fibroglandular portion consists of a few randomly located ductal segments and/or acini, and lymphocytes, surrounded by fiber bundles and elongated fibroblasts. Figure 5 illustrates the simulation of the predominantly fibroglandular portion of the pathology image. *First*, the locations for each ducts/acini and lymphocyte are selected; the spheroidal lumens of ducts/acini and the extent of lymphocytes are indicated (as light gray spherical areas on the left side of Fig. 5(a)). *Second*, positions and directions of fiber bundles and fibroblasts are automatically selected to follow equipotential lines calculated based upon the following assumptions:

1. The border between the adipose and fibroglandular regions (colored red in Fig. 5(a)) is kept at a given (e.g., positive) potential;
2. The locations of simulated ducts/acini and lymphocytes are kept at the opposite (e.g., negative) potential; and
3. The borders of the selected fibroglandular tissue region (colored blue in Fig. 5(a)) are at zero potential.

The potential values and their gradient are shown in Fig. 5(a) as colored lines and arrows, respectively. Examples of automatically placed fiber bundles and fibroblasts are shown as a connected series of small red ellipses in Fig. 5(b). This method currently does not simulate intracellular structures (e.g., nucleus, cytoskeleton, etc.); thus, our proof–of–concept example does not distinguish between collagen fibers and fibroblasts. Figure 5(b) shows a total of 5,438 simulated ellipsoidal fiber bundles and fibroblasts.

Finally, simulated ducts/acini are added, surrounded by layers of ellipsoidally shaped epithelial cells and flattened myoepithelial cells. Simulating lymphocytes completes the process of filling the predominantly fibroglandular portion of the pathology image, shown in Fig. 5(c).

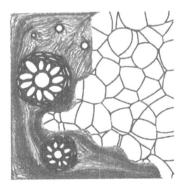

Fig. 6. A simulated pathology image, matching the region selected within the RS software breast phantom (Fig. 3). Included is a random collection of adipocytes (right) and randomly placed lymphocytes (upper left) and ducts/acini (central and lower left) surrounded by fiber bundles and fibroblasts (left). (No cell nuclei are currently simulated.)

Figure 6 shows the final version of the pathology image, produced by combining the simulated predominantly adipose and fibroglandular portions (shown in Figs. 4(b) and 5(c), respectively) of the selected RS phantom region (Fig. 3).

4   Discussion and Conclusions

We have presented a novel method for simulating breast tissue at the cellular level based upon recursive partitioning using octrees. This simulation method can be incorporated with our previously developed software phantoms at the macro/meso-scale, thus bridging the gap between the representation of the breast tissue in radiology and pathology images.

The proof-of-concept example (Fig. 6), shows the cellular scale anatomical structures within a small region selected within a RS breast phantom (Fig. 3). The selected region is extracted, resampled, and used as a mask for simulating predominantly adipose and predominantly fibroglandular tissue portions of the matching pathology image. The simulated tissue portions contain a random collection of adipocytes, as well as randomly placed ductal segments and/or acini, lymphocytes, collagen fiber bundles and fibroblasts. For comparison, Fig. 2 shows details of digitized clinical pathology images from the Department of Pathology at the University of Pennsylvania. Initial visual evaluation of synthetic pathology images has emphasized the realistic appearance of simulated adipocytes, fiber bundles and fibroblasts. A larger observer study by experienced clinical pathologists is currently undergoing.

The approach presented in this proof-of-concept example can be seen as a "zoom-in" of selected regions in the corresponding RS phantoms. For practical purposes, in the example presented it has been assumed that all the cells lay within the same plane of the pathology image. Our recursive partitioning simulation, however, does not require such a limitation; simulated structures (e.g., adipocytes, acini, collagen fibers, etc.) may be positioned at arbitrary 3D locations. This would allow the generation of successive pathology images at different depths, representing 3D pathology matched to the simulated RS phantom. The simulation of the whole breast volume at the cellular scale is not justifiable at the moment, due to the high data storage and transfer requirements. It might be considered, however, with further optimization of our anatomy simulation methods. Alternatively, optimized simulation might allow inclusion of more anatomical detail at the cellular scale (e.g., cell nuclei) to improve the realism of simulated pathology images.

Other directions for future research include the quantification of the spatial distributions for different cell types, corresponding to various parenchymal properties or clinical findings or local variations in breast parenchymal properties, to support realistic simulation of matched radiology and pathology images. Furthermore, the selection of appropriate coloring schemes for the matched pathology images could help represent a range of clinically used stains, for the same simulated cellular anatomy. The presented approach may be extended to simulate breast abnormalities at the cellular scale and enable their visualization in simulated radiological images. Such extended simulation can be used for discovery and virtual clinical trials [8] of image-based biomarkers for specific clinical breast findings.

Acknowledgments. This research was supported by a grant from the U.S. National Cancer Institute (R01 #CA154444), U.S. National Institute of General Medical Sciences (P20 GM103446) from the National Institutes of Health. The work was also supported in part by the US Department of Defense Breast Cancer Research Program (HBCU Partnership Training Award #BC083639), the US National Science Foundation (CREST grant #HRD-1242067), the US Department of Defense/Department of Army (Award #W911NF-11-2-0046). The authors thank Dr. Brad Keller for providing anonymized, previously collected pathology specimen, obtained as part of his Komen Postdoctoral Fellowship.

References

1. Pokrajac, D.D., Maidment, A.D.A., Bakic, P.R.: Optimized generation of high resolution breast anthropomorphic software phantoms. Med. Phys. **39**, 2290–2302 (2012)
2. Chui, J.H., Pokrajac, D.D., Maidment, A.D.A., Bakic, P.R.: Roadmap for efficient parallelization of breast anatomy simulation. In: Physics of Medical Imaging. SPIE, San Diego, CA, pp. 83134T83131–83110 (2012)
3. Chui, J.H., Pokrajac, D.D., Maidment, A.D., Bakic, P.R.: Towards breast anatomy simulation using GPUs. In: Maidment, A.D., Bakic, P.R., Gavenonis, S. (eds.) IWDM 2012. LNCS, vol. 7361, pp. 506–513. Springer, Heidelberg (2012)
4. Wellings, S.R., Jensen, H.M., Marcum, R.G.: An atlas of the subgross pathology of the human breast. J. Nat. Cancer Inst. **55**, 231–273 (1975)
5. Mendieta, C.G.: Power-assisted and ultrasound-assisted liposuction for gluteal sculpting. In: QMP's Plastic Surgery Pulse News. Quality Medical Publishing (2009)
6. Bakic, P.R., Pokrajac, D.D., De Caro, R., Maidment, A.D.: Realistic simulation of breast tissue microstructure in software anthropomorphic phantoms. In: Fujita, H., Hara, T., Muramatsu, C. (eds.) IWDM 2014. LNCS, vol. 8539, pp. 348–355. Springer, Heidelberg (2014)
7. Chui, J.H., Zeng, R., Pokrajac, D.D., Park, S., Myers, K.J., et al.: Two methods for simulation of dense tissue distribution in software breast phantoms. In: Physics of Medical Imaging. SPIE, Lake Buena Vista, FL, pp. 86680M86681–86610 (2013)
8. Maidment, A.D.: Virtual clinical trials for the assessment of novel breast screening modalities. In: Fujita, H., Hara, T., Muramatsu, C. (eds.) IWDM 2014. LNCS, vol. 8539, pp. 1–8. Springer, Heidelberg (2014)

Volumetric Breast Density Combined with Masking Risk: Enhanced Characterization of Breast Density from Mammography Images

Andreas Fieselmann[✉], Anna K. Jerebko, and Thomas Mertelmeier

Siemens Healthcare GmbH, Erlangen, Germany
andreas.fieselmann@siemens.com

Abstract. Automatic characterization of breast density can enable more personalized breast cancer screening work flows. In this work, we present a novel method to automatically characterize breast density in mammography images. Our method computes a volumetric density map and measures the relative volume of glandular tissue (VBD%). For critical cases when masking of small masses may be possible it additionally quantifies the masking effect of glandular tissue. VBD% and the masking risk combined provide a 4-point density score that correlates with the BI-RADS 5$^\text{th}$ edition guidelines. We evaluated our approach using a study with 32 radiologists and 2400 breast images (600 4-view FFDM exams). In a subset of 415 images identified as critical cases the accuracy to detect dense breasts (density categories c or d) increased as shown by the area under the curves (0.783 vs. 0.621). By taking masking risk into consideration our method provides a more comprehensive assessment of breast density.

Keywords: Mammography · Breast density · Masking · BI-RADS 5$^\text{th}$ edition

1 Introduction

Mammographic breast density refers to the amount of glandular tissue in the breast. A high breast density decreases sensitivity of mammography because masses may hide in the dense tissue areas. It is also considered to be an independent risk factor for breast cancer [1].

According to the BI-RADS 5$^\text{th}$ edition guidelines breast density is reported on a 4-points scale (a–d). Not only the amount of glandular tissue should be considered but also masking effects of glandular tissue should be taken into account [2].

Software-based analysis of breast density can provide reproducible and objective information. This information can be used to enable more personalized

A. Fieselmann—The concepts and information presented in this paper are based on research and are not commercially available.

A. Tingberg et al. (Eds.): IWDM 2016, LNCS 9699, pp. 486–492, 2016.
DOI: 10.1007/978-3-319-41546-8_61

breast cancer screening work flows, for example. To date, there are several approaches to automatically quantify breast density [3,4]. Some of them compute an area-based breast density as the fraction of the mammogram where glandular tissue is visible. Others follow an approach that measures the volume of glandular tissue in the breast and compute a volume-based breast density. Recently, there has been some work on quantifying masking effects in full-field digital mammogram (FFDM) [5–7].

In this work, we present a novel method for automatic assessment of breast density from FFDM similar to BI-RADS 5th edition guidelines. Our method measures volumetric breast density (VBD%). Additionally it analyzes the volumetric density map to determine the possibility that the glandular tissue may obscure small masses. Both steps are combined to report breast composition on a 4-point scale (a–d).

2 Materials and Methods

2.1 Volumetric Breast Density Measurement

To measure volumetric breast density we use a physical model of the image acquisition process and apply it to the unprocessed FFDM images [8]. This models assumes that the breast consists of glandular and fatty tissue with known energy dependent X-ray attenuation values. For each detector pixel we compute the amount of glandular tissue located above the pixel.

The total volume $\mathcal{V}_{\text{gl}}(u_i, v_j)$ of glandular tissue in the pyramid spanned by the x-ray focal spot and the 2D detector pixel at coordinates u_i $(i = 1, \ldots, N)$ and v_j $(j = 1, \ldots, M)$ is given by

$$\mathcal{V}_{\text{gl}}(u_i, v_j) = -\frac{A}{\mu_{\text{gl}}(E) - \mu_{\text{fat}}(E)} \times \ln\left(\frac{I(u_i, v_j)}{I_{\text{fat}}}\right). \tag{1}$$

A is the size of the detector pixel area projected onto a virtual plane in the center of the breast parallel to the detector, $\mu_{\text{gl}}(E)$ and $\mu_{\text{fat}}(E)$ are the energy-dependent attenuation values of fatty and glandular breast tissue, $I(u_i, v_j)$ is the measured intensity at pixel location (u_i, v_j).

I_{fat} is the intensity value that a breast consisting only of fatty tissue would have at this particular pixel location. As this value is not known it has to be determined from a reference region in the image. The reference region is based on geometrical constraints and the pixel value histogram. Note that use of Eq. 1 is an image-based approach for breast density estimation which does not require prior calibration scans [9].

The total amount of glandular tissue is the sum of the pixel-based, locally computed amount of glandular tissue and the summary value volumetric breast density (VBD%) is computed as

$$\text{VBD\%} = \frac{\sum_{ij} \mathcal{V}_{\text{gl}}(u_i, v_j)}{V_{\text{breast}}}. \tag{2}$$

In Eq. 2 the volume V_{breast} of the breast is determined using the known compressed thickness of the breast its projected surface area and a 3D shape model.

2.2   Masking Risk Analysis

In addition to computing the summary value VBD% we also calculate a masking risk score (m_{score}) from the volumetric density map $\mathcal{V}_{\text{gl}}(u_i, v_j)$. This score indicates the probability that small masses may be obscured due to locally accumulated glandular tissue.

We use the 2D distribution of the glandular tissue $\mathcal{V}_{\text{gl}}(u_i, v_j)$ as basis for the computation of m_{score}. The motivation for this metric is as follows. The same volume of glandular tissue can lead to different masking effects depending on how the volume is distributed. For example, if the glandular tissue is distributed homogeneously in the whole breast masking risk is low. However, if all glandular volume is accumulated in one place masking risk is high.

To compute m_{score} we first determine the connectivity of glandular tissue using morphological operations on N_l different levels of the density map.

Processing one level of the map consists of the following steps. We threshold $\mathcal{V}_{\text{gl}}(u_i, v_j)$ at value T_l ($l = 1, \ldots, N_l$) to obtain a binary image. This binary image shows all pixels that have a certain minimum amount of glandular tissue located above the pixel area. Small areas of locally accumulated glandular tissue are not considered as a masking risk. These areas are removed by applying morphological opening with a disc-shaped structuring element of radius R_l. After morphological opening the resulting area A_l is computed.

m_{score} is finally determined from the A_l values using a weighted sum with coefficients c_l as

$$m_{\text{score}} = f\left(\frac{1}{N_l} \sum_{l=1}^{N_l} c_l A_l\right) \qquad (3)$$

where

$$f(\rho) = 1 - \exp(-\alpha\rho) \qquad (4)$$

is a non-linear function that maps the output to a range from 0 % to 100 % given non-negative input values.

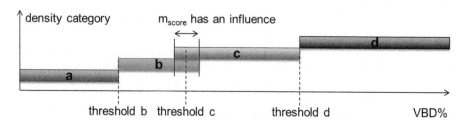

Fig. 1. Illustration showing how VBD% values are mapped to a 4-scale density score using VBD% threshold values. In a region around the VBD% thresholds of category b and c also the computed masking effect (m_{score}) influences the classification.

2.3   Density Score Classification

The breast image is classified on the 4-point scale (a–d) using fixed VBD% threshold values. The m_{score} additionally affects the classification in a certain VBD% interval between categories b and c (Fig. 1). I.e., in the majority of cases the VBD% threshold values alone determine the density score. For cases that are in a critical region between the non-dense (a,b) and dense (c,d) categories the classification is based on VBD% and m_{score}.

2.4   Reader Study

We evaluated automated breast density classification with our method in comparison with visual assessment by radiologists. 600 anonymized 4-view full-field digital mammography exams (mean age 57.3 ± 4.5 years, mean compressed breast thickness 52.7 ± 13.0 mm) were randomly selected from the ethics-committee approved Malmö Breast Tomosynthesis Screening Trial [10]. FFDM images had been acquired using a Mammomat Inspiration (Siemens Healthcare) mammography system.

32 MQSA-certified US radiologists were randomly allocated to three groups of 9, 10 and 13 radiologists each. The 600 exams were divided into 3 sets of 200 exams. Each group of radiologists had to rate the exams of one of the three sets on the 4-point breast density scale according to the criteria defined in the BI-RADS 5th edition guidelines [2]. In particular, the masking of glandular tissue should be taken into account as described in the guidelines.

The panel majority vote (PMV) per exam was compared to the software-determined density score (SDS). Simple agreement and weighted kappa value [11] were computed using R statistics software version 3.1.1 (R Foundation for Statistical Computing, Vienna, Austria). VBD% threshold values for the 4 density categories were determined by 10-fold cross-validation.

Table 1. Breast density assessment on 4-view exam level from radiologists (PMV) and software (SDS).

	PMV a	PMV b	PMV c	PMV d
SDS a	41	22	0	0
SDS b	55	190	19	0
SDS c	1	59	142	10
SDS d	0	0	27	34

3   Results

Examples of density maps and computed masking risks maps are shown in Fig. 2. Colors in the center and right images indicate different threshold levels applied to the volumetric density map.

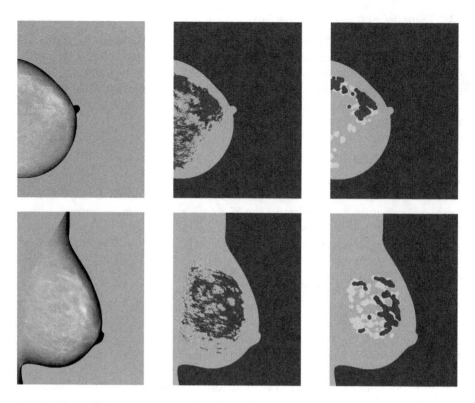

Fig. 2. Two examples for volumetric density maps (left), intermediate (center) and final (right) masking risk maps after morphological processing.

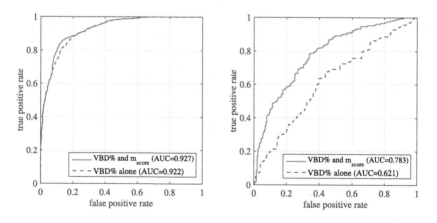

Fig. 3. ROC curves for dense breast ($\geq$ category c) classification with and without use of m_{score} computed from all 2400 images (left) and from subset of 415 critical images (right) in which VBD% is near the category c threshold.

Overall agreement between the PMV of the radiologists and the software density score is 67.8 % (weighted kappa = 0.76). A confusion matrix with detailed results is shown in Table 1. The software shows lowest sensitivity with PMV a ratings (42 %) and considerable higher sensitivity with PMV b (70 %), PMV c (76 %) and PMV d (77 %) ratings.

The performance of our method with and without the use of m_{score} in the classification of dense breasts ($\geq$ category c) is shown in Fig. 3 for the whole data set of 2400 images and for a subset of 415 images where the VBD% value was close to the category c threshold.

4   Discussion and Conclusion

Classification of dense breasts is important for personalized screening. The performance to classify dense breasts breast is lower in the subset of 415 critical cases than in the whole set of 2400 images. This can be attributed to the fact that the subset contains only cases whose VBD% value is close to the threshold value for category c. However, the performance increases substantially when m_{score} is introduced as an additional parameter. In this case area under the curves (AUC) increases from 0.621 to 0.783.

Evaluated on the whole set there is only a mild AUC performance increase when using m_{score} (AUC increases from 0.922 to 0.927). In the ROC curve the effect of m_{score} is visible at a distinct position that reflects the VBD% threshold for category c.

In agreement with the BI-RADS 5th edition guidelines our algorithm quantifies the volume of glandular tissue and analyzes the masking risk of glandular tissue. Including masking risk as an additional parameter increases accuracy to classify critical cases but does not help to classify simpler cases (category a or d cases).

To conclude, combining percentage volumetric breast density with masking risk assessment provides a more comprehensive characterization of breast density to aid personalized screening.

Acknowlegements. The authors would like to thank Magnus Dustler, Pontus Timberg and Sophia Zackrisson for supporting evaluation of the methods using data from the Malmö Breast Tomosynthesis Screening Trial (MBTST).

References

1. Boyd, N.F., Guo, H., Martin, L.J., Sun, L., Stone, J., Fishell, E., Jong, R.A., Hislop, G., Chiarelli, A., Minkin, S., Yaffe, M.J.: Mammographic density and the risk and detection of breast cancer. N. Engl. J. Med. **356**(3), 227–236 (2007)
2. Sickles, E.A., D'Orsi, C.J., Bassett, L.W. et al.: *ACR BI-RADS*® Atlas, Breast *Imaging Reporting and Data System*, chap. ACRBI-RADS® Mammography, 5th edn. American College of Radiology, Reston, VA (2013)

3. Ng, K., Lau, S.: Vision 20/20: mammographic breast density and its clinical applications. Med. Phys. **42**(12), 7059–7077 (2015)
4. He, W., Juette, A., Denton, E.R.E., Oliver, A., Martí, R., Zwiggelaar, R.: A review on automatic mammographic density and parenchymal segmentation. Int. J. Breast Cancer **2015**, Article ID 276217, 31 pages (2015)
5. Mainprize, J.G., Wang, X., Ge, M., Yaffe, M.J.: Towards a quantitative measure of radiographic masking by dense tissue in mammography. In: Fujita, H., Hara, T., Muramatsu, C. (eds.) IWDM 2014. LNCS, vol. 8539, pp. 181–186. Springer, Heidelberg (2014)
6. Kallenberg, M.G.J., Lilholm, M., Diao, P., Petersen, P.K., Holland, K., Karssemeijer, N., Igel, C., Nielsen, M.: Assessing breast cancer masking risk with automated texture analysis in full field digital mammography. In: Proceedings 101st Scientific Assembly and Annual Meeting of the Radiological Society of North America (RSNA 2015) (2015)
7. Holland, K., van Gils, C.H., Wanders, J.O.P., Mann, R.M., Karssemeijer, N.: Quantification of mammographic masking risk with volumetric breast density maps: how to select women for supplemental screening. In: Proceedings SPIE Medical Imaging: Physics of Medical Imaging, vol. 9785, p. 97850I (2016)
8. van Engeland, S., Snoeren, P.R., Huisman, H., Boetes, C., Karssemeijer, N.: Volumetric breast density estimation from full-field digital mammograms. IEEE Trans. Med. Imaging **25**(3), 273–282 (2006)
9. Lu, B., Smallwood, A.M., Sellers, T.A., Drukteinis, J.S., Heine, J.J., Fowler, E.E.E.: Calibrated breast density methods for full field digital mammography: a system for serial quality control and inter-system generalization. Med. Phys. **42**(2), 623–636 (2015)
10. Lång, K., Andersson, I., Rosso, A., Tingberg, A., Timberg, P., Zackrisson, S.: Performance of one-view breast tomosynthesis as a stand-alone breast cancer screening modality: results from the Malmö Breast Tomosynthesis Screening Trial, a population-based study. Eur. Radiol. **26**(1), 184–190 (2016)
11. Cohen, J.: Weighted kappa: nominal scale agreement with provision for scaled disagreement or partial credit. Psychol. Bull. **70**(4), 213–220 (1968)

Comparison of Four Breast Tissue Segmentation Algorithms for Multi-modal MRI to X-ray Mammography Registration

E. García[1(✉)], A. Oliver[1], Y. Diez[2], O. Diaz[1],
A. Gubern-Mérida[3], X. Lladó[1], and J. Martí[1]

[1] Institute of Computer Vision and Robotics, University of Girona, Girona, Spain
egarcia@eia.udg.edu
[2] Tokuyama Laboratory GSIS, Tohoku University, Sendai, Japan
[3] Radboud University Medical Center, Nijmegen, The Netherlands

Abstract. Breast MRI to X-ray mammography registration using patient-specific biomechanical models is one challenging task in medical imaging. To solve this problem, the accurate knowledge about internal and external factors of the breast, such as internal tissues distribution, is needed for modelling a suitable physical behavior. In this work, we compare four different tissue segmentation algorithms, two intensity-based segmentation algorithms (Fuzzy C-means and Gaussian mixture model) and two improvements that incorporate spatial information (Kernelized Fuzzy C-means and Markov Random Fields, respectively), and analyze their effect to the multi-modal registration. The overall framework consists on using a density estimation software (Volpara^{TM}) to extract the glandular tissue from full-field digital mammograms, meanwhile, a biomechanical model is used to mimic the mammographic acquisition from the MRI, computing the glandular tissue traversed by the X-ray beam. Results with 40 patients show a high agreement between the amount of glandular tissue computed for each method.

1 Introduction

Tissue segmentation has been an open problem in medical imaging for decades. In breast imaging, this problem is of particular importance for cancer screening due to the fact that breast density is being established as an important risk factor. Accurate knowledge of the internal tissue of the breast could provide information to radiologist to localize suspicious areas within the breast.

Magnetic Resonance Imaging (MRI), X-ray mammography and Breast Ultrasound are the most common imaging modalities used to early detection and diagnosis of breast diseases in women. X-ray mammography is considered as the gold standard in the early diseases detection. However, the 2D-projection hinders locating suspicious lesions within the uncompressed breast and the sensitivity is limited in women with dense breast. Sometimes, MRI or ultrasound scans are acquired to overcome those issues. In fact, radiologists have found that the combination of these modalities leads to a more accurate diagnosis and management

© Springer International Publishing Switzerland 2016
A. Tingberg et al. (Eds.): IWDM 2016, LNCS 9699, pp. 493–500, 2016.
DOI: 10.1007/978-3-319-41546-8_62

of the breast diseases [11] and researchers have focused their efforts on developing algorithms to fuse the information of the different imaging modalities, taking into account the position of the patient and the loading conditions of the breast during the imaging acquisition [4,8,9].

To fuse the information between MRI and X-ray mammograms, researchers have developed algorithms using patient-specific biomechanical models. During the multi-modal registration process, the biomechanical model is used to mimic the mammographic acquisition, compressing the model and projecting internal tissues from the MRI to a 2D space. However, the limited resolution of the MRI scanner makes almost impossible to get a voxel entirely composed by a single (adipose or glandular) tissue. In this case, the partial volume effect of the voxels must be taken into consideration.

This paper aims to analyze the impact of the tissue segmentation (in particular, of the glandular tissue) during the multi-modal registration. Segmentation algorithms are divided into two categories, parametric, those which assume that the intensity histogram follows a probability distribution (usually the Gaussian distribution), and non-parametric, which classify the voxels using just the intensity of the image, such as K-means or Fuzzy C-means [1].

In our experimental results, first of all, we use the commercial software Volpara^{TM} to extract the glandular tissue from the X-ray mammograms. These obtained density maps are considered as the ground truth of our problem. On the other hand, we use a biomechanical model to mimic the mammographic acquisition from the MRI and to compute the amount of glandular tissue traversed by the X-ray beam at each voxel. Four different segmentation algorithms are used to determine the glandular tissue in the MRI: a Fuzzy C-means (FCM) segmentation and a Gaussian-mixture model provided by the Expectation-Maximization algorithm, and two methods that incorporate spatial prior information to them: the Kernelized Fuzzy C-means and the EM-Markov Random Fields, respectively. Global and local measures are used to quantitatively analyze the obtained results.

The rest of this document is organized as follows: Sect. 2 introduces Volpara^{TM}, the MRI segmentation and the biomechanical model used for multimodal registration, Sect. 3 shows the experimental evaluation, while Sect. 5 discusses the main findings of this paper.

2   Methodology

2.1   Volpara^{TM} Density Maps

To compute the spatial distribution of breast glandular tissue from mammograms, we used the commercial software Volpara^{TM}. The basis of Volpara^{TM} software can be found in the work of Highnam et al. [7].

The starting point is to find an area within the mammogram which is entirely adipose (fatty) tissue. This area (P_{fat}) is used as a reference level to compute the thickness of glandular tissue (h_d) at each pixel (x, y) of the mammogram. The

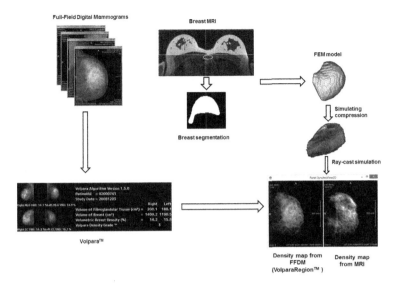

Fig. 1. Scheme of the process to generate the density maps. On the left, from the mammography using the Volpara^{TM} software, while on the right, departing from the MRI.

density map has a resolution equal to 638×765 pixels (0.28×0.28 millimeters per pixel).

In addition to local measures, Volpara^{TM} computes the volume of the glandular tissue, integrating the $h_d(x, y)$ values over the entire mammogram, the breast volume, using the area of the mammogram and the recorded breast thickness, and finally, the breast density and the Volpara Density Grade (VDG), a value, between 1 and 4, comparable to the BI-RADS rating for global breast density [3].

2.2 Generating the Density Map from MRI

In order to generate a density map from breast MRI comparable with the one provided by Volpara^{TM}, the acquisition conditions observed in mammography have to be reproduced. Figure 1 shows the scheme of the process to generate a density map. Firstly, each breast is separated from the rest of the body in the MRI volume. Subsequently, the breast is represented as a 3D model which is compressed simulating the mammographic acquisition and finally projected into a 2D plane using a ray-casting approach. This final projection is the density map obtained from the MRI.

Segmentation. Firstly, image inhomogeneities are corrected using the N4 bias field correction algorithm [15]. The 3D breast MR volume is segmented from the background and separated from the rest of the body using a probabilistic Atlas approach, a methodology similar to the one presented by Gubern-Mérida et al. [5].

Subsequently, internal tissues are further segmented using the FCM [2] and the EM algorithms. We complete this information using two methods that incorporate spatial prior information into them: the Kernelized Fuzzy C-means [17] and the Markov Random Fields, which provides spatial consistency to the Gaussian model. The main reason to use these two algorithms is to avoid the misclassification of skin voxels and uncorrected bias field regions close to the pectoral muscle. Finally, the membership of the voxel to belong to the glandular tissue class is stored, as a 3D density-probabilistic map of the whole MRI volume.

Mammographic Acquisition Simulation. The breast surface mesh and a secondary mesh, belonging to the glandular tissue (voxels with membership higher than 0.5), are extracted from the MR images by means of the marching cubes algorithm. Previously, a morphological operation closes the internal tissue, avoiding small isolated regions within the biomechanical breast model. The tetrahedral mesh is extracted using the open-source package tetgen [13], getting a high number of elements (approx. $100,000$).

The stress-strain relationship is approximated by a nearly incompressible, isotropic and hyperelastic neo-Hookean model for each tissue, using the corresponding Young's modulus measured by Wellman [16] (adipose tissue $E_{fat} = 4.46$ kPa and glandular tissue $E_{gland} = 15.1$ kPa at $Strain = 0.0$ [14]). The breast-body interface is fitted to a linear surface and the nodes belonging to this surface are allowed to slide in the parallel direction to the compression paddle displacement [6]. The simulation is performed by means of the software NiftySim v.2.3.1 [10], using a frictionless contact model to simulate the compression paddle. The necessary information to reproduce the mammographic acquisition (breast thickness, view angle, source-to-detector distance, etc.) is extracted from the DICOM header of the corresponding mammogram.

Finally, a ray-casting algorithm [12], accelerated by a GPU implementation, is used in conjunction with the compressed breast model, to simulate the mammographic geometry. The amount of glandular tissue traversed by each X-ray photon at different locations of the receptor is computed as the length of the ray multiplied by the membership of the traversed voxel.

2.3   Image Registration

After getting the compressed breast image, the biomechanical model is displaced to align as much as possible both density maps, using a Hill-Climbing optimization algorithm (3D/2D registration). The optimization process consists in finding the maximum Dice overlap coefficient between the real mammogram and the projected one. This map is the one that will be quantitatively compared to the map obtained with the Volpara^{TM} software.

3   Experimental Results

3.1   DataSet

The dataset used was acquired at the Radboud University Medical Centre (Nijmegen, The Netherlands) between April 2005 and September 2009, and contains 40 pre-contrast T1 MR images and 80 CC mammograms from 40 women. Patients were selected according to their VDG, choosing 10 patients for each density class. The 40 patients were aged 29 to 59 (mean: 40.91 ± 8.57).

The MRI scanner used was a 1.5 Tesla Siemens scanner (Magnetom Vision, Magnetom Avanto and Magnetom Trio) with dedicated breast coil (CP Breast Array, Siemens, Erlangen). Regarding the mammographic device, the images were acquired by either a GE Senographe 2000D or GE Senographe DS, according to the standard clinical settings. Both studies were acquired in the same day.

3.2   Results

To evaluate our result, each density class is taken independently. Moreover, the parameter of the FCM was set to 2 based on our initial experiments.

Global and local measures are combined to evaluate the agreement between the density maps. On one hand, global measures consist in computing the mutual information (MI) between both density maps and the distance between density maps histograms. On the other hand, local measures were obtained computing the statistics (mean and entropy) of the density maps difference.

Figure 2 shows the results obtained when computing the mutual information between Volpara density maps and the ones obtained from the MRI detailed for each density class and when using the four segmentation algorithms: Fuzzy C-means (FCM), Gaussian mixture models (EM), Kernelized FCM (KFCM) and Markov Random Fields (EM+MRF). We can see that the mutual information measure is higher in denser classes. Moreover, the performance is similar for all

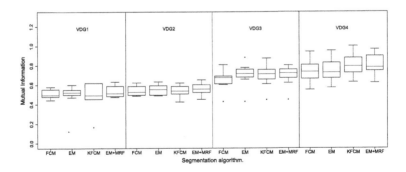

Fig. 2. Mutual information between histograms detailed for each density class (ordered in increasing density class). Higher values indicate a better agreement between the maps.

the algorithms, although adding spatial information provides better results in the densest class.

The histogram of the density maps allows to measure, in a global way, the amount of glandular tissue traversed by the X-ray beam during the projection. Due to the optimization performed we expected the density maps obtained from the mammogram (Volpara^{TM}) and from the MRI to be similar. Figure 3 shows the Euclidean distance between them. According to this measure, EM seems to perform better than FCM, specially in fatty breasts. Spatial information does not provide a significant increase of the algorithms performance.

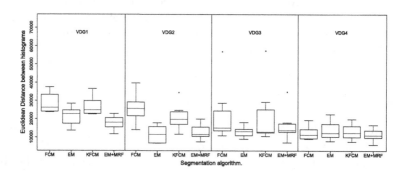

Fig. 3. Euclidean distance between histograms detailed for each density class. Lower values indicate a better agreement between the maps.

Finally, we calculate the point-to-point differences between density maps in order to extract local information of the divergences. In general, statistics extracted from the difference maps show a high similarity between results. For instance, the results of the mean of the difference density maps are shown in Fig. 4. We also observed that the entropy of the difference of the density maps decreases for denser breasts. Regarding algorithms, FCM performs better than EM according to this measure, although the use of spatial information helps to minimize the differences, increasing drastically the performance of the EM algorithm.

4   Discussion

Local distribution and the pattern of glandular tissue provide information to radiologist for risk assessment in localized areas. Comparing those measures from different image modalities (MRI and X-ray mammography) could help to improve the co-localization of these areas in a 3D-space. Our results show a high similarity between the amount of glandular tissue computed from each modality.

Comparing the intensity-based segmentation algorithms used on MRI, the Gaussian mixture model provided better results according to the global criteria while provided worse results according to the local measures. This is mainly

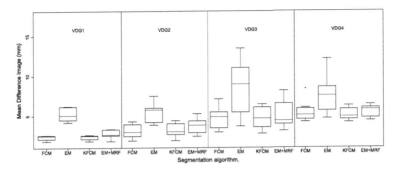

Fig. 4. Mean of the difference density maps detailed for each density class. Lower values indicate a better agreement between the maps.

due to inaccuracies introduced during the multi-modal registration. Moreover, our experiments have shown that the spatial information aids the segmentation and improves the obtained density maps. We also observed that the N4 MRI bias-field correction provided better results in denser breasts.

5   Conclusions

In this paper we analyzed the impact of four tissue segmentation algorithms during the multi-modal registration of breast MRI to X-ray mammography. Two of them consider only the gray intensity levels in the images while the others incorporated spatial information to improve segmentation results. The density maps obtained from this registration are then quantitatively compared with the corresponding maps obtained from the Volpara^{TM} software in the full-field digital mammograms.

Results show a high agreement between density maps. However, inaccuracies during the registration or the over-/underestimation of glandular tissue for each voxel reduce the accuracy of results. Further work will include a more robust multi-modal registration approach.

Acknowledgement. This research has been partially supported from the Ministry of Economy and Competitiveness of Spain, under project references TIN2012-37171-C02-01 and DPI2015-68442-R, and the FPI grant BES-2013-065314.

References

1. Baluwala, H., Sanghani, P., Malcom, D., Nielsen, P., Nash, M.: Comparison of fibroglandular tissue segmentation algorithms in breast MRI. In: Harz, M. et al. (ed.) Workshop MICCAI Breast Image Analysis, pp. 105–112 (2015)
2. Bezdek, J., Pal, M., Keller, J.: Fuzzy Models and Algorithms for Pattern Recognition and Image Processiong. Kluwer Academic Publishers, Dordrecht (1999)

3. Damases, C., Brennan, P., Mello-Thoms, C., McEntee, M.: Mammographic breast density assessment using automated volumetric software and breast imaging reporting and data system (BIRADS) categorization by expert radiologist. Acad. Radiol. **23**(1), 70–77 (2015)

4. Dietzel, M., Hopp, T., Ruiter, N., Zoubi, R., Runnebaum, I.B., Kaiser, W.A., Baltzer, P.A.T.: Fusion of dynamic contrast-enhanced magnetic resonance mammography at 3.0T with X-ray mammograms: pilot study evaluation using dedicated semi-automatic registration software. Eur. J. Radiol. **79**(2), 98–102 (2011)

5. Gubern-Mérida, A., Kallenberg, M., Platel, B., Mann, R., Martí, R., Karssemeijer, N.: Volumetric breast density estimation from full-field digital mammograms: a validation study. PLoS One **9**(1), e85952 (2014)

6. Han, L., Hipwell, J., Tanner, C., Taylor, Z., Mertzanidou, T., Cardoso, J., Ourselin, S., Hawkes, D.: Development of patient-specific biomechanical models for predicting large breast deformation. Phys. Med. Biol. **57**(2), 455–472 (2012)

7. Highnam, R., Brady, S.M., Yaffe, M.J., Karssemeijer, N., Harvey, J.: Robust breast composition measurement - Volpara^{TM}. In: Martí, J., Oliver, A., Freixenet, J., Martí, R. (eds.) IWDM 2010. LNCS, vol. 6136, pp. 342–349. Springer, Heidelberg (2010)

8. Hopp, T., Ruiter, N.V.: 2D/3D registration for localization of mammographically depicted lesions in breast MRI. In: Maidment, A.D.A., Bakic, P.R., Gavenonis, S. (eds.) IWDM 2012. LNCS, vol. 7361, pp. 627–634. Springer, Heidelberg (2012)

9. Hopp, T., Duric, N., Ruiter, N.: Image fusion of ultrasound computer tomography volumes with X-ray mammograms using a biomechanical model based 2D/3D registration. Comput. Med. Imaging Graph **40**, 170–181 (2015)

10. Johnsen, S., Taylor, Z.A., Clarkson, M., Hipwell, J., Modat, M., Eiben, B., Han, L., Hu, Y., Mertzanidou, T., Hawkes, D.J., Ourselin, S.: NiftySim: a GPU-based non-linear finite element package for simulation of soft tissue biomechanics. J. Comput. Assist. Radiol. Surg. **10**(7), 1077–1095 (2014)

11. Malur, S., Wurdinger, S., Moritz, A., Michels, W., Schneider, A.: Comparison of written reports of mammography, sonography and magnetic resonance mammography for preoperative evaluation of breast lesions, with special emphasis on magnetic resonance mammography. Breast Cancer Res. **3**(1), 55–60 (2001)

12. Roth, S.: Ray casting for modeling solids. Comput. Graph. Image Process. **18**(2), 109–144 (1982)

13. Si, H.: Tetgen, a Delaunay-based quality tetrahedral mesh generator. ACM Trans. Math. Softw. **41**(2), 1–36 (2015)

14. Tanner, C., Degenhard, A., Schnabel, J., Smith, A.C., Hayes, C., Sonoda, L., Lach, M., Hose, D., Hill, D., Hawkes, D.: A method for the comparison of biomechanical breast models. IEEE Workshop MMBIA **2001**, 11–18 (2001)

15. Tustison, N., Avants, B., Cook, P., Zheng, Y., Egan, A., Yushkevich, P., Gee, J.: N4ITK: improved N3 bias correction. IEEE Trans. Med. Imaging **29**(6), 1310–1320 (2010)

16. Wellman, P.: Tactile imaging. Ph.D. thesis, Cambridge, MA, Harvard University's Division of Engineering and Applied Sciences (1999)

17. Wu, Z., Xies, W., Yu, J.: Fuzzy C-means clustering algorithm based on kernel method. In: Proceedings Fifth International Conference on Computational Intelligence and Multimedia Applications, ICCIMA 2003, pp. 49–54. IEEE (2003)

3D Total Variation Minimization Filter for Breast Tomosynthesis Imaging

Ana M. Mota$^{(\boxtimes)}$, Nuno Oliveira, Pedro Almeida, and Nuno Matela

Faculdade de Ciências, Instituto de Biofísica E Engenharia Biomédica,
Universidade de Lisboa, Campo Grande, 1749-016 Lisbon, Portugal
`ammota@fc.ul.pt`

Abstract. The purpose of this work was to implement and evaluate the performance of a 3D Total Variation (TV) minimization filter for Poisson noise and apply
it to 3D digital breast tomosynthesis (DBT) data. The value of Lagrange multiplier
(λ) to be used in filter equation has a direct relationship with the results obtained.
Some preliminary studies about λ values were done.

A Mammographic Accreditation Phantom Model 156 was acquired and its
biggest tumor-like mass and cluster of microcalcifications were used for image
quality assessment. The proposed methodology was also tested with one clinical
DBT data set.

For 3D filter performance analysis: a reduction of 41.08 % and 38.60 % in 3D
TV was achieved when a constant or variable λ value is used over slices, respectively. Either for constant or variable λ, the artifact spread function was improved,
when compared to the unfiltered data. For the in-plane analysis: when constant λ
is used, a reduction of 37.02 % in TV, an increase of 47.72 % in contrast to noise
ratio (CNR) and a deterioration of 0.15 % in spatial resolution were obtained. For
a variable λ, a reduction of 37.12 % in TV, an increase of 42.66 % in CNR and
an improvement of 18.85 % in spatial resolution were achieved. A visual inspection of unfiltered and filtered clinical images demonstrates the quantitative values
achieved with the phantom, where areas with higher noise level become smoother
while preserving edges and details of the structures (about 43 % of TV reduction).

Both quantitative and qualitative analysis performed in this study confirmed
the relevance of this approach in improving image quality in DBT imaging.

Keywords: Digital breast tomosynthesis · Total variation minimization · Image
processing

1 Introduction

Breast cancer has been recognized as a major public health problem. It is the most
common type of cancer diagnosed among women worldwide, being one of the leading
causes of cancer death [1]. Approved by Food and Drug Administration five years ago
[2], Digital Breast Tomosynthesis (DBT), has been widely referred to as a possible
modality to replace Digital Mammography in the screening programs [3–5]. With DBT,
2D projections acquired over a limited angular range are reconstructed into a 3D volume
data, using approximately the same dose of two mammograms [6]. The angular limit

© Springer International Publishing Switzerland 2016
A. Tingberg et al. (Eds.): IWDM 2016, LNCS 9699, pp. 501–509, 2016.
DOI: 10.1007/978-3-319-41546-8_63

and low dose projections result in low statistics and high noise level in the reconstructed images. Besides, the presence of blur caused by out-of-plane structures is also a predominant issue in DBT imaging.

Some filters, such as Hanning [7, 8] or Butterworth [9, 10], can be applied in order to minimize noise level in DBT images. However, although these filters allow a reduction of image noise, there is a degradation of spatial resolution. Thus, their application has to be mediated by a compromise between noise minimization and spatial resolution preservation.

Total Variation (TV) based minimization algorithms have been investigated in image denoising field and the results are encouraging [11–17]. These algorithms have the ability to simultaneously preserve edges and reduce noise level. TV is a quantity that characterizes how smoothly the intensity of an image is changing and it increases significantly in the presence of noise. TV minimization algorithm was originally introduced in 1992 (ROF model), where the TV of a 2D image is minimized subject to constraints involving Gaussian noise statistics [18]. There are some studies addressing 2D TV minimization (with Poisson or Gaussian noise models) [19–22]. However, only few are about 3D TV minimization [23–26]. In the present work, our aim was to implement a method to reduce DBT data noise and to evaluate its 3D performance. For this we tested the approach of directly solving the 3D TV minimization problem, based on ROF model for Poisson noise. We applied this digital filter to real DBT data (phantom and clinical) and carried out visual and quantitative analysis.

2   Method

2.1   Acquisition and Reconstruction

A Mammographic Accreditation Phantom Model 156 by Gammex was acquired to perform image quality assessment. It was used a Siemens Mammomat Inspiration system that makes 25 low dose acquisition within a limited angular range of approximately 50°. The acquired data was reconstructed with the iterative image reconstruction algorithm Algebraic Reconstruction Technique (ART), with a constant relaxation coefficient of 0.20 (this choice was made based on previous studies – scientific paper under approval) and finalized after convergence iteration (7th), using IDL from Exelis with a voxel size of $0.34 \times 0.34 \times 1.00 \, \text{mm}^3$. Clinical DBT data set from an anonymous patient (with microcalcifications (MCs) and some dense regions) was obtained with the same equipment and reconstructed under the same conditions as the phantom.

2.2   Image Analysis

For phantom image analysis, quantitative and qualitative comparisons were performed between unfiltered and filtered reconstructed images. For an in-plane analysis, contrast to noise ratio (CNR) and full width at half maximum (FWHM) of one microcalcification were used. For the 3D quantitative analysis, the artifact spread function (ASF) was determined. For both cases the respective TV values were calculated and compared.

For CNR, a circular region of interest (ROI) over a selected feature (mass) at its in-focus plane and another over the background were drawn. CNR was calculated with Eq. (1):

$$CNR = \frac{\mu_F - \mu_B}{\sigma_B} \tag{1}$$

Where μ_F and μ_B stand for the mean pixel values in ROI over the feature and background, respectively; and σ_B stands for standard deviation in background ROI.

FWHM of a Gaussian curve fitted to the point spread function of one microcalcification was considered as an indicator of spatial resolution.

To quantify the magnitude of the ghosting artifacts [27], the ASF was calculated as:

$$ASF(z) = \frac{CNR(z)}{CNR(z_0)} \tag{2}$$

where $CNR(z_0)$ and $CNR(z)$ are the CNR measured at the in-focus (z_0) and off-focus (z) slice location of the real feature, respectively.

For a better visualization, in qualitative analysis, the results obtained for unfiltered and filtered images are presented in terms of smaller images containing only masses or MCs. Variations in clinical image quality were evaluated based on the visualization of a slice containing a good view of a microcalcification and a dense region.

2.3 Formulation of TV Minimization Algorithm

Our unconstrained problem (Eq. (3)) is composed by a regularization term that is the TV function and a fidelity term corresponding to the assumed noise model (Poisson).

$$\min_{u} \left\{ TV(u) + \lambda(u - f \ln u) \right\} \tag{3}$$

f and u are the original and denoised image, respectively, and $TV(u)$ is the TV of denoised image. λ is the Lagrange multiplier, also called as regularization or fitting parameter since it controls image regularization, between removing noise and preserving edges. TV values were determined according to Eq. (4).

$$TV(u) = \sum_{i=1}^{m} \sum_{j=1}^{n} \sum_{k=1}^{p} \sqrt{(\Delta_x u_{i,j,k})^2 + (\Delta_y u_{i,j,k})^2 + (\Delta_z u_{i,j,k})^2} \tag{4}$$

where $u_{i,j,k}$ is the intensity value of voxel (i, j, k), with $i = \{1, \ldots, m\}$, $j = \{1, \ldots, n\}$, $k = \{1, \ldots, p\}$ and $m \times n \times p$ the volume data dimensions. Δ_x, Δ_y and Δ_z are the discretization of the horizontal, vertical and z (perpendicular to the reconstruction plane) derivatives, respectively.

Equation (5) was obtained in order to solve the problem of Eq. (3).

$$0 = \frac{\lambda}{u_{i,j,k}}(u_{i,j,k} - f_{i,j,k}) - \left[\Delta_x^- \frac{\Delta_x^+ u_{i,j,k}}{\sqrt{\varepsilon^2 + (\Delta_x^+ u_{i,j,k})^2 + (\Delta_y^0 u_{i,j,k})^2 + (\Delta_z^- u_{i,j,k})^2}} \right.$$

$$+ \Delta_y^- \frac{\Delta_y^+ u_{i,j,k}}{\sqrt{\varepsilon^2 + (\Delta_x^- u_{i,j,k})^2 + (\Delta_y^+ u_{i,j,k})^2 + (\Delta_z^0 u_{i,j,k})^2}} \quad (5)$$

$$\left. + \Delta_z^- \frac{\Delta_z^+ u_{i,j,k}}{\sqrt{\varepsilon^2 + (\Delta_x^0 u_{i,j,k})^2 + (\Delta_y^- u_{i,j,k})^2 + (\Delta_z^+ u_{i,j,k})^2}} \right]$$

Here $\Delta_x^+, \Delta_x^-, \Delta_y^+, \Delta_y^-, \Delta_z^+, \Delta_z^-$, denote forward (+) and backward (−) one-sided differences in x, y and z directions, respectively; $\Delta_x^0, \Delta_y^0, \Delta_z^0$ indicate central difference in x, y and z directions, respectively; and $\varepsilon > 0$ is a small parameter to remove the derivative singularity when u is locally constant. This formulation is valid only for interior points. Boundary conditions were defined as in Ref. [18] but adapted for 3D data. To solve Eq. (5) for u, a routine was implemented and integrated in IDL.

λ is a determinant parameter to control the algorithm performance. For that reason, after filter implementation, some preliminary studies about λ were done. For phantom images, in a first stage, λ values (constant for all slices) from 10 to 200 were tested and the value which allowed a better filter performance in terms of 3D TV minimization was selected. We know λ depends on data noise and the latter is related with σ_B [22]. In a second stage, σ_B values were measured for each slice and the respective λ that minimize the TV were estimated and applied to each slice during the 3D minimization algorithm.

The TV minimization filter was applied to the clinical slices after reconstruction. After a comprehensive study with λ values (constant for all slices) ranging from 10 to 200, the λ value which enables the greater minimization of TV was chosen and the resultant image is shown.

3 Results

3.1 3D Filter Performance

The results for 3D TV values obtained with λ ranging between 10 and 200 (constant for all slices) are presented in Fig. 1.

We can see that the $\lambda = 80$, constant for all slices, is the one which allows the minimum 3D TV.

σ_B values measured for each slice ranged from a minimum of 1038.838 to a maximum of 1543.767, yielding λ values approximately between 120 and 75, respectively. The results obtained for 3D TV minimization with $\lambda = 80$ and variable λ for each slice are summarized in Table 1.

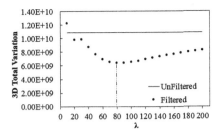

Fig. 1. 3D TV values for phantom unfiltered and filtered data plotted as a function of λ values.

Table 1. TV values obtained for the unfiltered and filtered data with λ = 80 and variable λ over slices. The variation in percentage between the unfiltered and filtered values is also presented.

	Unfiltered	Filtered	Variation (%)
3D TV (λ = 80)	1.086E+10	6.399E+09	−41.08
3D TV (λ Var.)		6.669E+09	−38.60

Table 2. Summary of the results of TV, CNR and spatial resolution obtained for the unfiltered and filtered phantom data with λ = 80 and variable λ over slices.

	TV	CNR	Spatial resolution (mm)
Unfiltered	2.320E+08	2.137	0.691
Filtered (λ = 80)	1.461E+08	4.088	0.692
Variation (%)	−37.02	47.72	0.15
Filtered (λ Var.)	1.459E+08	3.727	0.561
Variation (%)	−37.12	42.66	−18.81

To evaluate the filter influence in the image blur in z direction, the ASF for unfiltered and filtered data with λ = 80 and variable λ over slices is presented in Fig. 2.

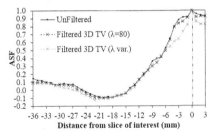

Fig. 2. ASF, plotted as a function of distance from slice of interest, for unfiltered and filtered data with λ = 80 and variable λ over slices.

3.2   In-Plane Filter Performance

Table 2 summarizes the in-plane results of TV, CNR and spatial resolution obtained for the phantom unfiltered and filtered data with $\lambda = 80$ and variable λ over slices. These values were calculated in a slice of interest containing both mass and MCs.

3.3   Qualitative Image Analysis

Images of a mass and a cluster of MCs are presented in Figs. 3 and 4, respectively. Figures (a), (b) and (c) are the unfiltered and filtered images with $\lambda = 80$ and variable λ, respectively. For clinical data, $\lambda = 60$ was chosen as the one which enables the greater minimization of 3D TV (about 43 %). In Fig. 5, clinical images of the same slice without (Fig. 5(a)) and with filter (Fig. 5(b)) are illustrated.

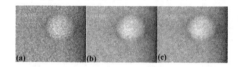

Fig. 3.   Images of an unfiltered (a) and filtered mass with $\lambda = 80$ (b) and variable λ (c).

Fig. 4.   Images of an unfiltered (a) and filtered cluster of MCs with $\lambda = 80$ (b) and variable λ (c).

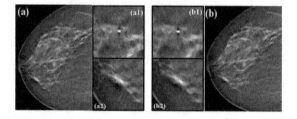

Fig. 5.   Reconstructed clinical images of the central unfiltered slice (a) and filtered (b) with $\lambda = 60$. Zoom in of one microcalcification (a1 and b1) and one dense zone (a2 and b2).

4   Discussion

A digital filter for 3D TV minimization in DBT was presented. It was based on the ROF model but for Poisson noise and three-dimensional data. This approach solves the minimization problem in a fast and straight-forward step, not being time-consuming. Each application of the filter is done in ~ 43 s. With the present work, we were able to implement the 3D filter and our analysis was focused on the obtained results when λ is constant and variable over slices. The filter has more influence in the TV and CNR values than in the spatial resolution values. Despite of λ being constant or variable between slices, the objectives of reducing 3D TV and increasing CNR were achieved.

In Fig. 1 we can see some oscillations for λ values bellow 30. For these lower values, λ is not able to ensure the fidelity term (which ensures the proximity between the unfiltered and filtered data) has enough weight in Eq. (3) to keep the fundamental information of initial data. Therefore, those values shouldn't be included in the analysis.

With $\lambda = 80$ we could achieve the minimum 3D TV, with a reduction of 41.08 % when compared with the 3D TV value of unfiltered data. With λ changing between slices this reduction was about 38.60 % (Table 1). This difference can be justified by the fact that, when a λ value is estimated in order to achieve the minimum TV in each slice, this may not correspond to the minimum global TV (3D). For some slices, λ values were estimated to be above 80. Consequently, the denoising effect will be smaller and this will be translated into a higher value of 3D TV. Either for $\lambda = 80$ or variable λ values over slices, the ASF was improved, when compared with the unfiltered data (Fig. 2). However, a better result for ASF was achieved when λ values are adjusted specifically for each slice.

About the in-plane results (Table 2), for $\lambda = 80$ a reduction of 37.02 % in TV, an increase of 47.72 % in CNR and a deterioration of 0.15 % in spatial resolution were obtained. As the variation observed for spatial resolution is very small, we can conclude that the definition of small structures is preserved. For a variable λ over slices, a reduction of 37.12 % in TV, an increasing of 42.66 % in CNR and an improvement of 18.85 % in spatial resolution were obtained. For the CNR analysis it is important to keep in mind that the empiric relation used between σ_B and λ was based in the TV minimization for each slice. Which means it wasn't based on the CNR maximization. As TV was calculated for the entire slice and CNR was determined only for the interest feature and background, the minimum TV may not correspond to the maximum CNR.

Zooming in in the mass (Fig. 3), we can see the effect of increasing CNR for both cases. On the other hand, observing the MCs cluster in Fig. 4, we observe that that the small details are preserved. In summary, with $\lambda = 80$ constant for all slices, the results for 3D TV and CNR were better. For a variable λ over slices we could achieve a higher reduction in the TV of the slice of interest and a better ASF.

Regarding clinical data, a reduction in 3D TV of about 43 % was achieved with $\lambda = 60$ (constant for all slices). The slice images in Fig. 5 are in accordance with this reduction. Comparing Fig. 5(a) with Fig. 5(b) it is quite visible that areas with higher noise level become smoother while preserving edges and details of the structures.

Some factors, such as voxel size could influence the results obtained. Smaller voxels represent a higher noise level (less information). On the other hand, smaller voxels also represent lower variability among voxels. Thus, the filter behavior and λ values will vary according to voxel size. Also, TV minimization does not solve imaging effects originated from variations in radiation energy, since it affects mainly image contrast level. The optimization of computation time, as well as, optimization of λ values and direct comparison with other filters should be considered in future work. This study has the advantage of analyzing real phantom and clinical images. Taking into account the preliminary results presented, we conclude that application of 3D TV denoising to DBT data is a very promising technique and allows a wide field of research in the future.

Acknowledgments. This work was supported in part by Fundação para a Ciência e a Tecnologia - Portugal (projects Pest-OE/SAU/IU0645/2013, Pest-OE/SAU/IU0645/2014 and PTDC/BBB-IMG/3310/2012).

References

1. Siegel, R.L., Miller, K.D., Jemal, A.: Cancer statistics, 2015. CA Cancer J. Clin. **65**(1), 5–29 (2015)
2. U.S. Food and Drug Administration (FDA) (2011). http://www.fda.gov/Radiation-EmittingProducts/MammographyQualityStandardsActandProgram/FacilityCertificationand Inspection/ucm114148.htm. Accessed May 2015
3. Sechopoulos, I.: A review of breast tomosynthesis. Part I. The image acquisition process. Med. Phys. **40**(1), 014301 (2013)
4. Brandt, K.R., et al.: Can digital breast tomosynthesis replace conventional diagnostic mammography views for screening recalls without calcifications? A comparison study in a simulated clinical setting. AJR Am. J. Roentgenol. **200**(2), 291–298 (2013)
5. Kopans, D.B.: Digital breast tomosynthesis from concept to clinical care. AJR Am. J. Roentgenol. **202**(2), 299–308 (2014)
6. Timberg, P., et al.: Impact of dose on observer performance in breast tomosynthesis using breast specimens. In: Proceedings of SPIE 6913, Medical Imaging: Physics of Medical Imaging (2008)
7. Zhao, B., Zhao, W.: Three-dimensional linear system analysis for breast tomosynthesis. Med. Phys. **35**(12), 5219–5232 (2008)
8. Zhao, B., et al.: Experimental validation of a three-dimensional linear system model for breast tomosynthesis. Med. Phys. **36**(1), 240–251 (2009)
9. Das, M., et al.: Evaluation of a variable dose acquisition technique for microcalcification and mass detection in digital breast tomosynthesis. Med. Phys. **36**(6), 1976–1984 (2009)
10. Das, M., et al.: Penalized maximum likelihood reconstruction for improved microcalcification detection in breast tomosynthesis. IEEE Trans. Med. Imaging **30**(4), 904–914 (2011)
11. Ertas, M., et al.: An iterative tomosynthesis reconstruction using total variation combined with non-local means filtering. BioMed. Eng. OnLine **13**(1), 65 (2014)
12. Feng, Y., et al.: Improved reconstruction of non-cartesian magnetic resonance imaging data through total variation minimization and POCS optimization. Conf. Proc. IEEE Eng. Med. Biol. Soc. **2009**, 2676–2679 (2009)
13. Jonsson, E., Huang, S.-C., Chan, T.: Total variation regularization in positron emission tomography. Department of Mathematics. UCLA. http://citeseerx.ist.psu.edu/viewdoc/summary?doi=10.1.1.35.4447
14. Joshi, S.H., et al.: MRI resolution enhancement using total variation regularization. Proc. IEEE Int. Symp. Biomed. Imaging **2009**, 161–164 (2009)
15. Nett, B., et al.: Tomosynthesis via total variation minimization reconstruction and prior image constrained compressed sensing (PICCS) on a C-arm system. Proc. Soc. Photo Opt. Instrum. Eng. **6913**, nihpa92672 (2008)
16. Sidky, E.Y., et al.: A constrained, total-variation minimization algorithm for low-intensity x-ray CT. Med. Phys. **38**(S1), S117–S125 (2011)

17. Zhiqiang, C., et al.: A limited-angle CT reconstruction method based on anisotropic TV minimization. Phys. Med. Biol. **58**(7), 2119 (2013)
18. Rudin, L.I., Osher, S., Fatemi, E.: Nonlinear total variation based noise removal algorithms. Physica D: Nonlinear Phenom. **60**(1–4), 259–268 (1992)
19. Le, T., Chartrand, R., Asaki, T.: A variational approach to reconstructing images corrupted by poisson noise. J. Math. Imaging Vis. **27**(3), 257–263 (2007)
20. Velikina, J., Leng, S., Chen, G.-H.: Limited view angle tomographic image reconstruction via total variation minimization, In: Proceedings of the SPIE 6510, Medical Imaging 2007: Physics of Medical Imaging, 14 March 2007. doi:10.1117/12.713750
21. Sawatzky, A., Brune, C., Müller, J., Burger, M.: Total variation processing of images with poisson statistics. In: Jiang, X., Petkov, N. (eds.) CAIP 2009. LNCS, vol. 5702, pp. 533–540. Springer, Heidelberg (2009)
22. Mota, A.M., et al.: Total variation minimization filter for DBT imaging. Med. Phys. **42**(6), 2827–2836 (2015)
23. Sidky, E.Y., et al.: Practical iterative image reconstruction in digital breast tomosynthesis by non-convex TpV optimization. In: Proceedings of the SPIE 6913, Medical Imaging 2008: Physics of Medical Imaging, 18 March 2008. doi:10.1117/12.772796
24. Sidky, E.Y., et al.: Enhanced imaging of microcalcifications in digital breast tomosynthesis through improved image-reconstruction algorithms. Med. Phys. **36**(11), 4920–4932 (2009)
25. Ertas, M., et al.: Digital breast tomosynthesis image reconstruction using 2D and 3D total variation minimization. Biomed. Eng. Online **12**, 112 (2013)
26. Seyyedi, S., Yildirim, I.: 3D digital breast tomosynthesis image reconstruction using anisotropic total variation minimization. Conf. Proc. IEEE Eng. Med. Biol. Soc. **2014**, 6052–6055 (2014)
27. Wu, T., et al.: A comparison of reconstruction algorithms for breast tomosynthesis. Med. Phys. **31**(9), 2636–2647 (2004)

Variations in Breast Density and Mammographic Risk Factors in Different Ethnic Groups

Elaine F. Harkness[1,2,3(✉)], Fatik Bashir[4], Philip Foden[5],
Megan Bydder[2], Soujanya Gadde[2], Mary Wilson[2],
Anthony Maxwell[1,2,3], Emma Hurley[2], Anthony Howell[2,6],
D. Gareth Evans[2,7], and Susan M. Astley[1,2,3]

[1] Centre for Imaging Sciences, Institute of Population Health,
University of Manchester, Stopford Building, Oxford Road,
Manchester M13 9PT, UK
Elaine.F.Harkness@manchester.ac.uk
[2] Genesis Breast Cancer Prevention Centre and Nightingale Breast Screening
Centre, University Hospital of South Manchester NHS Trust, Wythenshawe,
Manchester M23 9LT, UK
[3] The University of Manchester, Manchester Academic Health Science Centre,
University Hospital of South Manchester NHS Foundation Trust, Wythenshawe,
Manchester M23 9LT, UK
[4] Manchester Medical School, University of Manchester, Stopford Building,
Oxford Road, Manchester M13 9PT, UK
[5] Centre for Biostatistics, Institute of Population Health,
University of Manchester, Oxford Road, Manchester M13 9PT, UK
[6] The Christie NHS Foundation, Withington, Manchester M20 4BX, UK
[7] Genomic Medicine, Manchester Academic Health Sciences Centre,
University of Manchester and Central Manchester Foundation Trust,
Manchester M13 9WL, UK

Abstract. This study investigates variations in mammographic density by ethnic group in women attending the NHS breast screening programme in Greater Manchester. Density was estimated using Volpara[TM] and Quantra[TM]. Data was analysed for 651 Asian/Asian British, 416 Black/Black British, 394 Jewish origin, 181 'Mixed', 700 'Other' and a random sample of 10,000 women who declared their ethnic origin as White (British or Irish). Age ranged from 46–84 years and mean BMI was 27.4 kg/m^2. Fibroglandular volume (Volpara[TM]) was highest in women of Black/Black British origin (59.4 cm^3) and lowest in Asian/Asian British women (47.9 cm^3). After adjusting for a number of hormonal and other factors the magnitude of the difference between groups decreased, however, there were still a number of statistical differences between groups. Ethnic differences in mammographic density and personal factors may subsequently contribute to differences in breast cancer incidence.

Keywords: Digital · Mammogram · Breast density · Ethnicity · Breast screening

© Springer International Publishing Switzerland 2016
A. Tingberg et al. (Eds.): IWDM 2016, LNCS 9699, pp. 510–517, 2016.
DOI: 10.1007/978-3-319-41546-8_64

1 Introduction

Differences in breast cancer incidence, mortality and survival across different ethnic groups are well documented. In the UK, the age-standardised rates for breast cancer incidence amongst White females range from 122 to 126 per 100,000, while the rate is significantly lower for Asian (60 to 92 per 100,000) and Black females (69 to 108 per 100,000) [1]. The proportion of women diagnosed with breast cancer under the age of 50 years is significantly higher amongst Black (46%) compared to White women (18%) [2], and Black ethnicity has been found to be a significant independent predictor of poor prognosis in young Black women compared to White women [3].

Mammographic density is an independent risk factor for breast cancer [4], and has been shown to be associated with an increased risk of breast cancer in some ethnic groups (Caucasians, African-Americans and Asian-Americans) but not in others (Asian and Asian American populations) [5]. Women of Jewish Ashkenazi descent have also been shown to have a genetic susceptibility to breast cancer [6] and a recent study has demonstrated that these women may have a unique set of genetic variants or environmental risk factors that also increase mammographic density [7].

However, whether these associations are confounded by other risk factors for breast cancer, such as age, body mass index and hormonal factors is still unclear. The aim of this study was to investigate the relationship between automated breast density measures (Volpara^{TM} and Quantra^{TM}), personal risk factors for breast cancer, and ethnicity.

2 Methods

Women attending routine breast screening between October 2009 and April 2015 as a part of the Greater Manchester National Health Service Breast Screening Programme (NHSBSP) were invited to take part in the Predicting Risk Of Cancer At Screening (PROCAS) study. Approximately 58,000 women consented to participate in PROCAS and also provided additional information on risk factors for breast cancer by completing a 2-page questionnaire at the time of screening. For this study women had to have information in relation to their ethnicity and mammographic density data as measured by Volpara^{TM} and Quantra^{TM}. Women with breast cancer diagnosed at time of entry to PROCAS or with a previous diagnosis of breast cancer were excluded. A total of 2342 women met the inclusion criteria and recorded their ethnicity as non-white, a further 10,000 women were randomly selected from those of white ethnic origin. Ethical approval for the study was given by the North Manchester Research Committee (09/H1008/81).

Ethnicities: Options available for ethnicity on the questionnaire were as follows: White (British or Irish), Black or Black British (African or Caribbean), Asian or Asian British (Bangladeshi, Indian, Pakistani, Chinese), Mixed (White and Black African/Asian/Black Caribbean), Jewish origin, Jewish Ashkenazi and Other (with an option to specify). For the purposes of this research those who reported their ethnic origin as Jewish or Jewish Ashkenazi were combined.

Mammographic breast density measurements were performed on all screening mammograms at entry to PROCAS using Volpara^{TM} version 1.5.0 and Quantra^{TM}

version 2.0. Outputs from Volpara^{TM} and Quantra^{TM} included fibroglandular volume (cm^3) and percentage density. Volpara^{TM} values are calculated as the mean across four mammographic views, while Quantra^{TM} is based on the maximum value for each breast.

Categorical variables were compared using Chi-square tests. One-way analysis of variance (ANOVA) was used to examine the relationship between ethnicity and individual risk factors for continuous variables, and the log of the density measures. Log of the density measures was used due to the positive skew of the data. Pairwise comparisons for each ethnic group were performed using Scheffe's test. Analysis of covariance (ANCOVA) was used to examine the relationship between the log of density measures and ethnicity after adjusting for other risk factors found to be statistically different across ethnic groups in the one-way ANOVAs. Pairwise comparisons for each ethnic group were performed using the Bonferroni correction. Due to the relatively large proportion of women with missing BMI values (8%) we imputed BMI values for these women based on the mean of the ethnic group to which they belonged. To account for the number of comparisons results were considered statistically significant if p < 0.01.

3 Results

Of the 12342 women in the study 10,000 were White, 651 Asian or Asian British, 416 Black or Black British, 394 Jewish, 181 Mixed and 700 'Other'. Age ranged from 46 to 84 years and the mean BMI was 27.4 kg/m^2.

Descriptive statistics for the study population by ethnic group are shown in Tables 1 and 2. One-way ANOVA showed there were statistically significant differences across the groups for all factors in Table 1 (p < 0.001). Jewish women were significantly older than all other ethnic groups, White women also tended to be significantly older than other ethnic groups (except Jewish). Black women had a significantly higher BMI than all other groups, with the exception of Mixed, however Black women were also more likely to have information missing for BMI (25%) compared to other groups (4–13% missing). Jewish women had a significantly lower BMI compared to all other ethnic groups. Age at menarche was significantly younger for Jewish women compared to White, Asian or Asian British women, however, their age at birth of first child was significantly older than all groups, except for the 'other' group. Age at menopause was significantly younger for Black women compared to White, Jewish and 'Other' women.

Results from the comparisons of categorical variables by ethnic group are presented in Table 2 (χ^2 < 0.001 for all comparisons). Jewish women were most likely to have ever used HRT (41%) and Asian women least likely (15%). The number of women with children ranged from 83% in the 'Other' and Mixed groups to 92% in Asian women. The proportion of postmenopausal women at entry to PROCAS ranged from 44% in Black to 67% in Jewish women, and the proportion who reported having had a hysterectomy ranged from 15% in Asian women to almost 30% in the Mixed group.

Table 1. Risk factors by ethnic group

Ethnicity	Age	BMI (kg/m^2)	Age at menarche	Age first child	Age at menopause
N	12342	11369	12074	10750	6181
	Mean (SD)	Mean (SD)	Mean (SD)	Mean (SD)	Mean (SD)
White	57.1 (7.3)	27.5 (5.5)	12.9 (1.7)	24.5 (5.1)	47.9 (5.8)
Asian or Asian British	54.6 (6.4)	27.0 (5.9)	13.2 (1.6)	25.0 (5.2)	48.1 (5.1)
Black or Black British	54.2 (6.7)	29.5 (5.8)	13.3 (3.2)	24.1 (5.8)	46.3 (5.8)
Jewish	58.5 (7.4)	25.7 (5.1)	12.6 (1.6)	26.2 (5.0)	48.9 (5.9)
Mixed	54.5 (6.5)	28.2 (5.6)	13.0 (1.8)	23.1 (5.3)	48.1 (5.9)
Other	55.5 (6.5)	27.3 (6.2)	12.8 (1.6)	26.1 (5.7)	48.4 (5.4)
All groups	**56.8 (7.2)**	**27.4 (5.6)**	**12.9 (1.7)**	**24.6 (5.2)**	**48.0 (5.8)**

Table 2. Risk factors by ethnic group

Ethnicity	HRT ever used (%)	Parous (%)	Postmenopausal (%)	Hysterectomy (%)
White	34.9	87.7	61.3	23.5
Asian or Asian British	15.1	92.0	50.4	15.4
Black or Black British	14.2	84.1	44.0	26.0
Jewish	40.9	86.5	67.3	24.6
Mixed	26.0	83.4	49.2	29.3
Other	24.4	83.1	53.6	16.3
All groups	**32.6**	**87.4**	**59.7**	**22.8**

One-way ANOVA showed there were statistically significant differences across the ethnic groups for all density measures ($p < 0.001$). Univariate associations for Volpara^{TM} and Quantra^{TM} are presented in Table 3. Black women had the highest fibroglandular volume while Asian women had the lowest (54.5 cm^3 and 42 cm^3 respectively for Volpara^{TM}, 107.5 cm^3 and 75.6 cm^3 respectively for Quantra^{TM}). On the other hand percentage density was highest for Jewish women (7.1 and 12.5% for Volpara^{TM} and Quantra^{TM} respectively) and lowest for white women (5.5 and 10.5% for Volpara^{TM} and Quantra^{TM} respectively). There were a number of significant differences in these measures between ethnic groups (see Table 3).

In the ANCOVA we adjusted for ethnicity, age, BMI, age of menarche, number and age of birth of first child (no children, 14–19, 20–24, 25–29, 30–34, 35+), menopausal status, HRT use (never/ever) and hysterectomy (yes/no). Results from the ANCOVA

Table 3. Volpara density measures by ethnicity (mean; 95% CI)

Ethnicity[1]	Mean (95% CI) gland volume (cm^3)	Mean % (95% CI) density
	Volpara™	
White (a)	44.5 (44.1–44.9)^c	5.5 (5.4–5.6)^{b,d,f}
Asian or Asian British (b)	42.8 (41.3–44.3)^{c,d}	6.3 (6.0–6.6)^a
Black or Black British (c)	54.5 (52.3–56.7)^{a,b,f}	5.8 (5.5–6.1)^d
Jewish (d)	48.2 (46.0–50.6)^b	7.1 (6.7–7.5)^{a,c}
Mixed (e)	48.9 (45.6–52.4)	6.0 (5.5–6.6)
Other (f)	46.9 (45.2–48.6)^c	6.3 (6.0–6.6)^a
All groups	45.0 (44.7–45.4)	5.7 (5.6–5.7)
	Quantra™	
White (a)	87.8 (86.7–88.8)^{b,c}	10.5 (10.4–10.6)^d
Asian or Asian British (b)	75.6 (72.4–79.5)^{a,c,f}	10.5 (10.1–11.0)^d
Black or Black British (c)	107.5 (101.6–113.7)^{a,b,d,f}	11.1 (10.7–11.6)
Jewish (d)	87.2 (82.2–92.6)^c	12.5 (11.9–13.2)^{a,b}
Mixed (e)	92.2 (84.4–100.8)	11.0 (10.8–11.6)
Other (f)	87.1 (83.2–91.1)^{b,c}	11.2 (10.8–11.6)

[1]Superscripts indicate groups that are statistically significantly different (p < 0.01). For example, fibroglandular volume (cm^3) for white women is statistically significantly lower than (c) Black or Black British and (d) Jewish women.

models showed that ethnicity was significantly associated with all density measures (p < 0.001). Figure 1 shows the unadjusted and adjusted means by ethnic group. For volpara gland volume the unadjusted and adjusted means were similar for Black women, in all other groups gland volume increased with the largest increase in Jewish women (unadjusted 48.2 cm^3, adjusted 54.2 cm^3). After adjusting for variables that differed between ethnicities (Tables 1 and 2) a number of significant differences between ethnicities remained. Black and Jewish women had a significantly higher volpara gland volume than the White, Asian and Other groups. For volpara percent density the largest differences between the unadjusted and adjusted means occurred for the Black, White and Mixed women (Fig. 1b). White women had a significantly lower percent density (6.0%) than all other groups except for the Mixed group. Similar trends were seen for Quantra gland volume, with the exception being in Black women where unadjusted gland volume decreased from 107.5 cm^3 to 100.9 cm^3 after adjusting for other risk factors (Fig. 1c) which was only statistically significantly different from Asian women. Like the results for Volpara a number of significant differences remained between the ethnic groups after adjusting for other factors.

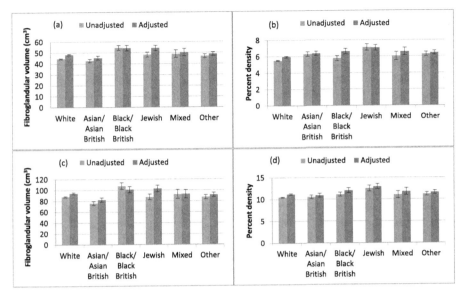

Fig. 1. Unadjusted and adjusted density measures by ethnicity for (a) Volpara FGV (b) Volpara % density (c) Quantra FGV and (d) Quantra % density (Color figure online)

4   Discussion

This study examines the relationship between key breast cancer risk factors and ethnicity, as well as the relationship between ethnicity and mammographic density. A number of factors examined differed by ethnic group including age, BMI, age at menarche, menopausal status, age at menopause, HRT use and parity. Women of Black ethnic origin had the highest Volpara gland volume compared to White, Asian and 'Other' women. On the other hand percent density for this group was not significantly different to the majority of ethnic groups and this may reflect the larger BMI values recorded within this group.

The findings in relation to women of Jewish origin are also of interest, Jewish women reported the highest proportion of HRT use, however, they were also significantly older than all other ethnic groups. Jewish women also tended to have a younger age of menarche, but a higher age of birth of first child. Women of Ashkenazi Jewish origin have a known genetic susceptibility to breast cancer [6] and a recent study has reported high mammographic density in Jewish women of Ashkenazi descent after adjusting for a number of factors. In the current study, the adjusted mean for Volpara gland volume was similar to that of Black women which was significantly higher than the White, Asian and 'Other' groups. Jewish women also had the highest levels of percentage density which are likely to reflect the lower BMI within this group.

It is unlikely that women attending the screening programme are representative of those in Greater Manchester as a whole. It is well known that women of non-White ethnic origin, in particular Asian women, are less likely to attend for breast screening and attendance rates are also lower amongst more deprived areas [8], although there may be differences by age due to immigration patterns in the population.

Ethnicity, and other factors were self-reported in PROCAS and a number of women reported their ethnicity as 'Other' it would be interesting to look at this group in further detail. There were also missing data on a number of other factors. For BMI, due to variations across the groups, we imputed values based on the mean of the particular ethnic group women belonged to. It may be that a different method of imputation may have been more appropriate, however analysis with and without imputation produced similar adjusted means for each outcome and therefore reflects some robustness in the method. As a result of the missing data the number of women included in the final model will be smaller than those originally reported within each ethnic group, overall less than 10% were omitted from the final model for this reason.

Due to the large study size a number of significant outcomes would be expected, and it is also appropriate to consider the clinical relevance of the results. For those women in ethnic groups with higher mammographic density it may be possible to increase awareness of certain risk factors, such as HRT use, or to introduce preventative measures, such chemopreventive therapy or lifestyle interventions.

5   Conclusion

Mammographic density varies between different ethnic groups and these differences persist even after adjustment for a number of factors. Differences in mammographic density in ethnic groups may subsequently contribute to differences in breast cancer incidence, mortality and/or survival.

Acknowledgements. We acknowledge the support of the National Institute for Health Research (NIHR) and the Genesis Prevention Appeal for their funding of the PROCAS study. We would like to thank the women who agreed to take part in the study and the study staff for recruitment and data collection. We also thank Hologic Inc. for providing Quantra^{TM} and Matakina Technology Limited for providing Volpara^{TM}. This paper presents independent research funded by the National Institute for Health Research (NIHR) under its Programme Grants for Applied Research programme (reference number RP-PG-0707-10031: "Improvement in risk prediction, early detection and prevention of breast cancer"). The views expressed are those of the author(s) and not necessarily those of the NHS, the NIHR, or the Department of Health.

References

1. Cancer Research UK: Breast cancer incidence (invasive) statistics (2016). http://www.cancerresearchuk.org/health-professional/cancer-statistics/statistics-by-cancer-type/breast-cancer/incidence-invasive. Accessed 31 Mar 2016
2. Lawrence, G., Kearins, O., Lagord, C., Cheung, S., Sidhu, J., Sagar, C.: The Second All Breast Cancer Report, Focussing on Inequalities – Variation in Breast Cancer Outcomes with Age and Deprivation. National Cancer Intelligence Network (2009)

3. Copson, E., Maishman, T., Gerty, S., Eccles, B., Stanton, L., Cutress, R.I., Altman, D.G., Durcan, L., Simmonds, P., Jones, L., Tapper, W.: POSH study steering group and Eccles D. Ethnicity and outcome of young breast cancer patients in the UK: the POSH study. Brit. J. Cancer **110**, 230–241 (2014)

4. Valerie, A., McCormack, V., dos Santos Silva, I.: Breast density and parenchymal patterns as markers of breast cancer risk: a meta-analysis. Cancer Epidemiol. Biomark. Prev. **15**(6), 1159–1169 (2006)

5. Vachon, C.M., van Gils, C.H., Sellers, T.A., Ghosh, K., Pruthi, S., Brandt, K.R., Pankratz, V.S.: Mammographic density, breast cancer risk and risk prediction. Breast Cancer Res. **9**, 217 (2007). doi:10.1186/bcr1829

6. Struewing, J.P., Hartge, P., Wacholder, S., Baker, S.M., Berlin, M., McAdams, M., Timmerman, M.M., Brody, L.C., Tucker, M.A.: The risk of cancer associated with specific mutations of BRCA1 and BRCA2 among Ashkenazi Jews. New Engl. J. Med. **336**(20), 1401–1408 (1997)

7. Caswell, J.L., Kerlikowske, K., Shepherd, J.A., Cummings, S.R., Hu, D., Scott Huntsman, S., Ziv, E.: High mammographic density in women of Ashkenazi Jewish descent. Breast Cancer Res. **15**, R40 (2013)

8. Jack, R.H., Møller, H., Robson, T., Davies, E.A.: Breast cancer screening uptake among women from different ethnic groups in London: a population-based cohort study. BMJ Open **4**, e005586 (2014)

Virtual Tools for the Evaluation of Breast Imaging: State-of-the Science and Future Directions

Predrag R. Bakic[1(✉)], Kyle J. Myers[2], Stephen J. Glick[2], Andrew D.A. Maidment[1], and The members of AAPM Task Group 234[1,2]

[1] Department of Radiology, University of Pennsylvania, Philadelphia, PA, USA
Predrag.Bakic@uphs.upenn.edu
[2] U.S. Food and Drug Administration, Silver Spring, MD, USA

Abstract. The beginning of this century saw the development of simulation methods for the evaluation of breast imaging, motivated by the limitations of conventional clinical trials. This has led to the formation of AAPM Task Group on Virtual Tools for the Validation of 3D/4D X-ray Breast Imaging Systems (TG234), gathering researchers from academia, industry, and government, interested in the development, testing, and adoption of these tools. TG234 is currently finalizing its report. The report has been designed as an experiential guide through the steps of simulating breast anatomy, image acquisition, image interpretation, and analysis. TG234 activities include disseminating the idea of virtual clinical trials through numerous focused conference sessions and AAPM annual meeting symposia. This paper reflects our desire to initiate wider discussion about the future directions in the development of virtual tools for the design and evaluation of novel breast imaging systems.

Keywords: Mammography · Digital breast tomosynthesis · Breast imaging simulation · Anthropomorphic phantoms · Virtual clinical trials · Model observers

1 Introduction

Modern x-ray breast imaging systems are complex, with designs based upon a multitude of modifiable parameters, all of which affect clinical performance. Conventional evaluation of these systems requires clinical imaging trials, which usually compare various image quality descriptors between repeated images of a large group of subjects acquired using different imaging systems (or different system parameters). Such studies are limited by their cost, duration, and the risk to participating subjects from repeated use of ionizing radiation.

An alternative approach based upon simulation of the complete breast imaging chain has been introduced in the last decade. The simulated components of the breast imaging chain include the object model (breast anatomy with or without simulated

---

The AAPM Task Group 234 roster is listed on https://www.aapm.org/org/structure/?committee_code=TG234.

abnormalities), the imaging process model (including the breast positioning, image acquisition, and post-processing or reconstruction of acquired images), and the interpretation of the image data using mathematical observer models. A generalized simulation pipeline is illustrated by Fig. 1. Such a simulation pipeline can be used to design and perform virtual clinical trials (VCTs), based upon performance metrics of specific tasks.

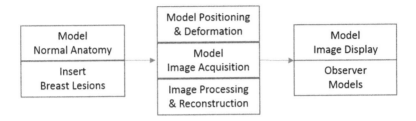

Fig. 1. Flow-chart of the breast imaging simulation for virtual evaluation.

Based upon the increasing interest in virtual evaluation of breast imaging systems, a dedicated Task Group on Virtual Tools for the Validation of 3D/4D X-ray Breast Imaging Systems (TG234) was founded by the American Association of Physicists in Medicine (AAPM) in 2012. [1] TG234 includes 24 researchers from academia, industry, and government agencies interested in the development, testing, and adoption of these tools.

The main task of TG234 is the preparation of a report, which is expected to be completed later in 2016. TG234 took an active role in disseminating the simulation approach and VCT concept throughout the breast imaging research community, by organizing focused symposia during the 2013 AAPM Annual Meeting in Indianapolis, IN [2], 2014 AAPM Annual Meeting in Austin, TX [3], and the upcoming 2016 AAPM Annual Meeting in Washington, D.C. [4], as well as by introducing a new AAPM abstract submission category related to the virtual evaluation of breast imaging. This has also motivated presentation at 2016 IWDM to provide a forum to review the task group activities and current challenges, the regulatory perspective on VCTs, and an opportunity to receive suggestions from the IWDM community about future directions of TG234.

2   State-of-the-Science of the Virtual Evaluation of Breast Imaging Systems

The TG234 report has been designed in the form of experiential guide, rather than prescriptions. It summarizes the state-of-the-science for the virtual evaluation of breast imaging systems, based upon the experience of the task group members' labs and discussions at our meetings and teleconferences. The report roughly follows the structure of the simulation pipeline, shown in Fig. 1, focusing on the steps of simulating breast anatomy, image acquisition, and interpretation.

2.1 Simulation of the Breast Anatomy (The Object Model)

The quality and realism of the simulated breast anatomy directly affects the validity of related VCTs, and at the same time critically influences the acceptance of the VCT concept in the research community. The TG234 report discusses two complementary views on phantom realism, which differ in the scope and range of the required tests of realism, namely:

1. *The task-based view* assumes that the realism depends on the specific tasks the phantom is designed for; therefore, the tests should be specific to individual evaluation tasks; and
2. *The reader-based view* assumes that the realism should be validated through radiologists' comprehensive visual assessment; thus, passing a so-called "fool-the-reader" test would warrant wide use of such assessed phantoms.

The report identifies various levels and types of realism validation, and reviews numerous examples of the realism validation from published simulation studies.

2.2 Simulation of the Breast Imaging Chain (The Imaging Acquisition Model)

Simulation of the image formation process by which the virtual phantom in object space is processed by each component of the imaging system, resulting in the detected data (synthetic images) is a necessary procedure in breast imaging VCTs. Acknowledging the complexity of the breast imaging process (which includes breast positioning and/or compression, acquisition, image pre-processing, post-processing and/or reconstruction), the TG234 report focuses primarily on the physics of projecting through computer simulated breast phantoms based upon the use of ray tracing or Monte-Carlo methods.

The effects of object discretization (i.e., phantom voxel size selection), and discrete or continuous simulation, are treated systematically, as parts of the imaging process simulation. To that end, we have introduced the simulation function, which depends on multiple parameters, some directly related to discretization and others not. The simulation function is used to compare the variation in the study endpoint introduced by different levels of discretization, against variations arising from other sources in the simulation.

2.3 Simulation of the Breast Image Interpretation

The last stage of a breast imaging VCT pipeline models the performance of a particular, relevant clinical task (e.g., lesion detection or the detection of micro calcification clusters), making use of the synthesized imaging data in either the projected data domain or following image reconstruction. This stage requires the selection and implementation of mathematical model observers. The task group report discusses possible performance tasks, choices for models for observers, and figures of merit for summarizing system performance. The report also reviews methods for estimating the uncertainty in a figure of merit, which is an essential component for hypothesis testing.

Finally, the TG234 report reviews the importance of VCTs from an industry perspective, based upon the experience of designing and utilizing the simulation methods during the development of breast imaging systems, as well as the potential use of computational modeling data in support of regulatory submissions. The U.S. Food and Drug Administration has issued draft guidance on the reporting of data from computational modeling studies in support of premarket submissions, and has made use of task-based evaluations using model observer studies in other imaging applications [5].

3 Challenges of Using Virtual Tools in Breast Imaging

Regular TG234 teleconferences and face-to-face task group meetings were instrumental in identifying the current challenges in breast imaging VCTs. These challenges have been included in the report to stimulate needed research in the field. As an illustration, here we briefly review two challenges related to the optimal selection of phantom voxel size and the training of model observers.

3.1 Optimal Size of the Phantom Voxels

Very early in the design of a VCT study, researchers are faced with the following question: *What size voxels should be used in simulation to ensure that the results are not dependent on the voxel size, or how finely should a numerical line integration routinely sample the phantom for stable integrals?* The answer is constrained by numerous factors related to various components of the breast imaging simulation flowchart (Fig. 1), including:

1. The size of the anatomical structure's detail that is being analyzed by the simulation study;
2. The trade-off between the discretization noise due to voxelizaton, and the image acquisition noise;
3. Practical limitations related to the computational time, data transfer time, and the memory storage for a given simulation platform; and
4. The accuracy required for the simulation study endpoint.
   These complex and even contradictory constraints cause the question of the optimal voxel size to persist up to the present, which will be acknowledged in the TG234 report.

3.2 Model Observer Training

Model observers are numerical algorithms that perform a task using the images resulting from the VCT simulation pipeline, which involves making decisions regarding the truth state of the virtual patient (lesion present vs. absent, for example). When the task–based performance of the model observer is determined for a large set of images, a summary figure of merit can be estimated that summarizes the quality of the imaging system for supporting that particular task.

All model observers make use of statistical properties of images, for example, the expected size or shape of the lesion, and the texture of the noise in the images. The challenge in training a model observer for a VCT study is that, for a particular simulated breast anatomy and lesion model, the size or shape of the lesion in an image will depend on the image acquisition geometry and reconstruction algorithm. Likewise, the noise texture will depend on image acquisition parameters and reconstruction method. Because VCTs are typically intended to compare multiple systems, or optimize system geometry parameters, a VCT must ensure that the model observer is well-suited for each system design or parameter combination. In other words, the model observer must be trained to be optimal for each set of system parameters, as these impact the model observer in terms of signal and noise characteristics in the resulting images. Training of the model observer involves simulation of an adequate number of subjects (breast anatomy and lesion characteristics) to ensure that the results of the VCT are stable (more training cases would not affect the VCT results). Hundreds or even thousands of simulated breasts can be used in a VCT study, in order to have confidence in the results or the investigation, allowing for adequate training of the model observer as well as data sets for testing once the model observer has been determined.

Two current challenges in the field of model observers are at the forefront of the field. The first is the development of methods for establishing that a model observer approximates ideal observer performance, which tells the investigator the best possible task performance that can be achieved given the data from the imaging system under evaluation. The second challenge is the need for recommendations on model observer designs that reliably predict human performance across a range of acquisition system parameters and reconstruction algorithms for 3D breast imaging systems so that the need for validation of new VCT studies against human data is reduced or eliminated.

4   Future Directions for the Virtual Evaluation of Breast Imaging

Following the report submission, the TG234 charge will be modified, redefining the focus of the Task Group. Anticipated future developments can be related to the extension of the VCT approach in several potential directions, including supporting other breast imaging modalities, a wider range of spatial scales, and the translation (or generalization) of the VCT concept to the imaging of other organs and diseases.

4.1   Virtual Evaluation of Other Breast Imaging Modalities

The original TG234 charge was focused on the evaluation of 3D/4D x-ray breast imaging, due to its widespread use in screening and diagnostic breast exams. Current digital breast phantoms are capable of supporting the simulation of other modalities and multi-modality studies, as the simulated breast anatomical structures are associated with various physical properties, matching the modality to be evaluated (Fig. 2). [6–8] The Penn open-source tissue simulation method builds software phantoms capable of synthesizing x-ray, MRI, and ultrasound images of the same simulated anatomy; it has been used to compare breast density estimates from mammography and ultrasound tomography. [6] Based on the segmentation of clinical breast CT data, Duke University has generated 100 phantoms capable of simulating a variety of breast imaging modalities. [7] In another recent example, a new open-source software tool was developed by Graff, to generate multimodality digital breast phantoms for use in the evaluation of both x-ray and MRI systems. [8] Of particular interest in the future, is the potential to perform virtual evaluation of systems for molecular imaging and radiomics analysis.

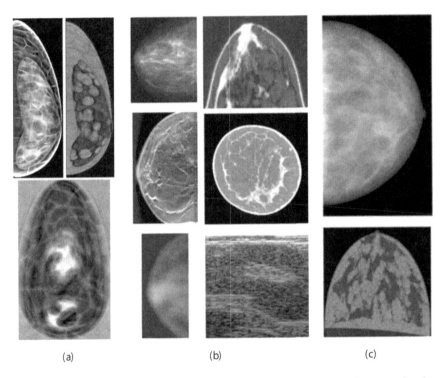

(a)   (b)   (c)

Fig. 2. Illustration of simulated multimodality images of computer breast phantoms, developed at (a) the University of Pennsylvania (modified from [6]), (b) Duke University (modified from [7]), and (c) FDA (modified from [8]).

4.2   Extending the Range of Spatial Scales in Breast Imaging Virtual Validations

Current digital breast phantoms are focused primarily on the anatomical scales visualized in clinical x-ray images of the breast. Recent progress in digital pathology and the close relationship between radiology and pathology, emphasize the need for simulating breast tissue at both radiologic and pathological scales. This introduces novel challenges to the virtual validation approach in terms of the computation speed, storage and transfer of simulated data, and the appropriate testing of phantom realism over the wide range of scales.

An example of recent efforts in the simulation of breast tissue at the radiologic and pathological scales has been reported by the researchers from the X-ray Physics Lab at the University of Pennsylvania. [9].

5   Conclusion

VCTs in breast imaging are increasingly being accepted by researchers in academia, industry, and government as an efficient preclinical approach to evaluate novel imaging system and image processing methods. This development is made evident by the growing body of published work, numerous conference sessions dedicated to VCTs, and the activities of the AAPM Task Group on Virtual Tools for 3D/4D X-ray Breast Imaging Validation (TG234).

This paper review the activities of the Task Group, current challenges related to the development and use of the virtual tools for breast imaging, and potential future directions of TG234.

Acknowledgment. The authors acknowledge the financial support and assistance from the AAPM for TG234 teleconferences and face-to-face meetings, and the Mini-Symposium on Virtual Clinical Trials held during the 2016 IWDM in Malmo, Sweden.

References

1. AAPM Task Group No. 234: Task group on virtual tools for the evaluation of new 3D/4D breast imaging systems (2012). http://www.aapm.org/org/structure/?committee_code=TG234
2. Bakic, P.R., Myers, K.J., Reiser, I., Kiarashi, N., Zeng, R.: Virtual tools for validation of x-ray breast imaging systems. Med. Phys. **40**, 390 (2013)
3. Myers, K.J., Bakic, P.R., Abbey, C.K., Kupinski, M., Mertelmeier, T.: Virtual tools for validation of x-ray breast imaging systems. Med. Phys. **41**, 446–447 (2014)
4. Myers, K.J., Bakic, P.R., Graff, C., Das, M., Avanaki, A.N.: Recent advances in virtual tools for validation of 3D/4D breast imaging systems (TG234). Med. Phys. (2016)
5. Vaishnav, J.Y., Jung, W.C., Popescu, L.M., Zeng, R., Myers, K.J.: Objective assessment of image quality and dose reduction in CT iterative reconstruction. Med. Phy. **41**, 071904 (2014)
6. Bakic, P.R., Li, C., West, E., Sak, M., Gavenonis, S.C., et al.: Comparison of 3D and 2D breast density estimation from synthetic ultrasound tomography images and digital mammograms of anthropomorphic software breast phantoms. In: Pelc, N.J., Samei, E., Nishikawa, R.M. (eds.) SPIE Medical Imaging: Physics of Medical Imaging, p. 79610Z (2011)
7. Segars, W.P., Veress, A.I., Wells, J.R., Sturgeon, G.M., Kiarashi, N., et al.: Population of 100 realistic, patient-based computerized breast phantoms for multi-modality imaging research. In: Whiting, B., Hoeschen, C., Kontos, D. (eds.) Physics of Medical Imaging: SPIE, p. 90331 (2014)
8. Graff, C.G.: A new, open-source, multi-modality digital breast phantom. In: Kontos, D., Flohr, T., Lo, J.Y. (eds.) Physics of Medical Imaging SPIE, p. 978309 (2016)
9. Bakic, P.R., Pokrajac, D.D., Batiste, R.C., Feldman, M.D., Maidment, A.D.: Simulation of breast anatomy: bridging the radiology-pathology scale gap. In: Tingberg, A., Lang, K. (eds.) International Workshop on Breast Imaging - IWDM. Springer, Malmo, Sweden (2016)

A Measure of Regional Mammographic Masking Based on the CDMAM Phantom

Benjamin Hinton[1(✉)], Serghei Malkov[1], Jesus Avila[1], Bo Fan[1], Bonnie Joe[1],
Karla Kerlikowske[2], Lin Ma[2], Amir Mahmoudzadeh[1], and John Shepherd[1]

[1] Department of Bioengineering, UC-San Francisco, San Francisco, CA, USA
bhinton@berkeley.edu
[2] Department of Epidemiology and Biostatistics, UC-San Francisco, San Francisco, CA, USA

Abstract. Detectability of invasive cancerous lesions in mammography is diminished in breasts with dense and complex fibroglandular tissue. If masking were locally quantified in mammograms, radiologists could potentially use this information to clear the region using targeted adjuvant screening techniques. We present a method to quantify localized masking using a model observer to detect virtual objects of varying thickness and size convoluted into the clinical mammogram. Contrast detail curves are used to create an Image Quality Factor (IQF) at high resolution throughout the breast. We report on preliminary findings of how IQF is related to measures of breast density and textural complexity in a cohort of women who experienced screening detected and interval (masked) cancers. This measure of masking using a localized contrast detail curve approach should provide a means to target adjuvant screening resources for faster and more effective determination of cancer status for women with dense breast.

Keywords: Breast density · BI-RADS · Interval cancer · CDMAM · Model observer · Mammography · Sensitivity · Masking · Detectability

1 Introduction

Interval cancers are defined as cancers diagnosed between normal screening mammogram intervals. Although there are several reasons for interval cancer to occur, one important category of interval cancers are those that were large enough to be detected at the time of screening but were masked by overlapping dense and spatially complex tissue. Masking delays treatment and potentially increases cancer mortality. Masked interval cancers often are larger than screening detected cancers and of a more advanced stage once discovered [1]. The ability to detect these tumors in women with dense breasts is diminished by 10–20 % compared to women with fatty breasts.

There has been much progress in describing the qualities of breast tissue including automated measures of breast density and texture [2–6]. Although masking can influence measures of breast cancer risk, there is a highly significant and independent relationship of breast density and cancer risk even after excluding masking effects [7]. Most breast density studies have been related to these direct associations to breast cancer [8]. Little

© Springer International Publishing Switzerland 2016
A. Tingberg et al. (Eds.): IWDM 2016, LNCS 9699, pp. 525–531, 2016.
DOI: 10.1007/978-3-319-41546-8_66

study has related breast density to masking. Kerlikowske showed that interval cancers would be most likely to occur in dense breast [9].

We do know that mammographic masking is related to low contrast between lesions and the surrounding and overlapping tissue. Contrast is lowered from surrounding tissue having a density similar to the lesion. It is also lessened by the complicated nature of the density referred to as the texture. Mainprize, et al. proposed the hypothesis that masking could be quantified using a normalized noise power spectrum of the mammography system [10]. The authors showed that this masking measure was correlated to volumetric breast density and density categories.

Our approach is to directly measure the contrast of objects that represent cancer lesions in each woman's mammogram. Our hypothesis is that a direct measure of masking will be more universal than picking a functional hypothesis. Our approach is based on the well-established CDMAM phantom (version 3.4). CDMAM phantoms are mammography phantoms with gold disks of various thicknesses and diameters and are widely used to characterize contrast and detail capabilities of mammography systems. The aim of this pilot study was to first demonstrate the technique of creating virtual gold disks based on the CDMAM phantom to simulate breast lesions and show how the contrast detail characteristics related to relevant measures of density and texture in women with and without interval cancer. We show how the disk attenuations can be simulated and develop a model observer based on the gold disks of the CDMAM phantom.

2   Subjects and Methods

In this pilot study, we first derive our virtual CDMAM approach and then validate our method against actual CDMAM results. We then show how the virtual CDMAM can be convoluted into clinical mammograms. We derive local contrast detail curves and the associated IQFs and display these values as a "masking map" showing regions with high and low masking. We then demonstrate the approach in a pilot study of clinical mammograms of women.

Subjects: Mammograms (N = 31) from a previous study were used. All mammograms were acquired on Hologic Selenia full-field mammography systems (Hologic, Inc, Bedford, MA).

Simulating CDMAM Disks: To simulate the attenuation of the gold disks from the CDMAM phantom in mammography images, we modeled the X-ray source spectra using header information for kVp, mAs, anode material, and filtration. The spectral input to the breast was generated using Boone et al. [11]. We then estimate the spectral output from the breast tissue after estimating the pixel-by-pixel breast density using the SXA program [2] and attenuations for adipose and fibroglandular tissue from the NIST XCOM program (http://www.nist.gov/pml/data/xcom/) [11]. The gold disk attenuations of diameters and thicknesses similar to the CDMAM phantom were estimated using similar methods. Spatial noise was assumed to be much larger than X-ray statistical noise and thus the X-ray noise was neglected in the current model. In this current model, scatter was not taken into account but will be incorporated in future models. Before inserting the disk virtually, the disk was blurred according to the modulation transfer function (MTF) of the system [12]. The final spectral X-ray output was then summed with and without the gold disks.

Determining Detectability: At this time all analysis of detectability is being performed on the "For Processing" images. We introduced our signal detection algorithm by creating a non-prewhitening matched filter (NPWMF) which has been done in several signal detection studies [13]. The test statistic to determine if the signal is detectable for the NPWMF is as follows, where g_2 is the mean of the signal-present image, g_1 is the mean of the signal-absent image, and g is the test image.

$$\lambda_{NPW(g)} = \left(\bar{g}_2 - \bar{g}_1\right)' g \tag{1}$$

To calculate this test statistic, we set the test search area of our image as a fixed diameter ($\sqrt{2}*D$) larger than the diameter of the gold disk in question, as done in previous studies [14].

Tuning Test Statistic: The threshold of detectability test statistic was determined by varying the threshold test statistic to minimize the least squared distance between the contrast detail curves produced from n = 10 CDMAM images analyzed with CDMAM Analyzer software (Version 1.5.5) and of the contrast detail curves produced from inserting our virtual discs into a blank region of the CDMAM images. This provides a measure of detectability in an untextured region, although it has been noted that detectability decreases in textured zones [15]. The CDMAM images were taken using a Hologic Selenia full-field mammography system (Hologic, Inc, Bedford, MA), at 29 kVp and 120.6 mAs.

Creating Masking Map: We calculated this test statistic for each thickness and diameter of the CDMAM phantom in our region of interest (ROI) to determine the minimum detectable thickness for each diameter of the phantom. The results of this can be presented as a contrast detail curve. To produce values on our masking map we calculated the Image Quality Factor (IQF) of each contrast detail curve as an indicator of the overall masking of that ROI, where the highest values correspond to the highest detectability [15]:

$$IQF = n \left/ \sum_{i=1}^{n} C_{i,min} D_i \right. \tag{2}$$

Where n is the number of diameters tested and $C_{i,min}$ is the smallest thickness detectable corresponding to a gold diameter D_i. The diameters used in this IQF measurement range in size from 0.06 mm up to 1 cm to simulate a range of lesion sizes. This IQF value was then calculated for every pixel throughout the breast and was displayed throughout the breast to create our masking map.

Once our masking map was created with these IQF values, they were examined and compared with the actual screening mammogram. We then compared the mean IQF values in each breast with the BIRADS density category to look for any trends.

3   Results

The women used in this study were on average 52 years old, had a height of 64.3 in., weighed 146.5 lb, and had an average BMI of 24.9. 54 % of the women had children previously, and 51 % of the individuals had stopped menstruation. Of the subjects, N = 2 were in BIRADS Density category A, N = 13 in category B, N = 14 in category C, and N = 2 were in category D.

Tuning the test statistic in our software produced threshold thickness values and contrast detail curves within the estimated threshold thickness range for human detectability that were produced from running the CDMAM Analyzer 1.5.5 program for the 10 different CDMAM phantom scans.

IQF values and a regional masking map of these values were produced for each individual. A masking map for one such individual is shown in Fig. 1, along with the raw unprocessed mammogram that we did the analysis on Lower IQF values correspond to darker regions on the masking map, which mean there is more mammographic masking.

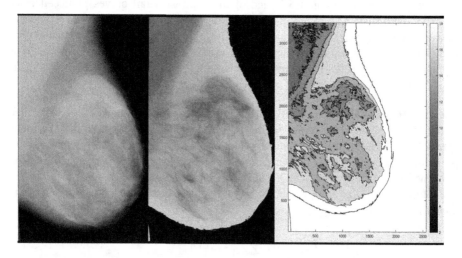

Fig. 1. Mammogram (raw, unprocessed) (left) and greyscale masking maps (center) of image quality factor of the different regions of a breast. Lower values correspond to lower IQF values and less detectability. At right, a greyscale contour map is shown to of the IQF

IQF values range from 10 to 20. The mean IQF value in these samples was 15.5 with a standard deviation of 0.8. Figure 2 summarizes the mean IQF values between the different BI-RADS density classification categories. In general, the less dense classifications had higher mean IQF values in the breast. This indicates that the IQF value differentiates between regions of high breast density and low breast density.

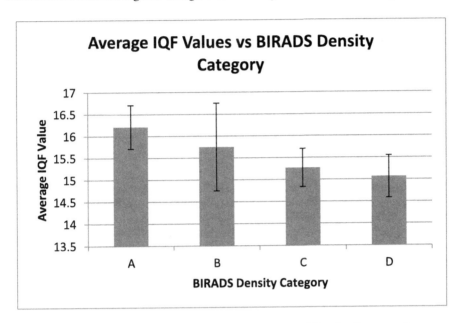

Fig. 2. Relationship between Average IQF values and BIRADS Density Category. One can see that the higher density categories have lower average IQF value. (A) The breasts are almost entirely fatty. (B) There are scattered areas of fibroglandular density. (C) The breasts are heterogeneously dense, which may obscure small masses. (D) The breasts are extremely dense, which lowers the sensitivity of mammography

4   Discussion

This study demonstrated how regional maps of mammographic masking based on the CDMAM phantom can be achieved. Images of masking maps indicated that high density areas and breasts tend to have lower IQF values than low density regions and breasts. This suggests that this preliminary masking value differentiates between dense and non-dense tissue and may hold value to determine regions of local masking.

Our study is at present a pilot study and had several limitations. Because the IQF value sums all threshold thicknesses thorough all diameters, it does not capture information about detectability at specific sizes that could be very useful to radiologists. Further, our threshold value was tuned on a blank background and to be more accurate we would need to tune this threshold on textured backgrounds, as that has been shown to affect detectability. We may alter this displayed value in the future to show detectability at different size ranges or to show the largest diameter disk that is still detectable. Further, this method has to date only been applied to unprocessed raw images. Further studies are needed using images as they are typically presented to the radiologist.

Dense regions of breasts have areas with different structures, tissues, and textures. As we develop this measure further, we plan to study how global and regional texture features affect the measures we produce. Lastly, our method currently simulates a gold disk, which has significant differences in texture and shape characteristics compared to lesions. This could affect the actual accuracy of the masking value, and in future iterations of this work we will examine modulating the shape (non-circular, irregular, etc.) and texture of the simulated lesion to be more similar to breast lesions.

It would be worthwhile to further study this IQF value, as it is likely correlated with texture features that may elucidate associations between mammographic texture features and mammographic masking. Further, it is hypothesized that mammographic masking is higher in cases of interval breast cancers compared to screen detected breast cancers, and future work includes calibrating the IQF feature to a probability of masking using women with interval and non-interval cancers.

Acknowledgements. I would like to thank the CBCRP for their generous grant that made this work possible under grant #21IB-0130. I would further like to thank the Shepherd Lab, Bo Fan, Jesus Avila, Bennett Ng, and the NSF GRFP for various types of support: This material is based upon work supported by the National Science Foundation Graduate Research Fellowship under Grant No. 1144247. Any opinion, findings, and conclusions or recommendations expressed in this material are those of the authors(s) and do not necessarily reflect the views of the National Science Foundation.

References

1. Tabar, L., Faberberg, G., Day, N., Holmberg, L.: What is the optimum interval between mammographic screening examinations? An analysis based on the latest results of the Swedish two-county breast cancer screening trial. Br. J. Cancer **55**(5), 547 (1987)
2. Shepherd, J., Herve, L., Landau, J., Fan, B., Kerlikowske, K., Cummings, S.: Novel use of single X-ray absorptiometry for measuring breast density. Technol. Cancer Res. Treat. **4**(2), 173–182 (2005)
3. Highnam, R., Sauber, N., Destounis, S., Harvey, J., McDonald, D.: Breast density into clinical practice. In: Maidment, A.D., Bakic, P.R., Gavenonis, S. (eds.) IWDM 2012. LNCS, vol. 7361, pp. 466–473. Springer, Heidelberg (2012)
4. Hartman, K., Highnam, R.P., Warren, R., Jackson, V.: Volumetric assessment of breast tissue composition from FFDM images. In: Krupinski, E.A. (ed.) IWDM 2008. LNCS, vol. 5116, pp. 33–39. Springer, Heidelberg (2008)
5. Manduca, A., Carston, M., Heine, J., Scott, C., Pankratz, V., Brandt, K., et al.: Texture features from mammographic images and risk of breast cancer. Cancer Epidemiol. Biomark. Prev. **18**(3), 837–845 (2009)
6. Nie, K., Chen, J., Hon, J., Chu, Y., Nalcioglu, O., Su, M.: Quantitative analysis of lesion morphology and texture features for diagnostic prediction in breast MRI. Acad. Radiol. **15**(12), 1513–1525 (2008)
7. Boyd, N., Dite, G., Stone, J., Gunasekara, A., English, D., McCredie, M., et al.: Heritability of mammographic density, a risk factor for breast cancer. N. Engl. J. Med. **347**(12), 886–894 (2002)

8. Eng, A., Gallant, Z., Shepherd, J., McCormack, V., Li, J., Dowsett, M., dos-Santos-Silva, I., et al.: Digital mammographic density and breast cancer risk: a case-control study of six alternative density assessment methods. Breast Cancer Res. **16**, 439 (2014)

9. Kerlikowske, K., Zhu, W., Tosteson, A., Sprague, B., Tice, J., Lehman, C., et al.: Identifying women with dense breasts at high risk for interval cancer: a cohort study. Ann. Intern. Med. **162**(10), 673–681 (2015)

10. Mainprize, J.G., Wang, X., Ge, M., Yaffe, M.J.: Towards a quantitative measure of radiographic masking by dense tissue in mammography. In: Fujita, H., Hara, T., Muramatsu, C. (eds.) IWDM 2014. LNCS, vol. 8539, pp. 181–186. Springer, Heidelberg (2014)

11. Boone, J., Fewell, T., Jennings, R.: Molybdenum, rhodium, and tungsten anode spectral models using interpolating polynomials with application to mammography. Med. Phys. **24**(12), 1863–1874 (1997)

12. Yip, M., Chukwu, W., Kottis, E., Lewis, E., Oduko, J., Gundogdu,O., et al.: Automated scoring method for the CDMAM phantom. In: Sahiner, B., Manning, D.J., (eds.), pp. 72631A–72631A-10 (2009). http://proceedings.spiedigitallibrary.org/proceeding.aspx?articleid=816030. [cited 2 Nov 2015]

13. Rico, R., Muller, S.L., Peter, G., Noel, A., Stines, J.: Automated scoring of CDMAM: a dose study. In: International Society for Optics and Photonics on Medical Imaging 2003, pp. 164–173 (2003). http://proceedings.spiedigitallibrary.org/proceeding.aspx?articleid=758494. [cited 2 Nov 2015]

14. Veldkamp, W.J.H., Thijssen, M.A.O., Karssemeijer, N.: The value of scatter removal by a grid in full field digital mammography. Med. Phys. **30**(7), 1712 (2003)

15. Grosjean, B., Muller, S.: Impact of textured background on scoring of simulated CDMAM phantom. In: Astley, S.M., Brady, M., Rose, C., Zwiggelaar, R. (eds.) IWDM 2006. LNCS, vol. 4046, pp. 460–467. Springer, Heidelberg (2006). http://link.springer.com/10.1007%2F11783237_62

A Statistical Method for Low Contrast Detectability Assessment in Digital Mammography

Chiara Spadavecchia[1,2], Raffaele Villa[1,2(✉)], Claudia Pasquali[1],
Nicoletta Paruccini[1], Nadia Oberhofer[3], and Andrea Crespi[1]

[1] Medical Physics Department, San Gerardo Hospital, ASST Monza, Monza, Italy
[2] University of Milan, Milan, Italy
`raffaele.vill@gmail.com`
[3] Medical Physics Department, Bolzano Hospital, Bolzano, Italy

Abstract. This study proposes a method to estimate low contrast detectability (LCD) applying a statistical method, based on the analysis of a uniform region. A dedicated test object was designed, made up of an acetate sheet equipped with a central uniform insert and an aluminium step wedge, allowing linear conversion from pixel values to millimeters of aluminium. A Matlab program for automated image analysis was developed. Phantom images were acquired on two different digital mammography systems. Reproducibility and sensitivity to exposure variations of the proposed method were investigated for different dose levels. Further the impact of scattering and attenuation on LCD was studied adding PMMA layers of variable thickness (2 to 7 cm) upon the acetate sheet during exposure in automatic exposure control modality. The statistical method turned out to be a reliable and rapid method for LCD evaluation. Applications include routine assessment of equipment performance for digital mammography systems.

Keywords: Low constrast detectability · Digital mammography · Quality assurance

1 Introduction

Performance assessment of digital mammography systems is commonly achieved using image quality metrics such as MTF (Modulation Transfer Function), NNPS (Normalised Noise Power Spectrum) and DQE (Detective Quantum Efficiency). These metrics provide a widely accepted method of characterising the physical performance of detector systems, but they generally do not include other fundamental elements of the imaging chain, such as scatter radiation. To provide a quantitative measure of image quality (IQ), low contrast detectability (LCD) is a fundamental parameter to be taken into account. Thus, the routine assessment and control of IQ is often evaluated in terms of threshold contrast visibility of details varying in diameter and contrast. Contrast detail curves,

© Springer International Publishing Switzerland 2016
A. Tingberg et al. (Eds.): IWDM 2016, LNCS 9699, pp. 532–539, 2016.
DOI: 10.1007/978-3-319-41546-8_67

displaying the minimum detected contrast for each detail diameter, are commonly used for reporting. A widespread phantom for IQ performance assessment of full field mammography systems is the CDMAM phantom (Artinis Medical Systems, The Netherlands). It embeds gold discs of 0.03–20 μm thickness and 0.06–2.00 mm diameter and is sandwiched between PMMA layers of variable thickness during image acquisition. Software packages have been developed in order to perform automated quantitative analysis of images produced with the CDMAM test object, in compliance with the European Guidelines Recommendations [1]. According to these recommendations, to increase reproducibility at least 16 CDMAM phantom images are required for each evaluation. This study proposes a method, based on statistical considerations [2], which allows to evaluate LCD from just a single image, overcoming the need of repeated exposures for each contrast detail curve. A dedicated test object was designed and assembled. The presented statistical method is based on the analysis of a uniform image region. A Matlab program for automated image analysis was developed. The performance of the LCD test object, in combination with the software analysis tool, was tested on two systems of different manufactures. The aim of this work was to investigate the feasibility of the statistical approach as assessment of LCD.

2   Materials and Methods

The next paragraphs explain the statistical approach supporting the method for LCD evaluation, followed by a description of the phantom designed and the dedicated analyser software. Set-up, image acquisition and analysis method are illustrated below.

2.1   A Statistical Method of Defining LCD

The statistical method adopted in this work was first presented by Chao et al. [2]. LCD is notably affected not only by the amount of noise, but also by the noise frequency spectrum. Hence the standard deviation σ of the pixel values in a homogeneous image is not by itself useful in determining LCD. However, considering several identical regions of interest (ROI) placed on a uniform background, each with a mean pixel value (PV) μ, the standard deviation of these means (σ_μ) is relevant when determining the LCD, since the ROI limits noise to the spatial frequencies of the object. According to the central limit theorem, σ_μ is normally distributed. Therefore a prediction on the detectability of an insert, identical in size with the considered ROI, can be made: an insert inside a homogeneous background is detectable with a 95 % confidence level if

$$\mu_{insert} - \mu_{bkg} > 3.29\sigma_\mu,$$

where μ_{insert} indicates the mean pixel value of the insert and μ_{bkg} the average of all μ_i for i ROIs of the same size as the insert under consideration (Fig. 1).

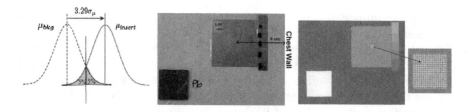

Fig. 1. Left: Normal distributions of ROIs in the background and in the low contrast object. The latter is detected with 95 % confidence level if the difference in the mean value of the two distributions is $3.29\sigma_\mu$; Center: a photo of the homemade phantom; Right: a schematic view of the LCD test object with an enlargement on the central 120*120 ROI divided in a matrix of subROIs

2.2   LCD Test Object

A dedicated phantom allowing application of the outlined method for LCD evaluation was designed (Fig. 1). It is made up of:

- an acetate sheet;
- a lead insert ($2 \times 2\,cm^2$, 0.5 cm thick), in lateral position;
- a central uniform aluminium region ($3 \times 3\,cm^2$, 0.49 mm thick);
- an aluminium step wedge, with increasing thicknesses from 0.20 to 1.00 mm (each step is $0.6 \times 0.8\,cm^2$).

The lead insert is useful to study scatter and veiling glare effects, whereas LCD assessment is carried out on the uniform central image area. LCD is obtained in terms of pixel value difference. The aluminium step wedge is meant for calibrating the image in terms of millimetres of aluminium (mm Al), thanks to the conversion from pixel value into mm Al.

2.3   Analyser Software

A Matlab code for automated analysis of LCD test object images was developed. After automatic identification of the uniform Al region, a square ROI (typically 120×120 pixels) is placed in the center. This ROI is divided into a subROIs-matrix, as shown in (Fig. 1). For each subROI, the mean pixel value μ_i is calculated, along with the standard deviation of these means σ_μ, according to the statistical method. The basic assumption of the statistical method, i.e. the normal distribution of μ_i, was evaluated both with Lilliefors and Jarque-Bera normality tests. The low contrast threshold LC_{th} necessary to detect an insert was estimated by multiplying σ_μ by 3,29. In order to express LC_{th} in terms of a more physical quantity, namely threshold Al thickness, image calibration in terms of mm Al has been performed. For that purpose square ROIs of 50px were placed on each step of the Al step wedge and linear regression between mean pixel value and Al thickness calculated for each image. These steps were repeated for several subROI sizes (24, 20, 15, 12, 10, 8, 6, 5, 4, 3 and 2 pixels).

This implies a variable numerosity of μ_i used for estimating σ_{mu}, depending on the considered subROI size. A contrast detail curve was determined, taking as detail size the product of subROI size (expressed in pixels) with pixel extension (in mm). To further quantify IQ, for each contrast detail curve a summarising figure of merit was used, the Inverse Image Quality Figure [3], calculated as:

$$IQF_{inv} = \frac{1}{\sum_i (diameter_i * threshold\_contrast_i)} \tag{1}$$

where diameter and threshold contrast refer to the contrast detail curve and the sum extends over all detail sizes.

2.4   Set-Up and Image Acquisition

Image were acquired with two digital mammography systems, MAMMOMAT Novation (Siemens, Germany) and Sectra MicroDose (Philips, The Netherlands). The uniform aluminium region was centered at 6 cm from the chest wall with the aluminium step wedge orthogonal to the anode-cathode axis. The proposed method was studied regarding reproducibility and sensitivity to changes in exposure settings. To investigate the reproducibility, five identical images of the test object were acquired on one system (Sectra MicroDose) with manual exposure setting (32 kVp, 0.73 mGy Average Glandular Dose (AGD)). To test the sensitivity to exposure settings variations, test object images were acquired on both systems in two ways: (a) with fixed high voltage (3 kVp) at various dose levels (0.29–1.13 mGy AGD), (b) with fixed Air Kerma at the detector surface at varying high voltage (32–38 kVp). Furthermore, to evaluate the effect of scatter and attenuation, a series of LCD test object images was produced in full automatic technique with PMMA slabs of variable thickness (2 cm to 7 cm) placed upon the phantom on both mammography systems.

2.5   Image Analysis

Image analysis was carried out on DICOM for processing images. Contrast detail curve plots were used to provide a first visual insight of detectability trend in low contrast small details. Overall IQF_{inv} value were calculated. Generally LC_{th} results were also analysed for each detail size separately, being the number of subROIs used for calculation subROI size dependent. To evaluate the methods reproducibility, five identical images acquired on the Sectra system were used. Varability was assessed in terms of standard deviation of the overall IQF_{inv} value and of LC_{th} for each detail size. For studying the influence of the initial squared ROI size on large detail reproducibility, the whole analysis was carried out for three different ROI side lengths: 120, 240 and 360 pixels. Increasing the ROI size reflects in increased subROI number used for σ_μ calculation. Additionally a multiple ROI analysis was undertaken with 5 or 9 ROIs (120 × 120 pixels).

The sensitivity of the method to changes in exposure settings (AGD and kVp) was both investigated through the analysis of the contrast detail curves obtained and IQF_{inv} score.

Table 1. Reproducibility of the statistical method through five images of the LCD test object (Sectra MicroDose).

Details(mm)	LCD(mmAl)	st.dev	CV%
1.2	0.0089	0.0012	13%
1	0.0098	0.0013	13%
0.75	0.0129	0.0008	6%
0.6	0.0166	0.0017	10%
0.5	0.0195	0.0013	7%
0.4	0.0241	0.0007	3%
0.3	0.0315	0.0009	3&
0.25	0.0368	0.0007	2%
0.2	0.0454	0.0012	3%
0.15	0.0574	0.0008	1%
0.1	0.0783	0.0014	2%
IQF_{inv}	9.7	0.4	4%

normality test failure		
$120 * 120$	$240 * 240$	$360 * 360$
7%	13%	17%

IQF_{inv} obtained from images with different PMMA thicknesses were compared in order to quantify the reduction of image quality due to increasing slab thicknesses, producing more scatter and attenuation. To further evaluate the effect of scatter and veiling glare, two ROIs (10×60 pixels) were drawn using images with PMMA slabs: the first one on the lead insert, close to its boundary edge, the second one on the background region. The average signal ratio of these two ROIs S_{lead}/S_{bkg} was analysed with respect to the PMMA thickness. Regarding the long term study also the image analysis was simplified, including only the statistical ROI analysis without the conversation in mm of aluminium.

3   Results and Discussion

3.1   Reproducibility of the Statistical Method

Table 1(a) reports one example of reproducibility analysis for the statistical method based on a squared 120×120 pixel ROI. IQF_{inv} data calculated on the five identical images showed a good reproducibility with a standard deviation of 4%. This is comparable with 5% IQF_{inv} uncertainty reported for automated analysis of CDMAM images [4]. The point by point analysis for each low contrast object (i.e. subROI size) outlined a good reproducibility for a wide range of detail dimensions with a standard deviation of calculated LC_{th} within 10%, except for the two largest details (>1.0 mm). The critical issue in LCD evaluation with large subROIs is strictly connected to the statistical method itself: for smaller inserts, LCD is derived from standard deviation σ_μ on many subROIs (up to 14440), while for 1.2 mm detail dimension it is calculated on 100 subROIs only. Data obtained with 240×240 or 360×360 pixel ROI showed better reproducibility of the method for larger insert. On the other hand, this implies a non-Normal distribution of mean values caused by spatial non-uniformity of the signal. On the other hand the amount of normality test failures increased using larger ROIs, resulting 7 %, 13 % and 17 % for 120, 240 and 360 pixels ROIs respectively. Larger ROIs in fact imply a non-Normal distribution of mean values μ_i caused by spatial non-uniformity (Table 1).

Table 2. Reproducibility of the statistical method: comparison among 1, 5 and 9 120×120 ROIs in terms of coefficient of variation

	Details (mm)										
	1.2	1	0.75	0.6	0.5	0.4	0.3	0.25	0.2	0.15	0.1
1 ROI	13 %	13 %	6 %	10 %	7 %	3 %	3 %	2 %	3 %	1 %	2 %
5 ROIs	4 %	5 %	5 %	3 %	2 %	1 %	1 %	1 %	2 %	1 %	1 %
9 ROIs	6 %	6 %	4 %	3 %	1 %	2 %	1 %	1 %	2 %	1 %	1 %

Table 2 compares the coefficients of variation corresponding to a multiple ROI analysis for 5 and 9 ROIs to the single ROI analysis. As the number of ROIs increased, the coefficient of variation decreased for each subROI size. The 5 ROIs variant turned out to be the best choice to improve reproducibility with acceptable processing times.

3.2 LCD for Different Acquisition Parameters

As expected, increasing AGD yielded to improved LCth for all detail sizes, as can be seen from the contrast detail curves in Fig. 2 (left). Quantitatively this was confirmed by the IQF_{inv} score, which almost doubled, varying AGD from 0.29 to 1.13 mGy (Fig. 2). The analysis of the contrast detail curves varying tube voltages showed an improvement of the LCD as the tube voltage decreased (Fig. 2 (right)).

Being known the trend of IQF_{inv} versus AGD, the uncertainty of the proposed method (4 %) allows a prediction on the sensitivity in terms of AGD (8 %). IQF_{inv} can also discriminate variations in kVp, thus, with AGD, it can be a relevant parameter for clinical optimization.

3.3 LCD for Different PMMA Thicknesses

The contrast detail curves in Fig. 3 show the expected worsening in image quality as PMMA thickness increases: the minimum contrast detected turned out to be larger. The analysis of IQF_{inv} parameter confirmed the results obtained through contrast detail curves analysis. IQF_{inv} increased with decreasing thickness: it almost doubled varying PMMA from 7 to 2 cm for both systems, as detailed in Fig. 4. The results obtained were explained by the increasing amount of scattering radiation due to PMMA growing thickness and the reduction of the overall contrast caused by the higher kVp, leading to a general worsening in detail visibility.

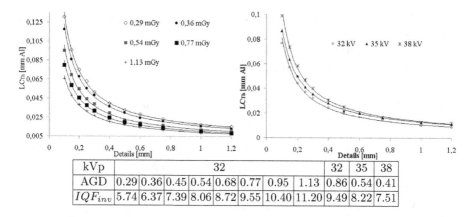

kVp	32								32	35	38
AGD	0.29	0.36	0.45	0.54	0.68	0.77	0.95	1.13	0.86	0.54	0.41
IQF_{inv}	5.74	6.37	7.39	8.06	8.72	9.55	10.40	11.20	9.49	8.22	7.51

Fig. 2. Contrast detail curve at different ADG (left) and different kVp (right).

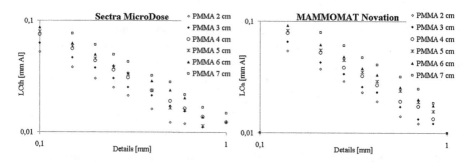

Fig. 3. Contrast detail curves for several PMMA thicknesses for Sectra MicroDose (left) and MAMMOMAT Novation (right). Data were plotted in logarithmic scale.

Regarding the scattering effect, the S_{lead}/S_{bkg} ratio resulted to be lower than 1 % for Sectra MicroDose. For MAMMOMAT Novation, S_{lead}/S_{bkg} increased as the PMMA thickness became higher: S_{lead}/S_{bkg} was 13.6 % and 29.4 % for 2 and 7 cm PMMA, respectively.

3.4   Use of the Statistical Method for LCD Assessment in Routine Quality Control

In our hospital every six month the CDMAM phantom with a 4 cm of PMMA is acquired according to European Guidelines Recommendations [1]. The evaluation of contrast-detail curves obtained with the statistical method above described has been included in a monthly routine quality assurance procedure over the last year to achieve a more frequent constancy control. It has been established to acquire a uniform image of 4 cm of PMMA. The analysis, possible in each uniform region, is carried out through the above described analyser software, without the conversion in millimetres of aluminium. Results show good accordance for small inserts and a worse one for larger diameters (CV larger than

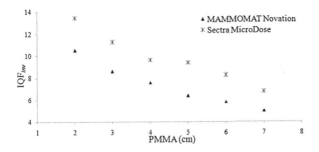

Fig. 4. IQF_{inv} values in function of different PMMA thicknesses.

10 %). As previously shown, the reliability of the analysis is affected by the different number of subROIs and could be improved evaluating LCD in 5 120 × 120 pixel ROIs on the central uniform aluminium region. The use of the LCD test object, not yet introduced in monthly routine quality assurance procedure, could also allow to obtain LCD curves in terms of millimetres of aluminium.

4   Conclusions

The presented statistical method combined with the use of a dedicated LCD test object demonstrated high reproducibility. It turned out to be a reliable and rapid method for low contrast threshold assessment. Also the overall image quality figure IQF_{inv} presented reliable scoring, thus being a valid approach in image quality assessment. Besides using the CDMAM phantom and automated analysis as routine quality control, the rapidity of the statistical method allows a less time-consuming approach for a quality control procedure as constancy performance. Further applications, for example to quality assessment of synthesized 2D images from digital breast tomosynthesis scans have to be investigated.

References

1. Perry, N.: European Guidelines for Quality Assurance in Breast Cancer Screening and Diagnosis, Supplement, 4th edn. Office for Official Publications of the European Communities, Luxembourg (2006)
2. Chao, E.H., Toth, T.L., Bromberg, N.B., Williams, E.C., Fox, S.H., Carleton, D.A.: A statistical method of defining low contrast detectability. Radiology **217**, 162 (2000)
3. Young, K.C., Cook, James J.H. Oduko, J.M., Bosmans, H.: Comparison of software and human observes in reading images of the CDMAM test object to asses digital mammography systems. In: Medical Imaging (2006)
4. Oberhofer, N., Paruccini, N., Moroder, E.: Image quality assessment and equipment optimisation with automated phantom evaluation in full field digital mammography (FFDM). In: Krupinski, E.A. (ed.) IWDM 2008. LNCS, vol. 5116, pp. 235–242. Springer, Heidelberg (2008)

Should We Adjust Visually Assessed Mammographic Density for Observer Variability?

Elaine F. Harkness[1,2,3(✉)], Jamie C. Sergeant[4,5], Mary Wilson[2], Ursula Beetles[2],
Soujanya Gadde[2], Yit Y. Lim[2], Anthony Howell[2,6],
D. Gareth Evans[2,7], and Susan M. Astley[1,3]

[1] Centre for Imaging Sciences, Institute of Population Health, University of Manchester,
Stopford Building, Oxford Road, Manchester, M13 9PT, UK
Elaine.F.Harkness@manchester.ac.uk

[2] Genesis Breast Cancer Prevention Centre and Nightingale Breast Screening Centre,
University Hospital of South Manchester NHS Trust, Wythenshawe, Manchester, M23 9LT, UK

[3] The University of Manchester, Manchester Academic Health Science Centre,
University Hospital of South Manchester NHS Foundation Trust, Wythenshawe,
Manchester, M23 9LT, UK

[4] Arthritis Research UK Centre for Epidemiology, Centre for Musculoskeletal Research,
Institute of Inflammation and Repair, Faculty of Medical and Human Sciences,
Manchester Academic Health Science Centre, University of Manchester, Oxford Road,
Manchester, M13 9PT, UK

[5] NIHR Manchester Musculoskeletal Biomedical Research Unit,
Central Manchester NHS Foundation Trust, Manchester Academic Health Science Centre,
Manchester, UK

[6] The Christie NHS Foundation, Withington, Manchester, M20 4BX, UK

[7] Genomic Medicine, Manchester Academic Health Sciences Centre,
University of Manchester and Central Manchester Foundation Trust, Manchester, M13 9WL, UK

Abstract. This study aimed to determine whether correcting for observer variability alters estimations of breast cancer risk associated with mammographic density. A case control design examined the relationship between mammographic density, measured by visual analogue scales (VAS), and the risk of breast cancer after correcting for observer variability. Mammographic density was assessed by two observers and average scores (V2) were adjusted to correct for observer variability ($V2_{ad}$). Two case-control sets were identified: (i) breast cancer detected during screening at entry and (ii) breast cancer detected subsequently. Cases were matched to three controls. In the first case-control set the odds ratio for breast cancer was 4.6 (95 %CI 2.8–7.5) for the highest compared to the lowest quintile of V2, and was attenuated for $V2_{ad}$ (OR 3.1, 95 %CI 1.9–4.8). Similar findings were observed for the second case-control set. Not adjusting for observer variability may lead to an overestimate of the risk of breast cancer.

Keywords: Digital · Mammogram · Breast cancer · Visual analogue scales (VAS) · Observer bias · Case-control study

© Springer International Publishing Switzerland 2016
A. Tingberg et al. (Eds.): IWDM 2016, LNCS 9699, pp. 540–547, 2016.
DOI: 10.1007/978-3-319-41546-8_68

1 Introduction

Several methods exist for measuring breast density, including visual assessment methods. One such method is the use of visual analogue scales (VAS) where individual observers score their perception of percentage density on a continuous scale from 0 to 100 % [1]. However, this visual assessment is subjective as different readers each have their own interpretation of the continuous scale which leads to inter-observer variability. By design, or otherwise, the case-mix seen by individual readers may also differ significantly, whereby some readers may only read mammograms with relatively low or high density. However, it is important to be able to draw conclusion across all entities independently of the particular subset of readers [2]. By correcting for observer variability, these differences may be taken into account.

Sperrin et al. (2013) describe a method to correct for inter-rater disagreement (or observer bias) for the general problem where observers assign scores on a continuous scale, using visual assessment of mammographic density as an example. The adjustment is performed in two stages: firstly by standardising the distributions of observer scores, to account for each observer's subjective interpretation of the continuous scale, by transforming all raters on to the same distribution; and secondly by correcting for case-mix differences between observers by exploiting pairwise information (i.e. where raters have read the same entity), comparing this with the first stage and adjusting for systematic differences that may be attributed to case-mix. This method gives a transformed average (V2$_{ad}$).

The aim of this study was to examine mammographic density rated using VAS, before (V2) and after (V2$_{ad}$) adjusting for observer variability, and to determine the relationship between V2 and V2$_{ad}$ and the association with a contemporaneous or future diagnosis of breast cancer.

2 Methods

Women were recruited as a part of the Predicting Risk Of Cancer At Screening (PROCAS) study [3]. Between October 2009 and April 2015 women in the Greater Manchester area invited for routine breast screening through the National Health Service Breast Screening Programme (NHSBSP) in the UK were also invited to take part in PROCAS. A total of 58,000 women consented to participate in PROCAS and provided additional information on risk factors for breast cancer by completing a 2-page questionnaire at the time of screening. Mammographic density at the time of screening was assessed by a number of methods, including VAS. Ethical approval for the study was given by the North Manchester Research Committee (09/H1008/81).

For all women recruited to the study before September 2013 a visual assessment of mammographic density was performed. The procedure used for the PROCAS study has previously been described [2]. Briefly mammographic density was recorded on a set of four horizontal 10-cm VAS, anchored at the ends with labels 0 % and 100 %, for each of the four radiographic views. Each mammogram was assessed independently by two readers from a pool of 18 readers, including consultant radiologists, advanced practitioner radiographers or breast physicians and who interpret at least 5000 mammograms per year. Assessors viewed batches of 20–50 sets of images on standardised monitors with each set of four views displayed in turn, and the corresponding VAS forms were completed. Assignment of assessors to batches was undertaken on a pragmatic basis according to availability of readers. The forms were scanned and VAS marks were automatically converted to percentages. Visually assessed density was calculated for each woman based on the average of the four radiographic views, which were then averaged between each pair of readers to form a single density score (V2).

All women in the PROCAS study with visual density assessments were used to calculate density corrected for observer variability (V2$_{ad}$) using code provided by Sperrin et al. (2013). The input file required patient identifier, rater identifier, mammographic view and VAS score. The code was run in R [4] and produced an output file containing the raw score (V2), a transformed average for the first stage (TA1) and a transformed average for the second stage (TA2).

We also conducted two case control studies to examine the relationship between V2 and V2$_{ad}$ and breast cancer risk. In the first case control study women diagnosed with breast cancer during screening at the time of entry to PROCAS were identified (first screen detected). Each case was matched to three controls with a negative screen at study entry and a further negative screen approximately three years later. Matching was performed on the basis of age (within a year), body mass index (BMI) group (< 25, 25–29.9, 30–39.9 and > 40 kg/m^2), menopausal status (premenopausal, perimenopausal, postmenopausal or unknown) and Homone replacement therapy (HRT) use (current versus never/ever). In the second case-control study, cases were identified as women with a negative screen at the time of study entry and were subsequently diagnosed with breast cancer at a further routine screen or between screens. Cases were each matched to three controls with a negative screen at study entry and a further negative screen approximately three years later. Matching was performed on the same factors as the first case-control set outlined above but also on year of mammogram.

Characteristics of cases and controls were compared using a Chi-square test for categorical data (menopausal status, HRT use, ethnic origin, and parity). Continuous variables (age, BMI) were compared by means of an unpaired sample t-test when the distribution was normally distributed or if not normally distributed by the Mann-Whitney U test. To examine the relationship between VAS and case control status conditional logistic regression was used due to the matched nature of the dataset. The final logistic regression models were also adjusted for breast volume and any other assessed factors that were statistically different between cases and controls.

3   Results

A total of 57,905 women were recruited to PROCAS, of which 51,733 (89 %) were recruited before September 2013 and 51,326 (99 %) of these had their mammographic density assessed visually and had a V2 and adjusted V2$_{ad}$ score. For V2 the median breast density was 24.4 % (interquartile range (IQR) 13.6 to 37.8 %) and the mean was 21.9 % (after normalisation) for V2$_{ad}$ the median breast density was 21.1 % (IQR 10.4 to 35.0 %) and the mean was 18.0 % (after normalisation).

The number of mammograms read by individual readers ranged from 161 for reader 1 to 16377 (16 % of total reads) for reader 10. Boxplots for the individual assessors are shown in Fig. 1 and illustrate the median, IQR and outliers for each reader based on their average VAS readings of the four mammographic views. The boxplots demonstrate wide variation in visual density assessment between readers, the median percentage density ranged from 2.3 % (IQR 1.1 to 9.5) in reader 1 to 38.3 % (IQR 29.5 to 46.5) in reader 8.

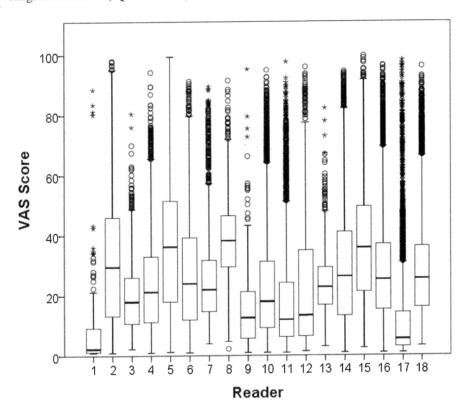

Fig. 1. Boxplots of the VAS distributions for individual readers based on the average of the VAS of four mammographic views (%)

Women with high mammographic density were classified as those above the 90th percentile of all PROCAS women with V2 scores. In total, 5139 women with a score greater than 51.25 % were classified as having high mammographic density using V2. The 90th percentile for $V2_{ad}$ was lower (49.52 %). Table 1 shows the number of women who would be reclassified using the 90th percentile to classify women as having high mammographic density for V2 and $V2_{ad}$. A similar number of women would be reclassified from high V2 to 'non-high' $V2_{ad}$ (870), as would 'non-high' V2 to high $V2_{ad}$ (863). Overall 49,453 (96.6 %) remain in the same category (Table 1).

Table 1. Women classified as having high mammographic density based on 90th percentiles for V2 ad V2$_{ad}$

	V2 $\leq$ 51.25 %	V2 > 51.25 %	Total
V2$_{ad}$ $\leq$ 49.52 %	45324	870	46194
V2$_{ad}$ > 49.52 %	863	4269	5132
Total	46187	5139	51326

3.1   Case-Control Study 1 – Cancers Detected at First Screen (FSDC)

There were a total of 366 women who had a breast cancer detected during their screen at entry to PROCAS, of these 320 had density assessed visually (the rest were recruited after September 2013). All cases were matched to three controls. Cases and controls were well-matched on the matching variables (age – mean 58 years, BMI – mean 28 kg/m^2, HRT use – 5 % current users, and menopausal status – 68 % post-menopausal) but there was a significantly lower proportion of controls of white ethnic origin compared to cases (91.3 % versus 94.5 % respectively, p = 0.003).

Figure 2 shows the associations with quintiles of V2 and V2$_{ad}$ for breast cancer after adjusting for ethnicity and breast volume. The odds ratio for developing breast cancer was 4.58 (95 % CI 2.80–7.47) for those in the highest quintile of V2 compared to those in the lowest quintile. Results were attenuated, but remained statistically significant, for V2$_{ad}$ with an odds ratio of 3.12 (95 % CI 1.89 – 4.81) for the highest compared to the lowest quintile.

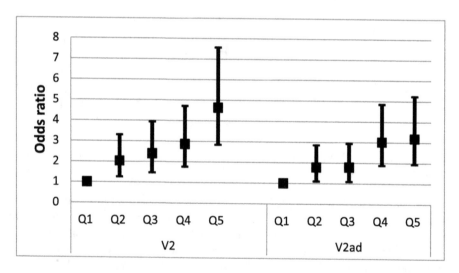

Fig. 2. First screen detected cancer odds ratios by quintiles of V2 and V2$_{ad}$

3.2 Case-Control Study 2 – Cancers with a Prior Negative Screening Mammogram (Priors)

For the second case control study there were a total of 338 women with a negative screen at entry to PROCAS who then went on to develop breast cancer at a subsequent screen or between screens. Of these, 336 women had visually assessed mammographic density for the negative screen at entry. Each case was matched to three controls. Cases and controls were well-matched on the matching variables (age – mean 60 years, BMI – mean 28 kg/m², HRT use – 11 % current users, menopausal status – 76 % postmenopausal), however more cases were nulliparous compared to controls (13.3 % compared to 9.7 % respectively, p = 0.02).

Figure 3 shows the associations for quintiles of V2 and $V2_{ad}$ for breast cancer risk after adjusting for breast volume and parity. The odds ratio for developing breast cancer was 4.54 (95 % CI 2.86–7.23) for those in the highest quintile of V2 compared to those in the lowest quintile. Similarly to the case control study of first screen detected cancers the results were attenuated, but to a lesser degree, and remained statistically significant after correction for observer variability with an odds ratio of 3.87 (95 % CI 2.39–6.28) for the highest compared to the lowest quintile of $V2_{ad}$.

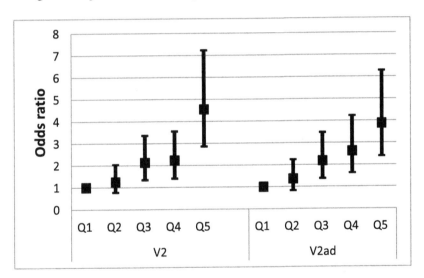

Fig. 3. Screen detected cancers with negative priors odds ratios by quintiles of V2 and $V2_{ad}$

4 Discussion

This study aimed to examine the effect of correcting for observer variability in visually assessed mammographic density, and to examine the relationship between V2 and adjusted $V2_{ad}$ and the association with current and future breast cancer status. VAS assessments of mammographic density were completed in the vast majority of women taking part in PROCAS (89 %). Assessments were made by 18 different readers, however the number of mammograms read and the case-mix of mammograms varied substantially. By applying the method proposed by Sperrin et al. (2013) we were able to correct for inter-rater variability (observer bias) in visually assessed mammographic density [2]. After adjusting for the differences between readers a similar number of women were reclassified from high to 'non-high' density and from 'non-high' to high density. We also examined the impact of the adjustment for rater variability on the association with breast cancer in two separate case control studies. In both case-control studies the unadjusted V2 density scores were significantly associated with an increased risk of developing breast cancer, and the risk was attenuated, but still statistically significant, after correcting for observer variability $V2_{ad}$. Thus adjustment for rater variability appears to yield more appropriate predictions for the risk of developing breast cancer, and by not adjusting for this particular type of variability there may be an overestimate of the relationship between mammographic density and breast cancer risk. Nevertheless, both adjusted and unadjusted estimates were statistically significantly associated with an increased risk of breast cancer, demonstrating an increased association with current or future breast cancer with increasing mammographic density as measured by VAS.

The strengths of this study include the large sample of women with visually assessed mammographic density scored by two independent readers. The method of adjusting for observer variability was performed on all women with V2 scores to provide a robust $V2_{ad}$ estimate. These adjusted estimates were then used for the smaller case control studies to examine the predictive ability of V2 and $V2_{ad}$ to differentiate cases and controls. One limitation of the study was that V2 and $V2_{ad}$ were performed on all mammograms (analogue and digital) in PROCAS whilst the smaller case control studies were based on those women with only digital mammograms. This may have had an influence on the results and is worth investigating further.

Whilst independent double reading of mammograms is standard practice in most NHSBSP centres in the United Kingdom it is not the standard approach adopted in many countries with most mammograms being read by only one reader. Furthermore, visual assessment of mammographic density is time consuming and impractical in the clinical setting. The advent of automated methods, such as Volpara^{TM} or Quantra^{TM}, for digital mammograms, means that mammograms can be assessed objectively, and there is evidence to suggest an association with the risk of breast cancer [5]. However, these methods do not enable readers to assess additional aspects of the mammogram such as texture and other features.

A further limitation of the current study is that it does not adjust for intra-observer variability or the discriminative ability of a given reader [2].

5   Conclusions

We examined the impact of adjusting for rater variability when mammograms were assessed by two readers using VAS in two separate case control studies. Unadjusted V2 density scores were significantly associated with an increased risk of developing breast cancer in both case control studies and the risk was attenuated, but still statistically significant, after correcting for observer variability $V2_{ad}$. By not adjusting for observer variability the odds ratios for breast cancer risk may be over-estimated.

Acknowledgements. We acknowledge the support of the National Institute for Health Research (NIHR) and the Genesis Prevention Appeal for their funding of the PROCAS study. We would like to thank the women who agreed to take part in the study and the study staff for recruitment and data collection. This paper presents independent research funded by the National Institute for Health Research (NIHR) under its Programme Grants for Applied Research programme (reference number RP-PG-0707-10031: "Improvement in risk prediction, early detection and prevention of breast cancer"). The views expressed are those of the author(s) and not necessarily those of the NHS, the NIHR, or the Department of Health.

References

1. Duffy, S.W., Nagtegaal, I.D., Astley, S.M., Gillan, M.G., McGee, M.A., Boggis, C.R., Wilson, M., Beetles, U.M., Griffiths, M.A., Jain, A.K., Johnson, J., Roberts, R., Deans, H., Duncan, K.A., Iyengar, G., Griffiths, P.M., Warwick, J., Cuzick, J., Gilbert, F.J.: Visually assessed breast density, breast cancer risk and the importance of the craniocaudal view. Breast Cancer Res. **10**(4), R64 (2008)
2. Sperrin, M., Bardwell, L., Sergeant, J.C., Astley, S., Buchan, I.: Correcting for rater bias in scores on a continuous scale, with application to breast density. Stat. Med. **32**, 4666–4678 (2013)
3. Evans, D.G.R., Warwick, J., Astley, S.M., Stavrinos, P., Sahin, S., Ingham, S., McBurney, H., Eckersley, B., Harvie, M., Wilson, M., Beetles, U., Warren, R., Hufton, A., Sergeant, J.C., Newman, W.G., Buchan, I., Cuzick, J., Howell, A.: Assessing individual breast cancer risk within the U.K. National Health Service Breast Screening Program: a new paradigm for cancer prevention. Cancer Prev. Res. **5**(7), 943–951 (2012)
4. R Core Team: R: a language and environment for statistical computing. In: R Foundation for Statistical Computing, Vienna, Austria (2012). ISBN: 3-900051-07-0. http://www.R-project.org/
5. Eng, A., Gallant, Z., Shepherd, J., McCormack, V., Li, J., Dowsett, M., Vinnicombe, S., Allen, S., dos-Santos-Silva, I.: Digital mammographic density and breast cancer risk: a case-control study of six alternative density assessment methods. Breast Cancer Res. **16**, 439 (2014)

Do Women with Low Breast Density Have Regionally High Breast Density?

Amir Pasha Mahmoudzadeh[1(✉)], Serghei Malkov[1],
Benjamin Hinton[1], Brian Sprague[3], Karla Kerlikowske[2],
and John Shepherd[1]

[1] Department of Radiology and Biomedical Imaging,
University of California, San Francisco, USA
AmirPasha.Mahmoudzadeh@ucsf.edu
[2] Departments of Medicine and Epidemiology and Biostatistics,
University of California, San Francisco, USA
[3] Department of Surgery, University of Vermont, Burlington, USA

Abstract. Average volumetric breast density has been found to be associated with interval cancers. The association is believed to be partly due to mammographic masking. We asked if regional density may be a more sensitive descriptor of masking than average density. In this work, we propose a new method to identify high density regions based on calibrating pixel-level volumetric breast density to Breast Imaging Reporting and Data System (BI-RADS) Version 4 categories. Local breast density was measured using the single-energy X-ray absorptiometry (SXA) technique. In 583 women undergoing screening mammography, we found percent fibroglandular volume ranges that corresponded to each BI-RADS category: 0–4.9 % (BI-RADS 1), 5.0–18.2 % (BI-RADS 2), 18.3–48.9 % (BI-RADS 3) and 49.0–100 % (BI-RADS 4). Women with an average BI-RADS 1 category had 21840 pixels (0.014 mm) breast area considered high density (category 4) compared to 186469 pixels (0.014 mm) in women with average BI-RADS 4 category. We conclude that some women with low breast density still have regions of high density that may mask breast cancers. These scores and localized density colorized maps may better help radiologists in the decision to utilize secondary adjuvant screening than whole breast BI-RADs scores.

Keywords: Breast density · Masking · BI-RADS · Mammography · FGV

1 Introduction

Interval cancers are defined in the NHSBSP (NHS Breast Screening Radiologists Quality Assurance Committee, 2005) as breast cancer diagnosed in the interval between scheduled normal screening. These interval cancers may occur for some reasons: The main reason is that the cancer was not detectable at the time of screening because was masked by overlapping dense and complex tissue. It is much easier to find these tumors in women with fatty breasts compared to women with dense breast and the ability to find these tumors with dense breast or complex tissue is decreased by 10–20 % compared to women with fatty breasts. Kerlikowske demonstrated that

© Springer International Publishing Switzerland 2016
A. Tingberg et al. (Eds.): IWDM 2016, LNCS 9699, pp. 548–553, 2016.
DOI: 10.1007/978-3-319-41546-8_69

interval cancers would most likely occur in dense breast [1]. The interval cancers usually are bigger than screening detected cancers and they are in advanced stage when discovered [2].

There has been a lot of work in automated measure of breast density and texture to describe the qualities of breast tissue [3–7]. Even after removing masking, there is an independent relationship of breast density and cancer risk [8]. Most of the study of breast density has been related to breast cancer risk [9] and there are few studies have been into relating breast density to masking.

In this study, we use a previously derived measure of localized breast density called single- energy X- ray absorptiometry, or SXA [3]. SXA compares the attenuation value of each image pixel to that of a reference phantom of a known density. Thickness is also accurately measured using the SXA phantom. We then calibrate the SXA density values to BI-RADS scores on a pixel level.

2   Methods

Using screening mammograms that contain a single-energy X-ray absorptiometry (SXA) phantom, we derived percent fibroglandular density for each image pixel. We calibrated these pixel breast density values to BI- RADS score using thresholds derived from whole breast average density and clinically-reported BI-RADS. We then assigned colors to these local categories to create localized scoring maps. This was performed in a subset of a large screening population. Prevalence of each BI-RADS category was determined by overall average Clinical BI-RADS score.

Subjects: Screening mammograms were collected along with serum and a breast health questionnaire as part of the San Francisco Mammography Registry (SFMR) and Vermont Breast Cancer Surveillance System from 2009–2013. These are two sites of the Breast Cancer Surveillance Consortium (BCSC). Only CC-view images were analyzed for this study. Women were selected at random from the overall screening population.

Mammography: All mammograms were acquired on Hologic Selenia full-field digital mammography systems (Hologic, Inc., Bedford, MA) that are within the BCSC. These systems are found at two sites in the San Francisco area (California Pacific Medical Center and University of California San Francisco) and at the University of Vermont Hospital. To be included, the mammograms had to contain the SXA phantom. This phantom has been in use since 2009 at these centers such that over 400,000 women and 4 million mammograms were available in the cohort. SXA breast density was analyzed using version 9.0 [10, 11].

We used the clinically-reported BI-RADS (4th edition) values as the reference value of density. To convert SXA fibroglandular volume to BI-RADS scores, we sorted all mammograms by density and found the cutoff densities that created categories of density with the same prevalence as the clinically-derived BI- RADS values.

Using the density-derive BI-RADS values, we assigned all pixels to one of four colors: Green = BI- RADS 1 (almost entirely fat), Yellow = BIRADS 2 (scattered fibroglandular density), Orange = BI-RADS 3 (heterogeneously density which could obscure detection of small masses), and Red = BI-RADS 4 (extremely dense).

Table 1. Demographics of women participating in mammography from 2009 to 2013.

	Cases	Controls
N	200	383
Mean age at mammogram (SD)	58.1 (11.8)	57.7 (11.5)
Mean BMI (SD)	25.07 (4.5)	25.1 (5.04)
Body mass index categories, kg/m^2		
<25	116 (58 %)	224 (58.5 %)
25–29	51 (25.5 %)	89 (23.3 %)
30–34	11 (5.5 %)	43 (11.3 %)
35+	8 (4 %)	14 (3.6 %)
Missing	14 (7 %)	13 (3.3 %)
Menopausal status		
Premenopausal	51 (25.5 %)	98 (25.5 %)
Postmenopausal	133 (66.5 %)	253 (66.2 %)
Missing	16 (8 %)	32 (8.3 %)
Age at 1st birth		
<30	77 (38.5 %)	169 (44.2 %)
None or >=30	123 (61.5 %)	214 (55.8 %)
Postmenopausal hormone therapy		
Missing	35 (17.5 %)	34 (8.9(%)
Yes	24 (12 %)	40 (10.5 %)
No	141 (70.5 %)	309 (80.6 %)
Race		
White	141 (70.5 %)	279 (72.8 %)
Non-white	59 (29.5 %)	104 (27.2 %)
BI-RADS breast density		
Almost entirely fatty (a)	19 (9.5 %)	58 (15.2 %)
Scattered fibroglandular densities (b)	59 (29.5 %)	171 (44.7 %)
Heterogeneously dense (c)	87 (43.5 %)	125 (32.6 %)
Extremely dense (d)	35 (17.5 %)	29 (7.5 %)

Images were created of the colorized images to study. Bar whisker plots were created to show the breast area of each density-derived BI- RADS for groups of women by clinically-derived BI-RADS.

3 Results

In total, we examined 583 sequentially acquired mammograms from 2009 to 2013. We found that the density cutoff values needed to match the frequency of the clinically-derived BI-RADS was 0–4.9 % (BI- RADS 1), 5.0–18.2 % (BI-RADS 2), 18.3–48.9 % (BI-RADS 3) and 49.0–100 % (BI-RADS 4). A summary of the demographic variables, risk factors, and other breast measures are shown in Table 1. Four example colorized images are shown in Fig. 1. We found as expected that the most prevalent

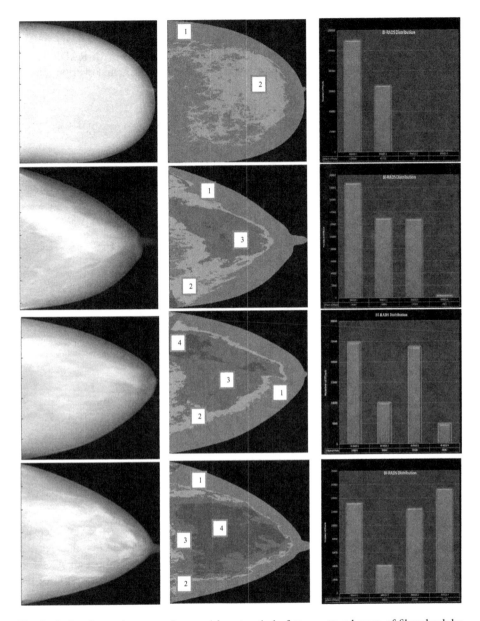

Fig. 1. Left column shows raw images (almost entirely fatty, scattered areas of fibroglandular, heterogeneously dense, extremely dense, respectively), the middle column shows colorized images based on volumetric breast density for each pixel (Green = BI-RADS 1, Yellow = BI-RADS 2, Orange = BI-RADS 3, Red = BI-RADS 4), the right column shows the number of pixels for each BI-RADS inside of breast. (Color figure online)

density-derived BI-RADS value was the clinically-derived value. However, there were a significant number of high density categories in women with low density breast. Figure 2 shows the bar-whisker representation of the distributions of BI-RADS values by Clinically-derived BI-RADS category. Also, Fig. 2 shows the actual distributions of areas for each score by group.

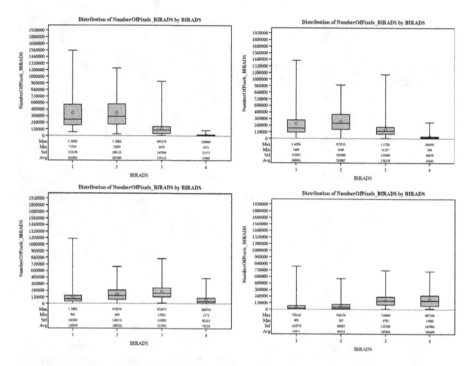

Fig. 2. (Top left) Group = BI-RADS 1, (Top right) Group = BI-RADS 2, (Bottom left) Group = BI-RADS 3, (Bottom right) Group = BI-RADS 4.

Our results show increase in volumetric breast density as BI-RADS density increased. Figure 1 (first row, middle column) shows green color is dominant in the breast (the number of pixels in BI-RADS 1 is higher than the number of pixels in BI-RADS 2,3 and 4 (first row, right column)). Figure 2 shows the distribution of the number of pixels of each BI-RADS density value across the population of women. As can be seen, women with BI-RADS 1 and 2 whole breast densities have virtually no BI-RADS 4 pixels.

4   Discussion and Conclusions

We have proposed and defined a method to represent localized breast density in terms of BI- RADS category. It was clear from our study that breast density is not a homogeneous values across the breast. Although we have yet to test our primary hypothesis, we now have a method where we can determine if masking is a regional effect and more prevalent in high density areas. We will proceed with future studies that will use interval cancers as a model for masked cancers versus mammographically detected screening cancers (non-masked cancers). We anticipate that interval cancers will be found predominantly in the BI-RADS 4 pixel regions. We conclude that automated, colorized pixel-specific volumetric density measures can be created and may be a useful tool in the study of masking and interval cancers.

References

1. Kerlikowske, K., Zhu, W., Tosteson, A.N., Sprague, B.L., Tice, J.A., Lehman, C.D., Miglioretti, D.L.: Identifying women with dense breasts at high risk for interval cancer: a cohort study. Ann. Intern. Med. **162**(10), 673–681 (2015)
2. Tabar, L., Faberberg, G., Day, N., Holmberg, L.: What is the optimum interval between mammographic screening examinations? An analysis based on the latest results of the Swedish two-county breast cancer screening trial. Br. J. Cancer **55**(5), 547 (1987)
3. Shepherd, J.A., Herve, L., Landau, J., Fan, B., Kerlikowske, K., Cummings, S.R.: Novel use of single X-ray absorptiometry for measuring breast density. Technol. Cancer Res. Treat. **4** (2), 173–182 (2005)
4. Highnam, R., Sauber, N., Destounis, S., Harvey, J., McDonald, D.: Breast density into clinical practice. In: Maidment, A.D.A., Bakic, P.R., Gavenonis, Sara (eds.) IWDM 2012. LNCS, vol. 7361, pp. 466–473. Springer, Heidelberg (2012)
5. Hartman, K., Highnam, R.P., Warren, R., Jackson, V.: Volumetric assessment of breast tissue composition from FFDM images. In: Krupinski, E.A. (ed.) IWDM 2008. LNCS, vol. 5116, pp. 33–39. Springer, Heidelberg (2008)
6. Manduca, A., Carston, M.J., Heine, J.J., Scott, C.G., Pankratz, V.S., Brandt, K.R., Sellers, T. A., Vachon, C.M., Cerhan, J.R.: Texture features from mammographic images and risk of breast cancer. Cancer Epidemiol. Biomarkers Prev. **18**(3), 837–845 (2009)
7. Nie, K., Chen, J.-H., Hon, J.Y., Chu, Y., Nalcioglu, O., Su, M.-Y.: Quantitative analysis of lesion morphology and texture features for diagnostic prediction in breast MRI. Acad. Radiol. **15**(12), 1513–1525 (2008)
8. Boyd, N.F., Dite, G., Stone, J., Gunasekara, A., English, D., McCredie, M., Giles, G., Tritchler, D.L., Chiarelli, A., Yaffe, M., et al.: Heritability of mammographic density, a risk factor for breast cancer. N. Engl. J. Med. **347**(12), 886–894 (2002)
9. Eng, A., Gallant, Z., Shepherd, J., McCormack, V., Li, J., Dowsett, M., Vinnicombe, S., Allen, S., dos-Santos-Silva, I.: Digital mammographic density and breast cancer risk: a case–control study of six alternative density assessment methods. Breast Cancer Res. **16**(5), 439 (2014)
10. Malkov, S., Wang, J., Kerlikowske, K., Cummings, S.R., Shepherd, J.A.: Single x-ray absorptiometry method for the quantitative mammographic measure of fibroglandular tissue volume. Med. Phys. **36**(12), 5525–5536 (2009)
11. Malkov, S., Wang, J., Shepherd, J.A.: Improvements to single energy absorptiometry method for digital mammography to quantify breast tissue density. In: Krupinski, E.A. (ed.) IWDM 2008. LNCS, vol. 5116, pp. 1–8. Springer, Heidelberg (2008)

Energy Dependence of Water and Lipid Calibration Materials for Three-Compartment Breast Imaging

Jesus Avila[1(✉)], Serghei Malkov[1], Maryellen Giger[2],
Karen Drukker[2], and John A. Shepherd[1]

[1] Department of Radiology and Biomedical Imaging, University of California,
San Francisco, CA 94115-0628, USA
jesus.avila@ucsf.edu
[2] Department of Radiology, University of Chicago, Chicago, IL, USA

Abstract. Approximately 75 % of biopsies performed in women with suspicious lesions are not found to have cancer. To reduce the number of false positive mammographic findings and the resulting biopsies, we have developed a combination of 3-compartment (lipid, water, protein) mammogram analysis and quantitative descriptors of lesions morphometry. The solution for lesion composition requires the calibration of dual energy mammogram attenuations to tissue equivalent standards. However, these phantom substitutes for actual breast tissue have inherent differences in energy-dependent X-ray characteristics that may lead to systematic errors in estimating composition. Here, we investigate the energy dependence of two biological materials (oil and water) to their phantom equivalents at different X-ray energies through both theoretical and empirical considerations. We first derived the relationship of the oil and water to the phantom materials at each energy and then compared to experimental measures. We found that the errors as large as 20 % in actual oil/water fraction when compared to the phantom materials at different energies. We conclude that calibrating breast composition to phantom materials at each dual-energy acquisition is not sufficient to ensure accuracy. A further basis transformation derived from bovine tissues greatly reduced these errors.

Keywords: Breast composition · Mammography · Three-compartment · Dual-energy

1 Introduction

Over a span of ten years, women who undergo annual mammograms have almost a 50 % chance of receiving a false positive diagnosis [1]. In the past two decades, studies have shown that women with higher breast density have a higher risk of developing breast cancer [2, 3]. In addition, these women are more prone to false positives because it is difficult to distinguish between normal features in dense breast and malignant lesions with conventional mammography [4].

Recently, Laidevant et al. developed a dual energy X-ray imaging method that uses a three-compartment model of the breast (3CB) to characterize tissue composition [5].

© Springer International Publishing Switzerland 2016
A. Tingberg et al. (Eds.): IWDM 2016, LNCS 9699, pp. 554–563, 2016.
DOI: 10.1007/978-3-319-41546-8_70

The 3CB method represents breast tissue as the equivalent composition of the phantom materials—Delrin, Plastic Water®, and machinable wax. The 3CB model is derived by acquiring three measurements: a low-energy image, a high energy image, and the total thickness of the breast at each pixel. By generating images of the lipid, water, and protein (LWP) content of the breast, it may be possible to get a characteristic signature of malignant and benign lesions. Drukker et al. recently used this technique in conjunction with breast morphometry features for classifying lesions and found that improved classification vs. either technique alone [6]. Additionally, Malkov et al. found compositional differences in lesion classifications [7]. There are some limitations of 3CB that need to be improved, however, for the technique to be reliable.

The 3CB technique relies on substitute materials for biological equivalents of lipid, water, and protein. However, errors will arise if the relationship between actual breast tissue compartments of lipid, water, and protein differ from the phantom materials in terms of the variables of image acquisition (kVp, filtration, anode material, etc.). The following corrections have been applied to the technique thus far: flat-fielding and initial intensity correction. Although these have shown some improvement, negative thicknesses in the protein as a result from errors in water and lipid estimates are still present.

In this study, we examine how well the phantom materials represent known quantities of biological materials of oil and water as a function of kVp setting used to create the 3CB images. We compare theoretical modeling to experimental measures to determine if a further basis set transformation is needed that is tube voltage dependent.

2   Methods

First, a theoretical approach was derived to show the dependence of thickness estimates on low energy (LE) selection. Following this, experimental work was performed on lipid and water substitute materials bathed in their biological equivalents. The typical 3CB technique was performed on these samples, which involves capturing a LE image, a high energy (HE) image, and measuring the total sample thickness. An additional LE image was taken to compare thickness estimates between the LE images. Next, a bovine experiment was performed to derive correction factors that are energy dependent to correct 3CB estimates. Finally, statistical analysis is performed to test the null hypothesis of no difference between the two thickness estimates of the LE images.

2.1   Theory

For monoenergetic sources, we have following equation for X-ray sources passing through the three lipid, water, protein materials:

$$I = I_0 e^{-(\mu_w(E)t_w + \mu_L(E)t_L + \mu_P(E)t_P)}$$

Or in the log-signal form:

$$A(E) = -\log\left(\frac{I}{I_0}\right) = (\mu_w(E)t_w + \mu_L(E)t_L + \mu_P(E)t_P)$$

The total thickness of the breast is composed of the three materials:

$$T = t_W + t_L + t_P$$

Acquiring two images at different monoenergies and using our total thickness equation we can write these equations in matrix form: $\boldsymbol{\mu t} = \boldsymbol{A}$, where

$$\boldsymbol{\mu} = \begin{bmatrix} \mu_{w,LE} & \mu_{L,LE} & \mu_{P,LE} \\ \mu_{w,HE} & \mu_{L,HE} & \mu_{P,HE} \\ 1 & 1 & 1 \end{bmatrix}, \boldsymbol{t} = \begin{bmatrix} t_w \\ t_L \\ t_P \end{bmatrix}, \boldsymbol{A} = \begin{bmatrix} A_{LE} \\ A_{HE} \\ T \end{bmatrix}$$

Solving for $\boldsymbol{t}$ we get $\boldsymbol{t} = \boldsymbol{\mu}^{-1}\boldsymbol{A}$.

Suppose that for each material, there is an error β_j between our substitute materials and their biological equivalents at particular low monoenergies, then

$$\mu'_{i,LE} = \beta_j\mu_{i,LE}$$

$$\Rightarrow A'_{LE} = \beta_1\mu_{w,LE}t_w + \beta_2\mu_{L,LE}t_L + \beta_3\mu_{P,LE}t_P = \alpha_1 A_{LE}, w, \text{ where}$$

$$\alpha_1 = \frac{\beta_1\mu_{w,LE}t_w + \beta_2\mu_{L,LE}t_L + \beta_3\mu_{P,LE}t_P}{\mu_{w,LE}t_w + \mu_{L,LE}t_L + \mu_{P,LE}t_P}$$

$$\Rightarrow \boldsymbol{t} = \begin{bmatrix} \beta_1\mu_{w,LE} & \beta_2\mu_{L,LE} & \beta_3\mu_{P,LE} \\ \mu_{w,HE} & \mu_{L,HE} & \mu_{P,HE} \\ 1 & 1 & 1 \end{bmatrix}^{-1} \begin{bmatrix} \alpha_1 A_{LE} \\ A_{HE} \\ T \end{bmatrix}$$

Let $\boldsymbol{t}'$ be a second estimate of LWP thicknesses at a different low monoenergy, LE'. For $\boldsymbol{t}'$ to have the same LWP thickness estimates, then $\boldsymbol{t}' - \boldsymbol{t} = 0$

$$\boldsymbol{t}' - \boldsymbol{t} = \begin{bmatrix} \beta'_1\mu_{w,LE'} & \beta'_2\mu_{L,LE'} & \beta'_3\mu_{P,LE'} \\ \mu_{w,HE} & \mu_{L,HE} & \mu_{P,HE} \\ 1 & 1 & 1 \end{bmatrix}^{-1} \begin{bmatrix} \alpha'_1 A_{LE'} \\ A_{HE} \\ T \end{bmatrix}$$

$$- \begin{bmatrix} \beta_1\mu_{w,LE} & \beta_2\mu_{L,LE} & \beta_3\mu_{P,LE} \\ \mu_{w,HE} & \mu_{L,HE} & \mu_{P,HE} \\ 1 & 1 & 1 \end{bmatrix}^{-1} \begin{bmatrix} \alpha_1 A_{LE} \\ A_{HE} \\ T \end{bmatrix}$$

We can see that only the first rows of each matrix need be equivalent for our estimates of LWP thicknesses to be equivalent; thus, if corresponding β_j and β'_j are not equivalent at different energies, then these will add error to the estimated LWP content of breast tissues.

2.2   Modeled LWP Estimates

NIST XCOM was used to derive the mass attenuation coefficients for the substitute materials and their biological equivalents. Chemical compositions were approximated for Plastic Water® LR and machinable blue wax. The LWP estimates were modeled using the derived monoenergetic estimates from above. The LWP content was estimated under two different conditions: (1) four samples composed of varying ratios of Plastic Water® LR and distilled water and (2) four samples composed of varying ratios of machinable blue wax and canola oil. Table 1 shows the thicknesses selected for each of the estimate.

Table 1. Thicknesses of substitute and biological equivalent materials for different LWP estimates.

Estimate #	Substitute material thickness (mm)	Biological equivalent thickness (mm)	Total thickness (mm)
1	0	30	30
2	10	20	30
3	15	15	30
4	20	10	30

2.3   Phantoms and Materials

Digital step wedge phantoms were machined from the two substitute materials, Plastic Water® LR and machinable blue wax (Fig. 1). Each phantom was placed in baths of distilled water and canola oil, respectively. Table 2 shows the densities of each material.

Table 2. Materials used for experiment and their densities.

Material	Density (g/ml)
Canola oil	0.920
Blue wax	0.914
Liquid water	1.000
Plastic water LR	1.008

A region of interest (ROI) was sampled on three of the phantom steps, and the thicknesses of these are as follows: 10, 15, and 20 mm. A fourth ROI was sampled where only liquid was present. Liquid was poured in their respective containers until the total thickness of material + liquid reached a uniform thickness of 30 mm (Fig. 2).

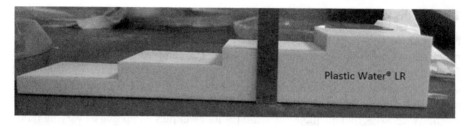

Fig. 1. The plastic water® LR digital step wedge phantom is shown. The thickness steps from left-to-right are 5, 10, 15, 20 mm. (Color figure online)

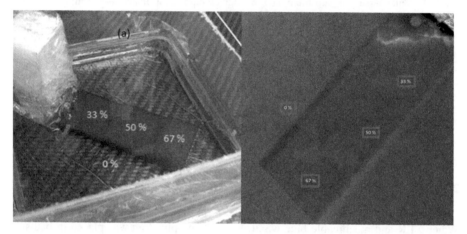

Fig. 2. The machinable wax digital step phantom bathed in canola oil is shown. (a) An optical image was taken to demonstrate experimental setup. (b) Four regions of interest of varying solid and liquid composition were sampled on the X-ray image. **_Percent_** $= 100 * \frac{solid}{solid + liquid}$. There are noisy regions in some of the ROI's, which are attributed to nonhomogeneous material compositions. We avoided these areas in our analysis. (Color figure online)

2.4   Containers

Plastic containers were prepared such that they did not interfere with the experiment, since the plastic material can attenuate the intensity of the X-rays. To remedy this, the bottom of each container was removed. In addition, a hole was cut on the container lids, and a thin plastic wrap (i.e., Glad ClingWrap) of negligible thickness (see estimate below) was used to seal the lid holes. The perforated lids were placed on the container, fastening the plastic wrap in place. The containers were imaged upside-down with the perforated lid as the bottom. After the liquids were poured, each container was inspected for leaks.

2.5 Estimate of the Change in Source Intensity Attributed to Plastic Wrap

Plastic wrap has a thickness $x = 12.5\,\mu m$ (micrometers) and is made from linear low-density polyethylene, which has a density $\rho = 0.915 - 0.925\frac{g}{cm^3}$. The mass attenuation coefficient μ decreases as energy (keV) increases. Using the worst case, $\rho = 0.925\frac{g}{cm^3}$ and $\mu = 2.088\frac{cm^2}{g}$ for 10 keV (10 keV, which is less than half of the lowest keV in this experiment). The percentage change from the source intensity I_0 is as follows:

$$100 * \frac{(I_0 - I)}{I_o} = 100 * \left(1 - e^{-\mu\rho x}\right) = 0.241\%$$

This indicates that plastic wrap attenuates less than 1 % of the source intensity; thus, we can expect errors in compositional differences attributable to the plastic wrap to be less than 1 %.

2.6 Imaging and Analysis

Low energy (LE) and high energy (HE) images were taken of the samples using a single Hologic Selenia full-field digital mammography system (Hologic, Inc., Bedford, MA). The samples were imaged at two different LE voltage levels, 27 and 30 kVp. The HE images were taken at 39 kVp. LE images were acquired under regular clinical screening mammography conditions. HE images were acquired with a Rhodium filter instead of Moly, and an additional 3 mm Aluminum filter was used. All images were acquired at the same exposure: 100 mAs. The total procedure is approximately 10 % more of the typical mammographic dose. All images were acquired at the same exposure: 100 mAs. The log-signals of the LE and HE images and the total thickness of the samples (30 mm) were used to estimate the total lipid, water, and protein content of each ROI. Two-sample t-tests were used to test significant difference between the estimated material content of the two LE levels for all composition percentages.

2.7 Bovine Calibration

Most of this procedure is described in detail in another article [8]. An affine transformation map was made from bovine samples to correct the LWP estimates for each kVp. The transformation is a basis set transformation from the substitute material space to the biological tissue (bovine) space. It is a matrix such that is applied to correct substitute material estimates as follows:

$$\begin{bmatrix} W' & L' & P' \end{bmatrix} = \begin{bmatrix} W & L & P \end{bmatrix} A(kVP), \quad where\ A = \begin{bmatrix} a_{11} & a_{12} & a_{13} \\ a_{21} & a_{22} & a_{23} \\ a_{31} & a_{32} & a_{33} \end{bmatrix},$$

and W, L, P are water, lipid, and protein estimates using a phantom derived from substitue materials

The coefficients for A were derived from known water, lipid, and protein compositions of a bovine phantom. A is estimated at each of the mammographic energies and is thus energy dependent: 25, 26, 27, 28, 29, 30, 31, 32, 39 kVp.

3 Results

Figure 3 shows a plot of the theoretical mass attenuations μ derived from XCOM. These values were derived for energies in the anticipated screening mammography range. Table 3 lists details about the theoretical mass attenuations derived for Fig. 3.

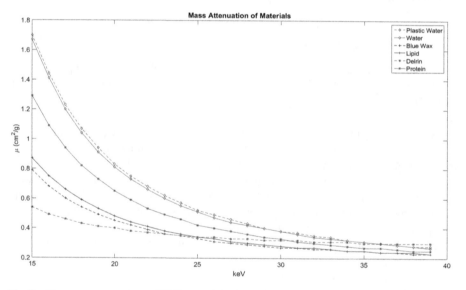

Fig. 3. The mass attenuations of 3CB materials. It can be seen how the substitute materials differ from their biological counterparts as a function of energy. Most notably, protein and Delrin vary the most at the lower energies.

The initial estimates using the 3CB technique for our experiment are shown in Fig. 4. The estimated lipid, water, and protein contents for the two experiments show significant differences between the two LE images at each ROI. The bovine-corrected estimates are shown in Fig. 5. Although these still are not accurate, they are consistent across all ROIs for both LE images. There are no significant differences between the two LE estimates at all ROIs.

Table 3. The materials used for the theoretical mass attenuation estimates. This lists the chemical compositions used for deriving the mass attenuations. Note: plastic water was derived from Ho and Paliwal [9]

Material	Composition	XCOM NIST chemical formula
Plastic water	8 % H, 67.22 % C, 2.4 % N, 19.84 % O, 2.32 % Ca, 0.13 % Cl	$H_{2137}C_{1507}N_{46}O_{334}Ca_{16}Cl$
Water	Distilled water	H_2O
Blue wax	65 % polyethylene, 35 % Stearic acid	$C_{38}H_{76}C_{18}H_{36}O_2$
Lipid	Fatty acid	$C_{55}H_{104}O_6$
Delrin	Polyoxymethylene plastic	CH_2O
Protein	Standard protein stoichiometry	$C_{100}H_{159}N_{26}O_{32}S$

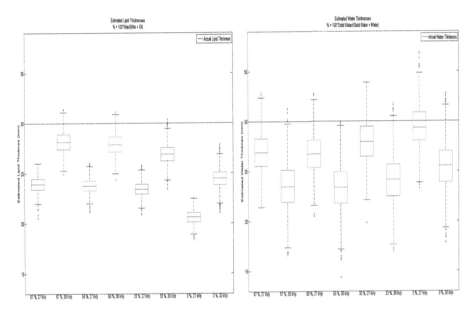

Fig. 4. The estimated lipid and water thicknesses for different regions of interest. (Left) This shows the estimated lipid thicknesses for two different LE's, 27 and 30 kVp. (Right) This shows the estimated water thicknesses. In both cases, one can see clear differences in the estimated thicknesses across all regions of interest between the two energy levels. All comparisons were significantly different at p < 0.001.

4 Discussion

Our theoretical analysis showed the conditions for which estimated lipid, water, and protein contents will be equivalent across varying keV for the monoenergetic case. If mass attenuation differences between substitute materials and their biological equivalents vary across keV, this will yield varying lipid, water, and protein estimates. The XCOM-derived mass attenuations show the differences between the substitute

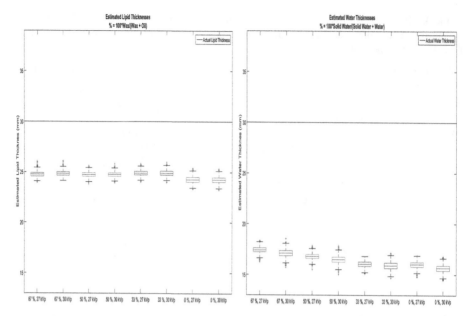

Fig. 5. The estimated lipid and water thicknesses for different regions of interest post bovine calibration. (Left) This shows the estimated lipid thicknesses for two different LE's, 27 and 30 kVp. (Right) This shows the estimated water thicknesses. In both cases, there is no significant difference between each LE estimate for each ROI.

materials and their biological equivalents. The largest differences can be seen for protein. One can see that the mass attenuation differences vary as a function of keV. We hypothesize that these differences attribute to the estimates in the lipid and water contents seen in Fig. 4, since other sources of systematic noise have been mollified. Applying a biological tissue calibration with a bovine phantom corrected the energy dependence error but an absolute thickness offset still remained.

One limitation in our study was that the bovine phantom for calibration did not have pure lipid or water compartments. This would imply that the affine transformation A does not cover these extrema. Consequently, we believe that this explains the offset seen in the estimated lipid and water contents in Fig. 5; both lipid and water were underestimated across all ROIs. Another limitation in this study was the chemical compositions used to derive blue wax (lipid substitute) and Plastic Water® mass attenuations. Best estimates were used for Plastic Water® found in literature [9]. The patent filing was used for blue wax, but the exact composition of which was not given, only varying quantities. We used their minimum estimate of polyethylene content and the rest we assumed to be stearic acid, a biological representative of lipid.

5 Conclusions

From the above analysis, it can be seen that the phantom materials are not good substitutes for biological materials at all energies, and their accuracy to biological materials differs by the imaging parameters (e.g. filters used and kVp). These parameters affect the mass attenuation coefficients of the substitute materials as a function of energy, and this could lead to inconsistent errors in LWP estimates when applying the 3CB technique. A calibration derived from biological tissues seemed to correct these errors.

References

1. Elmore, J.G., Barton, M.B., Moceri, V.M., Polk, S., Arena, P.J., Fletcher, S.W.: Ten-year risk of false positive screening mammograms and clinical breast examinations. N. Engl. J. Med. **338**, 1089–1096 (1998)
2. McCormack, V.A., dos Santos Silva, I.: Breast density and parenchymal patterns as markers of breast cancer risk: a meta-analysis. Cancer Epidem Biomar **15**, 1159–1169 (2006)
3. Boyd, N.F., Rommens, J.M., Vogt, K., Lee, V., Hopper, J.L., Yaffe, M.J., Paterson, A.D.: Mammographic breast density as an intermediate phenotype for breast cancer. Lancet Oncol. **6**, 798–808 (2005)
4. Lehman, C., White, E., Peacock, S., Drucker, M., Urban, N.: Effect of age and breast density on screening mammograms with false-positive findings. AJR Am. J. Roentgenol. **173**, 1651–1655 (1999)
5. Laidevant, A.D., Malkov, S., Flowers, C.I., Kerlikowske, K., Shepherd, J.A.: Compositional breast imaging using a dual-energy mammography protocol. Med. Phys. **37**, 164–174 (2010)
6. Drukker, K., Duewer, F., Giger, M.L., Malkov, S., Flowers, C.I., Joe, B., Kerlikowske, K., Drukteinis, J.S., Li, H., Shepherd, J.A.: Mammographic quantitative image analysis and biologic image composition for breast lesion characterization and classification. Med. Phys. **41**, 031915 (2014)
7. Malkov, S., Duewer, F., Kerlikowske, K., Drukker, K., Giger, M., Shepherd, J.: Compositional three-component breast imaging of fibroadenoma and invasive cancer lesions: pilot study. In: Fujita, H., Hara, T., Muramatsu, C. (eds.) IWDM 2014. LNCS, vol. 8539, pp. 109–114. Springer, Heidelberg (2014)
8. Malkov, S., Avila, J.I., Fan, B., Kerlikowske, K., Giger, M.L., Drukker, K., Drukteinis, J.S., Kazemi, L., Pereira, M., Shepherd, J.: Calibration procedure of three component mammographic breast imaging. In: Tingberg, A. (ed.) Breast Imaging, IWDM 2016, vol. 9699, pp. 211–218. Springer, Heidelberg (2016)
9. Ho, A.K., Paliwal, B.R.: Stopping-power and mass energy-absorption coefficient ratios for solid water. Med. Phys. **13**, 403–404 (1986)

Contrast-Enhanced Imaging

Development of Fully-3D CT in a Hybrid SPECT-CT Breast Imaging System

Martin P. Tornai[1,2,3(✉)], Jainil P. Shah[1,2], Steve D. Mann[1,4],
and Randolph L. McKinley[5]

[1] Department of Radiology, Duke University, Durham, NC 27710, USA
{martin.tornai,jainil.shah,steve.mann}@duke.edu
[2] Department of Biomedical Engineering, Duke University, Durham, NC 27705, USA
[3] Medical Physics Graduate Program, Duke University Medical Center, Durham,
NC 27710, USA
[4] Clinical Imaging Physics Group, Duke University, Durham, NC 27710, USA
[5] ZumaTek, Inc., Research Triangle Park, NC 27709, USA
rmckinley@zumatek.com

Abstract. This work describes initial measurements with the CT subsystem of
the assembled, fully-3D, hybrid SPECT-CT system for dedicated breast imaging.
The hybrid system, designed for clinical breast imaging, consists of fully-flexible
SPECT and CT subsystems, with each capable of 3D acquisition motions. The
SPECT subsystem employs a 16×20 cm^2 CZT detector with 2.5 mm pixellation,
is capable of viewing into the chest wall in addition to imaging the complete breast
volume, and has been extensively reported elsewhere. The polar tilting capability
of the CT subsystem has marked improvement in volumetric sampling while
eliminating cone beam artifacts due to the fully-3D acquisitions. The CT
subsystem can also view into the chest wall, while delivering <5 mGy total dose,
compared with a simple circular orbit breast CT. The CT subsystem consists of
a 0.4 mm focal spot x-ray tube with a rotating 14° W-anode angle, and a
40×30 cm^2 CsI(Tl) flat panel imager having 127 micron pixellation and 8.0 mm
bezel edge, placed on opposing ends of the completely suspended gantry. A linear
stage mechanism is used to tilt the suspended CT gantry up to ±15° in the polar
directions about the 3D center of rotation; the SPECT system is nestled inside the
suspended CT gantry, oriented perpendicular to the CT source-detector pair. Both
subsystems rest on an azimuthal rotation stage enabling truncated spherical
trajectories independently for each. Several simple and more complex 3D trajectories were implemented and characterized for the CT subsystem. Imaging results
demonstrate that additional off-axis projection views of various geometric phantoms and intact cadaveric breast, facilitated by the polar tilting yield more
complete breast-volume sampling and markedly improved iteratively reconstructed images, especially compared to simple circular orbit data. This is the first
implementation of a hybrid SPECT-CT system with fully-3D positioning for the
two subsystems, and could have various applications in diagnostic breast imaging.

Keywords: Breast CT · Cone beam CT · Hybrid · SPECT-CT

© Springer International Publishing Switzerland 2016
A. Tingberg et al. (Eds.): IWDM 2016, LNCS 9699, pp. 567–575, 2016.
DOI: 10.1007/978-3-319-41546-8_71

1 Introduction

For the past decade, three dimensional (3D) imaging modalities for dedicated computed tomography (CT) breast imaging have been investigated extensively [1], with a primary goal of overcoming the shortcomings of digital x-ray mammography. It is important to note that, as a still nascent technology, there is a rapidly ongoing evolution of breast CT. The evolution is similar to that for digital mammography, in that pixel size, which directly correlates with image resolution, is getting smaller. Smaller pixels mean finer resolution, and along with that comes an ability to distinguish finer features, such as the shape of calcifications. Neither clinically used planar digital detectors for mammography (smallest pixels sizes currently <60 µm), nor those same devices used in digital tomo-synthesis can currently distinguish different types of calcifications without object magnification. Furthermore, when a finer resolution digital detector is manufactured, it can readily be adapted for use in either digital mammography or quasi-3D tomosyn-thesis. The same pixel size reduction should be usable in dedicated breast CT, although the dataset sizes are considerably larger due to the fully tomographic acquisition required for breast CT, while only one image is needed in digital mammography, and up to 32 acquired images are currently used for tomosynthesis.

Moreover, dedicated breast CT provides better overall visualization of soft tissues due to the considerably higher intrinsic contrast differences in CT when overlapping tissue is removed with 3D imaging. This can really only be done accurately with more completely sampled volumetric data. So, while calcifications can be detected in breast CT, they are about as amorphous as those from digital mammography or tomosynthesis, but without the image distortions, and instead, with truly 3D localization of their distri-bution. Since calcifications alone cannot be used to identify true breast cancers [2], the advantage of diffuse soft tissue visualization with dedicated breast CT is poised to demonstrate its true ability to distinguish these features. In addition, there is no breast compression necessary with breast CT, unlike with both planar digital mammography and quasi-3D tomosynthesis (even with reduced compression). The high amount of structural overlap and patient discomfort due to compression are only some of the limi-tations of mammography and tomosythesis. Tomosynthesis does somewhat remove structural overlap in images, and has been shown to have a beneficial impact on disease diagnosis, but necessarily retains breast compression. Furthermore, the tomosythesis images are anisotropic, non-quantitative, and full of high-frequency artifacts. Thus, if clinical reader studies ultimately demonstrate that soft tissue detection and localization, in an artifact-free environment without multi-cross-planar blurring, rather than calcifi-cation detection, is required to detect malignant from benign disease in breast imaging, then breast CT has distinct advantages. The combination with molecular imaging using either single photon emission computed tomography (SPECT) or positron emission tomography (PET) offers even more opportunities and advantages.

To address the drawbacks of mammography and tomosynthesis, and to address the difficulty in diagnosing lesions close to the chest wall and axilla, we previously devel-oped independent CT and SPECT subsystems capable of fully-3D motions for dedicated breast imaging [3–5]. The fully-3D motions facilitated complex trajectories which elim-inate cone beam sampling artifacts in simple circular CT (and incomplete circular path tomosynthesis) and provide better sampling close to the chest wall for pendant breast imaging. We consequently combined the individual systems into a single hybrid system, such that the SPECT subsystem maintained its fully-3D acquisition capability, but the cone beam CT system was restricted to a simple circular orbit [6]. Phantoms were used to evaluate these systems extensively, and human clinical imaging studies were also performed [7, 8]. This limitation of the cone beam CT subsystem which could not tilt was eliminated with the redesign [9]. With both modalities capable of independently traversing complex acquisition trajectories around a common volume, the redesign effort yields a more complete hybrid system (Fig. 1).

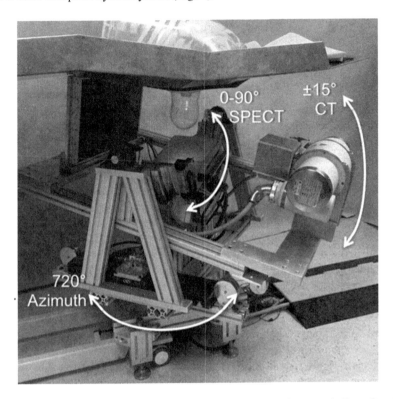

Fig. 1. Photograph of the new hybrid system in one position (with ranges indicated), with the SPECT subsystem nestled between the CT subsystem. Both imaging systems are underneath a fully-3D adjustable and radiopaque bed, which in this photograph supports a fillable anthropomorphic phantom, with a fillable pendant breast hanging in the common field of view.

On the one hand, an early aim was to develop a diagnostic CT system with which we could attenuation correct and also spatially localize the SPECT signals within the breast. On the other hand, the high quality breast CT scans in our prototypes [3, 4, 6] immediately indicated to us that the CT system could be used as a stand-alone system. The open geometry also lends itself to the inclusion of an onboard biopsy system, complete with 3D localization. Thus, the hybrid (one stop shop) system could be used as an early diagnostic, low dose CT system, and combined with an appropriate radioisotope tracer injection and non-invasive SPECT imaging could also be used (especially for those women for whom biopsy would be difficult, or if they refused biopsy) as another diagnostic line that should help increase the specificity for suspicious signals from the breast.

Thus, in an effort to improve the CT image quality to what we knew we could achieve in the stand alone breast CT system, in this work we have successfully mechanically integrated that fully-3D design for both the SPECT and CT subsystems (Fig. 1). Here, we present initial characterization and phantom measurement results from the CT subsystem in this hybrid SPECT-CT dedicated breast imaging system.

2   Materials and Methods

2.1   Design and Development

The individual subsystems were designed using *Solidworks* software (*Dassault Systems Solidworks Corp.*, Waltham, MA), and the parts were developed locally.

The CT subsystem consists of an x-ray source (model Rad-94, 0.4/0.8 mm focal spot size, rotating 14° W-anode, *Varian Medical Systems*, Salt Lake City, UT) a custom built 40×30 cm^2 CsI(Tl) flat panel detector with 127 μm pixellation (similar to *Varian* model Paxscan 4030E) [10], placed opposed on a gantry, with a source to image distance of 80 cm. This yielded a magnification of 1.57. The weight of the gantry is supported by heavy-duty bearings (model 6244K56, *McMaster-Carr*, Atlanta, GA) mounted on pivot posts manufactured using 80/20 bars. This CT gantry is in a suspended cradle, and allows tilting of the fixed-displacement source-detector pair (Fig. 1). A 25.00 cm travel linear stage (model ILS250CC, *Newport Corp*, Irvine, CA) was used to control the tilting motion by connecting a fixed length of cable underneath the gantry to pulleys, which reduce load and redirect the cable direction. This allows polar tilts of up to ±15.0° about the equator.

For the SPECT subsystem, a compact CZT gamma camera (model LumaGEM 3200S™, *Gamma Medica, Inc.*, Northridge, CA) is attached to a goniometer allowing 0–90° polar positioning about a pendant, uncompressed breast. Both subsystems are situated on top of a single rotation stage and move together azimuthally up to 720°, with the SPECT subsystem capable of moving in a complete 2π solid angle hemisphere, and the CT subsystem in a nearly 0.7π solid angle band on a sphere. The SPECT subsystem additionally has radius of rotation control using redesigned laboratory jacks (model M-EL120, *Newport Corp*).

Before initiating experiments, the linear stage-pulley mechanism was characterized to evaluate the relation between linear displacement and the degree of polar tilt. The linear stage has a motion range of ±12.50 cm; the linear displacement in both directions was incremented in 10.0 mm steps, and the corresponding polar tilt angle of the system was measured with a digital level (model Pro 3600, *Flexbar Machine Corp*). The measured linear displacement is used by the CT acquisition software to generate position coordinates in the complex orbits. Measurements were repeated 4 times, twice in each direction, to measure any hysteresis or discrepancy in the polar tilt angle of the system due to the linear motor.

2.2 Trajectories and Acquisitions

Various simple and complex trajectories were designed and implemented (Fig. 2): (1) a two-lobed sawtooth trajectory having equidistant polar and azimuthal increments, between $\pm 13°$ and over the $360°$, respectively; (2) two-lobed sinusoidal orbit (or "saddle") with maximum polar tilts of $\pm 13°$ over the full azimuthal direction; and (3) a 3-lobed sinusoid with maximum polar tilts of $\pm 13°$ over the full azimuthal direction. Simple circular orbits were also employed, mainly as a comparison to fixed-tilt breast CT systems: azimuthal circular orbits with (4) $0°$ fixed polar tilt ($AZOR_0$) and (5) $+13°$ fixed polar tilt on the system ($AZOR_{13}$) for all azimuthal angles.

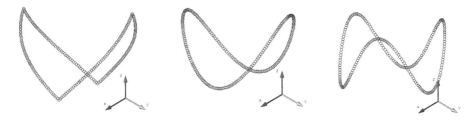

Fig. 2. Illustrations of 3 complex trajectories implemented and evaluated in this work: (LEFT) sawtooth, (MIDDLE) saddle or 2-lobed sinusoid, and (RIGHT) 3-lobed sinusoid. In these illustrations, each trajectory spans $\pm 13°$ polar tilt, symmetrically situated about a spherical surface of possible trajectories.

Uniformity corrections (gain, offset and defective pixel) were applied to the raw projection images using a *MATLAB* based graphical user interface. Projections were reconstructed using a well-established ordered subsets convex iterative reconstruction algorithm [11]. Reconstruction parameters were set to 5 iterations, 16 subsets, 0.254 mm voxels and $900 \times 900 \times 900$ grid size, which are standard acquisition parameters on the CT subsystem. No scatter or other beam hardening corrections were employed.

2.3 Phantoms and Cadaver Breast

For initial evaluation of tilted trajectories, a 10 cm inner diameter cylindrical phantom containing: (1) four Defrise disks in the top half (model ECT/MI-DEF/P *Data Spectrum Corp*, Durham, NC), and (2) the rod module from the Jaszczak resolution mini-rod phantom, was used (model ECT/STD/I, *Data Spectrum Corp*). The Defrise disks are made of 0.50 cm thick acrylic with 0.50 cm spacing between each disk; the cold rod phantom consists of 1.10–4.70 mm diameter acrylic rods spaced on twice their diameters. The phantom was positioned level, in the center of the detector field of view (FOV), and 240 projection images were acquired in 2×2 binning mode with the CT subsystem for all AZOR and complex trajectories.

Based on the results of the phantom testing, we also acquired our first images of a biological object: a fully intact cadaveric breast. The defrosted (room temperature) cadaveric breast tissue was kept moistened with mineral oil, and supported in a 700 mL plastic breast shaped bowl with plastic clips at the edges. An 8 mm nylon sphere was immersed into the breast tissue to provide an easily identifiable object within the volume. Using the same acquisition methods as above, a saddle scan was acquired of the cadaveric breast with bead implant.

3   Results

3.1   Polar Motion Evaluation

The linear motion calibration results illustrated that the multiply-measured polar tilt angles were within <0.02° variability. There is no apparent hysteresis in the system, due both to the high tension metal cables, as well as the sub-mm positioning reproducibility of the linear stage.

3.2   Initial Image Characterization with Simple & Complex Acquisitions

Representative coronal slices through the reconstructed volume show excellent resolution performance of the system regardless of the acquisition trajectory (Fig. 3). For all utilized orbits, the smallest 1.1 mm diameter rods are resolved almost identically to each other. However, sagittal slices reveal the sampling short comings of the simple circular AZOR orbits (Fig. 4). Cone beam sampling artifacts are clearly evident on the AZOR sagittal slices, especially at the Defrise disks due to insufficient sampling. The edges of the cylindrical support phantom are also compromised due to the blurring from the Defrise disks. On the other hand, the reconstructed images of the complex orbit data demonstrate completely eliminated cone beam sampling artifacts, the Defrise disks show no blurring, and uniform spacing between disks is easily seen.

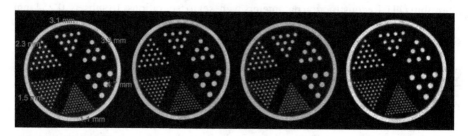

Fig. 3. Representative coronal images at the same slice level for each acquisition of the mini-rod phantom. Illustrated acquisitions are for (LEFT to RIGHT): AZOR0, sawtooth, saddle, and 3-lobed sinusoid. Result for AZOR13 was identical. Rod sizes are indicated. Images are plotted on the same gray scale.

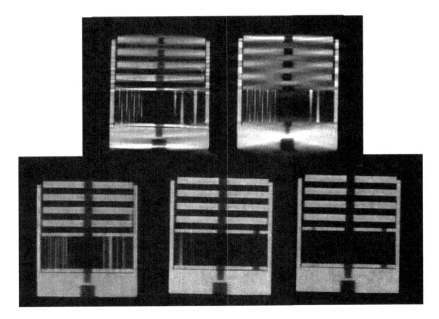

Fig. 4. Sagittal slices of the reconstructed Defrise + rod phantom within the cylinder support. (TOP) Simple circularly acquired data: (LEFT) AZOR0, (RIGHT) AZOR13. (BOTTOM) Complex acquisition data: (LEFT) sawtooth, (MIDDLE) saddle, (RIGHT) 3-lobed sinusoid. Data is acquired over 360° azimuth, with polar tilts and reconstruction parameters indicated in the text. Images are plotted on the same gray scale.

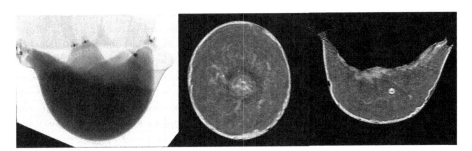

Fig. 5. (LEFT) Projection view of the cadaveric breast suspended in a plastic breast bowl, and secured with spring-loaded clips at the edges. The black diagonal shapes at the bottom are due to shadows from (LL) the SPECT camera and (LR) the radius positioning motor, but do not interfere with the breast. (MIDDLE and RIGHT) Representative reconstructed coronal and sagittal image slices through the breast, illustrating clearly distinguished skin (peripheral, light color), adipose (darker grey) and glandular (light interior colors) tissues throughout the breast. Central calcifications (distinct bright spots) are seen at the coronal slice level. Chest wall muscle tissue (lighter grey) is also seen in the sagittal view, at the posterior breast surface, above the visible implanted nylon bead.

3.3   Biological Breast Images

A projection image and slices through the reconstructed cadaver breast show excellent characteristic features of imaged biological tissue (Fig. 5). The projection image is relatively low contrast but has very fine resolution due to the magnification of the uncompressed object onto the detector FOV. The reconstructed images show clearly distinguished skin, adipose and glandular tissues throughout the breast. Central calcifications are seen at the coronal slice level in the 10 and 11 o'clock directions. Note also that there are some circular ring artifacts, since the reconstructed data had basic projection image corrections, but no image processing or cupping corrections (beam hardening or scatter) to optimize the image quality. Chest wall muscle tissue is seen in the sagittal view, at the posterior breast surface, above the implanted 8 mm nylon bead. Even the characteristic air centered hole in the nylon bead is easily recognizable.

4   Discussion

We have implemented a fully-integrated, fully-flexible SPECT-CT system successfully, with each subsystem having completely independent polar motions to enable more complete 3D sampling throughout the common FOV. This system was designed and constructed for dedicated breast imaging, and is the first fully-3D-capable dual-modality SPECT-CT system capable of human imaging that we are aware of. Results show that complex trajectories for the CT subsystem are both possible with this system, and yield qualitatively and quantitatively improved images compared to simple circular (tilted) breast CT acquisitions. The complex acquisition eliminates insufficient cone beam sampling artifacts present with simple circular acquisitions in the pendant breast imaging volume. We easily implemented 3 complex acquisitions, and were able to reconstruct both quantitative phantom and biological breast images. Some circular ring artifacts are present, and we believe that image quality can certainly be further improved. Though not shown in this work, we expect no changes to the SPECT results, since that system is nestled unobstructed within the fully-suspended cone beam CT subsystem. A multitude of other 3D trajectories are possible with this acquisition system along with the iterative reconstruction, and several will be investigated. Due to the open design of the system, many expansion options are possible, including addition of a biopsy unit as well as optical imaging for surface mapping or blood content analysis, with which other diagnostic information could be non-invasively obtained.

References

1. Glick, S.J.: Breast CT. Annu. Rev. Biomed. Eng. **9**, 501–526 (2007)
2. Harvey, J.A., Nicholson, B.T., Cohen, M.A.: Finding early invasive cancers: a practical approach. Radiology **248**(1), 61–76 (2008)
3. McKinley, R.L.: Development and characterization of a dedicated mammotomography system. Ph.D. thesis, Biomedical Engineering, Duke University (2006)

4. Madhav, P., Crotty, D., McKinley, R., Tornai, M.: Evaluation of tilted cone-beam CT orbits in the development of a dedicated hybrid mammotomograph. Phys. Med. Biol. **54**, 3659 (2009)
5. Brzymialkiewicz, C., Tornai, M., McKinley, R., Cutler, S., Bowsher, J.: Performance of dedicated emission mammotomography for various breast shapes and sizes. Phys. Med. Biol. **51**, 5051 (2006)
6. Madhav, P.: Development and optimization of a dedicated dual-modality SPECT-CT System for improved breast lesion diagnosis. Ph.D. thesis, Biomedical Engineering, Duke University (2010)
7. Mann, S.D., Perez, K.L., McCracken, E.K., Shah, J.P., Wong, T.Z., Tornai, M.P.: Initial in vivo quantification of Tc-99 m sestamibi uptake as a function of tissue type in healthy breasts using dedicated breast SPECT-CT. J. Oncol., 16 August 2012
8. Shah, J., Mann, S., Tornai, M.: Investigation the dependence of 2D and 3D scatter-to-primary ratios on breast density in clinical breast CT. Med. Phys. **39**, 3624–3625 (2012)
9. Shah, J.P., Mann, S.D., McKinley, R.L., Tornai, M.P.: Initial development of a nested SPECT-CT system with fully suspended CT sub-system for dedicated breast imaging. In: Proceeding of SPIE: Physics of Medical Imaging, pp. 90335O–90335O-6(2014)
10. Shah, J.P., Mann, S.D., Polemi, A.M., Tornai, M.P., McKinley, R.L., Zentai, G., Richmond, M., Partain, L.: Initial evaluation of a newly developed high resolution CT imager for dedicated breast CT. In: Maidment, A.D., Bakic, P.R., Gavenonis, S. (eds.) IWDM 2012. LNCS, vol. 7361, pp. 426–433. Springer, Heidelberg (2012)
11. Beekman, F.J., Kamphuis, C.: Ordered subset reconstruction for x-ray CT. Phys. Med. Biol. **46**, 1835 (2001)

Volumetric Breast-Density Measurement Using Spectral Photon-Counting Tomosynthesis: First Clinical Results

Erik Fredenberg[1]([⊠]), Karl Berggren[1,2], Matthias Bartels[3], and Klaus Erhard[3]

[1] Philips Health Systems, Mammography Solutions, Smidesvägen 5, 17122 Solna, Sweden
erik.fredenberg@philips.com
[2] Department of Physics, Royal Institute of Technology (KTH), 10691 Stockholm, Sweden
[3] Philips Research, Röntgenstrasse 24-26, 22395 Hamburg, Germany

Abstract. Measurements of breast density have the potential to improve the efficiency and reduce the cost of screening mammography through personalized screening. Breast density has traditionally been evaluated from the dense area in a mammogram, but volumetric assessment methods, which measure the volumetric fraction of fibro-glandular tissue in the breast, are potentially more consistent and physically sound. The purpose of the present study is to evaluate a method for measuring the volumetric breast density using photon-counting spectral tomosynthesis. The performance of the method was evaluated using phantom measurements and clinical data from a small population ($n = 18$). The precision was determined to be 2.4 percentage points (pp) of volumetric breast density. Strong correlations were observed between contralateral ($R^2 = 0.95$) and ipsilateral ($R^2 = 0.96$) breast-density measurements. The measured breast density was anti-correlated to breast thickness, as expected, and exhibited a skewed distribution in the range [3.7 %, 55 %] and with a median of 18 %. We conclude that the method yields promising results that are consistent with expectations. The relatively high precision of the method may enable novel applications such as treatment monitoring.

Keywords: Tomosynthesis · Breast density · Photon counting · Spectral imaging

1 Introduction

It is well established that breast density is directly correlated to the risk of developing breast cancer [1], and anti-correlated to the diagnostic accuracy of mammography [2]. Measures of breast density can therefore improve risk estimates and may enable personalized breast-cancer screening, which in turn has the potential to increase the sensitivity and minimize the cost of screening programs [3]. Other areas of application for breast-density measures include treatment monitoring and dose estimation.

Traditionally, breast density has been estimated from the areal fraction of the breast that is covered by fibro-glandular tissue in the mammogram, either visually (e.g. BI-RADS scoring) or automatically. Volumetric breast-density assessment methods measure the volumetric fraction of fibro-glandular tissue in the breast and are becoming

© Springer International Publishing Switzerland 2016
A. Tingberg et al. (Eds.): IWDM 2016, LNCS 9699, pp. 576–584, 2016.
DOI: 10.1007/978-3-319-41546-8_72

an established alternative to traditional methods because of a physically more meaningful interpretation and higher consistency [4].

A number of methods have been developed to measure the volumetric breast density [5–7]. Most often, additional information and assumptions are required in addition to the mammogram itself, such as the compression height [5, 6], a reference pixel value [7], and/or a breast model to take any thickness gradient into account [6], which add to the uncertainty of the measurement.

Two current trends in x-ray imaging of the breast are spectral imaging and tomosynthesis. Spectral imaging has been applied to measure breast density in two-dimensional (2D) mammograms [8, 9]. The technique can be expected to be more accurate than non-spectral methods because there is no need for additional assumptions or modelling. Tomosynthesis is three-dimensional (3D) imaging from a limited angular span. Coupled with spectral imaging, tomosynthesis has the potential to improve breast-density measurements in several respects, including improved precision and 3D localization.

Recently, a prototype system for spectral tomosynthesis has been developed by Philips Health Systems (Solna, Sweden), which is based on the same photon-counting technology that has previously been developed for 2D mammography [10]. In this study, we present a spectral breast-density measurement method developed for the photon-counting tomosynthesis system. The method is evaluated using phantom measurements and the first clinical data acquired with the system.

2   Materials and Methods

2.1   Spectral Photon-Counting Tomosynthesis System

The Philips MicroDose S0 is a prototype spectral photon-counting tomosynthesis system based on the Philips MicroDose SI 2D mammography system (Philips Health Systems, Sweden). The system comprises a tungsten-target x-ray tube with aluminum filtration, a pre-collimator, and an image receptor, all mounted on a rigid scan arm (Fig. 1, left). To acquire an image, the scan arm is rotated around a point below the patient support so that the tube-collimator-detector assembly is scanned across the object.

The image receptor consists of 21 photon-counting silicon strip detector lines with corresponding slits in the pre-collimator (Fig. 1, right). During the scan, each detector line will view each point in the object from a unique source-detector angle, and readouts from the 21 lines can therefore be used for 3D reconstruction. The width of the detector and the source-detector distance yield a tomographic angle of $\sim 11°$.

Photons that interact in the silicon strip detectors are converted to pulses with amplitude proportional to the photon energy [10]. A high-energy threshold sorts detected pulses into two bins according to energy, which enables spectral imaging. A low-energy threshold provides efficient rejection of electronic noise by discriminating against all pulses below a few keV. The multi-slit geometry rejects virtually all scattered radiation [11]. Low levels of electronic noise and scattered radiation improve the efficiency of tomosynthesis in general and of spectral tomosynthesis in particular.

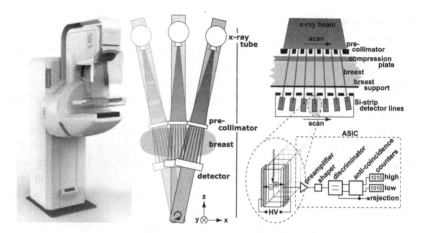

Fig. 1. Left: Photograph and schematic of the Philips MicroDose S0 prototype spectral tomosynthesis system. **Right:** The image receptor and electronics.

The 3D reconstruction was iterative (ART), but care was taken to minimize non-linear properties of the algorithm. In this first study we will not consider the 3D properties of the tomosynthesis reconstruction, but the reconstructed stack was summed over the depth direction to form a 2D image.

2.2 System Calibration and Spectral Breast-Density Measurement

X-ray attenuation of soft tissue in the mammographic energy range is approximately made up of only two interaction effects, namely photoelectric absorption and scattering processes [12]. Assuming known system properties, constant and known skin thickness, and known linear attenuation coefficients of adipose, glandular and skin tissue, acquisitions over two different energy ranges yield a non-linear system of equations with a unique solution for the thicknesses of adipose and glandular tissue. In practice, this equation is preferably solved with means of calibration because the system and reconstruction properties may be complex and partially unknown. A calibration phantom consisting of combinations of aluminum (Al) and polyethylene (PE) was manufactured for this purpose and imaged at each x-ray energy spectrum (i.e. each kVp) used in clinical practice. From this data set, a look-up table was produced to map image signal for the two energy bins to equivalent amounts of Al and PE. The calibrated Al and PE thicknesses were transferred to equivalent thicknesses of adipose and glandular tissue (attenuation according to Ref. [13]) by using a linear transfer function [14].

The images calibrated to adipose and glandular thicknesses were converted to total breast thickness (sum of adipose and glandular thicknesses) and volumetric breast density (thickness of glandular tissue over total thickness). We refer to these images as thickness and density maps. The average of the density map was taken as the volumetric breast density for the image. The mode (most common value) of the thickness map was used as a measure of breast thickness. We assumed 1.5 mm of skin on each side of the breast. The pectoralis muscle was segmented and excluded from all measurements.

2.3   Phantom Measurements and Clinical Measurements

Slabs of tissue-equivalent material (CIRS Inc., Norfolk, VA) in 57 different combinations were used to evaluate the precision of the breast-density measurement method. The thicknesses of CIRS adipose and glandular material were converted to equivalent thicknesses of adipose and glandular tissue according to Ref. [13] using a linear transfer function. These values were used as ground truth. Precision was defined as the standard deviation of the differences between measurements and ground truth.

A clinical study of photon-counting spectral tomosynthesis is ongoing at ImageRive, Geneva, Switzerland. Symptomatic patients are examined in two views (CC and MLO) using a MicroDose S0 system. All patients are asked to provide written informed consent prior to the examination. The study has been approved by SwissEthics. Data from the first $n = 18$ patients were included in the present study. One examination was excluded because of technical reasons, which yields a total of 68 measurement points (17 patients × 4 views).

The clinical data was evaluated in terms of: correlation between measured breast thickness and compression height (a strong correlation is expected); correlation between breast density and breast thickness (a weak anti-correlation is expected); the contralateral (left-right) breast density (a strong biological correlation is expected); the ipsilateral (CC-MLO) breast density (a strong correlation is expected).

3   Results

Figure 2 shows the measured volumetric density and thickness as a function of ground truth for the 57 phantom configurations. The precision of the density measurement was 2.4 percentage points (pp). The precision of the thickness measurement was 1.2 %.

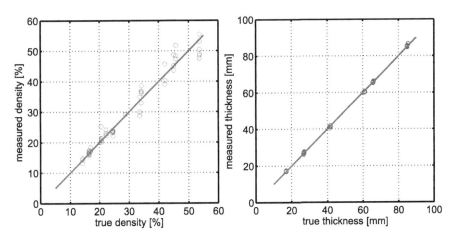

Fig. 2. Breast density (left) and thickness (right) as a function of ground truth from 57 phantom configurations. One-to-one lines are included for reference (red solid lines). (Color figure online.)

The left panel of Fig. 3 shows, as an example, the results from the first spectral mammogram that was acquired. The sum of the reconstructed stack, in right CC view, is shown to the left, and the thickness and density maps are shown to the right. This case had a density of 27 % and a thickness of 47.2 mm. The densities of the other three views of this patient (expected to be close to identical) were 27 % (left CC), 27 % (right MLO), and 28 % (left MLO). The thicknesses of the other three views (not necessarily identical) were 51.3 mm, 44.1 mm, and 44.4 mm.

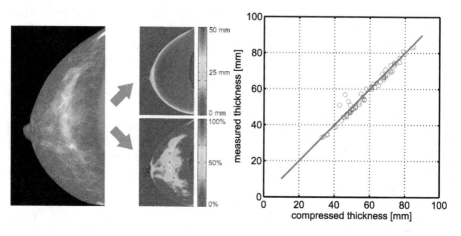

Fig. 3. Left: Illustration of the spectral breast-density measurement with the sum of the reconstructed stack, the density map, and the thickness map for a typical case in CC view. **Right:** Compression height as a function of measured breast thickness for 68 images. A one-to-one line (red) is included for reference. (Color figure online.)

The right panel of Fig. 3 shows the measured breast thickness (including the skin) as a function of the compression height reported by the system for all images of all patients (68 images in total). The correlation was strong with a Pearson correlation coefficient of $R^2 = 0.97$. There was a close-to constant offset of -0.7 mm.

Figure 4 shows the volumetric breast density, calculated from the 68 spectral mammograms, as a function of measured breast thickness. The data was fitted to a power function of the form $[\text{density}/\%] = 100 \times a \times [\text{thickness/mm}]^b$, where the coefficients were found to be $a = 121$ and $b = -1.58$. Also shown in Fig. 4 are histograms for the distributions of volumetric breast density and breast thickness. The range of densities was [3.7 %, 55 %], with a mean of 22 % and a median of 18 %. The range of thicknesses was [33, 83.5] mm, with a mean of 57.8 mm.

Figure 5 shows contralateral and ipsilateral volumetric breast-density scatter plots. The Pearson correlation coefficients were $R^2 = 0.95$ and $R^2 = 0.96$, respectively. The spread (one standard deviation) around the one-to-one lines were 3.1 pp and 2.8 pp, respectively.

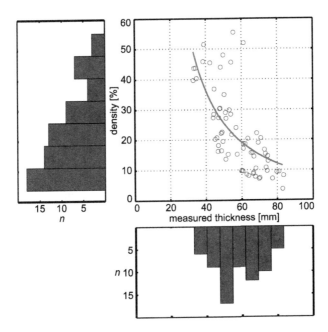

Fig. 4. Volumetric breast density from 68 spectral mammograms. The scatter plot shows the dependency on breast thickness, fitted to a power function (red line). The marginal histograms show projections along the axes of the scatter plot, i.e. distributions of densities and thicknesses. (Color figure online.)

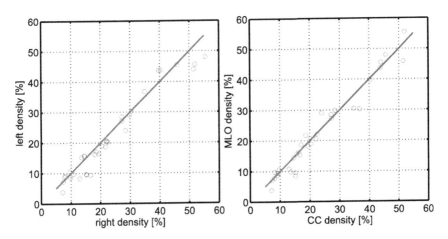

Fig. 5. Contralateral (left) and ipsilateral (right) breast density scatter plots. One-to-one lines (red) are included for reference. (Color figure online.)

4 Discussion

We make the following observations of the results in Sect. 3:

- There was a strong correlation between compression height and measured breast thickness (Fig. 3, right), which is physically sound. The constant offset of less than 1 mm is well within the expected accuracy of the compression paddle.
- As expected, the density was anti-correlated to breast thickness (Fig. 4).
- The distribution of breast densities (Fig. 4) was as expected; the distribution was skewed with mean and median close to 20 % and a range within [0 %, 100 %]. The distribution of breast thicknesses (Fig. 4) was also reasonable; the distribution appeared normal (or log-normal) with a mean close to 50 mm. The data are at this point too sparse for any further investigation of distribution statistics.
- The contralateral and ipsilateral correlation measures were relatively strong compared to non-spectral methods (e.g. $R = 0.864 \Rightarrow R^2 = 0.75$ in Ref. [15]).
- The ipsilateral correlation is in close agreement with previous results for 2D spectral mammography ($R = 0.99 \Rightarrow R^2 = 0.98$ in Ref. [16]). The difference is likely covered by differences in population, the lower experience of the clinical staff in positioning for tomosynthesis, and the limited amount of data in the present study.
- The ipsilateral correlation was stronger and the spread was lower compared to the contralateral measures, indicating that the contralateral variation was affected by biological factors in addition to technical factors such as positioning. We therefore expect the ipsilateral measures to be better indicators of system precision.
- In fact, the ipsilateral precision (2.8 pp) was in good agreement with the precision as determined by phantom experiments (2.4 pp). The deviation can be attributed to differences in positioning between CC and MLO views for the clinical images.
- The relatively high precision offered by spectral breast-density measurement may enable applications such as treatment monitoring, where subtle differences in density of typically a few pp indicate response to tamoxifen or raloxifene treatment [17].
- The spectral measurement algorithm presented here is relatively basic and improvements in precision can be expected by taking systematic variations in the spectral response, such as detector and x-ray tube temperature, into account.
- The study population included symptomatic women, which may have affected the results slightly, but we expect this contribution to be non-favorable. For instance, if a lesion were present in one breast, the contralateral correlation would be reduced.
- The present study marks an important and early step in our efforts to combine spectral imaging and tomosynthesis. The study does not cover the advantages that tomosynthesis may offer over 2D mammography for applications such as local breast density measurements, but such applications are part of ongoing research.

5 Conclusions

The method for measuring volumetric breast density using spectral photon-counting tomosynthesis was found to yield reasonable results on a small population of women. The precision of the method was determined to 2.4 percentage points (pp) on phantoms, a result that was corroborated by correlation in the clinical data. This relatively high precision (compared to non-spectral methods) may be useful to monitor changes in breast density on an individual basis, for instance in response to treatment.

Research is ongoing to further improve the precision of the method by using a more sophisticated spectral measurement algorithm. Future research will make use of the advantages offered by tomosynthesis for improved local breast-density measurements.

References

1. McCormack, V.A., dos Santos Silva, I.: Breast density and parenchymal patterns as markers of breast cancer risk: a meta-analysis. Cancer Epidemiol. Biomark. Prev. **15**, 1159 (2006)
2. Boyd, N.F., Guo, H., Martin, L.J., Sun, L., Stone, J., Fishell, E., Jong, R.A., Hislop, G., Chiarelli, A., Minkin, S., Yaffe, M.J.: Mammographic Density and the Risk and Detection of Breast Cancer. N. Engl. J. Med. **356**, 227–236 (2007)
3. Schousboe, J.T., Kerlikowske, K., Loh, A., Cummings, S.R.: Personalizing mammography by breast density and other risk factors for breast cancer: analysis of health benefits and cost-effectiveness. Ann. Intern. Med. **155**, 10–20 (2011)
4. Boyd, N.F., Rommens, J.M., Vogt, K., Lee, V., Hopper, J.L., Yaffe, M.J., Paterson, A.D.: Mammographic breast density as an intermediate phenotype for breast cancer. Lancet Oncol. **6**, 798–808 (2005)
5. Highnam, R., Pan, X., Warren, R., Jeffreys, M., Smith, G.D., Brady, M.: Breast composition measurements using retrospective standard mammogram form (SMF). Phys. Med. Biol. **51**, 2695–2713 (2006)
6. Gooßen, A., Heese, H.S., Erhard, K.: Automatic volumetric glandularity assessment from full field digital mammograms. In: Maidment, A.D., Bakic, P.R., Gavenonis, S. (eds.) IWDM 2012. LNCS, vol. 7361, pp. 753–760. Springer, Heidelberg (2012)
7. van Engeland, S., Snoeren, P.R., Huisman, H., Boetes, C., Karssemeijer, N.: Volumetric breast density estimation from full-field digital mammograms. IEEE Trans. Med. Imaging **25**, 273–282 (2006)
8. Ducote, J.L., Molloi, S.: Quantification of breast density with dual energy mammography: a simulation study. Med. Phys. **35**, 5411–5418 (2008)
9. Gooßen, A., Heese, H.S., Erhard, K., Norell, B.: Spectral volumetric glandularity assessment. In: Maidment, A.D., Bakic, P.R., Gavenonis, S. (eds.) IWDM 2012. LNCS, vol. 7361, pp. 529–536. Springer, Heidelberg (2012)
10. Fredenberg, E., Lundqvist, M., Cederström, B., Åslund, M., Danielsson, M.: Energy resolution of a photon-counting silicon strip detector. Nucl. Instrum. Methods Phys. Res. **613**, 156–162 (2010)
11. Åslund, M., Cederström, B., Lundqvist, M., Danielsson, M.: Scatter rejection in multislit digital mammography. Med. Phys. **33**, 933 (2006)
12. Alvarez, R.E., Macovski, A.: Energy-selective reconstructions in X-ray computerized tomography. Phys. Med. Biol. **21**, 733–744 (1976)
13. Johns, P.C., Yaffe, M.J.: X-ray characterisation of normal and neoplastic breast tissues. Phys. Med. Biol. **32**, 675–695 (1987)
14. Fredenberg, E., Dance, D.R., Willsher, P., Moa, E., von Tiedemann, M., Young, K.C., Wallis, M.G.: Measurement of breast-tissue x-ray attenuation by spectral mammography: first results on cyst fluid. Phys. Med. Biol. **58**, 8609–8620 (2013)
15. Gennaro, G., Highnam, R.: This is what volumetric breast density is. In: Poster at ECR 2013 (2013). doi: 10.1594/ecr2013/C-1033

16. Machida, Y., Tozaki, M., Yoshida, T., Saita, A., Yakabe, M., Nii, K.: Feasibility study of a breast density measurement within a direct photon-counting mammography scanner system. Jpn. J. Radiol. **32**, 1–7 (2014)
17. Li, J., Humphreys, K., Eriksson, L., Edgren, G., Czene, K., Hall, P.: Mammographic density reduction is a prognostic marker of response to adjuvant tamoxifen therapy in postmenopausal patients with breast cancer. J. Clin. Oncol. **31**, 2249–2256 (2013)

Texture Analysis of Contrast-Enhanced Digital Mammography (CEDM) Images

María-Julieta Mateos[1($\boxtimes$)], Alfonso Gastelum[2], Jorge Márquez[2], and Maria-Ester Brandan[1]

[1] Instituto de Física, Universidad Nacional Autónoma de México, 04510 Mexico City, Mexico
julieta8a3@gmail.com, brandan@fisica.unam.mx
[2] Centro de Ciencias Aplicadas y Desarrollo Tecnológico, Universidad Nacional Autónoma de México, 04510 Mexico City, Mexico
gastelum.strozzi@gmail.com,
jorge.marquez@ccadet.unam.mx

Abstract. A texture analysis aimed at finding correlations between textural descriptors and lesion diagnosis was applied to Contrast-Enhanced Digital Mammography (CEDM) subtracted images acquired under single-energy temporal subtraction modality using iodine-based contrast medium. The study, based on textural descriptors from Gray Level Co-occurrence Matrix (GLCM), included 68 CEDM images of 17 patients, 10 cancer and 7 benign, acquired 1 to 5 min after iodine injection. Seventeen GLCM descriptors were analyzed. Image processing consisted of geometric registration, logarithmic subtraction, and selection of regions-of-interest (adipose, glandular and lesion ROIs) by the radiologist. Results for lesion ROIs showed that homogeneity, normalized homogeneity, second-order inverse moment, energy and inverse variance were insensitive to the presence of iodine; a linear correlation existed between the sum mean and mean pixel value. Logistic regression showed that a linear combination of entropy and diagonal momentum discriminated between malignant and benign lesions with 79 % specificity, 93 % sensitivity and 87 % accuracy.

Keywords: Breast imaging · CEDM · Texture analysis · Contrast medium · Contrast enhanced digital mammography

1 Introduction

Early breast cancer detection through screening mammograms has been a factor in decreasing mortality. However, the technique has a high rate of false positives, and the sensitivity remains at about 70 %.

Contrast Enhanced Digital Mammography. Contrast-enhanced digital mammography (CEDM) is an acquisition technique that consists on the subtraction of radiological (digital) images of the breast after the administration of an iodinated contrast medium (CM). CEDM is based on the preferential iodine uptake by lesions that have developed angiogenesis, generally related to the growth and development of cancer.

A. Tingberg et al. (Eds.): IWDM 2016, LNCS 9699, pp. 585–592, 2016.
DOI: 10.1007/978-3-319-41546-8_73

The presence of a radiopaque CM at the lesion enhances its visualization by a radiological technique [1, 2].

Two modalities of CEDM have been developed: Dual-energy (DE) and single-energy temporal (SET). DE is based on the difference between linear attenuation coefficients due to acquisition with different X-ray spectra [3]. Images are acquired after the administration of the CM, at low- and high-energy (LE and HE), and they are subtracted applying an appropriate weighting factor [3, 4].

SET aims at visualizing the temporal changes of the CM. Images are acquired before and after the CM administration, and the pre-contrast image is subtracted from the post-contrast CM images. Subtracted SET images $I_{sub,t}$ are obtained as follows,

$$I_{sub,t} = \ln(I_{CM,t}) - \ln(I_0), \tag{1}$$

where I_0 is a mask image acquired before contrast medium injection and $I_{CM,,t}$ is acquired at time t after the CM administration. Before subtraction, images must be registered because patient motion is unavoidable. The temporal series of subtracted images grants the analysis of the CM dynamic behavior at the breast tissue.

In terms of the optimum X-ray spectrum for SET, HE exposures are chosen (ideally) above the 33.2 keV photoelectric K-edge to increase iodine conspicuity. The estimated mean glandular dose for the set of HE acquisitions is of the order of dose in a conventional mammography [1]. Independent CEDM studies have evaluated the relationship between CM uptake and lesion pathology (malignant or benign) [1, 5, 6].

CEDM Images Used in This Analysis: Our group conducted a recent study where the dynamic iodine uptake by lesions was quantified by the mean pixel value (MPV) within regions of interest (lesion, glandular an adipose tissue ROIs) and a possible correlation with pathology and microvessel density was investigated [6]. The images used in the present analysis were generated in that previous study [6]. This section recalls briefly their acquisition, processing and analysis.

Craneocaudal images of 26 participating patients with suspicious lesions, classified as BIRADS 4–5 (age rage 34–83), were acquired at the Mexican National Institute of Cancerology following a CEDM optimized protocol [3] for simultaneous DET and SET subtractions. In this section we refer to the SET images, which were the object of the present investigation on texture.

X-ray beams were produced by a clinical GE Senographe DS system, with 48 kV plus external 0.5 cm Al radiological parameters. First, the mask image was acquired and then, iodine-based CM (Optiray® 300, 300 iodine mg per ml) was injected at 4 ml/s using a mechanical injection system. CM images were acquired at 1, 2, 3, and 5 min after CM administration. Patients remained seated with their breast compressed in order to minimize motion. Acquisition lasted about 8 min. Diagnosis was established by core needle percutaneous biopsy under ultrasound and/or stereotactic guidance by a pathologist. `

A temporal series of subtracted images was obtained for each of 18 patients included in the study [6] by logarithmic subtraction of CM minus mask registered images. Registration was performed employing a transformation plugin for ImageJ which uses a rigid transformation and a moving least square optimization process.

Two parameters were evaluated to quantify the CM presence in subtracted images, the MPV at the lesion ROI and the lesion-to-healthy tissue contrast. Contrast was evaluated as MPV difference between lesion and glandular tissue ROIs. Dynamic curves for each of the parameters were obtained, classified and analyzed. No correlation was found between the image parameters (MPV, contrast, or type of dynamic curve for these two) and the pathology of the lesions or the density of microvessels. It was concluded [6] that CEDM improved the visibility of iodine irrigated lesions, which can help diagnosis, but probably the image analysis of such complex biological process as CM perfusion from angiogenic vessels required more complex tools than a MPV-analysis of ROIs.

Texture Analysis. Texture refers to the spatial distribution of intensity levels present in images. It is used to identify objects or regions of interest in images. Due to its potential, texture has been used in the study of mammographic images, to discriminate malignant from benign lesions [7, 8].

The GLCM is a discrete approximation to the distribution of joint probability for two gray levels occurrence at a certain distance and angle. We have chosen GLCM as the textural analysis tool in this work due to its statistical nature, which makes it robust to noise, and its probable potential to discriminate between malignant and benign lesions in breast images. In the work of Chan *et al.* [7] the GLCM descriptors: sum mean, correlation and energy were used to discriminate malignant lesions, achieving 89 % sensitivity and 76 % specificity. Lyra *et al.* [8] used the combination of first-order (based on gray level histograms) and second-order texture descriptors (based on GLCM) to classify malignant and benign lesions, achieving 84 % accuracy.

The purpose of this work has been to obtain texture descriptors for CEDM images acquired under a temporal modality (SET) [6], and determine their relation with the lesions pathology. Our hypothesis has been that, due to changes in vascularity, the diffusion of iodine through the breast results in textures detectable in radiological images, in accordance to the lesion malignancy or benignity.

2   Methods

2.1   Image Acquisition and Processing

As described above, the original (non-subtracted) SET images analyzed in this work were acquired during a previous work by our group [2, 6]; one of the patients was excluded from the present analysis due to poor quality of the subtracted images (main problem was motion between the acquisitions). Patient ID corresponded to the original numbering (1 to 26). Non-subtracted raw images ("for processing") of 17 patients were analyzed. Images were in DICOM format (16 bit), 1914×2294 pixels image size, 100 μm pixel size. Image processing consisted of geometric registration, subtraction, and selection of ROIs. In this analysis, the selected ROIs corresponded to adipose and glandular tissues, and the lesion.

Geometric Image Registration. For each patient the original images were registered with respect to their mask, employing a method automatically performing image feature extraction and maximizing their enhanced correlation coefficient [9], implemented in *Matlab R2013a*. In this study, an affine geometric transformation was employed, allowing for translation, rotation, shear and scaling of the images.

Image Subtraction. Subtraction followed Eq. (1), and a temporal series of four images per patient (at t = 1, 2 3 and 5 min) was obtained. Subtracted images were saved as float in TIFF format (32 bit). Figure 1 LEFT illustrates the subtraction method: (a) A mammogram acquired before the CEDM procedure and (b) a CEDM subtracted image are shown. In the CEDM image, the anatomical information has been strongly removed by subtraction.

Selection of the Regions-of-Interest. The participant radiologist selected adipose and glandular tissue ROIs in the mask, and the lesion ROI in the subtracted images.

2.2   Texture Analysis

Texture was analyzed computing the GLCM inside the ROIs. Typical ROIs diameter was 100 pixels. GLCM data were computed for 3, 5, 7 and 10 pixels (distance) and for $0°$, $45°$, $90°$ and $135°$ (angle). The selected distance to compute the GLCM was the one presenting the least angular dependence, which allowed an arbitrary angular selection. Distance $d = 3$ met this criterion, and the chosen orientation was $\theta = 0°$. The quantization levels (L) were reduced from 256 to 64, in order to simplify the GLCM calculation and avoid loss of detail. Figure 1 RIGHT shows a GLCM example.

The information contained in the subtracted images corresponds to the iodine presence, noise and registration artifacts. Pixels were divided in three categories, according to their intensity value: negative, positive, and out-positive. Negative intensity values were due to registration artifacts or noise. Positive intensity values cannot be identified or classified. Out-positive intensity values were those at least seven standard deviations greater than the average MPV of the lesion ROI, and thus considered to be registration artifacts. To increase the quality of the obtained information, negative and out-positive pixels were not included in the GLCM computation.

Based on the GLCM, seventeen texture descriptors (energy, entropy, contrast, correlation, dissimilarity, homogeneity, normalized homogeneity, second order inverse moment, variance, inverse variance, covariance, cluster tendency, cluster prominence, cluster shade, diagonal moment, sum mean and lacunarity) were calculated at each of the patient's ROIs. The temporal evolution of the GLCM, and of the descriptors, computed inside the ROIs were evaluated, as well as their sensitivity to (correlation with) the iodine presence.

Logistic Regression. The correlation between texture descriptors in the lesion ROIs (or combinations of them) and malignancy or benignity was analyzed by logistic regression.

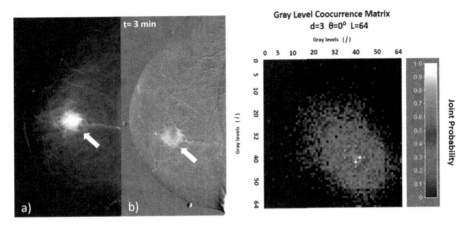

Fig. 1. LEFT: Images of patient 1. (a) Mammogram acquired before CEDM procedure. (b) CEDM image, 3 min after CM injection. Arrows signal the lesion. The patient had invasive ductal carcinoma with necrosis; the halo in image (b) can be associated to the necrotic process. RIGHT: GLCM computed with d = 3 pixels, $\theta = 0°$ and L = 64. The x-axis represents the j gray level, y-axis represents the i gray level. Each point in the matrix represents the joint probability $\{p_{i,j}\}$ of a pixel having intensity i and other pixel at d = 3 and $\theta = 0°$ having intensity j.

3   Results

The ten patients with malignant lesions had ductal carcinomas, 3 of them with necrosis, and 1 *in situ*. Among the 7 with benign lesions, 6 were fibroadenomas (one cellular fibroadenoma) and one microglandular adenosis.

CEDM Image Processing. The benefit of using a registration method based on an affine transformation (in opposition to the rigid transformation used previously [2, 6]) was evaluated by the ratio between intensity of pixels identified as registration artifacts and the total intensity of the image. For images registered with the affine transformation, the mean intensity ratio was 9 %, while for those registered with the rigid transformation the mean ratio was 87 %. However, the MPV computed within the ROIs in tissues of interest did not present statistically significant differences between both types of transformation.

Texture Analysis. The GLCM matrix showed temporal dependence due to the dynamic presence of iodine. The glandular and the adipose tissue ROIs were used as references, in order to compare with the temporal behavior of the lesion GLCM and texture descriptors.

Figure 2 refers to patient 23. Figure 2a shows the subtracted image at 3 min after injection, with the lesion ROI drawn. Figure 2(b–e) are intensity views of the lesion region as a function of time, with a false color scale. Temporal intensity changes due to the iodine distribution at the ROIs can be appreciated. Figure 2(f–i) are the GLCM matrices computed at the ROIs. These matrices were calculated rebinning to 64 gray levels. It can be observed that, for this patient, the intensity and the shape of elements within the GLCM are time-dependent.

The seventeen texture descriptors were calculated in 68 images (17 patients × 4 images each) in order to evaluate their time dependence, for the three types of ROI. Their possible correlation with the MPV was analyzed. The dynamic behavior of texture descriptors revealed those sensitive to the iodine presence and those uncorrelated with MPV. Also, it was found that uptake curves of different descriptors had no similarities between patients.

Figure 3a shows the diagonal moment descriptor at the ROIs of patient 7: The values for adipose and glandular tissues and the lesion are different, and they all present a time dependence. Figure 3b shows MPV for each ROI; for glandular tissue and the lesion, the MPV shows initial uptake followed by a plateau, while the MPV at the adipose tissue ROI remains small and constant. Figure 3c suggests no correlation (that is, their information is independent) between diagonal moment and MPV for this patient.

The analysis showed that the homogeneity, normalized homogeneity, second order inverse moment, and energy descriptors did not display dependence on time; also, parameter sum mean displayed a linear correlation with MPV. These were considered of no use to this investigation.

Logistic Regression. Logistic regression was applied to various combinations of texture descriptors; only those who offered dynamic information and were not correlated with MPV were considered. The linear combination of entropy and diagonal moment showed the best results predicting malignancy/benignity, with 78.6 % specificity, 92.5 % sensitivity and 86.8 % accuracy.

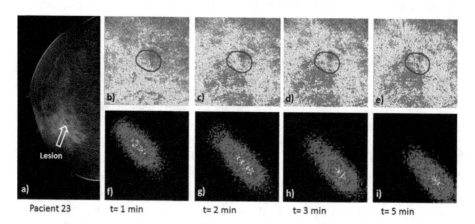

Fig. 2. Patient 23, her diagnosis was a fibroadenoma. (a) Subtracted image 3 min after CM injection. (b–e) Views of the lesion ROI in CEDM images. Colors represent intensities. (f–i) GLCM computed with information from the CEDM ROI of the lesion. Colors represent probabilities, same as in Fig. 1 RIGHT

Figure 4 shows results of the regression applied to a linear combination of entropy and diagonal moment. The x-axis represents the values of the linear combination of entropy and diagonal moment, the y-axis is the probability of malignancy; if the

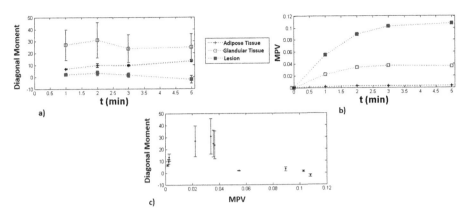

Fig. 3. Results for patient 7 (cellular fibroadenoma). (a) Diagonal moment values. (b) MPV calculated at the ROIs. (c) Diagonal moment values vs MPV.

probability is equal or greater than 0.5 it is classified as malignant and otherwise it is considered benign. Empty circles are the result of the regression and the solid circles represent the real diagnosis for each image. Black circles in top left and bottom right quadrants represent false negative (3) and false positive (6) cases, respectively.

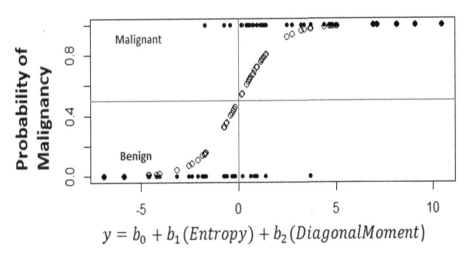

$$y = b_0 + b_1 (Entropy) + b_2 (DiagonalMoment)$$

Fig. 4. Logistic regression applied to the linear combination of entropy and diagonal moment, with parametrization values $b_0 = 21.4 \pm 6.3$, $b_1 = -2.3 \pm 0.7$ and $b_2 = -0.2 \pm 0.05$.

4 Discussion and Conclusions

Our hypothesis was that texture provided information on the lesion pathology, additional to the image intensity. This should manifest if texture parameters were not correlated with MPV in the lesion ROI, and if they presented time dependence. Among the considered texture descriptors, six were found not to add additional information to MPV. A linear combination of entropy and diagonal moment offered optimum discrimination between malignant and benign lesions. Entropy measures the randomness of the intensity levels; diagonal moment measures local changes in intensity.

This application of texture analysis to temporal series of CEDM images shows potential to improve the accuracy of breast cancer diagnosis. A larger study group of CEDM images is required to corroborate the usefulness of the proposed model.

Acknowledgements. We thank authors of Ref. [6] for agreeing to our use of yet unpublished data. UNAM-DGAPA IN105813 and IN107916 supported this work. We thank H Larreguy, ME Martínez and IM Rosado-Méndez for enriching discussions.

References

1. Dromain, C., Balleyguier, C., Muller, S., Mathieu, M.C., Rochard, F., Opolon, P., Sigal, R.: Evaluation of tumor angiogenesis of breast carcinoma using contrast-enhanced digital mammography. Am. J. Roentgenol. **187**, W528–W537 (2006)
2. Cruz-Bastida, J.-P., Rosado-Méndez, I., Pérez-Ponce, H., Villaseñor, Y., Galván, H.A., Trujillo-Zamudio, F.E., Benítez-Bribiesca, L., Brandan, M.-E.: Contrast optimization in clinical contrast-enhanced digital mammography images. In: Maidment, A.D., Bakic, P.R., Gavenonis, S. (eds.) IWDM 2012. LNCS, vol. 7361, pp. 17–23. Springer, Heidelberg (2012)
3. Rosado-Méndez, I., Palma, B.A., Brandan, M.E.: Analytical optimization of digital subtraction mammography with contrast medium using a commercial unit. Med. Phys. **35**, 5544–5557 (2008)
4. Smith, A.: The principles of contrast mammography. Hologic White Paper WP-00084-001 (2014). http://www.hologic.com
5. Diekmann, F., Freyer, M., Diekmann, S., Fallenberg, E.M., Fischer, T., Bick, U., Poellinger, A.: Evaluation of contrast-enhanced digital mammography. Eur. J. Radiol. **78**, 112–121 (2011)
6. Brandan, M.E., Cruz-Bastida, J.P., Rosado-Méndez, I.M., Villaseñor-Navarro, Y., Pérez-Ponce, H., Galván, H.A., Trujillo-Zamudio, F.E., Sánchez-Suárez, P., Benítez-Bribiesca, L.: A clinical study of contrast-enhanced digital mammography for dual-energy and temporal subtraction and the evaluation of blood and lymphatic angiogenesis, March 2016. (in revision)
7. Chan, H.P., Wei, D., Helvie, M.A., Sahiner, B., Adler, D.D., Goodsitt, M.M., Petrick, N.: Computer-aided classification of mammographic masses and normal tissue: linear discriminant analysis in texture feature space. Phys. Med. Biol. **40**, 857–876 (1995)
8. Lyra, M., Lyra, S., Kostakis, B., Drosos, S., Georgosopoulos, C., Skouroliakou, K.: Digital mammography texture analysis by computer assisted image processing. In: IEEE International Workshop on Imaging Systems and Techniques, pp. 73–76 (2008)
9. Evangelidis, G.D., Psarakis, E.Z.: Parametric image alignment using enhanced correlation coefficient maximization. IEEE Trans. Pattern Anal. **30**, 1858–1865 (2008)

Estimating Breast Thickness for Dual-Energy Subtraction in Contrast-Enhanced Digital Mammography: A Theoretical Model

Kristen C. Lau[✉], Raymond J. Acciavatti,
and Andrew D.A. Maidment

Department of Radiology, University of Pennsylvania,
Philadelphia, PA, USA
{Kristen.Lau,Raymond.Acciavatti,
Andrew.Maidment}@uphs.upenn.edu

Abstract. Dual-energy contrast-enhanced digital mammography (DE CE-DM) images the perfusion and vasculature of the breast using an iodinated contrast agent. High-energy (HE) and low-energy (LE) images of the breast are acquired; the DE image is obtained by a weighted logarithmic subtraction of the image pair. We hypothesized that the optimal DE subtraction weighting factor, w, is dependent on three parameters: breast thickness, kV, and filter material. We simulated the attenuation of x-rays through breasts of thicknesses ranging from 0.5 to 10 cm using different filter and kV combinations. The glandularity of the phantom for a given thickness was varied using different combinations of adipose and glandular tissues. We calculated the logarithm of the LE and HE signal intensities. For a given kV-filter pair, the signals decrease with increasing tissue thickness and glandularity. The DE weighting factor is thickness-dependent, and it decreases with increasing energy difference between the LE-HE kV pairs. These results facilitate the subtraction of tissue in the periphery of the breast, and aid in discriminating between contrast agent uptake in glandular tissue and subtraction artefacts.

Keywords: Breast · Dual-energy · Contrast-enhanced · Digital mammography · Glandularity · Software simulation

1 Introduction

Contrast-enhanced breast imaging is motivated by the observation that angiogenesis accompanies the development of cancer. Contrast-enhanced MRI (CE-MRI) is the current gold standard for imaging breast cancer perfusion and the characterization of lesions in the diagnosis of breast cancer. This imaging modality is also used to screen women who have a high risk of developing breast cancer. Although CE-MRI provides important information about the vasculature of breast lesions, it suffers from low spatial resolution when compared to conventional digital mammography (DM). For instance, microcalcifications are better visualized in DM than in CE-MRI.

Contrast-enhanced digital mammography (CE-DM) has emerged as an alternative to CE-MRI. An iodinated contrast agent is used in CE-DM to image the perfusion and

© Springer International Publishing Switzerland 2016
A. Tingberg et al. (Eds.): IWDM 2016, LNCS 9699, pp. 593–600, 2016.
DOI: 10.1007/978-3-319-41546-8_74

vasculature of the breast. CE-DM has great potential to improve the detection and diagnosis of breast cancer by combining morphologic and functional information on vascular kinetics in a single examination. It has the ability to acquire functional characteristics of breast lesions at a spatial resolution that is comparable to DM. Furthermore, CE-DM allows us to quantitatively assess the linear relationship between the attenuation coefficient and the concentration of contrast agent uptake. Contrast uptake by breast tissue is made more evident by dual-energy (DE) subtraction. In DE x-ray breast imaging, low-energy (LE) and high-energy (HE) images of the breast are acquired. The x-ray energies are chosen so that the k-edge of the contrast agent is in the range spanned by the LE and HE x-ray spectra, allowing us to distinguish between the linear attenuation coefficients of the soft tissue and contrast agent signals.

The goal of DE subtraction is to cancel the signal from the background breast tissue and to increase enhancement conspicuity. In addition, DE subtraction minimizes patient motion because the HE and LE image pairs are acquired almost simultaneously. The DE image is obtained by performing a weighted difference of the logarithms of the LE and HE images. The DE signal intensity S^{DE} is expressed as

$$S^{DE} = \ln(S^{HE}) - w * \ln(S^{LE}), \tag{1}$$

where w is the DE weighting factor, S^{HE} is the signal intensity of the HE image, and S^{LE} is the signal intensity of the LE image. The weighting factor, w, is calculated to eliminate the dependence of the DE signal on the glandular-adipose signal of the breast tissue, and it is expressed as

$$w = \frac{\mu_a^{HE} - \mu_g^{HE}}{\mu_a^{LE} - \mu_g^{LE}} = \frac{\ln(S_a^{HE}) - \ln(S_g^{HE})}{\ln(S_a^{LE}) - \ln(S_g^{LE})}, \tag{2}$$

where μ is the linear attenuation coefficient and the subscripts a and g represent adipose and glandular tissues, respectively. This is based on the work of Karunamuni and Maidment [1].

Current methods for DE subtraction do not consider compressed breast thickness, and a constant weighting factor is applied to the entire image. In our previous work, we developed a method for determining breast thickness and composition in DE CE-DM [2]. The motivation for our work arises from the difficulty in resolving contrast uptake at the boundaries of the breast in DE subtraction. A number of studies have noted the presence of subtraction artefacts in DE CE-DM [3, 4]. Yagil et al. [4] classify these artefacts into four categories: rim, ripple, axillary line, and skin-line artefacts.

We hypothesize that the optimal DE weighting factor is dependent on three different parameters: breast thickness, kV combination, and filter combination. Therefore, weighting factors near the periphery of the breast, where the breast is thinner, should be different from those in the centre. Methods for quantification of breast composition using DE mammography have been explored by Ducote and Molloi [5] and Laidevant et al. [6]. However, these methods require the use of a calibration phantom and do not quantitatively determine the breast thickness. By quantifying the breast thickness and composition as a function of position, we can optimize our DE subtraction by finding the optimal weighting factor at each pixel location.

2   Methods

Polyenergetic x-ray spectra were generated using simulation software developed by Boone and Seibert [7]. The software simulates x-ray spectra with a tungsten anode at 1 keV intervals using interpolating polynomials. X-ray energies were chosen so that the k-edge of iodine (33.2 keV) was in the range spanned by the LE and HE x-ray spectra. The kV, filter material, and filter thickness parameters used reflect those available on the prototype DE Hologic Selenia Dimensions imaging system (Table 1).

Table 1. Summary of parameters used in software simulation.

	Energy of Spectra (kV)	Filter	
		Material	Thickness (µm)
Low-Energy	25–35 kV	Aluminum	700
		Rhodium	50
		Silver	50
High-Energy	40–49 kV	Copper	200
		Copper	300

Breast tissue was modelled by simulating phantoms consisting of a uniform composition of glandular and adipose tissues. The thickness of the phantoms ranged from 0.5 to 10 cm, in 0.5 cm increments. The glandular-adipose composition of the phantom was varied in 10 % increments from 0 % glandularity to 100 % glandularity for a given thickness (Fig. 1).

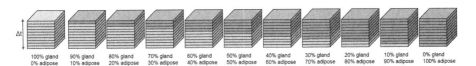

| 100% gland | 90% gland | 80% gland | 70% gland | 60% gland | 50% gland | 40% gland | 30% gland | 20% gland | 10% gland | 0% gland |
| 0% adipose | 10% adipose | 20% adipose | 30% adipose | 40% adipose | 50% adipose | 60% adipose | 70% adipose | 80% adipose | 90% adipose | 100% adipose |

Fig. 1. Example of a tissue phantom composed of adipose (red) and glandular (yellow) tissues (Colour figure online).

Given the incident number of photons, N_0, from an x-ray beam, the number of photons transmitted through a phantom, N_{ph}, at a specific energy bin, E, is given by the Beer-Lambert law as

$$N_{ph}(E) = N_0(E)e^{-(\mu_g m_g + \mu_a m_a)t_{ph}}, \tag{3}$$

where t_{ph} is the phantom thickness, μ is the linear attenuation coefficient, m is the percent tissue composition, and the subscripts a and g represent adipose tissue and glandular tissue, respectively. The glandular and adipose tissue compositions are related by

$$m_g + m_a = 1. \tag{4}$$

An energy-integrating selenium detector was modelled in our simulation, and the signal intensity of the phantom, S_{ph}, is determined by

$$S_{ph} = \sum_{}^{E_{max}} N_{ph}(E) * E * e^{-\mu_{Se} t_{Se}}, \tag{5}$$

where E_{max} is equal to the simulated tube potential, μ_{Se} is the linear attenuation coefficient of selenium, and $t_{Se} = 0.5$ mm is the thickness of the selenium. The DE signal intensity for each phantom was determined using the DE subtraction method detailed in Sect. 1.

3 Results and Discussion

The HE and LE spectra were generated using software simulation; the spectra were normalized by the mAs. A total of 145,200 phantoms were simulated in our study. Results from the tissue phantom simulation were plotted parametrically. The mean logarithmic HE intensity values, $\ln S^{HE}$, were plotted against the mean logarithmic LE intensity values, $\ln S^{LE}$ (Fig. 2). The mean logarithmic LE and HE signal intensities vary with phantom thickness and glandularity. For a given kV-filter pair, the mean logarithmic LE and HE signals decrease with increasing tissue thickness, and they also decrease linearly with increasing glandularity for a given thickness. A linear fit was modelled for each thickness. The mean r^2 for the linear fits is 0.999, indicating that a linear model is appropriate. It is important to note that the DE weighting factor, w, is represented graphically as the slope, $\frac{\Delta(\ln S^{HE})}{\Delta(\ln S^{LE})}$, of the linear fit. Therefore, it is relevant to calculate the weighting factor as a function of breast thickness.

It is shown upon closer inspection that for a given kV-filter pair, the slopes of these linear fits are not parallel. The weighting factor, w, was plotted three-dimensionally as a function of LE and HE (Fig. 3). Each surface represents a constant tissue thickness. The weighting factor changes with tissue thickness and kV pair. We previously showed that DE subtraction has the purpose of projecting a two-dimensional LE-HE signal pair down to a single value, and each thickness has a distinct DE signal [2]. The DE signal is unique for each thickness because DE subtraction intrinsically encodes breast thickness information when using the common weighting scheme designed to eliminate the signal between glandular and adipose tissues.

It is worth noting that there is a region of convergence between the different thickness surfaces. This is further illustrated in Fig. 4. The behaviour of the thickness surfaces can be divided into three different regions. The two surfaces represent tissues of different thickness; the red surface represents a thicker breast than the blue surface. Region I represents the situation in which the thickness surfaces converge. This indicates that the linear fits as a function of breast thickness of $\ln S^{HE}$ versus $\ln S^{LE}$ are parallel. Therefore, the weighting factor is constant for LE-HE kV pairs in this region. Region II represents the situation in which the fits converge to the left. Thus, the weighting factor decreases with increasing thickness. Region III represents the situation in which the fits converge to the right. This indicates that the weighting factor increases with increasing thickness. DE subtraction is simplified in Region I as only a single

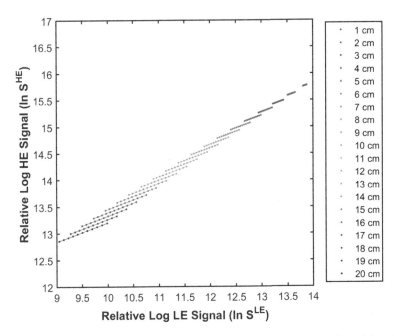

Fig. 2. Signal intensities for simulated breast tissue phantoms at thicknesses from 0.5 to 10 cm. Results are shown for a 30 kV/Rh 50 μm (LE) and 49 kV/Cu 300 μm (HE) pair (Colour figure online).

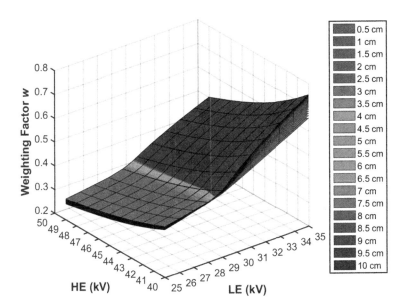

Fig. 3. DE weighting factor, w, as a function of HE and LE at a constant thickness. Results are shown for a 30 kV/Rh 50 μm (LE) and 49 kV/Cu 300 μm (HE) pair (Colour figure online).

w value is needed. However, a residual signal from the variations in breast thickness is still preserved. By contrast, regions II and III require a different weighting factor and a thickness correction as a function of thickness.

We then determined the range of DE values spanned by the linear fits of the thickest and thinnest phantoms. To calculate this value, we first located the point along the 5 cm linear fit that represented 50 % adipose/50 % glandular tissue. Next, we found the normal to the line at that point, and measured the distance between where the normal intersected the 0.5 cm and 10 cm lines.

The DE range was plotted as a function of LE and HE (Fig. 5). The range increases with increases in the energy difference between the LE- HE kV pairs. A maximal range value is desired for DE subtraction because this facilitates our ability to distinguish between different tissue thicknesses. This corresponds to a minimal DE weighting factor, as seen in Fig. 3.

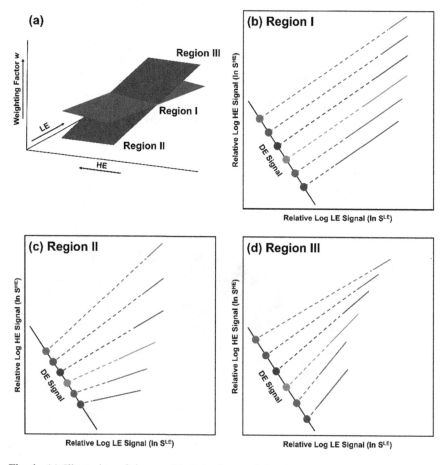

Fig. 4. (a) Illustration of the possible behaviours of signal intensity pairs projected onto DE signal space (black line) for a given kV pair and filter pair combination: (b) parallel, (c) converging, and (d) diverging (Colour figure online).

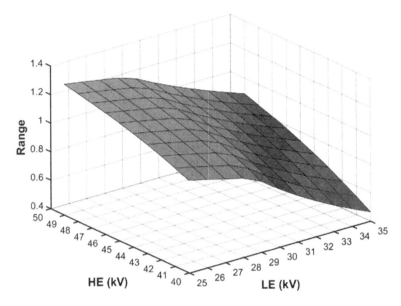

Fig. 5. Range as a function of HE and LE. Results are shown for a 30 kV/Rh 50 μm (LE) and 49 kV/Cu 300 μm (HE) pair (Colour figure online).

Upon closer inspection of the range, it can be shown that there is a set of optimal energy differences for a LE-HE kV pair. We plotted the range versus energy difference at a constant HE, and it can be seen that there is a region where the range value sharply increases. This set of kV differences corresponds to the same region where the range increases slowly in the plot of range versus energy difference at a constant LE. These results indicate that for a given HE or LE value, there is an optimal corresponding LE or HE value in order to determine tissue thickness (Fig. 6).

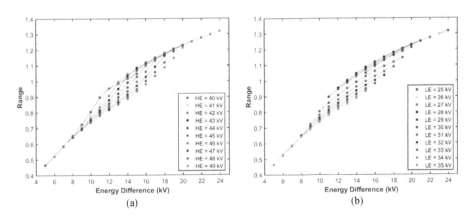

Fig. 6. Range as a function of energy difference at (a) constant HE and (b) constant LE. Results are shown for a 30 kV/Rh 50 μm (LE) and 49 kV/Cu 300 μm (HE) pair (Colour figure online).

4 Conclusions

We have developed a framework to determine breast tissue thickness and composition quantitatively in DE CE-DM. We have shown that breast thickness and composition can be predicted from the linear relationship between LE and HE signal intensities. This is possible because each tissue thickness has a distinct DE signal. Therefore, breast thickness is intrinsically encoded in DE subtraction when using the common weighting scheme to eliminate the signal between glandular and adipose tissues. This has implications for the weighting factor used in DE subtraction for a given thickness. We have also shown that the weighting factor, w, changes with thickness, kV of the spectra, and filter combination. In addition, we have shown that for a given HE or LE value, there is a corresponding LE or HE value that allows us to achieve an optimal range of values spanned by the thinnest and thickest phantoms. These results facilitate the subtraction of tissue in the periphery of the breast, and aid in discriminating between contrast agent uptake in glandular tissue and subtraction artefacts.

Acknowledgements. The project described is supported in part by Grant Number UL1RR024134 from the National Center for Research Resources. Support for R.J.A. was provided by the Postdoctoral Fellowship Grant PDF14302589 from Susan G. Komen®. The content is solely the responsibility of the authors and does not necessarily represent the official views of the funding agencies. This work is also supported in part by the Institute for Translational Medicine and Therapeutics' Transdisciplinary Program in Translational Medicine and Therapeutics.

References

1. Karunamuni, R., Maidment, A.D.A.: Search for novel contrast materials in dual-energy x-ray breast imaging using theoretical modeling of contrast-to-noise ratio. Phys. Med. Biol. **59**, 4311–4324 (2014)
2. Lau, K.C., Kwon, Y.J., Aziz, M.K., Acciavatti, R.J., Maidment, A.D.A.: Estimating breast thickness for dual-energy subtraction in contrast-enhanced digital mammography using calibration phantoms. In: Proceedings of SPIE 9783, Medical Imaging 2016 Physics Medical Imaging, vol. 9783 (2016)
3. Blum, K.S., Rubbert, C., Mathys, B., Antoch, G., Mohrmann, S., Obenauer, S.: Use of contrast-enhanced spectral mammography for intramammary cancer staging: preliminary results. Acad. Radiol. **21**, 1363–1369 (2014)
4. Yagil, Y., Shalmon, A., Rundstein, A., Servadio, Y., Halshtok, O., Gotlieb, M.: Challenges in contrast-enhanced spectral mammography interpretation: artefacts lexicon. Clin. Radiol. **71**, 450–457 (2016)
5. Ducote, J.L., Molloi, S.: Quantification of breast density with dual energy mammography: an experimental feasibility study. Med. Phys. **37**, 793–801 (2010)
6. Laidevant, A.D., Malkov, S., Flowers, C.I., Kerlikowske, K., Shepherd, J.A.: Compositional breast imaging using a dual-energy mammography protocol. Med. Phys. **37**, 164 (2010)
7. Boone, J.M., Seibert, J.A.: An accurate method for computer-generating tungsten anode x-ray spectra from 30 to 140 kV. Med. Phys. **24**, 1661–1670 (1997)

A Simulation Study on Spectral Lesion Characterization

Klaus Erhard$^{(\boxtimes)}$ and Udo van Stevendaal

Philips Research, Röntgenstr. 24-26, 22335 Hamburg, Germany
{klaus.erhard,udo.van.stevendaal}@philips.com

Abstract. Solitary, well-defined lesions are a common mammographic finding contributing more than 20 % of overall screening recalls. Discrimination of cystic from solid breast lesions therefore has the potential to reduce unnecessary recalls in mammography screening. A pre-clinical study, measuring the energy-dependent X-ray attenuation of tissue specimen and cystic fluid, revealed a measurable difference of the photon detection rate in the two energy bins of an energy-resolving photon-counting mammography system for these two tissue types. Based on these differences, a spectral lesion characterization algorithm has been developed, which estimates the lesion composition from spectral measurements in a lesion and a lesion-free reference region.

In this work, we present a simulation study to estimate the dependence of this lesion characterization algorithm on various types of uncertainties including the biological variation of cyst fluid and tumor tissue, variations in the mammographic background texture, and errors in the spectral measurements. The simulation study uses the receiver operating characteristics (ROC) for the task of identifying solid lesions ('positive result') to predict an expected area under the curve (AUC) and the specificity at the 99 % sensitivity level for a simulated screening population. The results of this simulation study are compared to those of a recently published pilot study.

Keywords: Spectral lesion characterization · Tissue characterization · Mammography · Spectral imaging · Breast lesion · Breast cyst

1 Introduction

Solitary, well defined lesions are a common mammographic finding. Probably benign mass lesions are contributing approximately 37 % of recalls for probably benign lesions at screening while the cancer rate is less than 2 % in this type of lesions [1]. Moreover, a large fraction of the lesions turn out to be simple cysts, which can easily be assessed with ultrasound and do not require further clinical evaluation [2]. Discrimination of cystic from solid breast lesions therefore has the potential to reduce unnecessary recalls in mammography screening reducing both the costs of the screening program as well as patient anxiety [3].

© Springer International Publishing Switzerland 2016
A. Tingberg et al. (Eds.): IWDM 2016, LNCS 9699, pp. 601–608, 2016.
DOI: 10.1007/978-3-319-41546-8_75

Spectral X-ray imaging [4] allows differentiation between given tissue types, provided their spectral absorption characteristics differ measurably. The discrimination of cystic from solid lesions was demonstrated to be technically feasible in a pre-clinical specimen study [5]. Based on the differences in the energy-dependent X-ray attenuation of cyst fluid and tumor tissue, a spectral lesion characterization algorithm has been developed [6] to translate these specimen results into clinical practice.

The evaluation of the accuracy and clinical performance of such a lesion characterization algorithm requires large and costly clinical trials for verification and validation. To obtain a first indication on the achievable sensitivity and specificity we have developed a method to estimate the expected outcome of the lesion characterization algorithm on a screening population with a simulation study. The presented simulation study investigates the dependence of the algorithm on various types of uncertainties including the biological variation of cyst fluid and tumor tissue, variations in the mammographic background texture, and errors in the spectral measurements. To this end, we use the receiver operating characteristics (ROC) for the task of identifying solid lesions ('positive result') to predict an expected area under the curve (AUC) and the specificity at the 99 % sensitivity level. For the simulation of a realistic screening population, a series of breast and lesion models have been generated using the empirical distribution of compression thickness and breast density derived from spectral mammograms, acquired on a Philips MicroDose SI system in a screening population. The results of this simulation study are compared to those of a recently published pilot study.

2   Methods

2.1   Breast and Lesion Model

The photo-electric and the Compton effect are the only absorption effects that occur in the relevant mammographic energy range for typical breast tissues. Therefore, the X-ray attenuation μ_X of a certain breast tissue type X at energy E can be decomposed [4] into a linear combination

$$\mu_X(E) = a_X^{\mathrm{Al}}\mu^{\mathrm{Al}}(E) + a_X^{\mathrm{PMMA}}\mu^{\mathrm{PMMA}}(E) \tag{1}$$

of the attenuation caused by two basis materials such as aluminum (Al) and poly-methylmethacrylat (PMMA) with material-specific constants a_X^{Al} and a_X^{PMMA}. These energy-dependent linear attenuation coefficients have been measured for adipose and glandular tissue [7,8]. More recently, the spectral decomposition of cyst fluid and tumor tissue has been measured on a spectral MicroDose prototype system [5]. The material coefficients, which have been used in this simulation study are listed in Table 1.

We are using the notation a_X^{Al} and a_X^{PMMA} with $X \in \{G, A, S, C, L\}$ for glandular, adipose, solid, cystic and lesion (cystic or solid) tissue, respectively. Let i denote an X-ray path through the breast, see Fig. 1 for a simplified illustration

Table 1. Attenuation coefficients – data origins: (1) Fit to [7] in (20–30 kV), (2) specimen measurements [5], (3) Calculated from elemental decomposition [8].

Tissue	a^{Al}/mm^{-1}	a^{PMMA}/mm^{-1}	
Glandular	0.0240	0.8522	(1)
Adipose	−0.0124	0.8425	(1)
Carcinoma	0.0291	0.8587	(2)
Cyst	0.0323	0.8118	(2)
Skin	0.0040	0.9521	(3)

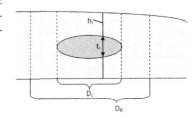

Fig. 1. Overview of the lesion model.

in parallel beam geometry. Assume that h_i, t_i, and g_i denote the local values of the breast height under compression, lesion thickness, and glandularity, i.e. the fraction of glandular tissue in a tissue sample composed of only adipose and glandular tissue.

Then, the X-ray attenuation along the path i can be simulated as

$$l_i^{Al}\mu^{Al}(E) + l_i^{PMMA}\mu^{PMMA}(E) = (h_i - t_i)\,g_i\mu_G(E) \tag{2}$$
$$+ (h_i - t_i)\,(1 - g_i)\,\mu_A(E)$$
$$+ t_i\mu_L(E)$$

or, using the vector notation $\boldsymbol{l}_i = (l_i^{Al}, l_i^{PMMA})$ and $\boldsymbol{a}_X = (a_X^{Al}, a_X^{PMMA})$ as

$$\boldsymbol{l}_i = (h_i - t_i)\,g_i\boldsymbol{a}_G + (h_i - t_i)\,(1 - g_i)\,\boldsymbol{a}_A + t_i\boldsymbol{a}_L. \tag{3}$$

2.2 Lesion Characterization Algorithm

For spectral lesion characterization we now aim at estimating the lesion composition $t_i\boldsymbol{a}_L$ from a pair of measurements $\boldsymbol{l}_i$. In the lesion-free reference region D_R, the lesion thickness is known to be zero. Hence, from (3) we can uniquely determine the compression height h_i as well as the glandularity g_i in D_R since the vectors $\boldsymbol{a}_A$ and $\boldsymbol{a}_G$ are linear independent.

From the measured height and glandularity values in the reference region D_R we are estimating its values inside the lesion region D_L. Glandularity values are estimated in D_R with harmonic interpolation by solving the Dirichlet boundary value problem for the Laplace equation in D_L. For interpolation of the breast height, a local breast shape model is adapted to the measured height values in the reference region [9,10]. Assuming a cyst-solid mixture of the lesion

$$t_i\boldsymbol{a}_L = t_{C,i}\boldsymbol{a}_C + t_{S,i}\boldsymbol{a}_S,$$

and using the interpolated height and glandularity estimates, we can now solve (3) inside D_L for the unknown cystic and solid tissue lengths $t_{C,i}$ and $t_{S,i}$, respectively. Finally, a cystic volume fraction can be computed via

$$CVF = \frac{\sum_{i \in D_L} t_{C,i}}{\sum_{i \in D_L} (t_{C,i} + t_{S,i})}$$

which defines the discriminating feature in the presented simulation study.

2.3   Simulation Parameters

For this simulation a set of 6813 spectral mammograms from a screening population, acquired on a Philips MicroDose SI system at Sodersjukhuset clinic,
Sweden, has been used to derive empirical distributions on the breast density
values and the compressed breast thickness. Volumetric breast density values
have been generated with a proprietary system application (Breast Density Measurement, Philips Digital Mammography Sweden AB, Solna, Sweden), which has
been clinically evaluated in [11]. The distribution of breast thickness within this
screening population is listed in Table 2 (left) together with the distribution of
volumetric breast density, classified into four categories (right). These values
have been used to populate the background tissue of a set of 2000 breast models, in which an additional spherical lesion with a uniformly distributed random
diameter between 5 and 60 mm has been embedded. The distribution of breast
thickness and breast density values within these 2000 breast models is illustrated
in Fig. 2. The lesion diameter has been restricted to be not larger than 60 % of
the breast thickness. With the forward model (3) and the attenuation coefficient
of Table 1, each of these 2000 breast models has then been used to simulate two
spectral mammograms, one with the lesion tissue modeled as cyst fluid and the
other with the lesion modeled as tumor tissue.

For each simulated spectral mammogram, a lesion characterization has been
performed assuming a cyst-solid lesion mixture model as described in Sect. 2.2.
To estimate the accuracy of the spectral lesion characterization in a clinical
setting, we investigate the receiver operating characteristic (ROC) for the task
of identifying a solid lesion ('positive' result) in this simulation study based on

Table 2. Distribution of breast thickness and density in the screening population.

Breast Thickness [mm]	Relative Frequency [%]
0-20	0.2
21-30	3.6
31-40	10.7
41-50	18.7
51-60	27.3
61-70	24.2
71-80	11.4
> 80	3.9

Volumetric Breast Density [%]	Relative Frequency [%]
0-25%	77.5
25-50%	16.2
50-75%	5.5
75-100%	0.7

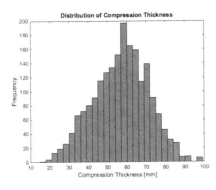
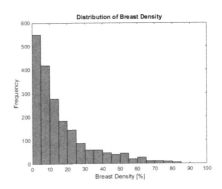

Fig. 2. Distribution of breast thickness and density used in the simulation.

the CVF discriminator. As a figure of merit, we use the area under the ROC-curve (AUC) together with the specificity at a 99 % sensitivity level, which takes into account that in a clinical setting only few solids should be mis-classified as cysts by the lesion characterization algorithm. Additional specificity values are reported for the 95 % and 90 % sensitivity levels.

3   Results

Biological Variation. In the first simulation, we are assuming a constant breast composition and breast height for each of the 2000 simulated breast models and allow for some biological variation in the lesion model. To this end, the spectral attenuation of the lesion has been chosen for each simulation randomly based on a Gaussian distribution, which has been fitted to the measurements reported in [5]. The probability density functions (PDF) for the cyst and tumor samples are indicated by elliptic iso-contour lines around the respective mean values in the left part of Fig. 3 while the 2×2000 random samples of the material decomposition coefficients $a_S^{Al,PMMA}$ of tumor tissue and $a_C^{Al,PMMA}$ of cyst fluid are illustrated with red and blue circles. The simulation includes a Poisson noise model corresponding to a mean glandular dose level of 0.7 mGy. The ROC curve of this simulation yields an area under the curve of 0.97 as depicted in the right image of Fig. 3. The specificity for identifying a solid lesion is given for this simulation by 29.0 %, 84.1 % and 96.2 % at the corresponding sensitivity levels of 99 %, 95 % and 90 %, respectively. This simulation sets an upper theoretical limit on the performance of the presented lesion characterization algorithm given the biological variation as observed in [5].

Glandularity Variation. In a second simulation experiment, we will investigate the degradation of the algorithm performance when allowing variations in the glandular background texture. To this end, the constant glandularity values of the previous simulation are refined by glandularity maps, which are

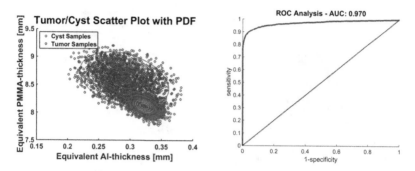

Fig. 3. Left: Scatter plot of the random samples of cyst and tumors in the Al/PMMA domain and normalized to a lesion size of 10 mm. Right: Corresponding receiver operating characteristic (ROC) curve. (Color figure online)

determined from the 6813 data sets of the screening population. The simulated lesions are placed randomly in these glandularity maps. This is indicated by the red circles in the left part of Fig. 4. The corresponding ROC curve, which is shown in the right image of Fig. 4, reveals an area under the curve of 0.968. In this case, the specificity is 31.2%, 78.9% and 93.6% at the corresponding sensitivity levels of 99%, 95% and 90%, respectively. Hence, a minor degradation of the performance of the lesion characterization algorithm due to errors introduced by the glandularity estimation in the lesion region D_L can be observed, but the results are still comparable to the theoretical limit established by the biological tissue variation.

Calibration Inaccuracy. Finally, we incorporate a model on the spectral calibration accuracy into the simulation study to investigate its impact on spectral lesion characterization. An uncertainty for the simulated Al and PMMA lengths is modeled in the random sampling process with a Gaussian distribution with

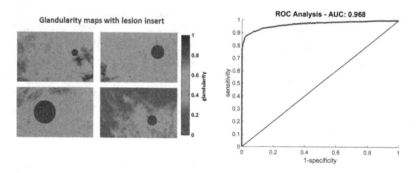

Fig. 4. Left: Four examples of glandularity maps determined from the screening population. The lesions vary randomly in size (red circle) and location within the mammograms. Right: Corresponding ROC curve. (Color figure online)

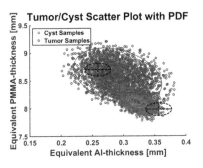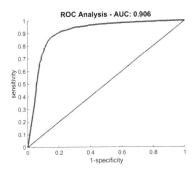

Fig. 5. Left: Scatter plot of cyst and tumors samples with black ellipses indicating the calibration inaccuracy. Right: Corresponding ROC curve. (Color figure online)

standard deviation σ of 5 % of the simulated Al and PMMA length. Additionally, the standard deviation of the Gaussian probability density function has been required to be at least 50 µm for drawing the Al and 500 µm for drawing the PMMA random calibration noise samples. The calibration inaccuracy is depicted by the black ellipses shown in the left image of Fig. 5. The corresponding ROC curve is further degrading as shown in the right image of Fig. 5 and yields an area under the curve of 0.906. The specificity is 25.8 %, 68.4 % and 81.1 % at the corresponding sensitivity level of 99 %, 95 % and 90 %, respectively. The impact of calibration inaccuracies are more dominant than the model assumption of the characterization algorithm itself. Therefore, improving the accuracy of the spectral material decomposition will be part of our future research.

4   Discussion

In this simulation study, the feasibility of discriminating cystic from solid lesions has been investigated to predict the outcome of spectral lesion characterization in a clinical setting. Using the cystic volume fraction as a single feature discriminator, a theoretical limit on the algorithm's accuracy was estimated with a specificity of 29 % at the 99 % sensitivity level and an AUC of 0.97 due to the biological variation of cystic and solid samples [5]. Minor degradations of the algorithm's performance are expected due to errors introduced by the glandularity estimation in the lesion region D_L. However, calibration inaccuracies have been identified as one major source of error in this simulation, which additionally decreased the AUC from 0.97 to 0.91 and the specificity from 29 % to 26 % at the 99 % sensitivity level. Errors in the breast height estimation have not been investigated in this simulation study and might additionally impact the performance of the algorithm, which will have to be investigated in the future.

The results of this simulation study compare well to a recently published clinical study on lesion characterization with a similar algorithm using a 2-feature discriminator [10]. The AUC of 0.91 is similar to the reported AUC value of 0.88 and within the 95 % confidence interval (CI) of 0.78-0.96. The specificity of

26 % at the 99 % sensitivity level is below the observed 56 % specificity (95 % CI: 33 %–78 %) and outside the 95 % confidence interval of the results published in this clinical study. This difference can be attributed to the use of a single feature discriminator in this simulation experiment compared to a 2-feature discriminator algorithm evaluated in [10]. Moreover, the biological variation of tumor tissue in an actual screening population might be less severe than modelled in this simulation study and reported in [5], where the tissue specimen were formalin-fixed prior to the spectral measurements.

References

1. Sickles, E.A.: Probably benign breast lesions: when should follow-up be recommended and what is the optimal follow-up protocol? Radiology **213**(1), 11–14 (1999)
2. Vizcano, I., Gadea, L., Andreo, L., Salas, D., Ruiz-Perales, F., Cuevas, D., Herranz, C., Bueno, F.: Short-term follow-up results in 795 nonpalpable probably benign lesions detected at screening mammography. Radiology **219**(2), 475–483 (2001)
3. Lauby-Secretan, B., Scoccianti, C., Loomis, D., Benbrahim-Tallaa, L., Bouvard, V., Bianchini, F., Straif, K.: Breast-cancer screening - viewpoint of the IARC working group. N. Engl. J. Med. **372**(24), 2353–2358 (2015)
4. Alvarez, R.E., Macovski, A.: Energy-selective reconstructions in x-ray computerized tomography. Phys. Med. Biol. **21**(5), 733–744 (1976)
5. Fredenberg, E., Dance, D.R., Willsher, P., Moa, E., von Tiedemann, M., Young, K.C., Wallis, M.G.: Measurement of breast-tissue x-ray attenuation by spectral mammography: first results on cyst fluid. Phys. Med. Biol. **58**, 8609–8620 (2013)
6. Erhard, K., Fredenberg, E., Homann, H., Roessl, E.: Spectral lesion characterization on a photon-counting mammography system. In: Proceedings of the SPIE, vol. 9033, p. 90331. SPIE (2014)
7. Johns, P., Yaffe, M.: X-ray characterisation of normal and neoplastic breast tissues. Phys. Med. Biol. **32**, 675 (1987)
8. Hammerstein, G.R., Miller, D.W., White, D.R., Masterson, M.E., Woodard, H.Q., Laughlin, J.S.: Absorbed radiation dose in mammography. Radiology **130**(2), 485–491 (1979)
9. Gooßen, A., Heese, H.S., Erhard, K.: Automatic volumetric glandularity assessment from full field digital mammograms. In: Maidment, A.D.A., Bakic, P.R., Gavenonis, S. (eds.) IWDM 2012. LNCS, vol. 7361, pp. 753–760. Springer, Heidelberg (2012)
10. Erhard, K., Kilburn-Toppin, F., Willsher, P., Moa, E., Fredenberg, E., Wieberneit, N., Buelow, T., Wallis, M.G.: Characterization of cystic lesions by spectral mammography: results of a clinical pilot study. Invest. Radiol. **51**, 340–347 (2016)
11. Machida, Y., Tozaki, M., Yoshida, T., Saita, A., Yakabe, M., Nii, K.: Feasibility study of a breast density measurement within a direct photon-counting mammography scanner system. Jpn. J. Radiol. **32**(9), 561–567 (2014)

Phase Contrast Breast Imaging

Contrast Detail Phantoms for X-ray Phase-Contrast Mammography and Tomography

Kristina Bliznakova[1(✉)], Giovanni Mettivier[2], Paolo Russo[2], and Ivan Buliev[1]

[1] Laboratory of Computer Simulations in Medicine,
Technical University of Varna, Varna, Bulgaria
{kristina.bliznakova,buliev}@tu-varna.bg
[2] Department of Physics "Ettore Pancini", University of Napoli and INFN Napoli, Naples, Italy
{mettivier,russo}@na.infn.it

Abstract. Primary goal of this study is to investigate the visibility of low-contrast details of different size on images obtained at conventional mammography unit, and at a monochromatic synchrotron radiation source, in absorption based and phase contrast imaging setups. For this purpose, three physical phantoms made of paraffin as a bulk material were used. They embedded various low contrast features. Single projection images were acquired with the GE Senographe mammography unit and at the beamline ID17, ESRF, Grenoble. Comparison of images showed that images obtained in a phase contrast mode have more visible details than the images acquired either in absorption mode at the synchrotron or at the conventional x-ray mammography unit. Analysis for δ and μ suggests that paraffin may be a suitable material for the manufacturing of tissue-mimicking phantoms dedicated to phase contrast applications. Results will be exploited in the development of a dedicated phantom for phase contrast imaging.

Keywords: Phase contrast · Breast phantoms · Phantom materials

1 Introduction

Phase-contrast (PhC) mammography and tomography are emerging alternative approaches to the absorption based mammography, digital breast tomosynthesis and breast computed tomography. Indeed, x-ray PhC imaging is a technique that is based not only on x-ray attenuation but also on the x-ray phase change related to diffraction and refraction effects during x-ray propagation in the tissue. The advancement in the development and the clinical implementation of this imaging technique is related to the development of new physical phantoms which correctly reflect the phase change characteristics of real breast tissues.

Nowadays, physical phantoms dedicated for testing the performance of x-ray breast imaging techniques are mostly suitable for absorption imaging. These physical phantoms reflect the photon absorbing and scattering properties of the various breast tissues, rather than their phase contrast properties. The analysis of tissue simulating materials used for breast imaging showed that the commonly used PMMA substitute exhibited δ greater than the fibroglandular tissue by ~12 % [1]. Although several materials exhibited

© Springer International Publishing Switzerland 2016
A. Tingberg et al. (Eds.): IWDM 2016, LNCS 9699, pp. 611–617, 2016.
DOI: 10.1007/978-3-319-41546-8_76

δ between that of adipose and fibroglandular tissue, there was an energy mismatch in terms of equivalent fibroglandular weight fraction between δ and μ for these materials. These results as well as the lack of up-to-date proper physical phantoms, cause the investigators to use tissue breast samples with and without breast cancers.

The aim of this investigation is related to the design and fabrication of suitable phantoms for x-ray breast imaging in absorption and phase-contrast modes, and to their test in a series of imaging studies with coherent monochromatic x-rays and with an incoherent polychromatic source.

2   Materials and Methods

2.1   Phantoms

Three physical phantoms that differ in their complexity were manufactured and used for the experimental work: (a) a homogeneous paraffin phantom of size 60 mm × 40 mm × 25 mm with three water spheres placed at different heights, (b) a phantom with 12 nylon wires with diameters between 0.08 mm and 0.4 mm embedded in a paraffin slab of size 60 mm × 60 mm × 20 mm, and (c) a paraffin phantom (60 mm × 60 mm × 28 mm) filled with water spheres. Photos of these phantoms are shown in Fig. 1.

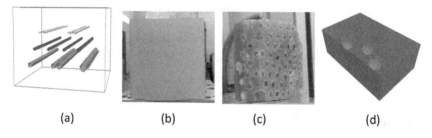

(a)   (b)   (c)   (d)

Fig. 1. Photographs and sketches of the physical phantoms used in the experimental work: (a) arrangements of the nylon fibers with diameters ranging from 0.08 mm to 0.40 mm; (b) phantom with nylon fibers embedded into a paraffin mixture; (c) water spheres embedded within a paraffin slab (d) paraffin phantom with 3 water spheres.

2.2   X-ray Imaging Systems

Images of the physical phantoms were acquired with a GE Senographe SD digital mammography unit featuring a detector with a pixel size of 0.1 mm × 0.1 mm and fully automatic exposure. The tube voltage was 28 kV (Mo/Rh), the source to detector distance was 660 mm, while the incident exposure depended from the phantom thickness (adjusted automatically). The three phantoms were also imaged at the ID17 ESRF [2]. The distance between the accumulation-ring source and the detector was about 155 m. The imaging protocol included acquisition of two images of each sample: one in PhC mode and one in absorption mode. To obtain a PhC image, the sample was placed approximately 11 meters far from the detector. To obtain pure attenuation type of images, the sample was moved as close as possible to the detector. Due to geometry limitations (mechanical construction of the sample carrying platform and the detector holder) the minimum distance was 17 cm. Changing the sample location, while keeping the detector position fixed with respect to the one of the source guaranteed the same x-ray beam properties, while obtaining the two different type of images.

At ESRF, the detector was a high resolution, fast readout low noise 'FReLoN' CCD camera with 2048×2048 pixels and pixel size of 47 μm $\times$ 47 μm.

3   Results and Discussion

Images of the paraffin phantom (Fig. 1d) with the three water spheres acquired with the three different setups are shown in Fig. 2a–c, along with corresponding normalized intensity profiles (Fig. 2d–f), taken across the images of the central sphere.

It can be observed that the images acquired with the dedicated mammography unit and the one acquired at the ID17 in absorption mode are similar in their visual appearance. The evaluation of the corresponding profiles that were taken across the middle sphere, however, shows signal enhancement at the edges of these spheres in the case of the synchrotron beam (SR) beam (Fig. 2b) compared to the conventional radiographic image (Fig. 2a). This is expected, since the use of SR beams results in sharper edges of the features on the images [3] mainly due to the slit geometry that results in scatter rejection as well as elimination of the soft x-rays that are present in the polychromatic spectrum of the conventional mammography unit. The image acquired in a PhC mode (Fig. 2c) shows much more details which were not visible in images acquired in absorption mode.

The water spheres in PhC images are characterized by improved contrast and visualization due to the edge enhancement as a consequence of the fringes around the details. At the same time, the small air bubbles are very well visualized in this PhC mode, while in contrary, they fail to be visualized on images acquired in absorption mode. This is well seen in the normalized intensity profiles, integrated vertically over four lines from the corresponding digital images. The visibility of object edge, calculated from these two profiles, as $V_{edge} = (S_{max} - S_{min})/(S_{max} + S_{min})$ [4], with S_{max} and S_{min} denoting the maximum and the minimum signal intensities, respectively, observed in the region of the sphere border was 12 % in PhC mode, while in the absorption mode, calculated only for the SR setup, this value was 2 %.

The benefits of the PhC effects are obviously in enhancing the borders between the different tissues. That is why a specific figure of merit is introduced (the edge contrast) and used to quantify the impact. For the used phantoms such enhancement is expected. In reality, the transition from healthy to malignant tissues is smoother and such a significant improvement would probably not be observed. This needs to be confirmed in practice and it is planned as a part of the currently running Maxima project [5]. For microcalcifications though, the PhC effect is expected to improve the detectability significantly.

Regions of interest from the radiographic images acquired from the paraffin phantom with the twelve nylon wires (Fig. 1a, b) are shown in Fig. 3a–c. It can be observed that

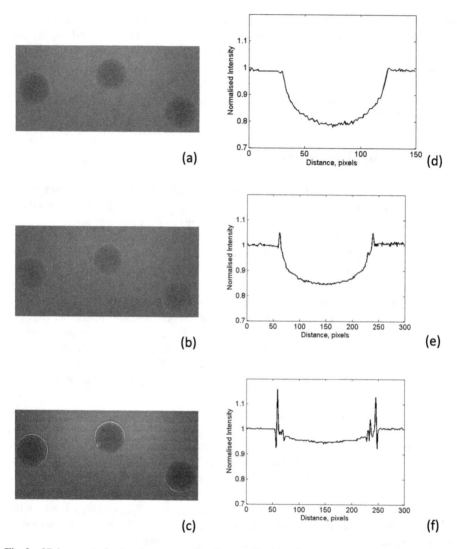

Fig. 2. 2D images (a, b, c) and corresponding line profiles (d, e, f) (taken across the middle sphere) of the paraffin slab with the three water-based spheres. The images were acquired with (a) a GE Senographe unit at 28 kV, and (b, c) at the ESRF beamline ID17 at 25 keV.

the visible nylon wires on the radiograph obtained from the conventional mammography system were these with a diameter between 0.25 mm and 0.4 mm (Fig. 3a). The image obtained at absorption mode on the SR facility shows improved visualization of these nylon wires as well as some other nylon wires were visible (Fig. 3b). Specifically, nylon fibers with diameters greater than 0.2 mm were well visualized. The nylon fibers with a diameter between 0.16 mm and 0.2 mm were slightly visible, while these with a diameter smaller than 0.16 mm were not visually depicted. The image, acquired in a PhC mode (Fig. 3c) is characterized with great nylon wire contrast improvement compared to the previous two images. All nylon wires were very well visualized. It should be noted that the incident dose was approximately equivalent in all cases. The quantitative analysis in terms of a comparison of profiles taken across the image confirms that the use of PhC setup results in higher image quality compared to the absorption setup realized either at SR facility or at conventional mammography units.

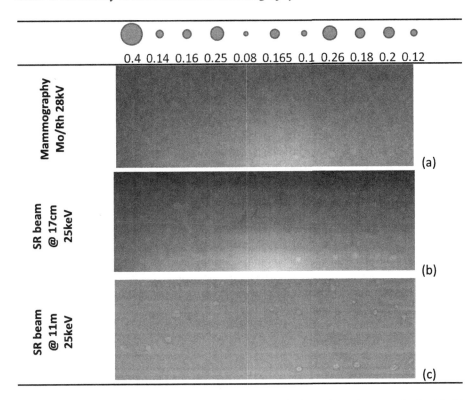

Fig. 3. Projection images of the paraffin phantom with the nylon wires acquired with (a) polychromatic 28 kVp Mo/Rh, and monochromatic 25 keV in (b) absorption and (c) PhC modes.

Figure 4 shows the comparison of 2D images obtained in absorption and PhC modes for the heterogeneous paraffin phantom shown in Fig. 1c. The visibility of the features, i.e. the water based spheres in the paraffin phantom and especially the edges are much improved in a PhC mode (Fig. 4c) compared to the images acquired in the absorption mode, which demonstrate similar visual appearance.

The design of this phantom included paraffin container filled with water spheres. The combination used in this phantom may be suitable for preparing physical phantoms dedicated to phase contrast studies.

Linear attenuation coefficient and refractive index decrement of paraffin-wax have been evaluated to be close to the corresponding coefficients of the adipose tissues for monoenergetic beam of 25 keV. The values for μ and δ are 0.3 cm^{-1} and 3.55×10^{-7}, respectively. Besides, the paraffin is handled more easily compared to other materials

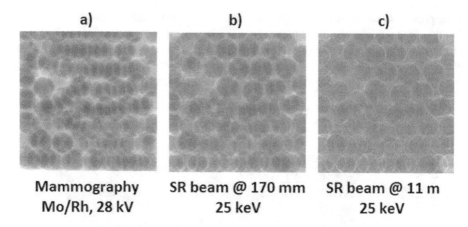

a)   b)   c)

Mammography   **SR beam @ 170 mm**   **SR beam @ 11 m**
Mo/Rh, 28 kV   **25 keV**   **25 keV**

Fig. 4. Projection images of the paraffin phantom with the nylon wires acquired with (a) polychromatic 28 kVp Mo/Rh, and monochromatic 25 keV in (b) absorption and (c) PhC modes.

like the epoxy resin with fewer defects that may be introduced during their manufacturing. Paraffin wax has an elemental composition of 15 % H and 85 % C, while the density is 0.93 g/cm^3. It can be used successfully to mimic the adipose in a physical phantom dedicated for phase contrast effects in future studies.

Development of a dedicated phantom for further research in this field is necessary. We are currently investigating the most appropriate materials to be used for the production of such a phantom. Amongst them are also epoxy resins, polylactide, leaf lard, as well as a mixture of epoxy and silver particles. Preliminary phantoms have been already developed (basic material is from lard-Fig. 5a, b and paraffin-Fig. 5c) and scanned at CT facility (Fig. 5, second row).

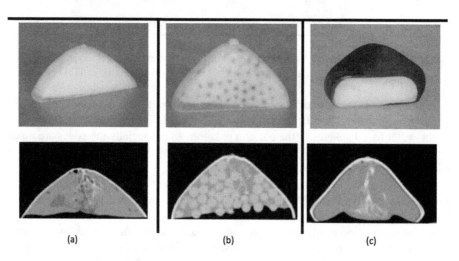

(a)   (b)   (c)

Fig. 5. In-house developed breast phantoms (upper row) and their tomograms shown in the second row.

Further development and optimisation of such phantoms will include the use of modelling and simulation. These approaches will accelerate the process of development of a suitable physical phantom for phase contrast imaging.

4   Conclusions

This paper presented a comparative study of images from ad-hoc phantoms obtained at conventional mammography unit and at SR facility in both, absorption and PhC mode. Comparison of 2D images showed that images obtained in a PhC mode depicts much more details than the images acquired in absorption mode at the synchrotron and the conventional x-ray mammography unit. Results will be exploited in the development of a dedicated phantom for phase contrast studies as well as for setting a future experimental setup for phase contrast tomosynthesis.

Acknowledgments. This research has been supported by Marie Curie Career Integration Grant within the 7th European Community Framework Programme, PHASETOMO (PCIG09-GA-2011-293846) and the MaXIMA project from the H2020-TWINN-2015. The ESRF (Grenoble, France) is acknowledged for the provision of beam time at ID17 and for financial support for four authors (K.B., I.B., G.M. and P.R.).

References

1. Vedantham, S., Karellas, A.: X-ray phase contrast imaging of the breast: analysis of tissue simulating materials. Med. Phys. **40**(4), 041906 (2013)
2. European Synchrotron Radiation Facility, ID17 - Biomedical Beamline Microbeam Radiation Therapy (MRT) Station (filtered white beam and pink beam)/Imaging and Therapy Station (monochromatic)
3. Malliori, A., Bliznakova, K., Sechopoulos, I., Kamarianakis, Z., Fei, B., Pallikarakis, N.: Breast tomosynthesis with monochromatic beams: a feasibility study using Monte Carlo simulations. Phys. Med. Biol. **59**(16), 4681–4696 (2014)
4. Pagot, E., Fiedler, S., Cloetens, P., Bravin, A., Coan, P., Fezzaa, K., Baruchel, J., Hartwig, J.: Quantitative comparison between two phase contrast techniques: diffraction enhanced imaging and phase propagation imaging. Phys. Med. Biol. **50**, 709–724 (2005)
5. MaXIMA: Three dimensional breast cancer Models for X-ray IMAging research, H2020-TWINN-2015 (No. 692097); 1/01/2016 - 31/12/2018. www.maxima-tuv.org

Image Quality and Radiation Dose in Propagation Based Phase Contrast Mammography with a Microfocus X-ray Tube: A Phantom Study

Roberta Castriconi[1,2]($\boxtimes$), Giovanni Mettivier[1,2], and Paolo Russo[1,2]

[1] Dipartimento di Fisica "Ettore Pancini",
Università di Napoli Federico II, Naples, Italy
[2] INFN Sezione di Napoli, Naples, Italy
{castriconi,mettivier,russo}@na.infn.it

Abstract. Digital mammography has limitations in sensitivity, in particular for patients with a dense breast. Phase contrast techniques (phase contrast mammography, PCM) might increase the tissue contrast for breast imaging. Propagation based PCM with a dedicated 0.1-mm-focal spot size mammography unit was investigated in past years, showing higher image quality in magnification PCM than in absorption based DM. In this work the authors investigated, using breast phantoms, the dependence of image quality on increasing mean glandular dose with a 0.007-mm-focal spot size W-anode microfocus X-ray tube. They compared PCM imaging (magnification $M \cong 2$) to absorption based contact imaging ($M \cong 1$) and then to phase retrieval for phase imaging, at low (40 kV) as well as high (80 kV) beam energy. Phase imaging shows higher image contrast for glandular masses and microcalcifications with MGD similar to one-view mammography. The phase contrast power spectrum assumes higher values than for absorption imaging. Possibility of dose reduction was suggested by the adoption of phase retrieval PCM.

Keywords: Phase contrast · Mammography · Mean glandular dose

1 Introduction

Digital mammography (DM) has limitations in sensitivity, in particular for patients with a dense breast. Indeed, in the mammographic energy range, tumor tissue has an attenuation coefficient at photon energy E, $\mu(E)$, close within a few percent to that of normal glandular tissue. The use of phase contrast techniques in DM (phase contrast mammography, PCM) might be viewed as a means of increasing the tissue contrast, relying on the energy dependent differences in the refractive index decrement, $\delta(E)$, of adipose, glandular and tumor breast tissues, rather than on glandular/tumor tissue contrast determined by differences in attenuation index $\beta(E) \propto \mu(E)/E$. Various techniques and contrast-generating effects have been proposed for PCM; they aim ultimately at retrieving the 3D phase map inside tissues via measurements of phase shifts ϕ (e.g. using X-ray grid interferometry), or phase-shift gradients $\nabla\phi$ (as in diffraction-enhanced imaging) or the transverse Laplacian of phase shift $\nabla^2\phi$ (as in propagation based

© Springer International Publishing Switzerland 2016
A. Tingberg et al. (Eds.): IWDM 2016, LNCS 9699, pp. 618–624, 2016.
DOI: 10.1007/978-3-319-41546-8_77

imaging) along ray paths drawn from the source through the object. The field of phase-contrast breast imaging has been reviewed recently [1]. The "superior sharpness" of the phase-contrast propagation based technique is due to the edge enhancement effect, so that the boundary of normal and tumor tissues may be better delineated with respect to the same mammogram acquired with the breast in contact with the detector [2]. This condition has been investigated in PCM with synchrotron radiation, which "… depicts normal structures and abnormal findings with higher image quality with respect to conventional digital mammography" [3]. For clinical applications, propagation based PCM with a dedicated 0.1-mm-focal spot size mammography unit has been investigated in past years [2], using a magnification factor, M, of 1.75, showing higher image quality in PCM than in absorption based DM. In this work, following a preliminary report [4], the authors investigated with breast phantoms the dependence on the calculated mean glandular dose (MGD) of image quality parameters in PCM with a 0.007-mm focal-spot size microfocus X-ray tube, in PCM imaging ($M \cong 2$) compared to absorption based contact imaging ($M \cong 1$) (i.e. in the absence of phase contrast effects) and then using phase retrieval for phase imaging, at low as well as high beam energy.

2   Methods

The authors' setup for propagation based PCM employs a microfocus X-ray tube (Hamamatsu L8121-03, 7 µm focal spot size, W anode, 1.58 mm Al additional filtration, 40 kV/250 µA or 80 kV/125 µA) and a CMOS CsI:Tl flat-panel detector (Hamamatsu C4792CA-002) with 50 µm pitch (Fig. 1a). 2D projection images were acquired at 40 and at 80 kV, of two mammographic phantoms (the homogeneous phantom CIRS BR50/50 014AD Fig. 2b, and the heterogeneous phantom CIRS BR3D 020 Fig. 2c). The first phantom is for quality control in mammography and the second phantom for breast tomosynthesis test. Given the magnifications and the focal spot size, the ratio L_{shear}/L_{coh} between the shearing length after the sample and the lateral coherence length of the incident beam, is between 10^{-3} and 10^{-2} for details of spatial frequency of 5 mm^{-1}: these values are $\ll 1$ and indicate that phase-contrast effects may be visible in the authors' setup [5] (Fig. 2). Images were acquired (a) with the phantom in contact with the detector (*absorption image* with magnification $M \cong 1$); (b) in a geometry with an image magnification $M \cong 2$ (*phase contrast image*). We retrieved the phase map (*phase image*) of the test objects (at 40 or at 80 kV) taken under phase contrast conditions, using the ANKAphase algorithm [6], assuming global homogeneity of the samples and uniformity of the ratio δ/β in the phantom volume. For phase retrieval, values of δ and β for 50/50 breast tissue were calculated from CSIRO CSS at the effective energies 28 keV and 42 keV (in 50/50 breast tissue) for the 40-kV and 80-kV beam spectra, respectively ($\delta/\beta \cong 2200$) (https://www.ts-imaging.net/Services/Simple/Default.aspx).

The effective energies were derived from attenuation measurements, which gave attenuation coefficient of BR50/50 of 0.369 cm^{-1} (40 kV) and 0.241 cm^{-1} (80 kV), respectively. The MGD calculated for a single exposure frame of the CIRS 014AD phantom was 0.00916 mGy (40 kV) or 0.0208 mGy (80 kV); values of 0.733 mGy/mGy (40 kV) and 0.968 mGy/mGy (80 kV) were assumed for the normalized glandular dose coefficient for 50/50 breast tissue. By taking the running sum of 100

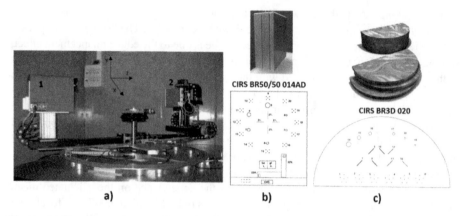

Fig. 1. (a) Experimental setup (1 – microfocus X-ray tube; 2 – CMOS flat panel detector). (b) Test object (CIRS 014AD), 5-cm BR50/50 thickness. (c) Test object (CIRS BR3D 020), 5-cm BR50/50 thickness. Both test objects contain a slab with details (microcalcification clusters, masses, fibers) of various size, as indicated in the corresponding schemes.

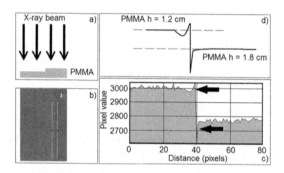

Fig. 2. Showing the presence of edge-enhancement effects in the experimental setup at 40 kV and $M \cong 2$. (a) Irradiation geometry; (b) phase-contrast radiography of the PMMA sharp step-edge; (c) average horizontal line profile across the ROI 1 indicated in (b), showing edge enhancement across the edge as shown by the black arrows; (d) schematization of the line profile indicating effects of phase contrast due to X-ray refraction at the edge boundary (Rayleigh scattering), slight Compton scattering toward the side of the thicker PMMA slab, and spectral energy dependence of the X-ray refraction towards the thinner side. Incident air kerma = 0.39 mGy. Pixel size = 0.050 mm.

consecutive flat-panel image frames the authors simulated the acquisition of variable-dose images up to a total MGD of 0.916 mGy (40 kV) and MGD = 2.208 mGy (80 kV), for as many as 100 dose values. For the CIRS BR3D phantom total doses of 2.9 mGy MGD ($M \cong 1$ or $M \cong 2$) and 1.6 mGy ($M \cong 2$) were used. Image quality parameters (CNR, dose normalized CNR, SNR) were evaluated in a region of interests (ROI) of 5-mm diameter, as a function of the MGD in both geometries: absorption imaging ($M \cong 1$) and phase contrast imaging ($M \cong 2$) at 40 and 80 kV. The same parameters were then evaluated for the retrieved phase maps. The CNR was evaluated for a detail with respect to the background BR50/50 material, as

$[\sqrt{2}(\mu_d - \mu_{bkg})/(s_d^2 + s_{bkg}^2)]$, where (μ, σ) indicate mean and standard deviation of pixel values in the ROI, respectively. The SNR was calculated as $[\sqrt{n}(\mu_d - \mu_{bkg})/\sigma_{bkg}]$, where n is the number of pixels in the ROI. Then, the 2D Power Spectrum (PS) of the images was calculated; the 1D radial profile extracted from this spectrum was compared in the various acquisition modalities.

3 Results

Figure 3 shows the CNR as a function of MGD for a 100 % fibroglandular rectangular area (5-mm detail thickness CIRS 014AD), as well as the CNRD = CNR/$\sqrt{MGD}$ and the SNR at 40 kV (a, c, e) and 80 kV (b, d, f), respectively. For both kilovoltages, at all

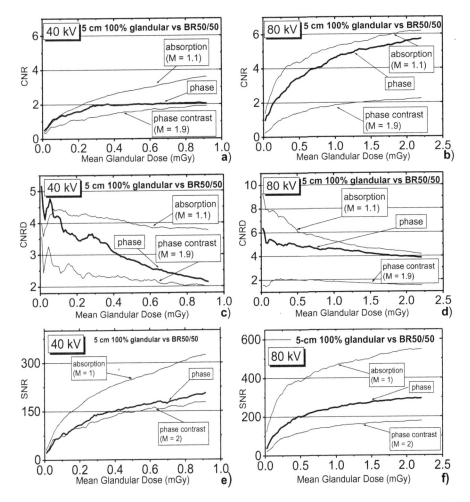

Fig. 3. CNR (a, b), CNRD (c, d) and SNR (e, f) as a function of MGD in a circular ROI of 5 mm diameter in CIRS 014AD phantom for 100 % fibroglandular rectangular area of (5-mm thick detail) vs. BR50/50 tissue at 40 kV (a, c, e) and 80 kV (b, d, f), respectively.

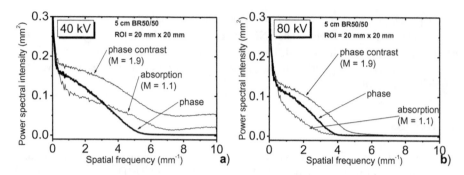

Fig. 4. Power spectrum in a square ROI of 20 mm side which contains rectangular areas of 100 % fibroglandular and 100 % of adipose tissue, at (a) 40 kV, and (b) 80 kV, respectively.

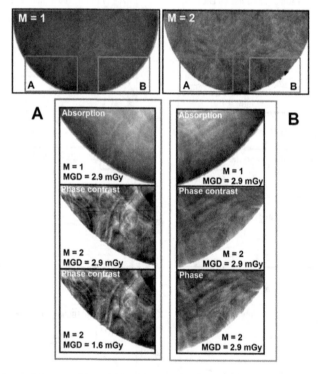

Fig. 5. 2D views of the test object BR3D 020 at different magnification, M (at 80 kV). Panel A and B show two regions of interest of the phantom at the same MGD value of 2.9 mGy for image with $M = 1$ and $M = 2$, as well as the same image with $M = 2$ acquired at a lower MGD value of 1.6 mGy. In panel B the same region B is viewed in absorption, in phase contrast and after phase retrieval, at constant MGD.

MGD values the image quality parameters are higher for absorption than for phase and phase contrast images, due to lower exposure on the detector at fixed MGD values. However, phase retrieval allows to reach higher CNR, CNRD and SNR than in raw phase contrast imaging. Figure 4a and b show the 1D Power Spectrum (evaluated in a square ROI of 20 mm side which contains rectangular areas of 100 % fibroglandular and 100 % of adipose tissue in CIRS 014AD) at 40 kV and 80 kV, respectively. The phase contrast PS is highest at both kilovoltages, revealing the role of edge-enhancement effect in phase contrast imaging. Up to 3 mm^{-1} the PS for phase images shows higher values than for absorption images, independently of kilovoltage. Figure 5 shows the different appearance of absorption based ($M \cong 1$) and phase contrast imaging ($M \cong 2$), at equal MGD values, with a higher conspicuity of masses; lowering the dose from 2.9 mGy to 1.6 mGy does not significantly alter the visibility of details in BR3D heterogeneous phantom (6.3 mm and 4.7 mm diameter spheroidal masses). As regards microcalcifications, they are visibile with higher contrast in phase contrast than in absorption imaging (Fig. 6a, b); moreover, for this heterogeneous BR3D mod. 020 BR50/50 breast phantom, the SNR for the largest masses (6.3 mm diameter) in phase contrast approaches that of absorption imaging, at increasing MGD values (Fig. 6c).

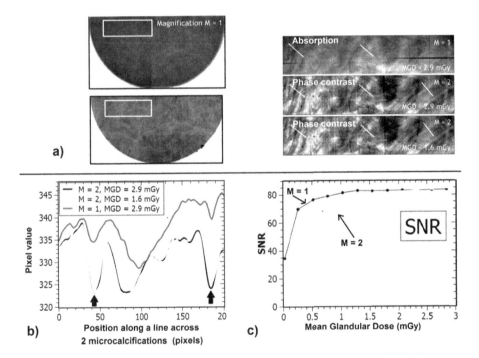

Fig. 6. Microcalcifications visibility in the CIRS BR3D phantom. (a) In the ROI indicated by the rectangles, images at $M \cong 2$ (phase contrast) reveal higher contrast of microcalcification clusters than at $M \cong 1$ (absorption). (b) Line profiles across two largest microcalcifications (CaCO$_3$ specks 0.4 mm size), whose position is indicated by the arrows. Higher contrast of microcalcifications is present at $M \cong 2$. (c) SNR as a function of the mean glandular dose. (Color figure online)

4 Conclusions

In conclusion, image quality parameters are higher for contact (absorption only) imaging rather than for phase contrast imaging and phase imaging, due to lower exposure on the detector, at any fixed value of MGD. The presence of the phase effects leads to an increase of the image contrast for model glandular masses and for microcalcifications with MGD similar to one-view mammography. This is in particular present for the locally heterogeneous phantom, where the presence of interleaved glandular and fat mimicking epoxy resin materials gives rise to better visibility of details in PCM than in contact imaging. The phase contrast power spectrum assumes higher values than for absorption imaging, revealing the role of edge-enhancement effects in phase contrast imaging. Phase contrast imaging with $M \cong 2$ magnification produces better visibility of mass and microcalcification details in a heterogeneous breast phantom, than with contact imaging ($M \cong 1$); moreover, phase contrast allowed to reduce the dose to the phantom without apparent deterioration of the detail visibility for masses and for microcalcifications.

References

1. Auweter, S.D., et al.: X-ray phase-contrast imaging of the breast—advances towards clinical implementation. Br. J. Radiol. **87**, 1–8 (2014)
2. Matsuo, S., Fujita, H., Morishita, J., Katafuchi, T., Honda, C., Sugiyama, J.: Preliminary evaluation of a phase contrast imaging with digital mammography. In: Krupinski, E.A. (ed.) IWDM 2008. LNCS, vol. 5116, pp. 130–136. Springer, Heidelberg (2008)
3. Longo, R., et al.: Clinical study in phase-contrast mammography: image-quality analysis. Philos. Trans. R. Soc. A **372** (2014). 2013.0025
4. Russo, P., et al.: Phase contrast mammography: a phantom study. In: Poster Presented at 8th Congress of AIFM, 16–19 November, Torino, Italy (2013)
5. Wu, X., Liu, H.: Clarification of aspects in in-line phase-sensitive x-ray imaging. Med. Phys. **34**, 737–743 (2007)
6. Weitkamp, T., et al.: ANKAphase: software for single-distance phase retrieval from inline X-ray phase-contrast radiographs. J. Synchrotron. Rad. **18**, 617–629 (2011)

Phase-Contrast Clinical Breast CT: Optimization of Imaging Setups and Reconstruction Workflows

Giuliana Tromba[1](✉), Serena Pacilè[1,2], Yakov I. Nesterets[3], Francesco Brun[1,2],
Christian Dullin[4], Diego Dreossi[1], Sheridan C. Mayo[3], Andrew W. Stevenson[3,5],
Konstantin M. Pavlov[6,7], Markus J. Kitchen[7], Darren Thompson[4,6],
Jeremy M.C. Brown[7], Darren Lockie[8], Maura Tonutti[9], Fulvio Stacul[9],
Fabrizio Zanconati[10], Agostino Accardo[2], and T.E. Gureyev[3,6,7,11]

[1] Elettra - Sincrotrone Trieste, Basovizza (Trieste), Italy
giuliana.tromba@elettra.eu
[2] Department of Engineering and Architecture, University of Trieste, Trieste, Italy
[3] Commonwealth Scientific and Industrial Research Organisation, Melbourne, Australia
[4] Department of Diagnostic and Interventional Radiology, University Hospital Göttingen,
Göttingen, Germany
[5] Australian Synchrotron, Melbourne, Australia
[6] School of Science and Technology, University of New England, Armidale, Australia
[7] School of Physics and Astronomy, Monash University, Melbourne, Australia
[8] Maroondah Breast Screen, Melbourne, Australia
[9] Department of Radiology, AOU - Trieste Hospital, Trieste, Italy
[10] Department of Medical Science-Unit of Pathology, University of Trieste, Trieste, Italy
[11] ARC Centre of Excellence in Advanced Molecular Imaging, School of Physics,
University of Melbourne, Parkville, Australia

Abstract. We present the outcomes of combined feasibility studies carried out at Elettra and Australian Synchrotron to evaluate novel protocols for three-dimensional (3D) mammographic phase contrast imaging. A custom designed plastic phantom and some tissue samples have been studied at diverse resolution scales and experimental conditions. Several computed tomography (CT) reconstruction algorithms with different pre-processing and post-processing steps have been considered. Special attention was paid to the effect of phase retrieval on the diagnostic value of the reconstructed images. The images were quantitatively evaluated using objective quality indices in comparison with subjective assessments performed by three experienced radiologists and one pathologist.

We show that the propagation-based phase-contrast imaging (PBI) leads to substantial improvement to the contrast-to-noise and to the intrinsic quality of the reconstructed CT images compared with conventional techniques as well as to an important reduction of the delivered doses, thus opening the way to clinical implementations.

Keywords: X-rays · Phase contrast · Computed tomography · Mammography · Synchrotron radiation · Breast CT

© Springer International Publishing Switzerland 2016
A. Tingberg et al. (Eds.): IWDM 2016, LNCS 9699, pp. 625–634, 2016.
DOI: 10.1007/978-3-319-41546-8_78

1   Introduction

In the current medical practice, two-dimensional (2D) X-ray mammography is the main examination for the diagnosis of breast cancer. Despite the great advances due to the introduction of more sensitive detectors and novel X-ray generators, the technique still produces a relatively high percentage of both false-positive and false-negative results [1].

The recently implemented digital tomosynthesis opened new perspectives for its ability to produce multiple 2D slices through the breast and reduces the camouflaging effect due to overlap of different tissue layers that takes place in projection X-ray imaging [2, 3]. However, the most attractive 3D approach remains computed tomography (CT). Breast CT has the important advantage to reduce the physical discomfort experienced by patients due to the painful compression of the breast in conventional mammography [4, 5] and to give a real 3D representation of the breast characteristics.

A few dedicated breast CT prototypes are in clinical use worldwide [6, 7] with very promising results. Similarly to conventional radiology, the main limit in this approach is the low absorption contrast between normal (fibrous) and abnormal tissue.

Phase-contrast techniques can have an important role in this framework. Feasibility studies [8] already showed the effectiveness of analyser-based CT (AB-CT) in the improved detection of tumours with a smaller radiation dose, compared to current clinical mammography. At the same time, recent studies [9–15] have shown that, alternative X-ray phase-contrast imaging methods, such as the propagation-based phase-contrast tomography (PB-CT), can deliver outcomes comparable to AB-CT in regards to image quality and dose, while being potentially simpler and cheaper to implement.

The aim of this work is to provide a path to clinical implementation of low-dose high-quality 3D mammographic imaging, which will result in improved breast cancer diagnosis, substantial reductions in radiation dose and removal of patient pain.

2   Materials and Methods

2.1   Experiments at the Australian Synchrotron

We have conducted in-line (propagation-based) phase-contrast CT imaging experiments [14] at the Imaging and Medical beamline (IMBL) of the Australian Synchrotron [16]. The detector used was a Hamamatsu CMOS Flat Panel Sensor C9252DK-14, utilised in partial scan mode, with the pixel size 100 μm $\times$ 100 μm, 1174 $\times$ 99 pixels (H $\times$ V) field of view and 12-bit output. The detector has a CsI scintillator directly deposited on a 2D photodiode array.

A specially designed and fabricated phantom was used in this experiment. The phantom consisted of a cylindrical block made of polycarbonate, with the diameter of 10 cm and the height of 2 cm, having eight irregularly located cylindrical holes of 1 cm diameter, each filled with different substances: glycerol, $CaCl_2$ 1 M, ethanol 35 v%, paraffin oil, water, fatty ham, meaty ham and fibrous ham. The sample was imaged with monochromatic X-rays at three energies: 38 keV, 45 keV and 50 keV. The sample rotation-axis to detector distance (sample-to-detector distance, for short), R2, was set to one of four values including 27 cm, 1 m, 2 m and 5 m.

CT data analysis (including pre-processing of data, CT reconstruction and optional post-processing) was carried out using X-TRACT software [17]. It is well acknowledged [11] that phase retrieval using an algorithm based on the homogeneous transport of intensity equation (TIE-HOM) [18] results, in general, in reduced noise in reconstructed CT slices while preserving the sharpness of the edges when used with a proper regularization (δ/β) parameter. We applied the TIE-HOM algorithm to projection data sets and subsequently carried out FBP CT reconstruction. In order to restrict the absorbed dose to values currently accepted for standard mammographic screening, we restricted the number of projections to 361 over 180°. The mean glandular doses (MGDs), D, per complete CT scans, were between 4.7 mGy and 10.8 mGy, depending on the imaging parameters.

2.2 Experiments at Elettra

In-line phase-contrast CT imaging experiments [13] have been carried out also at the SYRMEP imaging beamline of the Elettra synchrotron light source [19]. The detector used for low dose scans was a Dalsa Argus CCD TDI sensor with a pixel size of 27 μm and a maximum X-ray resolution up to 15 lp/mm. The detector used for the high resolution scans was a water-cooled CCD camera by Photonic Science, model VHR, 4008×2672 full frame, used in 2×2 binning mode (resulting in pixel size of 9 μm), coupled to a gadolinium oxysulfide scintillator placed on a fiber optic taper.

A large tissue specimen excised during a surgical mastectomy was scanned at high and low statistics using the Dalsa detector at 32 keV with a sample-to detector distance of 18 cm and 2 m. A centimeter size tissue sample containing a small lesion was scanned at higher resolution (using the Photonic Science detector) at 20 keV with sample-to-detector distances of 4 cm (simulating absorption), 30, 100 and 166 cm.

Datasets have been reconstructed using the SYRMEP Tomo Project (STP) in-house developed software [20] using several different reconstruction algorithms such as: Filtered Back Projection (FBP) [21], Simultaneous Iterative Reconstruction Technique (SIRT) [22], Simultaneous Algebraic Reconstruction Technique (SART) [23], Conjugate Gradient Least Squares (CGLS) [22], Equally Sloped Tomography (EST) [24], Total Variation (TV) minimization [25] and an iterative FBP algorithm [26]. Like for the Australian experiment a phase retrieval (phr) algorithm was applied prior to the actual reconstruction by processing each projection independently, in accordance with the TIE-HOM algorithm [18]. For each of the above approaches images were reconstructed with and without application of phase retrieval pre-processing.

2.3 Quantitative Evaluation of the Images: Objectives Quality Indexes and Radiological Assessment

Reconstructed images for the mastectomy sample were quantitatively evaluated using several full-reference and no-reference image quality assessment indexes [27]. Full references indexes require the definition of a certain 'reference image' that in our case is the one obtained by applying the FBP reconstruction algorithm to the high statistics scan using all available projections. The considered full reference indexes were: Mean Squared Error (MSE), Signal-to-Noise Ratio (SNR), Universal Quality Index (UQI) [28], Noise Quality Measure (NQM) [29] and Structural Similarity Index (SSIM) [27]. Apart from the MSE index, higher values of SNR, UQI, NQM and SSIM correspond to higher image quality.

The no-references indexes used were: the Contrast-to-Noise ratio (CNR), the Full Width Half Maximum (FWHM) and the dimensionless no-reference intrinsic quality characteristic Qs which incorporates both the noise propagation and the spatial resolution properties of a linear system [12, 30]. Since the evaluation of FWHM requires a well-defined image edge, this index was evaluated by considering the images of the polycarbonate phantom sample and analyzing the line profiles at the interface between the background and one of the details [13].

CT scans of the mastectomy sample, carried out at clinical dose, were also assigned with subjective radiological scores provided by three experienced radiologists and one pathologist who expressed a blind opinion about the recognition of the lesion borders and their spiculations, the visibility of small connective residues included in the adipose tissue, the perceived contrast and spatial resolution. A global score was given from 0, for the worst case to 4, for the best image, i.e. the above defined 'reference image'. On the basis of these scores, the images were then classified into three categories: no-diagnostic power (radiological score from 0 to 2), where the lesion characterization is difficult to be done; poor diagnostic power (radiological score higher than 2 to 3), i.e. it would be possible to diagnose the tumour but without an accurate evaluation of spiculations and/or connective residues existing in the tissue; and full diagnostic power (radiological score higher than 3), where all the relevant features are detectable and quantifiable.

3   Results

3.1   Outcomes from the IMBL Experiment

CT scans at the Australian Synchrotron were conducted at clinical doses and were focused to reveal the presence of phase effects, despite the large pixel size of the Hamamatsu detector widely used for conventional clinical imaging, and to evaluate the improvements of the image quality with respect to absorption images.

One reconstructed (using TIE-HOM phase retrieval with $\gamma = 1000$) CT slice from low photon statistics data (361 projections over 180°), corresponding to the X-ray energy of 38 keV, for four values of the sample-to-detector distance (0.27 m, 1 m, 2 m and 5 m) is shown in Fig. 1 together with its magnified fragments. Some quantitative image quality parameters, including the SNR per unit dose, $SNR/D^{1/2}$, and the intrinsic quality characteristic, $Qs = SNR/D^{1/2}/(Spatial\ resolution)$ [30], for four values of the propagation distance and using phase retrieval, are summarized in Table 1.

Table 1. Quality characteristics of CT slices reconstructed (using FBP) from phase-retrieved (using TIE-HOM).

Material	$R_2 = 0.27m^{b)}$		$R_2 = 1m$		$R_2 = 2m$		$R_2 = 5m$	
	SNR $/ D^{1/2}$ (mGy$^{1/2}$)	$Q_s \times 10^4$ (μm^{-1}mGy$^{1/2}$)	SNR $/ D^{1/2}$ (mGy$^{1/2}$)	$Q_s \times 10^4$ (μm^{-1}mGy$^{1/2}$)	SNR $/ D^{1/2}$ (mGy$^{1/2}$)	$Q_s \times 10^4$ (μm^{-1}mGy$^{1/2}$)	SNR $/ D^{1/2}$ (mGy$^{1/2}$)	$Q_s \times 10^4$ (μm^{-1}mGy$^{1/2}$)
Polycarbonate	1.73±0.02	122±1	3.46±0.03	217±2	4.71±0.04	283±2	6.98±0.06	402±3
Glycerol	2.54±0.02	179±2	5.33±0.04	333±3	6.84±0.06	406±4	10.01±0.09	576±5
CaCl₂ 1M	3.14±0.03	222±2	6.16±0.05	383±3	8.43±0.07	504±4	11.4±0.1	651±6
Ethanol 35v%	1.81±0.02	128±1	3.66±0.03	232±2	4.67±0.04	280±2	6.73±0.06	385±3
Paraffin oil	1.83±0.02	127±1	3.58±0.03	221±2	4.64±0.04	274±2	6.64±0.06	374±3
Water	2.23±0.02	156±1	4.43±0.04	276±2	5.88±0.05	353±3	8.18±0.07	469±4
Meaty ham	2.21±0.02	157±1	4.44±0.04	289±2	6.15±0.05	387±3	7.90±0.07	463±4

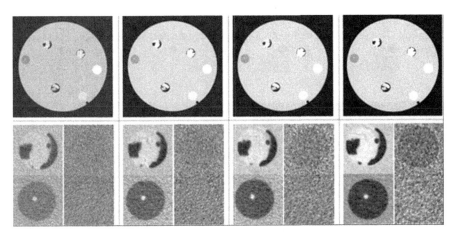

Fig. 1. Effect of phase retrieval on FBP CT reconstruction. The sample-to-detector distance, from left to right: 0.27 m, 1 m, 2 m and 5 m. Estimated Mean Glandular Doses (MGD) were 8.2 mGy, 8.2 mGy, 9.3 mGy and 10.8 mGy, respectively.

3.2 Outcomes from the Elettra Experiment

The first experiment conducted at Elettra was aimed at evaluating and optimizing the effects of phase contrast and phase retrieval in the detection of small malignant lesions in breast tissue specimens. For these purposes, high resolution scans (using the Photonic Science detector) have been performed at different propagation distances and the benefits of applying phase retrieval algorithm for the image quality have been evaluated in comparison with the absorption images. An example is shown in Fig. 2, where a representative slice of the tissue specimen obtained from the scan in absorption modality (a) is compared with the corresponding slice resulting from the phase-contrast scan obtained from phase-retrieved data; delivered doses were 4.8 and 5.8 Gy respectively.

In a quantitative images evaluation, a 20-fold improvement of the image quality-characteristic Qs was found in the phase-retrieved image, which is equivalent to 400-fold reduction of X-ray dose at the same image quality. The second experiment carried

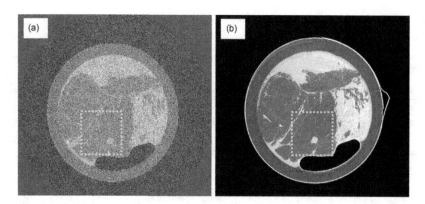

Fig. 2. Representative slice of the tissue specimen from absorption CT scan reconstructed with FBP (a) and phase contrast scan reconstructed with FBP after application of phase retrieval (b). The yellow box highlights a region with a suspect satellite lesion. (Color figure online)

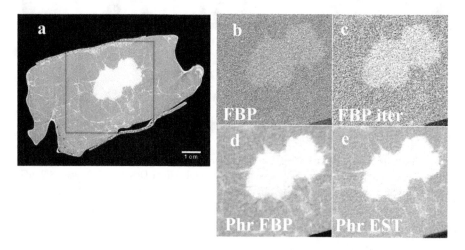

Fig. 3. Reference image for the mastectomy sample (a) and reconstructed images obtained with conventional FBP (b), Iterative FBP (c), Phr + Iterative FBP (d), Phr + EST algorithm (e).

out at Elettra was focused on low-dose CT scans using the Dalsa detector. The purpose of this experiment was to optimize the reconstruction workflow and perform a quantitative comparison of images obtained with different approaches, taking into account, with particular attention, the radiologist's point of view. The considered reference image for the mastectomy sample, including a malignant lesion of about 3 cm with irregular edges, blurred margins and spicules, is shown in Fig. 3a.

This image was obtained at high dose, so that all the features are very well outlined. The red square indicates the region-of-interest (ROI) used for the image quality assessment. The low-dose CT scan, acquired at a MGD of about 1.5 mGy, was then considered, several reconstruction approaches were applied and the respective ROIs were compared. Figure 3b, c show the slices obtained with conventional FBP and Iterative FBP algorithms, respectively, and were assigned by the radiologists to the 'No diagnostic power' class. Slices in Fig. 3d, e were obtained by applying the phase-retrieval pre-processing prior to the Iterative FBP and EST reconstruction respectively: both of them were evaluated in the 'full diagnostic power' class.

The correlation between the objective indexes and the radiological scores obtained for the same sample slice using different reconstruction workflows is shown in Fig. 4. In general, most of the image quality scores are in a good agreement with the radiological assessment, in particular the SSIM trend is the closest one.

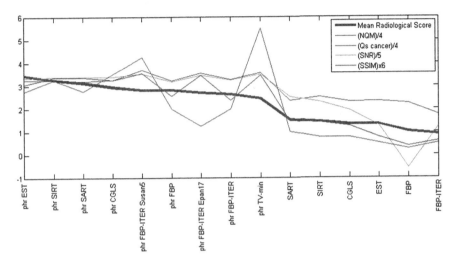

Fig. 4. Correlation between the radiological scores and various image quality indexes (Color figure online)

4   Discussion

Propagation-based phase-contrast CT with the application of phase retrieval using the TIE-HOM method with proper regularization (δ/β) parameter allows one to convert phase-contrast CT images into direct analogues of absorption CT images, while substantially increasing contrast-to-noise ratio without excessive image blurring. In fact, while a slight blurring effect induced by the application of phase retrieval can be perceived, the adoption of high resolution detectors (finer than the ones adopted in the nowadays clinical practice) and the significant benefits in terms of contrast and noise still supports the propagation-based CT approach. This conclusion is also validated by the qualitative evaluation performed by the radiologists. It was observed that the radiological assessment prefers, in all the cases, phase-retrieved images.

When comparing the performance of the same reconstruction algorithm with and without the application of phase retrieval (e.g. SIRT vs. phr SIRT), bigger values (indicating better quality) for the quality indexes like MSE, NQM and SNR were obtained, and similar trend was also found for the considered no-reference indexes CNR and Qs.

Strong improvement of CNR with phase retrieval was found particularly in the high resolution scans: for the small breast tissue specimen, a CNR value of up to 20 times bigger than in conventional CT was obtained at the same radiation dose.

At low dose, the application of phase retrieval makes the CT reconstruction much more effective. An example is shown in Fig. 3, where images reconstructed using FBP iterative algorithm without phase retrieval (Fig. 3c) are considered as having 'no diagnostic power', while the one obtained with the application of phase-retrieval pre-processing (Fig. 3d) has a high clinical quality ('full diagnostic power'). By increasing the propagation distances to several meters, phase effects can be revealed even by a detector with relatively large pixel sizes (of the order of 100 μm), like in the case of Hamamatsu detector. As detectors with larger pixel sizes typically have higher detective quantum efficiency (DQE), compared to high-resolution X-ray detectors, the use of long propagation distances can become a valid possibility to reduce the radiation dose. It has to be pointed out that for this assumption an adequate spatial coherence of the source is required to avoid penumbral blurring: this is the case of synchrotron beamlines as well as last generation microfocus X-ray sources or compact sources.

5   Conclusions

The use of phase contrast and phase retrieval results in significant improvement in the quality of X-ray images of breast tissue. This has been demonstrated in the low-dose scans by evaluating several different quality indexes and considering the radiological assessment.

Low-dose phase-contrast CT images can be obtained with a conventional flat-panel detector having relatively large pixels if large propagation distances are implemented.

The outcomes of this study provide practical guidelines for the optimization of image processing workflows not only for synchrotron-based phase-contrast tomography but can be extended to new generator-based phase-contrast setups (gratings, coded aperture) or compact sources.

References

1. Pisano, E.D., Hendrick, R.E., Yaffe, M.J., Baum, J.K., Acharyya, S., Cormack, J.B., Hanna, L.A., Conant, E.F., Fajardo, L.L., Bassett, L.W., D'Orsi, C.J., Jong, R.A., Rebner, M., Tosteson, A.N.A., Gatsonis, C.A.: Diagnostic accuracy of digital versus film mammography: exploratory analysis of selected population subgroups in DMIST. Radiology 246, 376–383 (2008)
2. Ciatto, S., Houssami, N., Bernardi, D., Caumo, F., Pellegrini, M., Brunelli, S., Tuttobene, P., Bricolo, P., Fantò, C., Valentini, M., Montemezzi, S., Macaskill, P.: Integration of 3D digital mammography with tomosynthesis for population breast-cancer screening (STORM): a prospective comparison study. Lancet Oncol. 14, 583–589 (2013)

3. Pisano, E.D., Yaffe, M.J.: Breast cancer screening should tomosynthesis replace digital mammography? JAMA **311**(24), 2488–2489 (2014)
4. De Groot, J.E., Branderhorst, W., Grimbergen, C.A., den Heeten, G.J., Broeders, M.J.: Towards personalized compression in mammography: a comparison study between pressure- and force-standardization. Eur. J. Radiol. **84**(3), 384–391 (2015)
5. Papas, M.A., Klassen, A.C.: Pain and discomfort associated with mammography among urban low-income African-American women. J. Community Health **30**(4), 253–267 (2005)
6. Prionas, N.D., Lindfors, K.K., Ray, S., Huang, S.Y., Beckett, L.A., Monsky, W.L., Boone, J.M.: Contrast enhanced dedicated breast CT: initial clinical experience. Radiology **256**, 714–723 (2010)
7. O'Connell, A.M., Karellas, A., Vedantham, S.: The potential role of dedicated 3D breast CT as a diagnostic tool: review and early clinical examples. Breast J. **20**, 592–605 (2014)
8. Zhao, Y., Brun, E., Coan, P., Huang, Z., Sztrókay, A., Diemoz, P.C., Liebhardt, S., Mittone, A., Gasilov, S., Miao, J., Bravin, A.: High-resolution, low-dose phase contrast X-ray tomography for 3D diagnosis of human breast cancers. Proc. Nat. Acad. Sci. **109**(45), 18290–18294 (2012)
9. Diemoz, P.C., Bravin, A., Langer, M., Coan, P.: Analytical and experimental determination of signal-to-noise ratio and figure of merit in three phase-contrast imaging techniques. Opt. Express **20**, 27670–27690 (2012)
10. Gureyev, T., Mohammadi, S., Nesterets, Y., Dullin, C., Tromba, G.: Accuracy and precision of reconstruction of complex refractive index in near-field single-distance propagation-based phase-contrast tomography. J. Appl. Phys. **114**(14), 144906 (2013)
11. Nesterets, Y.I., Gureyev, T.E.: Noise propagation in X-ray phase-contrast imaging and computed tomography. J. Phys. D Appl. Phys. **47**(10), 105402 (2014)
12. Gureyev, T.E., Mayo, S.C., Nesterets, Y.I., Mohammadi, S., Lockie, D., Menk, R.H., Arfelli, F., Pavlov, K.M., Kitchen, M.J., Zanconati, F., Dullin, C., Tromba, G.: Investigation of the imaging quality of synchrotron-based phase-contrast mammographic tomography. J. Phys. D Appl. Phys. **47**, 365401 (365418 pp) (2014a)
13. Pacilè, S., Brun, F., Dullin, C., Nesterets, Y.I., Dreossi, D., Mohammadi, S., Tonutti, M., Stacul, F., Lockie, D., Zanconati, F., Accardo, A., Tromba, G., Gureyev, T.E.: Clinical application of low-dose phase contrast breast CT: methods for the optimization of the reconstruction workflow. Biomed. Opt. Express **6**, 3099–3112 (2015)
14. Nesterets, Y.I., Gureyev, T.E., Mayo, S.C., Stevenson, A.W., Thompson, D., Brown, J.M., Kitchen, M.J., Pavlov, K.M., Lockie, D., Brun, F., Tromba, G.: A feasibility study of X-ray phase-contrast mammographic tomography at the Imaging and Medical beamline of the Australian Synchrotron. J. Synchrotron Radiat. **22**, 1509–1523 (2015)
15. Longo, R., Arfelli, F., Bellazzini, R., Bottigli, U., Brez, A., Brun, F., Brunetti, A., Delogu, P., Di Lillo, F., Dreossi, D., Fanti, V., Fedon, C., Golosio, B., Lanconelli, N., Mettivier, G., Minuti, M., Oliva, P., Pinchera, M., Rigon, L., Russo, P., Sarno, A., Spandre, G., Tromba, G., Zanconati, Z.: Towards breast tomography with synchrotron radiation at Elettra: first images. Phys. Med. Biol. **61**, 1634–1649 (2016)
16. Stevenson, A.W., Mayo, S.C., Hausermann, D., Maksimenko, A., Garrett, R.F., Hall, C.J., Wilkins, S.W., Lewis, R.A., Myers, D.E.: First experiments on the Australian Synchrotron Imaging and Medical beamline, including investigations of the effective source size in respect of X-ray imaging. J. Synchrotron Radiat. **17**, 75–80 (2010)
17. Gureyev, T.E., Nesterets, Y., Ternovski, D., Thompson, D., Wilkins, S.W., Stevenson, A.W., Sakellariou, A., Taylor, J.A.: Toolbox for advanced X-ray image processing. Proc. SPIE **8141**, 1–14 (2011)

18. Paganin, D., Mayo, S.C., Gureyev, T.E., Miller, P.R., Wilkins, S.W.: "Simultaneous phase and amplitude extraction from a single defocused image of a homogeneous object. J. Microsc. **206**(1), 33–40 (2002)

19. Tromba, G., Longo, R., Abrami, A., Arfelli, F., Astolfo, A., Bregant, P., Brun, F., Casarin, K., Chenda, V., Dreossi, D., Hola, M., Kaiser, J., Mancini, L., Menk, R.H., Quai, E., Quaia, E., Rigon, L., Rokvic, T., Sodini, N., Sanabor, D., Schultke, E., Tonutti, M., Vascotto, A., Zanconati, F., Cova, M., Castelli, E.: The SYRMEP beamline of Elettra: clinical mammography and bio-medical applications. AIP Conf. Proc. **1266**, 18–23 (2010)

20. Brun, F., Pacilè, S., Accardo, A., Kourousias, G., Dreossi, D., Mancini, L., Pugliese, R.: Enhanced and flexible software tools for X-ray computed tomography at the Italian synchrotron radiation facility Elettra. Fundamenta Informaticae **141**(2–3), 233–243 (2015)

21. Kak, A.C., Slaney, M.: Principles of Computerized Tomographic Imaging. IEEE Press, New York (1988)

22. Van der Sluis, A., Van der Vorst, H.: SIRT- and CG-type methods for the iterative solution of sparse linear least-squares problems. Linear Algebra Appl. **130**, 257–303 (1990)

23. Gordon, R., Bender, R., Herman, G.: Algebraic reconstruction techniques (ART) for three-dimensional electron microscopy and X-ray photography. J. Theor. Biol. **29**, 471–476 (1970)

24. Miao, J., Frster, F., Levi, O.: Equally sloped tomography with oversampling reconstruction. Phys. Rev. B **72**, 052103 (2005)

25. Tang, J., Nett, B.E., Chen, G.: Performance comparison between total variation (TV)-based compressed sensing and statistical iterative reconstruction algorithms. Phys. Med. Biol. **54**, 5781–5804 (2009)

26. Myers, G.R., Thomas, C.D.L., Paganin, D.M., Gureyev, T.E., Clement, J.G.: A general few-projection method for tomographic reconstruction of samples consisting of several distinct materials. Appl. Phys. Lett. **96**, 021105 (2010)

27. Wang, Z., Bovik, A.C., Sheikh, H.R., Simoncelli, E.P.: Image quality assessment: from error visibility to structural similarity. IEEE Trans. Image Process. **13**, 600–612 (2004)

28. Wang, Z., Bovik, A.C.: A universal image quality index. IEEE Signal Proc. Let. **9**, 81–84 (2002)

29. Damera-Venkata, N., Kite, T.D., Geisler, W.S., Evans, B.L., Bovik, A.C.: Image quality assessment based on a degradation model. IEEE Trans. Image Process. **9**, 636–650 (2000)

30. Gureyev, T.E., Nesterets, Y.I., De Hoog, F., Schmalz, G., Mayo, S.C., Mohammadi, S., Tromba, G.: Duality between noise and spatial resolution in linear systems. Opt. Express **22**, 9087–9094 (2014)

Improving Breast Mass Segmentation in Local Dense Background: An Entropy Based Optimization of Statistical Region Merging Method

Shelda Sajeev$^{(\boxtimes)}$, Mariusz Bajger, and Gobert Lee

School of Computer Science, Engineering and Mathematics,
Medical Device Research Institute, Flinders University,
Adelaide, SA 5001, Australia
{shelda.sajeev,mariusz.bajger,gobert.lee}@flinders.edu.au

Abstract. In this paper, an optimization algorithm, utilizing a component measure of entropy, is developed for automatically tuning segmentation of mammograms by the Statistical Region Merging technique. The aim of this paper is to improve the mass segmentation in dense backgrounds. The proposed algorithm is tested on a database of 89 mammograms of which 41 have masses localized in dense background and 48 have masses in non-dense background. The algorithm performance is evaluated in conjunction with six standard enhancement techniques: Adjustable Histogram Equalization, Unsharp Masking, Neutrosophy based enhancement, standard CLAHE, Adaptive Clip Limit CLAHE based on standard deviation and Adaptive Clip Limit CLAHE based on standard entropy measure. For a comparison study, same experiments are performed using Fuzzy C-means Clustering technique. The experimental results show that the automatic tuning of SRM segmentation has the potential to produce an accurate segmentation of masses located in dense background while not compromising the performance on masses located in non-dense background.

Keywords: Statistical Region Merging · Dense background · Enhancement · Entropy · Segmentation · Mammography

1 Introduction

Mammography is the most common screening tool available for early breast cancer detection [1]. A number of factors may contribute to cancers being undetected at screening. One of these is the density of breast tissues, which can be dense (fibrous) or non-dense (fat). Fatty tissues appear as dark regions in a mammogram, while fibroglandular tissues (including masses) appear as white areas. Masses located in fibroglandular tissues (dense background) are particularly difficult to detect even for experienced radiologists [7]. This study focuses on delineation of breast masses in local dense background.

ⓒ Springer International Publishing Switzerland 2016
A. Tingberg et al. (Eds.): IWDM 2016, LNCS 9699, pp. 635–642, 2016.
DOI: 10.1007/978-3-319-41546-8_79

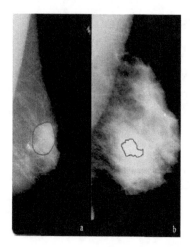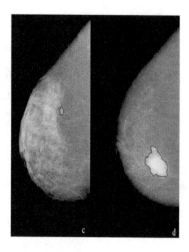

Fig. 1. Examples of mammograms showing masses in local dense and local non dense background. Left panel (a and b) shows mass in local dense background where (a) is BIRADS II and (b) is BIRADS IV and right panel (c and d), mass in local non dense background where (c) is BIRADS III and (d) is BIRADS I.

The local dense background is the density of an immediate background environment of the mass which is not the same as Breast Imaging Reporting and Data System (BI-RADS) classification which measures the overall breast density. Figure 1 shows an example of mass in local dense and non dense background. It is evident from the mammograms (See Fig. 1 left panel (a and b)) that the mass is hardly visible and the boundaries are very hard to detect in local dense background.

2   Related Works

Computer-aided diagnosis/detection (CAD) have been developed to help in improving the detection of breast cancer [12] and facilitating radiologists in making informed clinical decisions. Although CAD improves the detection rate, sensitivity is lower in dense breast [14].

Image segmentation is a crucial step in the automatic detection of masses. This study focus is to base segmentation on sound statistical image analysis that can help in extracting good features for detection and classifying lesions in local dense background. The Statistical Region Merging (SRM) [13] method which is based on probabilistic properties of distributions from the theory of concentration was adopted for breast mass segmentation in local dense background. SRM method belongs to the family of region growing and merging techniques but it views the image segmentation as an inference problem.

The SRM technique, first introduced by Nock and Nielsen [13] for segmentation of natural scenes, has also proved its potential for producing efficient and usable segmentation in medical image analysis. Celebi et al. [8] applied SRM for border detection in dermoscopy images to help with skin cancer detection. Bajger et al. [4] demonstrated the potential of SRM for 3D segmentation of CT images. Lee et al. [11] used SRM for temporal mammographic data analysis. Caon et al. [6] used SRM segmentation for the production of voxel models of anatomy for CT dosimetry. The above studies show that SRM-based techniques can be successfully applied to many challenging tasks in medical image segmentation.

The SRM algorithm requires choosing of one parameter Q, which controls the coarseness of the segmentation. The value of Q has to be determined prior and its choice is critical for an accurate mass segmentation. Finding the best value of Q is a challenging task and only partial solutions were reported. Bajger et al. [4,5] showed that, it is possible to restrict Q to an interval but no optimal choice of Q was suggested. In this study, an entropy based optimization technique is developed for automatically tuning the Q value of SRM segmentation.

3   Entropy Optimized SRM

3.1   Statistical Region Merging

In SRM segmentation, Q is a parameter whose value has to be set by the user. This parameter quantifies the statistical complexity of the image and hence controls the granularity of the SRM segmentation. Smaller Q values result in under segmentation and high Q values produces over segmentation. In applications using SRM technique, a fixed value of Q is selected empirically for a class of images with the result that is often far from the optimal one for some members of the class. Hence it is critical to select a Q value in such a way that objects of interest are well segmented. In this paper, the Q value is selected automatically for each image by optimizing a measure of local and global image entropy.

3.2   Entropy

The approach used in this paper (Eq. 1) utilizes an entropy measure of effectiveness of an image segmentation introduced in [16]. For image I, the total image entropy H is defined as

$$H(I) = H_l(I) + H_r(I). \tag{1}$$

In Eq. (1), $H_l(I)$ measures the global image disorder called *layout entropy*. Usually this number increases with the number of components. It is defined by the following formula

$$H_l(I) = -\sum_{j=1}^{N} \frac{|A_j|}{|A|} \log \frac{|A_j|}{|A|},$$

where $|A|$ is the area of the whole image and $|A_j|$ is the area of the j-th segmented component.

The second term $H_r(I)$, called *region entropy*, measures the uniformity within components. The region entropy decreases when the number of regions increases and is given by the formula

$$H_r(I) = \sum_{j=1}^{N} \frac{|A_j|}{|A|} H_\mu(A_j),$$

where $H_\mu(A_j)$ is the entropy of attribute μ for component A_j. In [16], luminance was used as the attribute μ. In this work, μ is the intensity value of the image pixel. Denoting by M_j the set of values associated with feature μ in component A_j and by $L_j(m)$ the number of pixels in component A_j with value m for feature μ, the entropy of component A_j is expressed as

$$H_\mu(A_j) = - \sum_{m \in M_j} \frac{L_j(m)}{|A_j|} \log \frac{L_j(m)}{|A_j|}.$$

3.3   Optimizing SRM Segmentation

For optimizing the value of the parameter Q, each mammogram was segmented using SRM technique for a specified range of values of Q. Then for each value of Q, the entropy of the segmented image was computed using the formula in (1). The value of Q resulting in maximum difference in entropy was selected as an optimal one. The range for Q was selected empirically (50:10:300). The detailed flow-chart of the proposed technique is shown in Fig. 2.

4   Materials and Methods

For this study, the mammograms were enhanced with six standard enhancement techniques: Adjustable Histogram Equalization [3], traditional Unsharp Masking (UM), Neutrosophy based enhancement [9], standard CLAHE, ACL-CLAHE based on standard deviation [2], ACL-CLAHE based on standard measure of entropy. The optimized by our method SRM technique was applied to 6 versions of enhanced image and to the original (un-enhanced) image. To compare the performance of automatically optimized SRM segmentation, another popular segmentation algorithm, Fuzzy C-Means Clustering (FCM), with 10 seeds, was selected. FCM with 10 seeds was found performing better than FCM optimized by the proposed method. Like SRM, FCM was also applied to 6 enhanced images and the original image.

4.1   Dataset

For this study, images were selected from the publicly available Digital Database for Screening Mammography (DDSM) [10]. The database has 41 images with malignant mass in local dense background, for a fair comparison 48 images

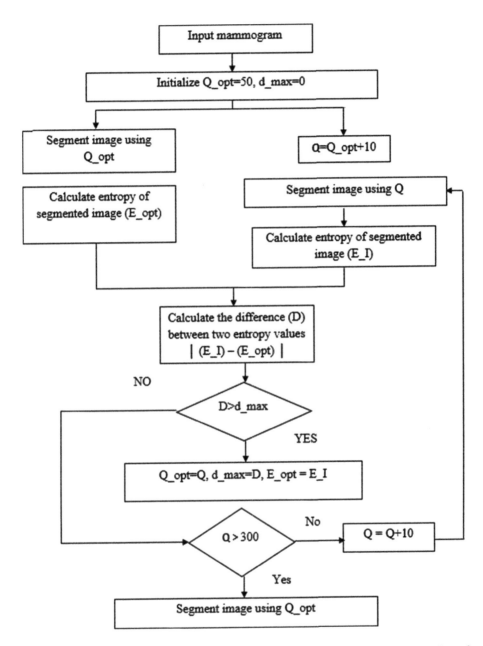

Fig. 2. Flow-chart for proposed entropy based optimization of SRM segmentation of mammograms.

with mass in local non dense background were also included in the study making the total 89. The annotations provided in the DDSM database do not always indicate a tight boundary for the masses. Therefore, one of the authors (S.S) have manually marked the core mass contours as directed by an experienced radiologist in mammography. These contours were used as ground truth to evaluate the performance of our method. Images were down sampled by 8 to reduce the computational time.

4.2   Mass Candidate Selection

In this study, a suitable criterion for measuring the quality of the segmentation of mass-like regions is to compute how well the union of all reasonable components which overlap the annotated region fits the annotation. By a reasonable component is meant a component with at least 60 % of its area residing within the annotated region and with Dice index more than 20 %.

4.3   Performance Evaluation

Results of SRM and FCM segmentation were assessed against the ground truth. A number of measures can be used to quantify the results. Dice Index is one of the most popular similarity measures for sets and is used in this study. Let X and Y be two sets to be measured, the Dice index is defined as

$$DICE(X,Y) = \frac{2\,|\,X \cap Y\,|}{|X| + |Y|} \tag{2}$$

The Dice index values ranges between 0 and 1, where 0 indicates no overlap between the sets and 1 indicates the segmentation output and ground truth overlap perfectly (are identical).

5   Results and Discussion

Table 1 shows the performance comparison of SRM and FCM for mass segmentation using Dice index. It also shows the parameter values used for enhancements techniques. The result shows that the proposed SRM parameter tuning algorithm has the potential to produce effective mass segmentation without any preprocessing (enhancement). For un-enhanced image the SRM outcome outperformed FCM outcome by 24 % for masses in dense background and by 15 % for masses in non dense background. Furthermore, for Adjustable HE, UM and neutrosophy based enhancement, SRM technique also outperformed FCM by 24 %, 27 % and 14 %, respectively for masses in dense background. For masses in non dense background, SRM showed an increase of segmentation accuracy by 7 %, 11 %, 10 %, respectively. The CLAHE group (standard CLAHE, ACL-CLAHE using standard deviation and entropy) results are comparable for both SRM and FCM techniques.

Table 1. Performance of SRM and FCM segmentation on 6 standard enhancement techniques and un-enhanced image for both mass in dense background (41 images) and non-dense background (48 images). Column 3 and 4 are the percentage of the number of images whose Dice index is greater than 0.5. The corresponding number of images is shown in brackets.

Mass in dense background			
Approach	Paramater value	FCM	SRM
original (no enhancement)	no	66 %(27)	**90 %(37)**
Adjustable HE [3]	sigma(0.5)	71 %(29)	95 %(39)
UM	scaling factor(0.7)	63 %(26)	90 %(37)
neutrosophic [9]	alpha(0.85) beta(0.85)	61 %(25)	75 %(30)
CLAHE	clip-limit(0.012) block-size(64)	93 %(38)	88 %(36)
ACL-CLAHE-std [2]	block-size(64)	93 %(38)	83 %(34)
ACL-CLAHE-entropy [15]	Automatic tuning	**95 %(39)**	**95 %(39)**
Mass in non-dense background			
Approach	Paramater value	FCM	SRM
original (no enhancement)	no	83 %(40)	**98 %(47)**
Adjustable HE [3]	sigma(0.3)	83 %(40)	90 %(43)
UM	scaling factor(0.5)	85 %(41)	96 %(46)
neutrosophic [9]	alpha(0.85) beta(0.85)	88 %(42)	98 %(47)
CLAHE	clip-limit(0.01) block-size(64)	98 %(47)	94 %(45)
ACL-CLAHE-std [2]	block-size(64)	96 %(46)	81 %(39)
ACL-CLAHE-entropy [15]	Automatic tuning	**96 %(46)**	**98 %(47)**

6   Conclusion

A method for automatically determining the SRM parameter value for each image individually using a measure of component entropy is proposed. A number of image enhancement techniques were used in conjunction with optimized SRM method. For performance comparison FCM method was used. It has been found that the optimized SRM technique achieved superior results without the need of prior image enhancement.

Acknowledgments. The authors would like to thank Dr. Peter Downey, clinical radiologist of BreastScreen SA for validating the core mass contours and valuable comments and discussions.

References

1. World Health Organization (WHO): WHO position paper on mammography screening. World Health Organization (WHO), Geneva (Switzerland) (2014)
2. Abbas, Q., Celebi, M.E., Garcia, I.F.: Breast mass segmentation using region-based and edge-based methods in a 4-stage multiscale system. Biomed. Sig. Process. Control **8**(2), 204–214 (2013)

3. Arici, T., Dikbas, S., Altunbasak, Y.: A histogram modification framework and its application for image contrast enhancement. IEEE Trans. Image Process. **18**(9), 1921–1935 (2009)

4. Bajger, M., Lee, G.N., Caon, M.: 3D segmentation for multi-organs in CT images. Electron. Lett. Comput. Vis. Image Anal. **12**(2), 13–27 (2013)

5. Bajger, M., Ma, F., Williams, S., Bottema, M.: Mammographic mass detection with statistical region merging. In: 2010 International Conference on Digital Image Computing: Techniques and Applications, pp. 27–32. Syndey (2010)

6. Caon, M., Sedlar, J., Bajger, M., Lee, G.: Computer-assisted segmentation of CT images by statistical region merging for the production of voxel models of anatomy for CT dosimetry. Australas. Phys. Eng. Sci. Med. **37**(2), 393–403 (2014)

7. Castellano, C.R., Nunez, C.V., Boy, R.C., et al.: Impact of mammographic breast density on computer-assisted detection (CAD) in a breast imaging department. Radiologia **53**, 456–461 (2011)

8. Celebi, M.E., Kingravi, H.A., Iyatomi, H., et al.: Border detection in dermoscopy images using statistical region merging. Skin Res. Technol. **14**(3), 347–353 (2008)

9. Guoa, Y., Cheng, H.D.: New neutrosophic approach to image segmentation. Pattern Recogn. **42**, 587–595 (2009)

10. Heath, M., Bowyer, K., Kopans, D., et al.: The digital database for screening mammography. In: Proceedings of the Fifth International Workshop on Digital Mammography, pp. 212–218. Medical Physics Publishing (2001)

11. Lee, G.N., Bajger, M.: Statistical temporal changes for breast cancer detection: a preliminary study. In: Fujita, H., Hara, T., Muramatsu, C. (eds.) IWDM 2014. LNCS, vol. 8539, pp. 635–642. Springer, Heidelberg (2014)

12. Morton, M.J., Whaley, D.H., Brandt, K.R., et al.: Screening mammograms: interpretation with computer-aided detection prospective evaluation. Radiology **239**, 204–212 (2006)

13. Nock, R., Nielsen, F.: Statistical region merging. IEEE Trans. Pattern Anal. Mach. Intell. **26**(11), 1452–1458 (2004)

14. Oliver, A., Freixenet, J., Marti, J., Perez, E., Pont, J., Denton, E., Zwiggelaar, R.: A review of automatic mass detection and segmentation in mammographic images. Med. Image Anal. **2**, 87–110 (2010)

15. Sajeev, S., Bajger, M., Lee, G.: Segmentation of breast masses in local dense background using adaptive clip limit-CLAHE. In: 2015 International Conference on Digital Image Computing: Techniques and Applications (DICTA), DICTA 2015, pp. 669–676. IEEE (2015)

16. Zhang, H., Fritts, J.E., Goldman, S.A.: An entropy-based objective evaluation method for image segmentation. In: Proceedings of SPIE: Storage and Retrieval Methods and Applications for Multimedia, vol. 5307, pp. 38–49 (2004)

Simulations and Virtual Clinical Trials

System Calibration for Quantitative Contrast-Enhanced Digital Breast Tomosynthesis (CEDBT)

Melissa L. Hill[1(✉)], James G. Mainprize[1], and Martin J. Yaffe[1,2]

[1] Physical Sciences, Sunnybrook Research Institute, Toronto, ON, Canada
melissa.hill.sri@gmail.com
[2] Department of Medical Biophysics, University of Toronto, Toronto, ON, Canada

Abstract. In contrast-enhanced (CE) breast imaging, lesion contrast agent content may be diagnostic, relating to vascularization and tumour angiogenesis. However, factors in CE digital breast tomosynthesis (DBT) such as incomplete angular sampling, beam hardening and scatter can confound quantitative measurement. We propose system calibration to improve CEDBT quantitative potential. Fifteen projection images of an iodine calibration phantom, with various breast-equivalent compositions, thicknesses and lesion locations, were acquired over 40°, and reconstructed using SART. A separate breast-equivalent phantom with iodinated spherical lesions was imaged to test quantification accuracy. Excellent linearity between voxel signal and iodine concentration was achieved in the calibration data. In test phantom cases, lesion signal faithfully represented the true iodine concentration, but with wide confidence intervals for small lesions. While promising, it remains to be determined whether the iodine quantification accuracy is sufficient for lesion differentiation, and whether lesion shape, position, and non-uniform breast tissue would impair this estimation.

Keywords: Contrast-enhanced · Tomosynthesis · Mammography · Iodine · Quantitative imaging

1 Introduction

Clinical evaluation of contrast-enhanced digital mammography (CEDM) has demonstrated great promise for its application in a diagnostic setting to characterize breast lesions and to improve their detection [1, 2]. In dual-energy (DE) CEDM, an intravenous injection of an iodinated contrast agent is made and then low-energy and high-energy projection images are acquired of the compressed breast [3]. Single-energy (SE) CEDM has also been proposed in which one image acquisition is made before contrast injection, and then one, or more (temporal CEDM), images are acquired post-contrast [4]. In both techniques, contrast-enhancement is anticipated in subtracted images in areas of greater vascularization, or regions expressing tumour angiogenesis, where the agent preferentially leaks from the vasculature. Diagnosis is made based on lesion morphology and the presence of iodine enhancement [1]. Currently, judgement of contrast-enhancement is made subjectively because in the projection images contrast agent present in superimposed normal tissue outside the plane of the lesion interferes with lesion measurement

© Springer International Publishing Switzerland 2016
A. Tingberg et al. (Eds.): IWDM 2016, LNCS 9699, pp. 645–653, 2016.
DOI: 10.1007/978-3-319-41546-8_80

[4, 5]. In tomosynthetic imaging, a more direct relationship between iodine contrast-enhancement and tumour angiogenesis is expected [6].

Contrast-enhanced digital breast tomosynthesis (CEDBT) and CE dedicated breast CT (CE bCT) have each been favourably tested in clinical pilot studies [2, 7]. The potential of CE bCT for quantitative lesion measurement [7] and vascular assessment has been demonstrated, however, concern remains over tissue coverage [8]. Given its similar acquisition geometry to conventional DM, CEDBT has good tissue coverage, but reconstructions are quasi-3D due to limited angular sampling, and as such the voxel values are only semi-quantitative. Nonetheless, investigators have shown that by using system calibration, DBT voxel values can be corrected to vary linearly with object attenuation in a laboratory setting [9].

We believe that diagnosis made with quantitative CEDBT would have greater accuracy than the current clinical CEDM. In this research, similar principles of system calibration used in conventional DBT are applied to CEDBT to allow for estimates of lesion iodine concentration from reconstructed slice images.

2 Methods

The study performed here is intended to be a proof-of-concept rather than a clinic-ready calibration of a commercial system, and as such was carried out on an experimental bench-top system operated in SE mode for practical purposes. Compared to DE, this approach is simpler to calibrate as it limits the parameters required for optimization (*e.g.* x-ray spectra, DE algorithm) and correction (*e.g.* x-ray scatter, beam hardening and detector response for different spectra). However, we suggest that the approach employed here can be translated to a DE system, and effective methods for scatter correction in DE CEDBT have been described in the literature [10].

2.1 Image Acquisition and Reconstruction

The bench-top imaging system was equipped with a mammographic x-ray tube (GE DMR v.2) and a flat-panel detector (GE Senographe 2000D). The source-to-detector distance was 66 cm, with a 4 cm detector-to-pivot distance. Each DBT acquisition consisted of 15 projection images, equally spaced over a 40° extent. High-energy images were acquired at 49 kV [Rh/(1 mm Al + 0.3 mm Cu)] and 38 mAs/projection. For a 5 cm 50/50 breast, this would yield a total mean glandular dose of ~4.3 mGy for a SE CEDBT exam. Images were gain and offset corrected. An interval of at least 1 min between acquisitions minimized lag and ghosting, such that these effects contributed an uncertainty of only 0.03 mg/ml iodine between DBT sets.

Reconstruction was performed using a simultaneous algebraic reconstruction technique (SART) algorithm at $0.4 \times 0.4 \times 1$ mm^3 voxel size, with the number of slices selected according to the phantom thickness, plus 1 cm extra margin [11].

The calibration phantom consisted of 1 cm thick iodinated-epoxy samples with 0.0, 0.2, 0.5, 1.0 and 2.0 mg/ml iodine concentration [12]. Two samples of each concentration were loaded in a 2 cm thick PMMA frame machined with 1 cm deep channels for repeatable sample positioning, shown in Fig. 1(a). At the acquisition x-ray energies, epoxy was estimated to be equivalent to 64 % fibroglandular, and PMMA equivalent to 96 % fibroglandular based on comparison with a stepwedge of breast-equivalent materials of several compositions (CIRS Inc., Norfolk, VA) included in the image.

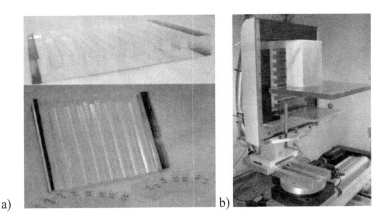

Fig. 1. (a) Two views of a 2 cm thick PMMA calibration frame with 1 cm deep channels to hold 1 cm iodinated-epoxy samples (bottom); and (b) experimental imaging set-up with calibration frame overlaid by breast tissue-equivalent plastic.

Calibration images were acquired with the PMMA frame alone (0 cm) and overlaid with 1 cm, 2 cm, 3 cm and 5 cm thicknesses of 100 % adipose, 50/50, and 100 % fibroglandular breast-equivalent plastic (CIRS Inc., Norfolk, VA), as shown in Fig. 1b. To study the effect of lesion depth, the frame was placed on top of 5 cm of 50/50-equivalent plastic for one calibration, but was placed directly on the detector cover in all other instances. For each of 14 composition-thickness combinations, two samples of equal iodine concentration were placed end-to-end in a single positioner row (see Fig. 2), and with the positioner fixed in place, were moved to adjacent rows between each of five CEDBT acquisitions. The five reconstructed volumes were in turn subtracted from each other, generating 10 image combinations per composition-thickness. This resulted in 140 subtracted volumes, from which one central slice that intersected all iodinated samples was analyzed for calibration.

Subtracted CEDBT reconstructions of a 6 cm thick BR12 breast-equivalent phantom with iodinated spherical lesions from 4 to 9.5 mm diameter at 0.5, 1.0 and 1.5 mg/ml, imaged and reconstructed under matching conditions to the present calibration, were used to test iodine quantification accuracy. A full description of phantom properties, and experimental conditions was presented at a previous IWDM meeting [13], but an important design feature is lesion channels at multiple phantom heights, filled with either water or dilute iodine. Quantification of only one lesion channel was analyzed here, such that other channels contributed to background signal non-uniformity. Measurement uncertainty of lesion iodine concentration in the test phantom was estimated to be about 5 %.

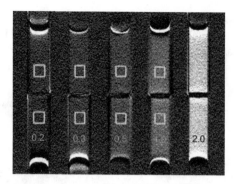

Fig. 2. Example central slice from a subtracted CEDBT volume with ROI placement shown. Sharply bright and dark regions arise from subtraction of iodinated samples of slightly different lengths. The effective iodine concentrations after subtraction are indicated in mg/ml.

From a single CEDBT slice for each iodine concentration, lesion voxel signal uncertainty was estimated by computing the standard deviation of the means of 10 background regions of interest (ROI), with the same size, and adjacent to lesion ROI.

2.2   Image Analysis and Calibration

Square 15×15 voxel ROI were selected within a central slice of subtracted CEDBT reconstructions (Fig. 2). The mean ROI signal and standard deviation among 10 (0.2, 0.3, 0.8, 1.5 and 1.8 mg/ml) to 20 (0.5, 1.0 and 2.0 mg/ml) independent sample measurements, were measured for each imaging condition. Calibration curves were calculated by a weighted least squares fit of voxel signal versus iodine concentration.

In test phantom volumes, circular ROI were selected within lesion central slice images (Fig. 3) by setting ROI diameter equal to the diameter at the FWHM of the in-plane lesion signal. Estimates of the iodine concentration were made in these test cases by linearly interpolating the appropriate calibration curves.

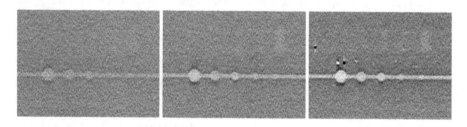

Fig. 3. Test case central slices from subtracted CEDBT volumes with, from left to right, 0.5, 1.0 and 1.5 mg/ml iodine in a lesion channel. Identical technique factors and DBT geometry to the calibration were used for acquisition, as described in Ref. [13].

3 Results

In Table 1, the slope, y-intercept and R^2 values are reported for all calibration curves. The calibration data for 100 % adipose, 50/50 and 100 % fibroglandular materials at equal thicknesses were not significantly different (see Table 1), so for clarity, only the zero thickness, and 50/50 composition data are plotted in Fig. 4. Central slices were selected for analysis from reconstruction volume heights of 19 mm and 69 mm for the 'bottom', and 5 cm 'top' frame positions, respectively.

Table 1. Summary of weighted least-squares CEDBT iodine calibration. Standard deviations of the slope and y-intercept are indicated. Figure 4 plots the 0 cm and 50/50 calibration curves.

Material	Thickness (cm)	Slope (mm^{-1} ml/mg 10^{-4})	Y-intercept (mm^{-1} 10^{-4})	R^2
None	0	6.16 ± 0.08	0.15 ± 0.08	0.999
Fat	1	4.40 ± 0.04	0.04 ± 0.04	1.000
50/50	1	4.41 ± 0.04	0.06 ± 0.05	0.999
Fibroglandular	1	4.41 ± 0.01	0.02 ± 0.01	1.000
Fat	2	3.42 ± 0.06	0.08 ± 0.07	0.998
50/50	2	3.34 ± 0.06	0.14 ± 0.07	0.998
Fibroglandular	2	3.43 ± 0.05	0.07 ± 0.06	0.999
Fat	3	2.83 ± 0.11	0.20 ± 0.12	0.992
50/50	3	2.73 ± 0.10	0.28 ± 0.12	0.992
Fibroglandular	3	2.86 ± 0.09	0.19 ± 0.10	0.994
Fat	5	2.15 ± 0.12	0.27 ± 0.15	0.980
50/50	5	2.20 ± 0.08	0.23 ± 0.09	0.993
Fibroglandular	5	2.22 ± 0.09	0.16 ± 0.09	0.989
50/50 (calib @ top)	5	2.58 ± 0.12	0.21 ± 0.11	0.986

Table 2. Iodine concentration 95 % confidence intervals calibrated from test phantom CEDBT slice lesion signal, organized by experimental iodine concentration (± 5 %) and lesion diameter.

Lesion diameter (mm)	$[I]_{calib}$ (mg/ml)		
	0.5 mg/ml	1.0 mg/ml	1.5 mg/ml
9.5	(0.44, 0.69)	(1.01, 1.35)	(1.42, 1.86)
7.4	(0.32, 0.63)	(0.85, 1.20)	(1.15, 1.62)
5.0	(0.23, 0.66)	(0.73, 1.15)	(0.93, 1.49)
4.0	(0.28, 0.83)	(0.53, 1.12)	(0.98, 1.72)

Iodine quantification results for three test phantom iodine concentrations are listed in Table 2 in terms of their calibrated 95 % confidence intervals (CI), $[I]_{calib}$. Subtracted slices at 38 mm height were used for analysis. To account for phantom material differences, the 6 cm BR12 phantom was estimated to be equivalent to 5.9 cm 50/50 plastic, while the calibration frame (1 cm PMMA, 1 cm epoxy) was estimated to be equivalent to 2.3 cm of 50/50 material. Thus, the 50/50 calibration slope values in Table 1 were linearly interpolated over effective thicknesses of 2.3 to 7.3 cm, for an estimated slope of 2.57×10^{-4} mm^{-1} ml/mg at 5.9 cm. Further, to account for differences in calibration

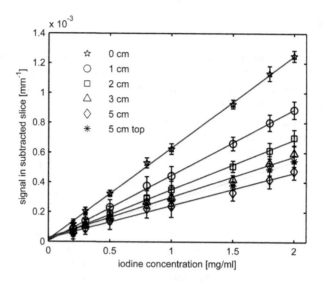

Fig. 4. CEDBT iodine voxel signal calibration as a function of concentration for 0, 1, 2, 3 and 5 cm of 50/50 CIRS plastic placed on top of a 2 cm calibration frame. The data, '5 cm top' was acquired with the calibration frame on top of the 5 cm of material. Linear least-squares fits to the data are shown as black lines (gray for '5 cm top'), extrapolated to 0 mg/ml iodine.

and test case slice heights, this value was scaled by the ratio of the '5 cm top'-to-'5 cm bottom' slopes (see Table 1) interpolated to 38 mm height, yielding 2.74×10^{-4} mm^{-1} ml/mg. Given that the 50/50 material y-intercepts were the same within error for all thicknesses and frame placements, the 3 cm 50/50 value was used for calibration since its effective thickness was closest to the test phantom thickness.

4   Discussion and Conclusions

The excellent calibration curve linearity in Fig. 4 demonstrates that there was good repeatability between CEDBT image acquisitions, and that the iodinated samples have good accuracy. Further, the curves all pass through the origin within a 95 % CI, so the data appear physical, and are expected to be adequate for the desired calibration.

In Fig. 4, increasing breast thickness resulted in lower iodine signal. The greater amounts of scatter and beam hardening at greater breast thicknesses are well known to reduce object contrast in this manner. However, the fact that the different breast-equivalent tissue compositions did not result in significantly different signal at equal phantom thickness is likely due to the operation of image subtraction in SE CEDBT. At equal thicknesses the differences between amounts of scatter and attenuation are already small [14, 15], but after subtraction only their effects on the iodine signal remain. No effect was measurable at the small iodine concentrations studied here.

Good agreement is seen in the Table 2 comparison of true test case iodine concentrations and calibrated 95 % CI. However, there is generally more uncertainty for smaller lesion sizes. The test phantom was not completely uniform, with several other channels present in other slice planes, filled with either water or diluted contrast agent. Due to incomplete angular sampling, some out-of-plane signal from these non-uniformities can result in relatively greater noise for the smallest lesions compared to largest lesions. Also, even at the largest lesion size, the estimated iodine concentration is only known to within about 0.4 mg/ml. It would be necessary to study whether this degree of accuracy is sufficient for diagnostic use, and whether true breast 'anatomical noise' [16], or the presence of other lesions within the breast, would substantially increase uncertainty compared to the limited simulated background non-uniformity.

Other limitations of this work include a narrow investigation of the effect of lesion height, shape, position and DBT imaging parameters. Only one test was carried out where the position of the calibration frame was varied relative to the detector. While Fig. 4 demonstrates that the effect of lesion slice height was small, a superior calibration could likely be achieved by including a greater number of slice positions. Also, it is known that differences in object frequency content contribute to variations in the artifact spread function. [17] This effect could be important for both lesion shape and heterogeneity of normal breast tissue. A square calibration object was used here, while testing was carried out with spherical lesions. Although there was good agreement between the calibration and truth in Table 2, it would be helpful to understand whether the calibration would have similar performance for other lesion morphologies, such as spiculated or regional enhancements. Furthermore, uniform, rectangular phantom backgrounds were used for both calibration and testing. Variations in uncancelled normal breast tissue signal may affect lesion voxel values given the signal spread throughout DBT reconstructed volumes. The breast shape and lesion position will also each likely affect iodine quantification, due to scatter correction limitations [10], and small differences in beam hardening. For practical purposes only one set of technique factors and acquisition geometry were tested, but in the clinic, technique factors will likely be selected according to a woman's breast characteristics, and angular extent or number of projections could be varied. It is anticipated that separate iodine calibrations would be required for each acquisition parameter variation. Finally, the reconstruction algorithm is known to affect the voxel values. [17] For example, changing the number of SART iterations, or the use of a direct reconstruction approach (*e.g.* FBP) where filtration can modify the signal, would require separate calibration.

This work demonstrated that CEDBT images can be calibrated so that the voxel signal is directly related to the lesion iodine concentration. It is important to note that even in an ideal laboratory setting, the calibration is laborious with many factors to account for. Further work will be required to determine whether normal variations in patient anatomy and lesion presentation can be adequately addressed, and whether the achievable CEDBT quantification accuracy has diagnostic potential.

Acknowledgments. This work was conducted with the support of the Ontario Institute for Cancer Research through funding provided by the Government of Ontario. The authors thank Michael Kempston for his contributions.

References

1. Fallenberg, E.M., Dromain, C., Diekmann, F., Engelken, F., Krohn, M., Singh, J.M., Ingold-Heppner, B., Winzer, K.J., Bick, U., Renz, D.M.: Contrast-enhanced spectral mammography versus MRI: Initial results in the detection of breast cancer and assessment of tumour size. Eur. Radiol. **24**, 256–264 (2014)
2. Chou, C.-P., Lewin, J.M., Chiang, C.-L., Hung, B.-H., Yang, T.-L., Huang, J.-S., Liao, J.-B., Pan, H.-B.: Clinical evaluation of contrast-enhanced digital mammography and contrast enhanced tomosynthesis-comparison to contrast-enhanced breast MRI. Eur. J. Radiol. **84**, 2501–2508 (2015)
3. Lewin, J.M., Isaacs, P.K., Vance, V., Larke, F.J.: Dual-energy contrast-enhanced digital subtraction mammography: feasibility. Radiology **229**, 261–268 (2003)
4. Jong, R.A., Yaffe, M.J., Skarpathiotakis, M., Shumak, R.S., Danjoux, N.M., Gunesekara, A.: Contrast-enhanced digital mammography: initial clinical experience. Radiology **228**, 842–850 (2003)
5. Dromain, C., Balleyguier, C., Muller, S., Mathieu, M.-C., Rochard, F., Opolon, P., Sigal, R.: Evaluation of tumor angiogenesis of breast carcinoma using contrast-enhanced digital mammography. Am. J. Roentgenol. **187**, W528–W537 (2006)
6. Hill, M.L., Liu, K., Mainprize, J.G., Levitin, R.B., Shojaii, R., Yaffe, M.J.: Pre-clinical evaluation of tumour angiogenesis with contrast-enhanced breast tomosynthesis. In: Maidment, A.D., Bakic, P.R., Gavenonis, S. (eds.) IWDM 2012. LNCS, vol. 7361, pp. 1–8. Springer, Heidelberg (2012)
7. Prionas, N.D., Lindfors, K.K., Ray, S., Beckett, L.A., Monsky, W.L., Boone, J.M.: Contrast-enhanced dedicated breast CT: initial clinical experience. Radiology **256**, 714–723 (2010)
8. He, N., Wu, Y.-P., Kong, Y., Lv, N., Huang, Z.-M., Li, S., Wang, Y., Geng, Z., Wu, P.-H., Wei, W.-D.: The utility of breast cone-beam computed tomography, ultrasound, and digital mammography for detecting malignant breast tumors: a prospective study with 212 patients. Eur. J. Radiol. **85**, 392–403 (2016)
9. Shafer, C.M., Samei, E., Lo, J.Y.: The quantitative potential for breast tomosynthesis imaging. Med. Phys. **37**, 1004–1016 (2010)
10. Lu, Y., Peng, B., Lau, B.A., Hu, Y.-H., Scaduto, D.A., Zhao, W., Gindi, G.: A scatter correction method for contrast-enhanced dual-energy digital breast tomosynthesis. Phys. Med. Biol. **60**, 6323–6354 (2015)
11. Andersen, A.H., Kak, A.C.: Simultaneous algebraic reconstruction technique (SART): a superior implementation of the ART algorithm. Ultrason. Imaging **6**, 81–94 (1984)
12. Hill, M.L., Mainprize, J.G., Mawdsley, G.E., Yaffe, M.J.: A solid iodinated phantom material for use in tomographic x-ray imaging. Med. Phys. **36**, 4409–4420 (2009)
13. Hill, M.L., Mainprize, J.G., Yaffe, M.J.: Sensitivity of contrast-enhanced digital breast tomosynthesis to changes in iodine concentration during acquisition. In: Krupinski, E.A. (ed.) IWDM 2008. LNCS, vol. 5116, pp. 643–650. Springer, Heidelberg (2008)
14. Boone, J.M., Lindfors, K.K., Cooper, V.N., Seibert, J.A.: Scatter/primary in mammography: comprehensive results. Med. Phys. **27**, 2408–2416 (2000)
15. Johns, P.C., Yaffe, M.J.: X-ray characterisation of normal and neoplastic breast tissues. Phys. Med. Biol. **32**, 675–695 (1987)

16. Hill, M.L., Mainprize, J.G., Carton, A.-K., Muller, S., Ebrahimi, M., Jong, R.A., Dromain, C., Yaffe, M.J.: Anatomical noise in contrast-enhanced digital mammography. Part I. Single-energy imaging. Med. Phys. **40**, 051910 (2013)
17. Hu, Y.-H., Zhao, B., Zhao, W.: Image artifacts in digital breast tomosynthesis: investigation of the effects of system geometry and reconstruction parameters using a linear system approach. Med. Phys. **35**, 5242–5252 (2008)

Rapid Generation of Structured Physical Phantoms for Mammography and Digital Breast Tomosynthesis

Lynda Ikejimba[✉], Christian Graff, and Stephen Glick

Division of Imaging, Diagnostics, and Software Reliability,
OSEL/CDRH/FDA, Silver Spring, USA
{Lynda.Ikejimba,Christian.Graff,
Stephen.Glick}@fda.hhs.gov

Abstract. Nonuniform phantoms are needed in order to fully characterize the impact of anatomical structures on system performance in mammography and digital breast tomosynthesis (DBT). In this work, a new type of textured physical phantom is presented, compatible for use in both 2D and 3D applications. The breast phantom was first modeled analytically, and then fabricated using inkjet printing onto parchment paper and slide transparencies. A radiographic ink solution was synthesized with 350 mg/mL iohexol and pigmented ink. The effective linear attenuation coefficient (μ_{eff}) of the parchment paper alone (0.078 ± 0.003 mm^{-1}) was found to be very close to that of a 70 % adipose, 30 % fibroglandular tissue mixture (0.078 ± 0.004 mm^{-1}). The μ_{eff} of the parchment paper with iodine (0.010 ± 0.005 mm^{-1}) was close to that of 100 % fibroglandular tissue (0.11 ± 0.004 mm^{-1}). This new parchment and iodine phantom has strong potential for use in imaging studies.

Keywords: Breast phantom · Anthropomorphic · Iodine · Linear attenuation

1 Introduction

Physical breast phantoms remain a cornerstone for the effective evaluation and quality control (QC) of clinical imaging systems, such as full field digital mammography (FFDM) and digital breast tomosynthesis (DBT). In mammography, a planar radiograph is taken, and the resulting 2D image contains superposing tissue from various depths in the breast. However, the standard evaluation phantoms consist of a layer of inserts against a uniform backgrounds, which do not reflect the true structure of the breast [1, 2]. In DBT, a series of projection radiographs are acquired and reconstructed to create a 3D volume. Since DBT uses a limited number of angular projections, the resulting volume is undersampled and suffers from out of plane artifacts. Additionally, because the aforementioned phantoms were originally designed for use with 2D systems, they may not capture aspects of 3D imaging that may be of interest, such as the axial spread function or partial volume artifacts. An important component of measuring performance could then incorporate the extent to which out-of-plane structures are

© Springer International Publishing Switzerland 2016
A. Tingberg et al. (Eds.): IWDM 2016, LNCS 9699, pp. 654–659, 2016.
DOI: 10.1007/978-3-319-41546-8_81

suppressed. For these reasons, it is of great interest to use a structured 3D phantom in both FFDM and DBT evaluation.

Work has been done to create physical breast phantoms with nonuniform texture. Such phantoms may be based on patient histology [3], consist of acrylic spheres [4], or contain other complex arrangements of glandular and adipose tissues [5, 6] and fabrication using additive manufacturing techniques [6]. Typically, these phantoms also follow the same power law properties of the breast. However, some drawbacks to these phantoms include resolution limitations, cost, and the time to produce each one. In this work, we develop a new type of 3D phantom that can model random anatomy and can be quickly fabricated from inkjet printing.

2   Materials and Methods

2.1   Virtual Modeling of Breast Phantom

The in silico breast phantom was procedurally generated using a recently described model [7] developed in our group. The procedure can be summarized as follows: An anthropomorphic uncompressed breast shape was created based on a series of parameters controlling breast volume and surface curvature. A skin layer and nipple were generated to cover the surface of the breast shape. The interior of the breast was segmented into fat regions and glandular compartments based on a random Voronoi segmentation. Within each glandular compartment a ductal tree with terminal duct lobular units were generated. Cooper's ligaments were created using a network of random Perlin-noise perturbed surfaces. Perlin noise interpolates randomly generated gradient directions across multiple length scales. This type of noise is commonly used to procedurally generate textures reminiscent of the randomness found in nature. In this work we have created fat lobules with random shapes by perturbing the surface of a base spheroid with Perlin noise tuned to qualitatively resemble fat lobule surface variability observed in vivo. A vascular tree was grown using random branching structures emanating from a muscle layer at the base of the breast phantom. This model was digitized with voxels of 120 μm, which was adequate for the present application. To model compression, a tetrahedral mesh was generated, with each element assigned either glandular or fat elastic properties based on the voxels contained within the element. A linear elasticity finite element method was used to model compression of the breast to a thickness of 30 mm. For the present study, this thickness was selected to represent a smaller breast, but in practice a breast of any thickness could be created.

All breast surfaces are defined analytically so there is no inherent limitation to voxel size or total breast volume. For efficient computation it is necessary to store the entire phantom in memory during generation, which imposes a practical limit on the total number of voxels in the phantom. For an average size breast, 40 micron voxels are achievable on a computer with at least 8 GB of RAM. The computational time scales with the number of voxels, so time constraints can also impose practical limits on voxel or breast size.

2.2   Printing of Physical Phantom

The virtual phantoms were realized through inkjet printing with radiopaque ink onto a thin material base. The radiopaque ink was created by mixing 350 mg/mL iohexol (Omnipaque, GE Healthcare, Princeton, NJ) with pigmented ink (InkThrift, Vermont PhotoInkjet) in a solution of 25 % iohexol and 75 % ink. The solution was inserted via syringe into refillable inkjet cartridges. Using this solution, the virtual phantom was then printed slice by slice at the nominal resolution of 120 µm or 210 dpi. The phantom was printed onto several types of material. The first was 70 µm thick parchment paper with a silicone coating. The second was 120 µm thick slide transparency (C-Line). The final was a 100 µm thick "organic" paper. The background material would serve as the adipose-only component of the breast, while the glandular components are overlaid with the printed ink. Since each printed sheet corresponds anatomy at a different depth of the virtual breast, the composite physical phantom can be used in 3D imaging modalities. Fiducial markers were placed on each slice of the virtual model to assist with aligning the pages.

Because each slice of the phantom is printed on a single sheet of paper, the final height of the printed stack can be affected by the thickness of the paper. For example, the 120 µm paper will yield a stack closer to 30 mm. However, for thinner paper the final stack height may be slightly less than 30 mm.

2.3   Image Acquisition

For validation of the materials used, the attenuation properties of the phantom materials were compared with those from six tissue equivalent chips of known glandular density ranging from 0 % glandularity (100 % adipose) to 100 % glandularity (CIRS, Norfolk, VA). Phantoms images were acquired on a clinical mammography system (Hologic Lorad Selenia, Bedford, MA). A target/filter combination of molybdenum/molybdenum was used to examine the material properties under typical mammographic beams. The source to imager distance was 660 mm, using an a-Se direct detection imager with 70 µm pixel pitch. Images were processed only for gain map correction.

The effective linear attenuation coefficient μ_{eff} was calculated from Beer's law. To obtain the incident exposure, an open field image was acquired without the phantom. In addition, to determine the dark field offset an acquisition was made with zero exposure onto the detector; this offset was then used to correct both the phantom and open field images prior to numerical calculations. Finally, the effect of scatter was also measured from the air gap method. Images of the phantom are presented in Fig. 1 as (a) a slice through the binary digital model, (b) a picture of the physical realization, with a side view of the stack thickness inset, and (c) a radiograph with Mo/Mo at 28 kVp. For demonstration purposes, the images in Fig. 1(b), (c) represent only a subset of the stack, with duplicate prints of some slices to enhance visibility.

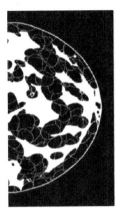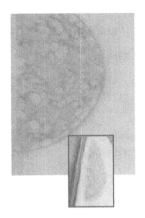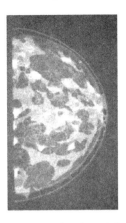

Fig. 1. Fabrication of physical phantom. The phantom was (a) designed as a virtual model, (b) realized through printing and (c) x-rayed on a mammographic system.

3   Results and Discussion

The effective linear attenuation coefficient was measured for the tissue chips of known glandular fraction, and data are provided in Fig. 2. Results were found to be in good agreement with published data [6]. At 28 kVp, the attenuation coefficients of the chips were plotted against their percent glandular density. The relationship was determined to be linear, and the equation of fit provided a correspondence between the effective linear attenuation coefficient and an approximate glandular fraction, for a given beam condition. Error bars on the estimates are from the pixel variance and slight variability in sample thickness. This linear mapping was then used to determine an equivalent glandular density for the parchment paper, transparency slides, and organic paper. Scatter was measured through the air gap method, and determined to have a small effect (<7 %) on the calculated attenuation values.

Results are plotted in Fig. 3 of the μ_{eff} and estimated glandular density for the six tissue equivalent chips and sheets of material, obtained with Mo/Mo at 28 kVp. For a given material sample, the μ_{eff} is given on the left axis and the equivalent percent glandular density, derived from the linear regression equation, is give on the right axis. The column labeled "100 % G" denotes the chip of 100 % glandular density, "70 % G" the 70 % glandular density, and so on. The column labeled "BR12" corresponds to a sample of the BR12 consistency testing material, equivalent to 47 % glandular/53 % adipose. An estimated glandular density below zero indicates the material is less dense than adipose tissue. The results show that the μ_{eff} of the parchment paper alone, 0.078 ± 0.003 mm^{-1}, was very close to that of the 30 % glandular chip, 0.078 ± 0.004 mm^{-1}. For the fibroglandular component, the μ_{eff} of the parchment with iodine was approximately 0.010 ± 0.005 mm^{-1}, compared to the 100 % glandular chip with 0.11 ± 0.004 mm^{-1}. The slide transparency was equivalent to about 100 % glandularity on its own, and was much higher with the addition of iodine. Similarly, the approximate glandular density of the paper alone exceeded 100 %, and with iodine was almost 175 %.

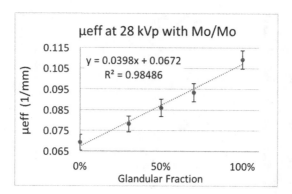

Fig. 2. Mapping of μ_{eff}. The μ_{eff} was computed for each material at a specific tube voltage. Linear regression was applied to determine the relationship between the x-ray attenuation coefficients and the percent glandularity of the materials.

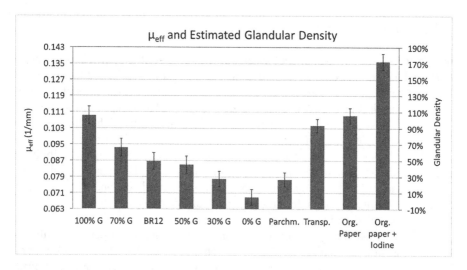

Fig. 3. μ_{eff} and glandular density of sheet materials and tissue chips. The linear attenuation coefficients of the phantom materials were compared with those of known glandular density.

Phantom printing is a promising area of active research, particularly with the use of additive manufacturing techniques. However, current additive manufacturing techniques have limited feasibility due to the high cost of the printing machine and inks, along with a small selection of desirable materials. The method presented in this study, however, uses readily available materials to produce a cheap and fully customizable 3D structured phantom with realistic material properties.

The results of the analysis showed that the parchment paper and iodine ink can be used to create a phantom with similar x-ray properties as breast tissue glandular tissue, under the beam conditions considered. Because the phantom is not limited to two materials, it is possible to print other anatomical features of interest, such as lesions or microcalcifications (MC). Additionally, because the model resolution is arbitrary, a smaller voxel size may be selected to better resolve microcalcifications smaller than 120 µm. Once created, these features can be easily inserted into and removed from the phantom by printing the mass or MC over multiple sheets and simply replacing select slices within the original phantom. The phantom can also be modeled with blood vessels, thus the modeling of iodine uptake through the breast arterial system would also be possible. While an analytical virtual phantom is used here, another benefit of the technique is that it is not limited to such models and can readily be applied with any type of voxelized phantom. The realism of the virtual model was not the primary focus of this work, and its appearance was not evaluated by radiologists. However, the present approach provides a method to print any virtual breast model using tissue equivalent materials.

4 Conclusions

Structured phantoms are necessary for evaluating 2D and 3D breast imaging systems. Existing phantoms can be expensive, time consuming to create, or limited in their anatomical realizations. In this work we demonstrated a unique technique for printing 3D physical breast phantoms with a radiographic ink and parchment paper. The x-ray attenuation properties of the ink and parchment allowed us to print glandular structures directly onto an adipose-like background. This method enables for the cheap, rapid creation of breast tissue-equivalent phantoms with great diversity.

References

1. McLelland, R., Hendrick, R.E., Zinninger, M.D., Wilcox, P.A.: The American college of radiology mammography accreditation program. AJR Am. J. Roentgenol. **157**, 473–479 (1991)
2. Thijssen, M.A.O., Bijkerk, K.R., Van der Burght, R.J.M.: Manual contrast-detail phantom Artinis CDMAM type 3.4. University Medical Center Nijmegen, Department of Radiology, The Netherlands, Utilisation Manual 2006 (2007)
3. Carton, A.K., Bakic, P., Ullberg, C., Derand, H., Maidment, A.D.: Development of a physical 3D anthropomorphic breast phantom. Med. Phys. **38**, 891–896 (2011)
4. Gang, G., Tward, D., Lee, J., Siewerdsen, J.: Anatomical background and generalized detectability in tomosynthesis and cone-beam CT. Med. Phys. **37**, 1948–1965 (2010)
5. Freed, M., Badal, A., Jennings, R.J., de las Heras, H., Myers, K.J., Badano, A.: X-ray properties of an anthropomorphic breast phantom for MRI and x-ray imaging. Phys. Med. Biol. **56**, 3513 (2011)
6. Kiarashi, N., Nolte, A.C., Sturgeon, G.M., Segars, W.P., Ghate, S.V., Nolte, L.W., Samei, E., Lo, J.Y.: Development of realistic physical breast phantoms matched to virtual breast phantoms based on human subject data. Med. Phys. **42**, 4116–4126 (2015)
7. Graff, C.G.: A new open-source multi-modality digital breast phantom. In: Medical Imaging 2016: Physics of Medical Imaging. Proceedings of SPIE, vol. 9783 (2016). doi:10.1117/12. 2216312

A Novel 3D Stochastic Solid Breast Texture Model for X-Ray Breast Imaging

Zhijin Li[1,2(✉)], Agnès Desolneux[1], Serge Muller[2], and Ann-Katherine Carton[2]

[1] CMLA, Ecole Normale Supérieure de Cachan, Cachan, France
zli@ens-cachan.fr, agnes.desolneux@cmla.ens-cachan.fr
[2] GE Healthcare, Buc, France
{jonathan.li,serge.muller,ann-katherine.carton}@ge.com

Abstract. Performance assessment of breast x-ray imaging systems through clinical imaging studies is expensive and may result in unreasonable high radiation doses to the patient. As an alternative, several research groups are investigating the potential of virtual clinical trials using realistic 3D breast texture models and simulated images from those models. This paper describes a mathematically defined solid 3D breast texture model based on the analysis of segmented clinical breast computed tomography images. The model employs stochastic geometry to mimic small and medium scale fibro-glandular and adipose tissue morphologies. Medium-scale morphology of each adipose compartment is simulated by a union of overlapping ellipsoids. The boundary of each ellipsoid consists of small Voronoi cells with average volume of 0.5 mm^3, introducing a small-scale texture aspect. Model parameters were first empirically determined for almost entirely adipose breasts, scattered fibro-glandular dense breasts and heterogeneously dense breasts. Preliminary evaluation has shown that simulated mammograms and digital breast tomosynthesis images have a reasonable realistic visual appearance, depending though on simulated breast density. Statistical inference of model parameters from clinical breast computed tomography images for the variety of fibro-glandular and adipose tissue distributions observed in clinical images is ongoing.

Keywords: Solid 3D breast texture model · Stochastic geometry

1 Introduction

Since clinical imaging studies are expensive and time consuming, there has been an increased research investment into less costly and more time-efficient simulation studies [1, Sect. 12.5]. Reliable simulation studies in the field of digital breast tomosynthesis (DBT), and more generally in 3D imaging of the breast, require a realistic numerical 3D anthropomorphic test object model, a realistic numerical image acquisition chain and task-based mathematical observer models.

Several numerical 3D anthropomorphic breast object models have been proposed [1–5]. Each model presents advantages and restrictions in terms of the visual realism of breast object images, the consistency between statistical features of test object and clinical images, and the potential to mimic the anatomical variability seen in real breast

A. Tingberg et al. (Eds.): IWDM 2016, LNCS 9699, pp. 660–667, 2016.
DOI: 10.1007/978-3-319-41546-8_82

images. These aspects may impact the model validity for certain performance assessment studies.

Pokrajac *et al.* [1, Sect. 12.3.1] and Mahr *et al.* [4] have proposed 3D breast phantoms with mathematically defined structures. To simulate medium scale adipose tissue compartments in the fibroglandular tissue, Pokrajac *et al.* employs a region growing scheme implemented as a Voronoi diagram with a specific norm associated with ellipsoidal shapes [1, Sect. 12.3.1]. Each adipose compartment is simulated as a single geometry controlled by a seed point. Simulation of small scale fibroglandular tissue is obtained by sub-compartmentalization of the adipose tissue compartments [2]. To simulate the medium scale adipose tissue in the fibroglandular tissue, Mahr et al. [4] uses uniformly distributed ellipsoids pointing towards the nipple with stochastic tilt-angles and the semi-axes lengths of the ellipsoids are uniformly distributed and empirically determined. Clusters of 0.5 to 1 mm diameter randomly distributed spheres are positioned at the end-point of each ductal tree terminal branch to mimic small scale structures in the fibro glandular tissue.

We propose an alternative 3D solid breast texture model inspired by the morphology of medium and small scale fibro-glandular and adipose tissue observed in clinical breast computed tomography (bCT) images (UC Davis database). The model admits a mathematical formulation using stochastic geometry theory, a branch of mathematics studying the distribution of random geometric objects. Each adipose compartment is modeled as a union of overlapping ellipsoids and the whole model is formulated as a spatial marked point process [6]. A small-scale texture aspect is introduced by replacing the smooth ellipsoid boundaries by Voronoi cells with average volume of 0.5 mm^3. The texture model allows for simulation of visually realistic 2D and 3D breast x-ray images and for providing a complete mathematical formulation.

2   Methodology

2.1   Materials and Input

The construction of our 3D solid breast texture model is based on the observations from segmented clinical bCT image datasets. Li et al. [1, Sect. 12.3.2] has shown that by projecting segmented clinical bCT image datasets, mammographic textures depicting realistic morphological variations perceived in clinical mammograms can be obtained. This observation offers a reasonable justification of using segmented bCT datasets as the ground truth for the construction of our breast texture model. By observing binary bCT images, it appears that each adipose compartment can be well approximated by a union of overlapping ellipsoids (Fig. 1a). Therefore the idea of our model is to create a system of ellipsoids whose union accurately exhibits the distribution and morphological characteristics of the medium scale adipose regions observed from segmented bCT datasets. To simulate the small scale texture aspect, we introduce small Voronoi cells at the boundaries of the ellipsoids, simulating irregular adipose compartment boundaries as observed in segmented clinical bCT datasets. Figure 1b illustrates this irregularity in a region of interest of a slice of binary clinical bCT volume. The low spatial resolution of binary bCT images (0.38 mm/pixel) is not the primary reason we simulated micro-texture by introducing adipose compartment boundary irregularity. In fact, histological images demonstrate that the adipose compartment boundary irregularity is real. Bakic *et al.* [2] already illustrated irregular variations around adipose compartments in microscopic breast histological images.

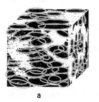 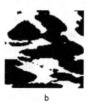

a   b

Fig. 1. a. Each adipose compartment in a binary clinical bCT volume can be seen as a union of several ellipsoids. b. An example illustrating irregular adipose compartment boundaries in a binary clinical bCT image region of interest of size 3×3 cm^2.

2.2 Model Construction Algorithm

The different steps to construct our 3D solid breast texture model are illustrated in Fig. 2 and the algorithm can be summarized as follows:

1. Given a voxelized texture cube W with voxel size v, uniformly generate N points, with N following a Poisson distribution of parameter $\lambda_0|W|$, where $|.|$ denotes the volume measure and λ_0 is a positive real number. This generates a realization of a homogeneous Poisson point process [6].
2. Generate a Voronoi diagram [6] using points obtained from step 1 as cell centers.
3. Independently from step 1 and step 2, create another set of points by drawing a realization of a spatial point process Φ_s in W with distribution $\mathbf{P}_s$. This set of points is named the seed points.
4. For each seed point i, assign a random ellipsoid $\text{Ell}_i(\theta)$ with parameter vector $\theta = (\varphi_1, \varphi_2, \varphi_3, La, Lb, Lc)$ having distribution Θ, where $\varphi_1, \varphi_2, \varphi_3$ are angles determining the orientation of the ellipsoid and La, Lb, Lc are the lengths of semi-axes. The ensemble of the seed point process and the ellipsoid parameters $\Xi = \{\Phi_s, \theta\}$ can be treated as a spatial marked point process [6] determined by the joint distribution of $\mathbf{P}_s$ and Θ.
5. Check each point x of step 1, if $x \in \bigcup_i \text{Ell}_i$, in other words, if it falls inside at least one ellipsoid, then assign all voxels of its corresponding Voronoi cell a value 0. Assign all other voxels value 1.

To demonstrate the impact of the irregular adipose compartment boundaries using small Voronoi cells on improved visual realism of simulated images, texture simulations were performed with smooth and irregular ellipsoid boundaries. Smooth boundaries were simulated by starting directly from step 3 and by modifying step 5 through simply assigning each time a voxel the value 0 if it falls inside at least one ellipsoid.

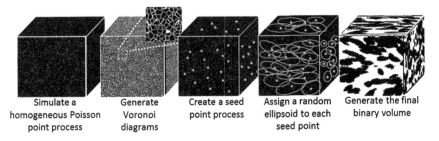

| Simulate a homogeneous Poisson point process | Generate Voronoi diagrams | Create a seed point process | Assign a random ellipsoid to each seed point | Generate the final binary volume |

Fig. 2. Different steps to construct the 3D solid breast texture model.

3 Simulation Results

For our preliminary simulation study, the seed point process Φ_s is set to be a homogeneous Poisson point process (*i.e.* all points are independently uniformly distributed). Parameters were empirically determined for almost entirely adipose breasts, scattered fibro-glandular dense breasts and heterogeneously dense breasts (Table 1). Figure 3 shows examples of regions of interest of simulated texture volume slices, mammograms and DBT reconstructed slices from realizations of 3D solid texture model for breasts of different densities. This figure also shows images created using segmented bCT datasets as reference. Mammograms and DBT projection images were simulated by virtually projecting the texture model using the previously described breast x-ray imaging simulator. DBT reconstructed slices were constructed by processing the projections using an in-house iterative reconstruction algorithm. Breast texture deformation to mimic breast compression during mammography and DBT image acquisition was not modeled. Preliminary evaluations on regions of interest of simulated mammograms and DBT reconstructed slices, similarly to those shown in Fig. 3, indicate a high visual realism compared to real clinical images.

Table 1. Model parameters used for the simulations shown in Fig. 3.

Parameters	Almost entirely adipose	Scattered fibro-glandular dense	Heterogeneously dense
W	$(5 \text{ cm})^3$ voxelized cube with isotropic voxels of size v between $(0.2 \text{ mm})^3$ and $(0.4 \text{ mm})^3$ to match bCT data resolution		
λ_0	2 mm^{-3} (i.e. the average volume of a Voronoi cell $= 0.5 \text{ mm}^3$)		
Φ_s intensity	$3.5 \times 10^{-3} \text{ mm}^{-3}$	$5 \times 10^{-3} \text{ mm}^{-3}$	$2.3 \times 10^{-3} \text{ mm}^{-3}$
La, Lb, Lc (in mm)	$\mu_{La} \sim N(7.4, 1.5)$ $\mu_{Lb}, \mu_{Lc} \sim N(4.5, 0.7)$	$\mu_{La} \sim N(6.4, 1.5)$ $\mu_{Lb}, \mu_{Lc} \sim N(2.5, 0.7)$	$\mu_{La} \sim N(6.4, 1.5)$ $\mu_{Lb}, \mu_{Lc} \sim N(2.5, 0.7)$
$\varphi_1, \varphi_2, \varphi_3$	Gaussians with means determined by a vector from the ellipsoid center to a predefined nipple. Standard deviations are $\frac{\pi}{12}$		

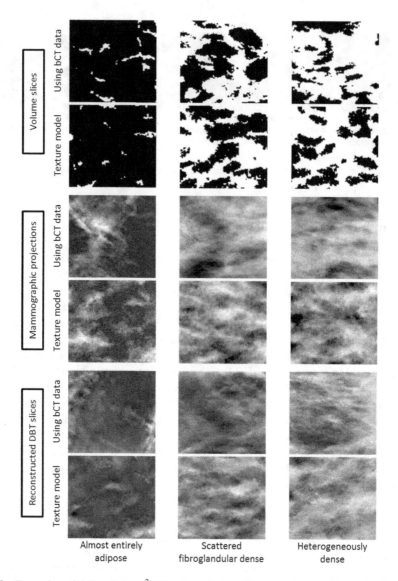

Fig. 3. Examples of 3.5 × 3.5 cm² ROIs in volume slices, mammographic projections and reconstructed DBT slices simulated starting from texture volumes and segmented clinical bCT data of different breast density

Figure 4 shows examples of regions of interest of simulated mammograms and DBT reconstructed slices from a breast texture volume according to a heterogeneously dense breast. Ellipsoids with smooth boundaries and ellipsoids with irregular boundaries introduced by small Voronoi are considered. These examples illustrate that irregular adipose compartment boundaries may improve visual realism of simulated images.

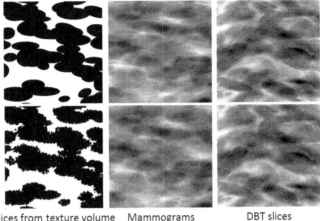

Slices from texture volume   Mammograms   DBT slices

Fig. 4. Slices through simulated breast texture volumes and regions of interest of corresponding mammograms and DBT reconstructed slices. Smooth ellipsoid adipose/glandular boundaries (top row) and irregular ellipsoid boundaries introduced by small Voronoi cells (bottom row) were simulated.

4   Realism Assessment Through Psycho-Physical Studies

A two-alternative forced choice (2AFC) experiment was performed to assess the visual realism of simulated DBT reconstructed images. Pairs of 3.5×3.5 cm^2 ROIs, extracted from images simulated from our texture model and clinical bCT data were displayed side-by-side. Images on the left always came from the clinical bCT data set, while images on the right had 50 % chance to be from the texture model and 50 % chance to be from clinical bCT data. The reader had to tell whether the image on the right was from the clinical bCT data set or from the texture model. Similar level of glandular density was maintained for each image pair. In total, 144 image pairs were presented; 52 pairs from almost entirely adipose breasts, 56 pairs from scattered fibro-glandular dense breasts and 36 pairs from heterogeneously dense breasts. Each image pair was displayed during 5 s, followed by the display of a uniform gray–level image for another 5 s; the readers were thus imposed to make a decision within 10 s.

A short training session with 10 image pairs of known ground truth was performed before the real experiment with no time constraint. Images were displayed on 5 M pixels grayscale portrait monitors (SMD 21500 G, Siemens AG; Munchen, Germany) at 100 % resolution. The reading distance was set to be one meter.

Four readers participated in the experiment, all GE Healthcare engineers. Reader 1, 2 and 3 have no prior knowledge of our texture model while reader 4 knows the algorithm of the texture model construction. The percentage of correct answers, Pc, was calculated as an indication for the realism of the simulated images from the texture model. Under the null hypothesis that images simulated from the model and clinical bCT images data cannot be distinguished, Pc = 0.5.

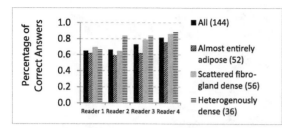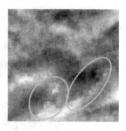

Fig. 5. Left: percentage of correct answers of 4 readers of the 2AFC experiment, calculated together for images of all density categories and separately for images of different density categories. Right: example of the quantification effect appearing like "small square blocks" in a 2×2 cm^2 ROI of one reconstructed DBT slice created from the texture model.

The left chart of Fig. 5 shows the Pc value of the four readers of the 2AFC experiments. Readers 1 and 2 had overall Pc values of 0.65 and 0.66, while reader 3 had a Pc value of 0.73 indicating that he could more easily distinguish texture images from clinical bCT images. Reader 4 had the highest Pc value of 0.82. He reported that he was able to infer simulated images from his prior knowledge of the intermediate steps of the model construction. Readers 1, 3 and 4 reported that they had observed a quantification effect appearing like "small square blocks" in some simulated images from the texture model, as illustrated in the right image of Fig. 5. When this effect was present, they used it as criterion to distinguish simulated images using the texture model from those using clinical bCT data. Reader 2 did not report the same primary criteria. This 'small square block artifact' can likely be attributed to the size of the Voronoi cells at the transition of glandular/adipose tissue. Table 2 reports Pc for each reader by type of breast density. The p-value indicates whether the reader was or was not able to differentiate simulated data from real data. The lower Pc values for almost entirely adipose breasts can be explained by the lower number of adipose/dense transitions, designed by Voronoi cells, in this type of breasts.

Table 2. Detection rate and p-values for each reader by type of breast ($p < 0.05$ means the reader was able to differentiate simulated data from real data).

	Almost entirely adipose			Scattered fibroglandular dense			Heterogenously dense			All		
	n = 52			n = 56			n = 36			n = 144		
Reader 1	31	0.60	p > 0.05	39	0.69	p < 0.05	24	0.66	p > 0.05	94	0.65	p < 0.05
Reader 2	30	0.58	p > 0.05	36	0.64	p < 0.05	30	0.83	p < 0.05	95	0.66	p < 0.05
Reader 3	32	0.62	p > 0.05	44	0.79	p < 0.05	30	0.83	p < 0.05	105	0.73	p < 0.05
Reader 4	39	0.75	p < 0.05	51	0.86	p < 0.05	32	0.89	p < 0.05	118	0.82	p < 0.05

5   Discussion and Conclusion

In this paper, we described a mathematically defined solid 3D breast texture model based on the analysis of segmented clinical breast computed tomography images. Our model is formulated as a spatial marked point process, exhibiting mathematical formulation.

Preliminary evaluations of simulated 2D and 3D breast x-ray images using a prototype of the solid breast texture model, with empirically determined parameters appear to have high visual realism compared with clinical images. To assess visual realism of synthetic DBT images simulated using our texture model, we performed a 2-AFC experiment involving four readers. This preliminary experiment results demonstrated that the model with empirical parameters can simulate fairly realistic DBT reconstructed images for almost entirely adipose breast types. The results also demonstrate that a quantification artifact, introduced by the size of the Voronoi cells at the transition of adipose/glandular tissue, reduces the realism of the texture model for higher density breasts. Using the empirically determined parameters, our current model is thus restricted to simulate a limited variability of breast tissue types encountered in real breasts. We will further address this limitation by fitting our model parameters to different breast types seen in the clinical bCT database.

Due to the stationarity of the seed point process which assumes no interactions between the ellipsoids, simulations of larger texture volumes results in reduced visual realism in simulated images. To address this, a point process with clustering interactions might be worth investigating.

Acknowledgements. We thank Dr. John Boone, University of Davis, for allowing us to use his large database of clinical bCT images. This study was partially funded by ANRT, under CIFRE convention N° 2013/1052.

References

1. Hendee, W.T.: Digital phantoms for breast imaging. In: Physics of Mammographic Imaging, Series Editor. CRC Press, Boca Raton (2012)
2. Bakic, P.R., Pokrajac, D.D., De Caro, R., Maidment, A.D.A.: Realistic simulation of breast tissue microstructure in software anthropomorphic phantoms. In: Fujita, H., Hara, T., Muramatsu, C. (eds.) IWDM 2014. LNCS, vol. 8539, pp. 348–355. Springer, Heidelberg (2014)
3. Chen, F., Bakic, P.R., Maidment, A.D.A., Jensen, S.T., Shi, X., Pokrajac, D.D.: Description and characterization of a novel method for partial volume simulation in software breast phantoms. IEEE Trans. Med. Imaging **34**(10), 2146–2161 (2015). doi:10.1109/TMI.2015.2424854
4. Mahr, D.M., Bhargava, R., Insana, M.F.: Three-dimensional in silico breast phantoms for multimodal image simulations. IEEE Trans. Med. Imaging **31**(3), 689–697 (2012). doi:10.1109/TMI.2011.2175401
5. Carton, A.-K., Grisey, A., de Carvalho, P.M., Dromain, C., Muller, S.: A virtual human breast phantom using surface meshes and geometric internal structures. In: Fujita, H., Hara, T., Muramatsu, C. (eds.) IWDM 2014. LNCS, vol. 8539, pp. 356–363. Springer, Heidelberg (2014)
6. Chiu, S.N., Stoyan, D., Kendall, W.S., Mecke, J.: Stochastic Geometry and Its Applications, 3rd edn. Wiley, Hoboken (2013)

OPTIMAM Image Simulation Toolbox - Recent Developments and Ongoing Studies

Premkumar Elangovan[1(✉)], Andria Hadjipanteli[2],
Alistair Mackenzie[2], David R. Dance[2,3], Kenneth C. Young[2,3],
and Kevin Wells[1]

[1] Centre for Vision, Speech and Signal Processing, University of Surrey,
Guildford GU2 7XH, UK
p.elangovan@surrey.ac.uk
[2] NCCPM, Royal Surrey County Hospital, Guildford, Surrey GU2 7XX, UK
[3] Department of Physics, University of Surrey, Guildford GU2 7XH, UK

Abstract. Virtual clinical trials (VCTs) are increasingly being seen as a viable pre-clinical method for evaluation of imaging systems in breast cancer screening. The CR-UK funded OPTIMAM project is aimed at producing modelling tools for use in such VCTs. In the initial phase of the project, modelling tools were produced to simulate 2D-mammography and digital breast tomosynthesis (DBT) imaging systems. This paper elaborates on the new tools that have recently been developed for the current phase of the OPTIMAM project. These new additions to the framework include tools for simulating synthetic breast tissue, spiculated masses and variable-angle DBT systems. These tools are described in the paper along with the preliminary validation results. Four-alternative forced choice (4-AFC) type studies deploying these new tools are underway. The results of the ongoing 4AFC studies investigating minimum detectable contrast/size of masses/microcalcifications for different modalities and system designs are presented.

Keywords: Digital breast tomosynthesis · 2D-mammography · Modelling · Simulation · 4AFC · Simulated masses · Breast phantom

1 Introduction

National breast cancer screening programs play a vital role in early detection and treatment of breast cancer in Western countries. The choice of imaging modality, or modalities, to be used in such screening programs is constantly reassessed and is still a source of debate [1]. With new modalities being introduced into the market and a wide choice of system designs available within each modality, evaluation by means of clinical trials becomes challenging as this conventional approach requires timescales that cannot keep pace with the rate of technological innovation. Recently, virtual clinical trials (VCTs) have started to be used for rapid pre-clinical evaluations of new modalities using modelling tools. This approach also provides a means to study the effects of various intrinsic design variations so as to optimize the design for the best screening performance.

© Springer International Publishing Switzerland 2016
A. Tingberg et al. (Eds.): IWDM 2016, LNCS 9699, pp. 668–675, 2016.
DOI: 10.1007/978-3-319-41546-8_83

The CR-UK funded OPTIMAM project is producing modelling tools for use in such VCTs [2]. The early phase of the project was predominantly focused on the design of simulation tools for 2D-mammography and narrow angle DBT systems. The framework included: (1) cancer simulation models (masses [3, 4] and microcalcification [5]); (2) a ray tracing tool (image acquisition); (3) image degradation model (scatter, noise and blur) [6, 7] and (4) manufacturer specific post-processing tools (image processing and reconstruction). The lesion simulation models were validated qualitatively by means of observer studies involving radiologists [3–5]. Models of image formation were validated quantitatively using image quality metrics [2, 6, 7].

In the current phase of the OPTIMAM project, these tools have been extended to include further modelling components for use in four-alternative forced choice (4-AFC) experiments. New tools include: (1) a tool for simulating 3D breast structure [8]; (2) a model for simulating spiculated lesions [9]; (3) simulation of DBT imaging using a wide-angle geometry and (4) a user interface for 4AFC studies. In this paper, we describe in detail the new additions to the OPTIMAM framework and provide some selected results of ongoing 4AFC studies [10, 11] that employ these tools.

2   Materials, Methods and Results

Figure 1 provides an illustration of the OPTIMAM simulation framework. New developments have been made in the simulation of tissues and imaging as described in following sections.

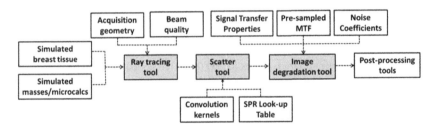

Fig. 1. OPTIMAM simulation framework [2]

2.1   Synthetic Breast Model

One of the important additions to the current phase of the OPTIMAM project is a synthetic breast model [8]. This allows insertion of synthetic pathology (masses or micro calcifications) in a more realistic manner, as prior work using template multiplication [3–5] led to realism issues [12] with intersecting anatomical features at certain anatomical locations. These issues have been particularly apparent when inserting masses into DBT image data. Using synthetic tissue allows pathology to be inserted by voxel replacement which produces greater levels of realism in the resulting images. The elements of normal breast tissue were simulated by first extracting various anatomical features from DBT images of patients.

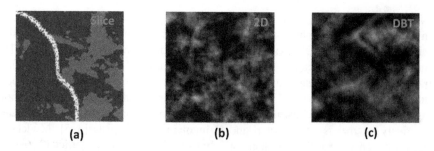

Fig. 2. (a) Cross-sectional slice from the breast model; (b) processed 2D image and (c) reconstructed DBT plane

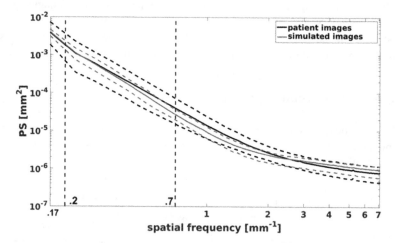

Fig. 3. Normalized power spectrum curves for 2D (blue, red dotted lines represent 5th and 95th percentiles) [8]. Vertical dashed lines indicate window of spatial frequencies recognized as being mainly attributable to image texture rather than other factors such as quantum noise (Color figure online)

The process starts by extracting glandular segments from DBT images using a region-growing method and subsequently decluttering the segments by applying a series of morphological operations. This process is repeated until a database of glandular segments is produced. An empty breast volume is created and then filled with fatty tissue. Glandular segments are then gradually added to the empty volume until the required glandularity has been achieved. A wireframe of blood vessels and Cooper's ligaments was produced by spline interpolation of in-focus landmarks produced by manual annotation of DBT image planes. The wireframe representation was then dilated to anatomically appropriate diameters and added to the breast volume containing the glandular matrix to simulate these anatomical components with high spatial frequencies. Figure 2 shows an example of a slice through the breast model and simulated 2D and DBT images of the model.

The breast model was validated by computing the power spectra of simulated images and comparing these with the spectra computed for real images. The methods described by Hill *et al.* [13] and Cockmartin *et al.* [14] were used for calculating the power spectrum of real and simulated images. A selection of 300 3 cm × 3 cm regions of interest in simulated images was used to calculate the power spectrum. The real image dataset contained 40 sets of patient images acquired using the Hologic Selenia Dimensions 3D breast tomosynthesis system (Hologic, Bedford, Massachusetts, USA). Figure 3 shows the mean power spectra of real and simulated 2D images. The curve for simulated images closely overlaps with that of real images.

Simulated 2D and DBT images of the breast model were interleaved with real images and presented to a team of experienced observers in an ROC study. The team comprised of 4 observers with an average breast screening experience of around 10 years. The average area under the curve (AUC) for 2D and DBT images were 0.53 ± .04 and 0.55 ± .07 respectively [8]. The results indicate that the observers had difficulty in differentiating real and simulated images.

2.2 Mass Simulation Model

In the early phase of the OPTIMAM project, irregular lesions were simulated by a fractal-growth process known as diffusion limited aggregation (DLA) [3, 4]. The appearance of such irregular simulated masses after insertion into clinical radiological images was found to be largely indistinguishable from real masses with similar appearance using an ROC paradigm. By changing the parametric prescriptions of the DLA growth model it was possible to simulate masses of different densities and appearances. In the current phase of the OPTIMAM project, this model has now been extended to simulate spiculated lesions [9]. Such lesions are characterized by linear structures branching from a central core. In order to simulate spicules with realistic appearance, in terms of curvature and distribution, various features were extracted from patient DBT images and used as a guideline for generating synthetic spicules. This was performed by (Fig. 4a) manually scrolling through DBT planes and marking the points at which spicule segments appear in-focus across a variety of different planes. 3D spline interpolation (Fig. 4b) was then used to connect the selected points to produce a 3D skeleton for each spicule. The resulting 3D "spicule skeletons" (Fig. 4c) were converted into thin horns (Fig. 4d) and placed on the surface of a DLA mass (Fig. 4e–f). Finally, the 3D geometric horns were filled up with fine fibrotic structures in order to provide the correct density and internal texture. This fibrotic characteristic can be observed in specimen X-ray images of real spiculated lesions. Some examples of simulated irregular and spiculated masses are shown in Fig. 5.

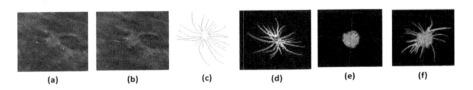

(a)   (b)   (c)   (d)   (e)   (f)

Fig. 4. Spiculated mass generation process [9]

For preliminary validation, a total of 13 simulated spiculated masses were inserted into 2D and DBT patient images and presented to an experienced breast radiologist (>15 years screening experience). The simulated images were interleaved with images containing real spiculated masses and presented blind to the radiologist for feedback. The radiologist rated 60 % of the simulated lesions in 2D and 50 % of the simulated lesions in DBT to be realistic. The radiologist was able to correctly identify all the 2D and DBT real images in the dataset.

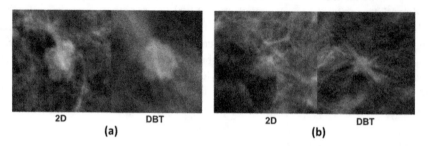

Fig. 5. Examples of (a) simulated irregular and (b) simulated spiculated masses

2.3   Image Degradation Model

In the early phase of the OPTIMAM project, we modelled the system acquisition and image degradation processes of narrow angle DBT systems, in particular the geometry and settings of the Hologic Selenia Dimensions 3D breast tomosynthesis system. The entire simulation framework was validated by simulating geometrically defined objects and quantitatively comparing the simulated images with real images of the same objects [2]. The process starts with the simulation of X-ray projections through a 3D voxelized phantom for a particular X-ray spectrum. Then, scatter estimated from a lookup table produced from Monte Carlo simulations [6] for different breast thickness/glandularity is added to the projections. Finally the appropriate noise and blur are added to the images using methods described in our previously published work [7].

In the present phase of the project we have extended these tools to simulate wide angle geometry such as that used by the Siemens Mammomat Inspiration (Siemens Healthcare, Erlangen, Germany) systems. The new system was characterized using standard techniques for measuring the pre-sampled MTF (modulation transfer function), NNPS (normalized noise power spectrum), STP (signal transfer properties), flat fielding correction map, focal spot size and focus motion. The increase in motion blur due to tube motion in the wide-angle DBT system was included in the simulations by elongating the focal spot along the direction of the tube motion. A detailed description of the image simulation procedure is given in our previously published work [2].

2.4   Ongoing 4AFC Studies

VCTs conducted during the early phase of the OPTIMAM project predominantly involved modification of real images to simulate the synthetic objects representative of cancers. Planned virtual clinical trials for the current phase of the project are aimed at using the 4AFC paradigm. AFC experiments can be used to examine the fundamental human signal detection response for a variety of stimuli. This paradigm has been previously used to compare and evaluate breast imaging modalities. The figure of merit for our 4AFC experiment is the minimum detectable contrast or object size which is defined as the value at which the observer makes 92.5 % correct decisions (d' of 2.5) for a given experimental condition. Two studies are currently underway, details and results are given below.

The objective of the first study is to consider the minimum detectable contrast in 2D-mammography and DBT systems for simulated masses and solid spheres. Masses and spheres of 5 mm diameter were simulated and inserted into synthetic breast models of different thicknesses at random depths. 2D and DBT (15° tube sweep/15 projections) images were produced for image acquisition and detector settings for the Hologic Selenia Dimensions 3D breast tomosynthesis system. Images were simulated with the inserted lesions having different contrast levels (1 % to 6 % in steps of .5%), resulting in 45 mass images and 15 sphere images per contrast level for both 2D and DBT. The contrast was varied by changing the attenuation properties of the inserted masses and spheres. The contrast was defined as the relative difference between background and target pixel intensity measured in the 2D image. Hologic image processing (Hologic LORAD FFDM Selenia V5.0) and reconstruction tools were used to post-process the images, which were then cropped to 3×3 cm^2 with the target in the center. The results of the mass/sphere 4AFC study are shown in Fig. 6a [10]. They indicate that the observers needed approximately twice the signal contrast to correctly identify a mass in 2D-mammography (0.094 ± .005) compared with DBT (0.040 ± .001). The differences were much bigger when spheres were used instead of simulated irregular masses. However, the minimum detectable contrast for spheres was much lower in both 2D-mammography (0.075 ± .008) and DBT (0.0074 ± .002) compared to simulated masses. This might be because of the regular geometry of spheres making them easy to spot in DBT images. The errors given are the standard errors in the average minimum detectable contrast from all the observers.

The objective of the second study is to determine the minimum detectable micro calcification diameter in breast images using 2D-mammography and narrow (15° tube sweep/15 projections) and wide (50° tube sweep/25 projections) angle DBT. The microcalcification clusters (5 calcs/2.5 mm cluster size) were produced containing microcalcifications of different sizes (100 μm to 500 μm in steps of 25 μm). These clusters were inserted in the middle of 6 cm thick synthetic breast models and 50 images per experimental condition were produced for each modality considered. The mean glandular dose to the breast was set to approximately 2.5 mGy in all three cases. Briona (Real Time Tomography, LLC, Philadelphia, USA) image processing and reconstruction tools were used to post process the images, and the images were cropped to 2.7×2.7 cm^2 with the target in the center. The results of the microcalcification cluster study are shown in Fig. 6b [11]. The results indicate that the minimum detectable microcalcification diameters for 2D-mammography, narrow angle DBT and wide angle DBT are 164 ± 5 μm, 210 ± 5 μm and 255 ± 4 μm respectively. The errors given are the standard errors in the average minimum detectable calcification diameter from all the observers. Currently, the mass/sphere 4AFC study is underway

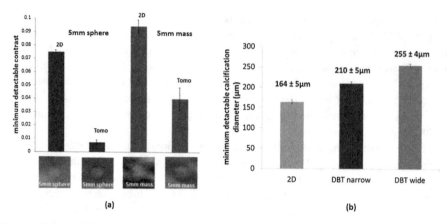

Fig. 6. Results of the 4AFC observer study for (a) lesion and sphere targets [10] and (b) microcalcification clusters [11]

for different mass sizes, and the microcalcification cluster size 4AFC study is underway for different heights and breast thicknesses.

3   Conclusions

Recent improvements to the OPTIMAM image simulation toolbox have been demonstrated. Much of the recent progress has come from improving the tissue/image simulation tools and adoption of the 4AFC paradigm for VCTs. The preliminary validation results of the tissue simulation model are very promising and encourage further development. The results of the 4AFC studies demonstrate the variations in detection performance for different types of targets and system designs. This highlights the potential of virtual clinical trials encouraging further studies.

Acknowledgements. This work is part of the OPTIMAM2 project funded by Cancer Research UK (grant, number: C30682/A17321). We are grateful for Hologic's assistance with the reconstruction. The authors thank colleagues at NCCPM, Dr. Vicky Cooke at the Jarvis Breast Screening Centre, Guildford and observers at St Georges Hospital, London for invaluable assistance.

References

1. Hevie, M.A., Chang, J.T., Hendrick, R.E., Banerjee, M.: Reduction in late-stage breast cancer incidence in the mammography era: implications for overdiagnosis of invasive cancer. Cancer **120**, 2649–2656 (2014)
2. Elangovan, P., Mackenzie, A., Diaz, O., Rashidnasab, A., Dance, D.R., Young, K.C., Warren, L.M., Shaheen, E., Bosmans, H., Bakic, P.R., Wells, K.: Development and validation of a modelling framework for simulating 2D-mammography and breast tomosynthesis. Phys. Med. Biol. **59**, 4275–4293 (2014)

3. Rashidnasab, A., Elangovan, P., Diaz, O., Mackenzie, A., Young, K.C., Dance, D.R., Wells, K.: Simulation of 3D DLA masses in digital breast tomosynthesis. In: Proceedings of SPIE, vol. 8668, p. 86680Y (2013)

4. Rashidnasab, A., Elangovan, P., Yip, M., Young, K.C., Dance, D.R., Wells, K.: Simulation and assessment of realistic breast lesions using fractal growth models. Phys. Med. Biol. **15**, 5613–5626 (2013)

5. Shaheen, E., De Keyzer, F., Bosmans, H., Dance, D.R., Young, K.C., Van Ongeval, C.: The simulation of 3D mass models in 2D digital mammography and breast tomosynthesis. Med. Phys. **41**, 081913-1-17 (2014)

6. Diaz, O., Dance, D.R., Young, K.C., Elangovan, P., Bakic, P.R., Wells, K.: Estimation of scattered radiation in digital breast tomosynthesis. Phys. Med. Biol. **59**, 4375–4390 (2014)

7. Mackenzie, A., Dance, D.R., Diaz, O., Young, K.C.: Image simulation and a model of noise power spectra across a range of mammographic beam qualities. Med. Phys. **41**, 12901–12914 (2014)

8. Elangovan, P., Dance, D.R., Young, K.C., Wells, K.: Generation of 3D synthetic breast tissue. In: Proceedings of SPIE, vol. 9783, p. 9783081-6 (2016)

9. Elangovan, P., Alrehily, F., Pinto, R.F., Rashidnasab, A., Dance, D.R., Young, K.C., Wells, K.: Simulation of spiculated breast lesions. In: Proceedings of SPIE, vol. 9783, p. 97832E1-5 (2016)

10. Elangovan, P., Rashidnasab, A., Mackenzie, A., Dance, D.R., Young, K.C., Bosmans, H., Segars, W.P., Wells, K.: Performance comparison of breast imaging modalities using a 4AFC human observer study. In: Proceedings of SPIE vol. 9412, p. 94121T1-7 (2015)

11. Hadjipanteli, A., Elangovan, P., Looney, P.T., Mackenzie, A., Wells, K., Dance, D.R., Young, K.C.: Detection of microcalcification clusters by 2D-mammography and narrow and wide angle digital breast tomosynthesis. In: Proceedings of SPIE, vol. 9783, p. 9783061-8 (2016)

12. Rashidnasab, A., Elangovan, P., Mackenzie, A., Dance, D.R., Young, K.C., Bosmans, H., Wells, K.: Virtual clinical trials using inserted pathology in clinical images: investigation and assumptions for local glandularity and noise. In: Proceedings of SPIE, vol. 9412, p. 94122D1-7 (2015)

13. Hill, M.L., Mainprize, J.G., Carton, A.K., Saab-Puong, S., Iordache, R., Muller, S., Jong, R. A., Dromain, C., Yaffe, M.J.: Anatomical noise in contrast-enhanced digital mammography. Part I. Single-energy imaging. Med. Phys. **40**, 051910 (2013)

14. Cockmartin, L., Bosmans, H., Marshall, N.W.: Comparative power law analysis of structured breast phantom and patient images in digital mammography and breast tomosynthesis. Med. Phys. **40**, 081920 (2013)

Impact of Clinical Display Device on Detectability of Breast Masses in 2D Digital Mammography: A Virtual Clinical Study

Alaleh Rashidnasab[1,2]([✉]), Frédéric Bemelmans[1], Nicholas W. Marshall[3], Tom Kimpe[4], and Hilde Bosmans[1,3]

[1] Department of Imaging and Pathology, KU Leuven, Leuven, Belgium
a.rashidnasab@ucl.ac.uk
[2] Institute of Nuclear Medicine, University College London, London, UK
[3] Department of Radiology, UZ Leuven, Leuven, Belgium
hilde.bosmans@uzleuven.be
[4] Barco, Kortrijk, Belgium
tom.kimpe@barco.com

Abstract. This work investigates the impact of advanced clinical displays on cancer detection in 2D digital mammograms using four-alternative-forced-choice (4AFC) and a dataset of images with inserted simulated lesions. Images were displayed on a standard monitor (Barco Coronis 5MP mammo) and an advanced monitor (Barco Coronis Uniti 12MP MDMC-12132). Ill-defined margin and spiculated mass models were inserted into mammographic regions of interest using a validated physics-based insertion framework. Experiments were conducted for mass size of 8–11 mm to 2–3 mm and density of 100 % to 70 % of glandular tissue with 142 trials per condition. Five medical physicists read the dataset on both monitors. Percentage correct (PC) of detected masses for average observer and 95 % confidence intervals were determined. Paired t-test and ANOVA analysis were performed. The observers had significantly better detection rates when the dataset was read on the advanced monitor compared to the standard monitor (3 % increase in overall PC, paired p-value = 0.0076).

Keywords: Clinical display · Virtual clinical trial · Detection · 2D digital mammography · Simulated lesions · DLA mass · Spiculated mass · 4AFC observer study

1 Introduction

New digital mammography technologies allow optimization of systems at different stages of acquisition, processing and display. Clinical trials are conventionally used to study these systems but they are time consuming and require collection of large patient datasets. Alternatively, a simulation approach that utilizes models of imaging system and realistic models of pathology that are then inserted into

© Springer International Publishing Switzerland 2016
A. Tingberg et al. (Eds.): IWDM 2016, LNCS 9699, pp. 676–683, 2016.
DOI: 10.1007/978-3-319-41546-8_84

normal mammograms or breast phantoms of systems with specific characteristics may overcome such limitations. Virtual clinical trials using such simulation tools can be conducted to evaluate and optimise mammography systems and detection rates in a fast and efficient manner. Moreover, virtual clinical trials allow investigation of a small part or a detail characteristic of an imaging chain that may not be feasible to test through clinical trials [1, 2].

It is in the virtual clinical trial motivational context that this study aimed to compare a new advanced clinical monitor (Barco Coronis Uniti 12MP MDMC-12132) with a standard 5 MP monitor (Barco Coronis 5MP mammo) in terms of breast mass detection in 2D mammograms. A comprehensive dataset was created using simulated mass models of validated realistic appearances inserted into mammographic regions of interest (ROIs) extracted from 2D digital mammograms. A validated physics-based insertion framework was utilised. The simulated images were read by human observers on both monitors in a 4-alternative forced choice (4AFC) study paradigm. The significance of difference in breast mass detection on the standard vs. advanced monitors was investigated. Furthermore, the detectability of breast masses on these monitors was compared for various factors: type, size and composition (density) of masses, and the glandularity of the background ROI.

2 Methods and Material

2.1 Simulated Dataset Generation

For the purpose of the study, raw normal mammograms of screening patients with compressed breast thickness of 40–49 mm were collected. The images were acquired on a Mammomat Inspiration Siemens system with 28 kV and W/Rh as target/filter combination. ROIs of 3×3 cm were extracted from these mammograms. A software tool determined the edge and the area within the breast for automatic extraction of ROIs. Using a volumetric breast density estimation tool (Volpara, Matakina, New Zealand [5]) the average density of each ROI was estimated. In total, 142 ROIs were selected to create signal-present images for the 4AFC study. This included 61 ROIs with low glandularity (<15 %), 61 ROIs with medium glandularity (15 %–30 %) and 20 ROIs with high glandularity (>30 %). For signal-absent images in the 4AFC study, a large pool of ROIs excluding the above 142 ROIs was created from the same mammograms and classified based on their average density.

Three-dimensional (3D) models of breast masses, developed and validated for realistic appearance in 2D mammograms [3, 4], were used for insertion into the selected 142 ROIs. Ill-defined margin mass models were generated using a fractal growth method known as diffusion limited aggregation (DLA) [3]. Spiculated mass models were simulated by segmenting contrast enhanced MRI breast lesions to use these volumes as the core of the mass, and subsequently growing the spicules from the core using an iterative branching algorithm [4]. A voxel size of 45 μm was used for the simulation of the masses. Five masses with ill-defined margin and five spiculated masses with initial size of 8–11 mm in the x-y plane were selected for the present study. Originally, a linear attenuation coefficient equivalent to 100 % glandular tissue was assigned to the mass models. To create masses of different sizes in present study, the original 10 masses were digitally scaled in all three dimensions to create masses of 6–8 mm, 4–6 mm and 2–3 mm in-plane size. In addition, to create masses of different density the original masses of 8–11 mm were systematically assigned with reduced linear attenuation coefficient to generate masses with 90 %, 80 % and 70 % of the glandular tissue composition. To determine a clinically relevant measure of the size of the simulated masses in the x-y plane, an expert radiologist was asked to measure the size of each original mass inserted in the same location in a very fatty 2D mammogram. The reason for this approach is linked to the generation of the model: spicules can be simulated very long and thin as defined by the user. However, the ultimate length of the spicules may not be clinically relevant due to the lack of physical ground for their creation. The threshold thickness for a spicule to be detected with mammography is not known.

A validated physics-based insertion framework [4] was used to insert simulated masses into selected ROIs. The insertion method accounted for the system geometry, polychromatic X-ray spectra, MTF and scatter of the imaging system being modelled (i.e. the Siemens Inspiration system). The local glandularity estimate from Volpara [5] was used to estimate the attenuation coefficient of the hypothetical breast tissue being replaced by the mass model. For each ROI, one original ill-defined margin mass and one original spiculated mass were randomly selected and inserted in the centre of two copies of the same ROI. Insertion in the same ROI was repeated for the more subtle versions of these masses (reduced size and less density) as shown in Fig. 1. Each ROI with inserted mass was then processed with the manufacturer's image processing software and used as signal present images for the 4AFC study.

Fig. 1. Example of insertion of an ill-defined margin mass in a given ROI: (top) original mass and reduced size masses from left to right for a constant mass density (100 % glandular tissue), (bottom) original mass and reduced density masses from left to right for a constant mass size (10 mm).

2.2   Clinical Displays Specifications

The standard monitor used in the experiment was a Barco Coronis 5MP mammo. This display has a 5 MP resolution and was set to the default monitor luminance value of $500\,cd/m^2$. The advanced monitor was a Barco Coronis Uniti 12MP MDMC-12132. This display system has a resolution of 12 MP (intended to replace a dual head display) and was set to the default monitor luminance value of $1000\,cd/m^2$. The advanced monitor has a number of improved specifications compared to the standard monitor. The advanced monitor has higher calibrated luminance ($1000\,cd/m^2$ versus $500\,cd/m^2$). Its optical design has been largely improved compared to the standard monitor. Specifically, the protective front glass of the advanced monitor has been optically bonded to the panel glass. This results into a significant reduction of undesired reflections inside the monitor, which improves MTF especially for small image features [6]. Both displays were calibrated to DICOM GSDF and compliance was verified by means of AAPMTG18 testing. During the entire study, periodic QA checks were also performed to continuously monitor compliance and no deviations were observed.

2.3   4AFC Study

Five medical physicists experienced in breast imaging participated in a series of 4AFC human observer studies to determine the detectability of breast masses in 2D digital mammograms for the two types of monitors under study. Two types of breast masses, four mass sizes (with constant density: 100 % glandular tissue) and four mass densities (with constant size: 8–11 mm) resulting in 16 conditions were investigated. For each condition, 142 trials were assessed per observer. For each 4AFC trial a signal-present image was randomly selected from the signal-present dataset. Three other images were then randomly selected from the pool of signal-absent images with similar local glandularity group as the signal-present image. Black and white concentric Toto circles were added on each ROI to emphasise that the mass is in the centre of the circle. Projections of the simulated masses were available as target clues during the study. A training session with targets of all conditions was provided prior to the main study to familiarize the observers with the task and use of the software. Each observer read a total of 2272 images in the dataset on the standard monitor in 4 sessions. After a three months gap, the study was repeated in the same manner with the same observers reading the images on the advanced monitor.

The percentages of correctly detected masses (PC) were determined for each observer as well as the average over all observers. Bootstrapping was used to calculate the 95 % confidence intervals. These PCs achieved on the standard monitor readings were then compared with the corresponding PCs achieved on the advanced monitor for all the images combined and each condition. ANOVA analysis was performed to study the effect of lesion size, density and background glandularity on the detectability performance of both monitors.

3   Results and Discussion

Figure 2 shows in blue the overall PC of average observer for all the images read on the standard monitor compared to the advanced monitor for all masses. On average, the advanced monitor had an overall increase in PC of 3 % compared to the standard monitor for all types of masses. The result of a paired t-test showed that the difference in PC was statistically significant (p-value = 0.0076, which is <0.05. Figure 2 also shows the overall PC for the subcategories of the masses. On average, the PC was increased by 3 % for ill-defined masses (in black) and 2 % for spiculated masses (in red) when images were read on the advanced monitor. The paired t-test showed the increase in PC was significant for both ill-defined margin and spiculated masses (p-value = 0.0406 and 0.0184, respectively).

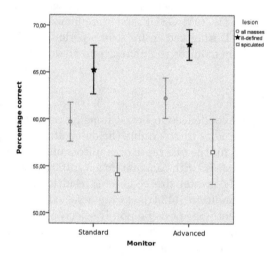

Fig. 2. Overall PC averaged over all observers for standard monitor vs. advanced monitor for all mass types (blue), ill-defined margin masses (black) and spiculated masses (red). Error bars show 95 % CI. (Color figure online)

Figure 3 shows observer averaged PC as a function of the mass size and density on the standard monitor and the advanced monitor for all types of masses combined. The percentage of correctly detected masses increases as the size of the mass increases as shown in Fig. 3a. The percentage of detected masses also increases as the density of the masses increases as shown in Fig. 3b. Present analysis now quantifies these known facts. The advanced monitor is outperforming the standard monitors as shown in the figures. The increase in detectability for the advanced monitor versus the standard monitor was significant for the masses of 4–6 mm group size. Also, the increase in PC was significant for the higher contrast masses, which were simulated with density of 90 % and 100 % of glandular tissue. The results were further subdivided into two types of masses (ill-defined margin and spiculated). PC differentiated for the type of mass as a

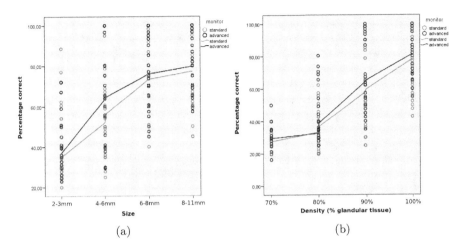

(a)   (b)

Fig. 3. All mass types: PC averaged over all observers for standard monitor vs. advanced monitor for all mass types as a function of (a) mass size (for a constant density), (b) mass density (for a constant size). Data points show PC values for the tested conditions. (Color figure online)

function of mass size is shown in Fig. 4a and for mass density in Fig. 4b. Similar PC trends were observed as in Fig. 3.

Figure 5 shows the observer study results subdivided into low, medium and high background glandularity groups used in the study. Figure 5a shows the PC as a function of size of the mass for each type of background glandularity, labeled for each monitor. An increasing trend in PC is clearly visible when the mass size increases for all three types of background glandularity. Higher PC values in lower glandularity backgrounds suggest that more masses were detected correctly when the mass (with a given attenuation coefficient) was inserted into a low glandularity background. Figure 5b similarly shows an increase in PC as the background glandularity decreases. PC also increases by increasing the density (attenuation coefficient) of mass for all three types of background glandularity indicating a higher detectability of lesions at a higher contrast.

ANOVA analysis showed that background has a significant effect on the detectability of the lesion. The percentage correct does significantly increase when the lesions are simulated in low background glandularity in comparison to high and medium background glandularity but the increase was not significant between insertion in medium and high glandular backgrounds. ANOVA analysis showed a significant increase in detectability as a function of size when mass was inserted in the high background glandularity. The advanced monitor had a significantly better detection for masses of different densities in all three types of background compared to the standard monitor.

This study suggests that more challenging masses may be detected when the images are displayed on the advanced monitor. In addition to this fact, the advanced monitor contains several productivity tools that are intended

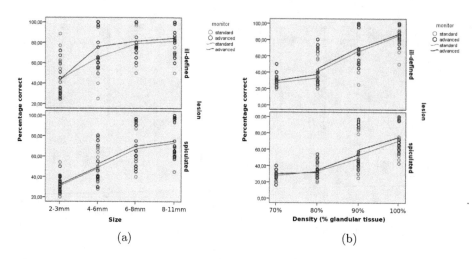

Fig. 4. Percentage correct differentiated for lesion type: PC averaged over all observers for standard monitor vs. advanced monitor for ill-defined and spiculated masses as a function of (a) mass size (for a constant density), (b) mass density (for a constant size). Data points show PC values for the tested conditions. (Color figure online)

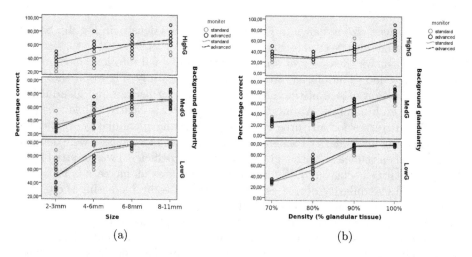

Fig. 5. Percentage correct differentiated for background type: PC averaged over all observers for standard monitor vs. advanced monitor for all masses inserted into high, medium and low glandularity background as a function of (a) mass size (for a constant density), (b) mass density (for a constant size). Data points show PC values for the tested conditions. (Color figure online)

to improve workflow efficiency and to reduce fatigue. It also has integrated SpotView image processing that allows the radiologist to focus better on subtle image features. For the purpose of this study we disabled these options on the advanced display, as our interest was to understand the potential improvement due to improved optical design and higher luminance. Present study did not investigate the reading time. Therefore, the reported results may not yet reflect the maximum capabilities of the advanced monitor. A virtual clinical trial with a search task using radiologists can further validate the benefit of the advanced monitor.

4   Conclusion

This work presents an example of partially virtual clinical study to investigate the impact of clinical display on cancer detection in 2D mammography. Previously developed and validated tools that simulate projections of lesion models into patient images were applied here to study display systems in an efficient way with paired statistics for maximal statistical power. The advanced display, Barco Coronis Uniti, performed with significantly higher PC rates (overall 3 % higher PC) compared to the standard monitor. Since the productivity tools and SpotView functionality on the advanced monitor were disabled in this study, the presented results may still underestimate the full potential of this monitor. The effect of extra functionalities is subject of an ongoing research.

References

1. Maidment, A.D.A.: Virtual clinical trials for the assessment of novel breast screening modalities. In: Fujita, H., Hara, T., Muramatsu, C. (eds.) IWDM 2014. LNCS, vol. 8539, pp. 1–8. Springer, Heidelberg (2014)
2. Elangovan, P., Warren, L.M., Mackenzie, A., Rashidnasab, A., Diaz, O., Dance, D.R., Young, K.C., Bosmans, H., Strudley, C.J., Wells, K.: Development and validation of a modelling framework for simulating 2D-mammography and breast tomosynthesis images. Phys. Med. Biol. **59**(15), 4275 (2014)
3. Rashidnasab, A., Elangovan, P., Yip, M., Diaz, O., Dance, D.R., Young, K.C., Wells, K.: Simulation and assessment of realistic breast lesions using fractal growth models. Phys. Med. Biol. **58**(16), 5613 (2013)
4. Shaheen, E., De Keyzer, F., Bosmans, H., Dance, D.R., Young, K.C., Van Ongeval, C.: The simulation of 3D mass models in 2D digital mammography and breast tomosynthesis. Med. Phys. **41**(8), 081913 (2014)
5. Highnam, R., Brady, S.M., Yaffe, M.J., Karssemeijer, N., Harvey, J.: Robust breast composition measurement - VolparaTM. In: Martí, J., Oliver, A., Freixenet, J., Martí, R. (eds.) IWDM 2010. LNCS, vol. 6136, pp. 342–349. Springer, Heidelberg (2010)
6. Coronis Uniti (MDMC-12133). www.barco.com/en/Products/Displays-monitors-workstations/Medical-displays/Diagnostic-displays/. Accessed 19 Apr 2016

Author Index

Printed in the United States
By Bookmasters